Men's Reproductive and Sexual Health throughout the Lifespan

Approximately 1 in 20 men have sperm counts low enough to impair fertility, but little progress has been made in answering fundamental questions in andrology or in developing new diagnostic tools or management strategies for infertile men. Many of these problems increase with age, leading to a growing population of men seeking help. To address this, there is a strong movement toward integrating male reproductive and sexual health care involving clinicians such as andrologists, urologists, endocrinologists, and counselors. This book will emphasize this integrated approach to male reproductive and sexual health throughout the lifespan. Practical advice on how to perform both clinical and laboratory evaluations of infertile men is given, as well as a variety of methods for medically and surgically managing common issues. This text ties together the three major pillars of clinical andrology: clinical care, the andrology laboratory, and translational research.

Douglas T. Carrell is Director of the Andrology and IVF laboratories at the Center for Reproductive Medicine in Minneapolis, MN, as well as Professor Emeritus of Surgery (Urology) and Human Genetics and the University of Utah.

Alexander W. Pastuszak is Assistant Professor of Surgery (Urology) in the Department of Surgery at the University of Utah School of Medicine in Salt Lake City, Utah.

James M. Hotaling is Associate Professor of Surgery (Urology) and Director of the Men's Health program at the University of Utah Center for Reproductive Medicine, Salt Lake City, Utah.

Men's Reproductive and Sexual Health throughout the Lifespan

An Integrated Approach to Fertility, Sexual Function, and Vitality

Edited by

Douglas T. Carrell
University of Utah

Alexander W. Pastuszak
University of Utah

James M. Hotaling
University of Utah

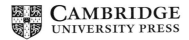

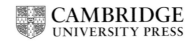

Shaftesbury Road, Cambridge CB2 8EA, United Kingdom

One Liberty Plaza, 20th Floor, New York, NY 10006, USA

477 Williamstown Road, Port Melbourne, VIC 3207, Australia

314–321, 3rd Floor, Plot 3, Splendor Forum, Jasola District Centre, New Delhi – 110025, India

103 Penang Road, #05–06/07, Visioncrest Commercial, Singapore 238467

Cambridge University Press is part of Cambridge University Press & Assessment, a department of the University of Cambridge.

We share the University's mission to contribute to society through the pursuit of education, learning and research at the highest international levels of excellence.

www.cambridge.org
Information on this title: www.cambridge.org/9781009197557

DOI: 10.1017/9781009197533

© Douglas T. Carrell, Alexander W. Pastuszak, and James M. Hotaling, 2023

This publication is in copyright. Subject to statutory exception and to the provisions of relevant collective licensing agreements, no reproduction of any part may take place without the written permission of Cambridge University Press & Assessment.

First published 2023

Printed in the United Kingdom by TJ Books Ltd, Padstow Cornwall

A catalogue record for this publication is available from the British Library.

Library of Congress Cataloging-in-Publication Data
Names: Carrell, Douglas T., editor. | Hotaling, James M., editor. | Pastuszak, Alexander W., editor.
Title: Men's reproductive and sexual health throughout the lifespan : an integrated approach to fertility, sexual function and vitality / edited by Douglas T. Carrell, James M. Hotaling, Alexander W. Pastuszak.
Description: Cambridge, United Kingdom ; New York, NY : Cambridge University Press, 2023. | Includes bibliographical references and index.
Identifiers: LCCN 2022030689 (print) | LCCN 2022030690 (ebook) | ISBN 9781009197557 (hardback) | ISBN 9781009197533 (epub)
Subjects: MESH: Infertility, Male–therapy | Genital Diseases, Male–therapy | Fertility–physiology | Reproductive Health | Sexual Health | Men's Health
Classification: LCC RC889 (print) | LCC RC889 (ebook) | NLM WJ 709 | DDC 616.6/921–dc23/eng/20221209
LC record available at https://lccn.loc.gov/2022030689
LC ebook record available at https://lccn.loc.gov/2022030690

ISBN 978-1-009-19755-7 Hardback

Cambridge University Press & Assessment has no responsibility for the persistence or accuracy of URLs for external or third-party internet websites referred to in this publication and does not guarantee that any content on such websites is, or will remain, accurate or appropriate.

Contents

List of Contributors vii
Preface xi

Section 1 An Introduction to Men's Health Care

1. **How Has Men's Health Changed over the Past Two Decades?** 1
   Dyvon T. Walker, Sriram V. Eleswarapu, and Amarnath Rambhatla

2. **The Business Landscape of Men's Health** 8
   James M. Weinberger and Jesse N. Mills

3. **Urologic Men's Health, the Internet, and Social Media** 16
   Adithya Balasubramanian, Kassandra E. Zaila, James M. Hotaling, and Jesse N. Mills

Section 2 The Biology of Male Reproduction and Infertility

4. **Current Understanding of the Physiology and Histology of Human Spermatogenesis** 23
   Chiara Capponi and Elena Vicini

5. **Male Reproductive Endocrinology** 34
   Christos Tsametis, George Kanakis, and Dimitrios G. Goulis

6. **Sperm Chromatin Packaging and the Toroid Linker Model** 54
   Hubert Szczygieł, Anna Ung, Hieu Nguyen, and W. Steven Ward

7. **Ejaculation and Sperm Transport: Physiology and Clinical Concerns** 61
   Christopher Koprowski, Garrick Greear, and Tung-Chin Hsieh

8. **Genetic Aspects of Male Infertility** 67
   Albert Salas-Huetos and Kenneth I. Aston

9. **The Mechanistic and Predictive Utility of Sperm Epigenetics** 76
   Timothy G. Jenkins

10. **Aging and Environmental Interactions with the Sperm Epigenome** 81
    Albert Salas-Huetos and Douglas T. Carrell

11. **The Effects of Aging on Male Fertility and the Health of Offspring** 87
    Alex M. Kasman, Francesco Del Giudice, and Michael L. Eisenberg

Section 3 Clinical Evaluation and Treatment of Male Infertility

12. **Office Evaluation of the Infertile Male** 97
    Kevin J. Campbell, John F. Sullivan, and Larry I. Lipshultz

13. **Medical Management of Male Infertility** 106
    Jason R. Kovac

14. **Surgical Management of Male Infertility** 113
    Jesse B. Persily, Sameer Thakker, and Bobby B. Najari

15. **Varicocele Repair in the Era of IVF/ICSI** 120
    Jessica N. Schardein, Alexander Pastuszak, and James W. Hotaling

16. **Implementing Genetic Testing of Male Infertility in the Clinic** 127
    Ahmad Majzoub, Chak Lam Cho, and Sandro C. Esteves

17. **Andrological Care of the Patient with Spinal Cord Injury** 135
    Christian Fuglesang S. Jensen, Jens Sønksen, and Dana A. Ohl

18. **Clinical Fertility Preservation Decision-Making for Prepubertal and Postpubertal Individuals with Male Gametes** 141
    Jerrine Morris, Heiko Yang, John Lindsey, and James F. Smith

19. **Mental Health Considerations in the Infertile Male and Couple** 154
    Elizabeth Grill

Section 4 Laboratory Evaluation and Treatment of Male Infertility

20 **The Modern Semen Analysis: Theory and Techniques of Ejaculate Examination** 159
Lars Björndahl

21 **The Future of Computer-Assisted Semen Analysis in the Evaluation of Male Infertility** 165
David Mortimer and Sharon T. Mortimer

22 **Reactive Oxygen Species and Sperm DNA Damage** 175
Lesley Haddock, Erica Gardiner, and Sheena E. M. Lewis

23 **Clinical Value of Sperm DNA Fragmentation Tests** 183
Armand Zini

24 **The Current Use of Sperm Function Assays** 191
Sara Marchiani and Elisabetta Baldi

25 **Sperm Selection in the Laboratory** 197
Denny Sakkas and Denis A. Vaughan

26 **Methods to Select Ejaculated, Epididymal, and Testicular Spermatozoa for Assisted Conception** 204
Sergey I. Moskovtsev, Michal Dviri, and Clifford L. Librach

27 **Optimal Sperm Selection in the ICSI Era** 210
Joshua Calvert, Darshan Patel, and James M. Hotaling

28 **Microfluidics for Sperm Sample Preparation and Sperm Identification** 218
Raheel Samuel, Haidong Feng, Hayden Brady, and Utpal Saha

29 **Practical Concerns for Patient Semen Banking** 224
Grace M. Centola

30 **The Potential Future Applications of In Vitro Spermatogenesis in the Clinical Laboratory** 229
Swati Sharma and Stefan Schlatt

31 **Spermatogonial Stem Cell Culture and the Future of Germline Gene Editing** 244
Xichen Nie, Jan-Bernd Stukenborg, and Jingtao Guo

Section 5 Medical and Surgical Management of Issues of Male Health

32 **Hypogonadism in the Male: Evaluation and Treatment** 251
Parviz K. Kavoussi and G. Luke Machen

33 **Selective Androgen Receptor Modulators in the Treatment of Hypogonadism and Men's Health** 264
John T. Sigalos, Dyvon T. Walker, and Larry I. Lipshultz

34 **Male Fertility and Testosterone Therapy** 269
Juan Andino and James M. Dupree

35 **Sleep and Men's Health** 279
Vanessa Peña, Taylor P. Kohn, and Larry I. Lipshultz

36 **Molecular Biology and Physiology of Erectile Function and Dysfunction** 289
James L. Liu, Arthur L. Burnett, and Amin S. Herati

37 **Evaluation of the Male with Erectile Dysfunction** 295
William T. Berg and Martin Miner

38 **Lifestyle Modifications for Erectile Dysfunction** 303
Jeffrey S. Edman, Jade Warner, and Amy M. Pearlman

39 **Medical and Surgical Management of Erectile Dysfunction** 308
Mohit Khera and Skyler Howell

40 **Surgical Management of Peyronie's Disease** 315
Aron Liaw and Faysal Yafi

41 **Medical Management of Benign Prostatic Hyperplasia** 323
Christopher Martin, Laurel Mast, and Stephen Summers

42 **Evidence-Based Management of Chronic Orchialgia and Chronic Prostatitis/Chronic Pelvic Pain Syndrome** 329
Sharon P. Lo and Kelli X. Gross

Index 337

Contributors

Juan Andino, Department of Urology, Michigan Medicine, University of Michigan, Ann Arbor, MI

Kenneth I. Aston, Department of Surgery, University of Utah School of Medicine, Salt Lake City, UT

Adithya Balasubramanian, Department of Urology, Weill Cornell Medical College, New York, NY

Elisabetta Baldi, Department of Experimental and Clinical Medicine, University of Florence, Italy

William T. Berg, Department of Urology, Renaissance School of Medicine, Stony Brook University, New York, NY

Lars Björndahl, Andrology Laboratory, ANOVA, Karolinska University Hospital and Department of Medicine, Karolinska Institutet, Stockholm, Sweden

Hayden Brady, Department of Mechanical Engineering, Weber State University, Ogden, UT

Arthur L. Burnett, The James Buchanan Brady Urological Institute and Department of Urology, Johns Hopkins University School of Medicine, Baltimore, MD

Joshua Calvert, Department of Urology, Vanderbilt University Medical Center, Nashville, TN

Kevin J. Campbell, Department of Urology, University of Florida College of Medicine, Gainesville, FL

Chiara Capponi, Department of Anatomy, Histology, Forensic Medicine and Orthopedic, Section of Histology, Sapienza University of Rome

Douglas T. Carrell, Andrology and IVF Laboratory, Division of Urology, Department of Surgery, University of Utah School of Medicine, Salt Lake City, UT

Grace M. Centola, Reproductive Laboratory and Tissue Bank Consultant

Chak Lam Cho, Department of Surgery, Union Hospital, Hong Kong and S. H. Ho Urology Centre, Department of Surgery, The Chinese University of Hong Kong

Francesco Del Giudice, Department of Maternal-Infant and Urological Sciences, Sapienza University of Rome; Policlinico Umberto I Hospital, Rome

James M. Dupree, Department of Urology, Michigan Medicine, University of Michigan Institute for Healthcare Policy and Innovation, Ann Arbor, MI

Michal Dviri, CReATe Fertility Centre, Toronto, Canada; Department of Obstetrics and Gynecology, University of Toronto, Canada

Jeffrey S. Edman, Department of Urology, University of Iowa Hospitals and Clinics, Iowa City, IA

Michael L. Eisenberg, Department of Urology and Department of Obstetrics and Gynecology, Stanford University School of Medicine, CA

Sriram V. Eleswarapu, Division of Andrology, Department of Urology, David Geffen School of Medicine at the University of California, Los Angeles

Sandro C. Esteves, ANDROFERT, Andrology and Human Reproduction Clinic; Division of Urology, Department of Surgery, University of Campinas (UNICAMP), Campinas,

List of Contributors

Brazil; Faculty of Health, Department of Clinical Sciences, Aarhus University, Denmark

Haidong Feng, Department of Mechanical Engineering, University of Utah, Salt Lake City, UT

Erica Gardiner, ExamenLab Ltd, Belfast, UK

Dimitrios G. Goulis, Unit of Reproductive Endocrinology, 1st Department of Obstetrics and Gynecology, Medical School, Aristotle University of Thessaloniki, Greece

Garrick Greear, Department of Urology, University of California, San Diego, La Jolla, CA

Elizabeth Grill, The Ronald O. Perelman and Claudia Cohen Center for Reproductive Medicine, Weill Cornell Medical College, New York, NY

Kelli X. Gross, Center for Reconstructive Urology & Men's Health, University of Utah School of Medicine, Salt Lake City, UT

Jingtao Guo, Division of Urology, Department of Surgery, University of Utah School of Medicine, Salt Lake City, UT

Lesley Haddock, ExamenLab Ltd, Belfast, UK

Amin S. Herati, The James Buchanan Brady Urological Institute and Department of Urology, Johns Hopkins University School of Medicine, Baltimore, MD

James M. Hotaling, Division of Urology, Department of Surgery, University of Utah School of Medicine, Salt Lake City, UT

Skyler Howell, McGovern Medical School, University of Texas Health Science Center at Houston, Houston, TX

Tung-Chin Hsieh, Department of Urology, University of California, San Diego, La Jolla, CA

Timothy G. Jenkins, Department of Physiology and Developmental Biology, Brigham Young University, Provo, UT

Christian Fuglesang S. Jensen, Department of Urology, Herlev and Gentofte Hospital, Herlev, Denmark

George Kanakis, Unit of Reproductive Endocrinology, 1st Department of Obstetrics and Gynecology, Medical School, Aristotle University of Thessaloniki, Greece; Department of Endocrinology, Athens Naval and Veteran Affairs Hospital, Greece

Alex M. Kasman, Department of Urology, Stanford University School of Medicine, CA

Parviz K. Kavoussi, Austin Fertility & Reproductive Medicine/Westlake IVF

Mohit Khera, Department of Urology, Baylor College of Medicine, Houston, TX

Taylor P. Kohn, The James Buchanan Brady Urological Institute and Department of Urology, Johns Hopkins University School of Medicine, Baltimore, MD

Christopher Koprowski, Department of Urology, University of California, San Diego, La Jolla, CA

Jason R. Kovac, Men's Health Center, Indianapolis, IN

Sheena E. M. Lewis, Faculty of Medicine, Health, and Life Sciences, Queen's University Belfast, UK

Aron Liaw, Department of Urology, University of California, Irvine

Clifford L. Librach, CReATe Fertility Centre, Toronto, Canada; Department of Obstetrics and Gynecology, Department of Physiology, and Department of Medicine, University of Toronto, Canada; Institute of Medical Sciences, University of Toronto, Canada

John Lindsey, Department of Urology, University of California San Francisco

Larry N. Lipshultz, Scott Department of Urology, Baylor College of Medicine, Houston, TX

James L. Liu, The James Buchanan Brady Urological Institute and Department of Urology, Johns Hopkins University School of Medicine, Baltimore, MD

Sharon P. Lo, Division of Urology, Department of Surgery, University of Utah School of Medicine, Salt Lake City, UT

List of Contributors

G. Luke Machen, Austin Fertility & Reproductive Medicine/Westlake IVF

Ahmad Majzoub, Department of Urology, Hamad Medical Corporation, Doha, Qatar; Weill Cornell Medicine – Qatar, Doha, Qatar

Sara Marchiani, Azienda Ospedaliero Universitaria Careggi, Florence, Italy

Christopher Martin, Division of Urology, Department of Surgery, University of Utah School of Medicine, Salt Lake City, UT

Laurel Mast, Division of Urology, Department of Surgery, University of Utah School of Medicine, Salt Lake City, UT

Martin Miner, Department of Family Medicine and Urology, Warren Alpert School of Medicine, Brown University, Providence, RI

Jesse N. Mills, Department of Urology, David Geffen School of Medicine at the University of California, Los Angeles

Jerrine Morris, Department of Obstetrics, Gynecology, and Reproductive Sciences, University of California San Francisco

David Mortimer, Oozoa Biomedical Inc., West Vancouver, Canada

Sharon T. Mortimer, Oozoa Biomedical Inc., West Vancouver, Canada

Sergey I. Moskovtsev, CReATe Fertility Centre, Toronto, Canada; Department of Laboratory Medicine and Pathobiology, University of Toronto, Canada

Bobby B. Najari, Department of Urology and Department of Population Health, New York University Grossman School of Medicine, New York, NY

Hieu Nguyen, Institute for Biogenesis Research, Department of Anatomy, Biochemistry & Physiology and the Department of Obstetrics, Gynecology & Women's Health, John A. Burns School of Medicine, University of Hawaii at Manoa, Honolulu, HI

Xichen Nie, Division of Urology, Department of Surgery, University of Utah School of Medicine, Salt Lake City, UT

Dana A. Ohl, Department of Urology, Michigan Medicine, University of Michigan, Ann Arbor, MI

Alexander W. Pastuszak, Department of Surgery, University of Utah School of Medicine, Salt Lake City, UT

Darshan Patel, Department of Surgery, University of Utah School of Medicine, Salt Lake City, UT

Amy M. Pearlman, Department of Urology, University of Iowa Hospitals and Clinics, Iowa City, IA

Vanessa Peña, The James Buchanan Brady Urological Institute and Department of Urology, Johns Hopkins University School of Medicine, Baltimore, MD

Jesse B. Persily, New York University Grossman School of Medicine, New York, NY

Amarnath Rambhatla, Vattikuti Urology Institute, Henry Ford Health, Detroit, MI

Utpal Saha, Department of Mechanical Engineering, University of Utah, Salt Lake City, UT

Denny Sakkas, Boston IVF, Waltham, MA

Albert Salas-Huetos, Department of Surgery, University of Utah School of Medicine, Salt Lake City, UT

Raheel Samuel, Department of Mechanical Engineering, University of Utah, Salt Lake City, UT; Advanced Conceptions Inc.

Jessica N. Schardein, Department of Urology, SUNY Upstate Medical University, Syracuse, NY

Stefan Schlatt, Center for Reproductive Medicine and Andrology, University of Münster, Germany

Swati Sharma, Center for Reproductive Medicine and Andrology, University of Münster, Germany

John T. Sigalos, Department of Urology, David Geffen School of Medicine, University of California, Los Angeles

James F. Smith, Department of Urology, Department of Obstetrics, Gynecology, and Reproductive Sciences, and Philip R. Lee Institute for Health Policy, University of California San Francisco

List of Contributors

Jens Sønksen, Department of Urology, Herlev and Gentofte Hospital, Herlev, Denmark

Jan-Bernd Stukenborg, NORDFERTIL Research Laboratory Stockholm, Childhood Cancer Research Unit, Department of Women's and Children's Health, Karolinska Institute and Karolinska University Hospital, Solna, Sweden

John F. Sullivan, Department of Urology, St James's University Hospital, Dublin, Ireland

Stephen Summers, Division of Urology, Department of Surgery, University of Utah School of Medicine, Salt Lake City, UT

Hubert Szczygieł, Institute for Biogenesis Research, Department of Anatomy, Biochemistry & Physiology and the Department of Obstetrics, Gynecology & Women's Health, John A. Burns School of Medicine, University of Hawaii at Manoa, Honolulu, HI

Sameer Thakker, Department of Medicine, New York University Grossman School of Medicine, New York, NY

Christos Tsametis, Unit of Reproductive Endocrinology, 1st Department of Obstetrics and Gynecology, Medical School, Aristotle University of Thessaloniki, Greece

Anna Ung, Institute for Biogenesis Research, Department of Anatomy, Biochemistry & Physiology and the Department of Obstetrics, Gynecology & Women's Health, John A. Burns School of Medicine, University of Hawaii at Manoa, Honolulu, HI

Denis A. Vaughan, Boston IVF, Waltham, MA; Department of Obstetrics and Gynecology, Beth Israel Deaconess Medical Center, Boston, MA; Department of Obstetrics, Gynecology, and Reproductive Biology, Harvard Medical School, Boston, MA

Elena Vicini, Department of Anatomy, Histology, Forensic Medicine and Orthopedic, Section of Histology, Sapienza University of Rome

Dyvon T. Walker, Division of Andrology, Department of Urology, David Geffen School of Medicine, University of California, Los Angeles

W. Steven Ward, Institute for Biogenesis Research, Department of Anatomy, Biochemistry & Physiology and the Department of Obstetrics, Gynecology & Women's Health, John A. Burns School of Medicine, University of Hawaii at Manoa, Honolulu, HI

Jade Warner, Carver College of Medicine, University of Iowa, Iowa City, IA

James M. Weinberger, Department of Urology, David Geffen School of Medicine at the University of California, Los Angeles

Faysal Yafi, Division of Men's Health and Reconstructive Urology, University of California, Irvine

Heiko Yang, Department of Urology, University of California San Francisco

Kassandra E. Zaila, Department of Urology, University of California Los Angeles

Armand Zini, Division of Urology, Department of Surgery, McGill University and OVO Fertility Clinic, Montreal, Canada

Preface

Our main motive in writing this book was to provide a comprehensive text tying together the three major pillars of clinical andrology: clinical care, the andrology laboratory, and translational research. While there are multiple texts that address these foundations in isolation, and some that address two topics together, there is not a comprehensive text that brings everything together from each of the pillars. Ultimately, if our goal is to improve patient care, we need to view all of these areas holistically.

Our second motivation for this book is the breathtaking and unprecedented advances in translational sciences that are occurring. The vaccine for COVID-19 is one such example. This vaccine was generated in silico in January 2020, just weeks after the sequence of the virus was released. The vaccine then became available less than a year later, an astounding accomplishment compared to prior efforts at making a viable vaccine, such as that for smallpox, which took 20 or more years. mRNA vaccines, and other technologies like them, are but one example of how translational sciences are revolutionizing both human health and, potentially, specific fields like reproductive medicine. It is with the spirit of anxious determination that we have compiled this book as a guide for future advances in the field of male reproductive health care.

Unfortunately, the study of male reproduction has lagged significantly behind the study of female reproduction. We often tell our patients that male infertility is at least 20 years behind our understanding of female infertility and perhaps as much as 30 years behind our molecular understanding of cancer. This book is really an attempt to weave together how translational research can impact both clinical care and advances in the andrology lab. We are hopeful that recent and future scientific advances in the care of both infertile men and those with sexual dysfunction will ultimately usher in a revolution akin to what IVF did for female infertility. The goal of this book is to provide an outline of what is known in the field and also, perhaps, a glimpse into what the future might hold.

To obtain our objectives, we have relied on the efforts of leading clinicians and scientists in the fields covered. We would like to sincerely thank all of the authors who contributed to this book, which has truly been a team effort. We hope that the readers will find this book valuable and will view it as a comprehensive text to deliver optimal care in the laboratory and the clinic with an eye toward future advancements.

Section 1 An Introduction to Men's Health Care

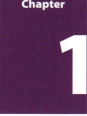

How Has Men's Health Changed over the Past Two Decades?

Dyvon T. Walker, Sriram V. Eleswarapu, and Amarnath Rambhatla

1.1 Introduction

Men's health has emerged as a distinct discipline within medicine and has experienced significant changes and advances within the last 20 years. Common medical conditions affecting men include heart disease, diabetes, hypertension, and kidney disease. Male-specific disorders include prostate and testicular problems, erectile dysfunction (ED), hypogonadism, and male factor infertility. In order to strike a balance for a healthy society, it is of equal importance to discuss issues related to the health of men as well as to that of women, and to understand the differences between them. In this chapter we aim to discuss how men's health has evolved over the past two decades and the role of the urologist in bringing men's health to the forefront. Just as the field has improved over the past 20 years, we expect that there will be significant gains over the next few decades quarterbacked by the urologist.

1.2 Health Disparities

Men's health disparities are differences in health outcomes that are determined by cultural, economic, and environmental factors associated with socially defined identities and group memberships [1]. More attention is needed toward addressing men's health and to optimize efforts to educate men regarding their healthcare needs. These health disparities are perhaps best exemplified by life expectancy and preventable disease.

Globally, the average male life expectancy at birth has increased from 65 years to approximately 70 years within the last two decades [2]. Despite this increase, there is not a single country where male life expectancy exceeds that of females, and by 2030 it is expected that male life expectancy will lag behind female life expectancy by at least seven years [3]. There are a number of reasons for gendered differences in life expectancy, including biological differences as well as cultural and behavioral ones linked to different social expectations of men and women. These social expectations include use of and access to health care. Males, for example, are more likely than females to die prematurely from noncommunicable and preventable disease, the major risk factors of which include tobacco use, unhealthy diets, and alcohol abuse.

Studies examining gender differences in preventive-care services have shown that men utilize general healthcare services as well as preventive-care services to a much lower degree than women. Specifically, it has been shown that men undergo blood pressure, cholesterol, dental checks, and also get the influenza vaccine in lower numbers compared to women [4]. Additionally, gender differences exist within specific health conditions, a phenomenon that can again be potentially explained by socioeconomic, environmental, genetic, and even physiological factors. The incidence of cardiovascular disease, for example, is higher in men than in women of similar age, a gender difference that is more prominent at a younger age and partly explained by the protective effects of sex hormones [5,6]. Furthermore, studies have demonstrated that men, compared to women, are more likely to be overweight or obese, more likely to consume fast food, high-sugar beverages, and alcohol, and are less likely to be knowledgeable about nutrition [7]. In order for some of these gender disparities to be understood, it is crucial to evaluate the primary motivators for men seeking physician evaluation and care.

1.3 Drivers for Seeking Health Care

It is estimated that 25% of men in the US population had no visits to the doctor in the past 12 months, compared with 12% of women, a difference that persists even after correcting for the use of healthcare services that are specific for women. This discrepancy in utilization has been present historically, and certainly over the last 20 years. It is thought to be influenced by a combination of variables, including mental distress, physical illness, perceived symptoms, poor subjective health, and propensity to use services. Women have higher levels of all of these variables, leading to the increased healthcare utilization among them [8].

Men commonly attribute their reluctance to visit a physician to busy schedules, fear of finding out something is wrong, and discomfort of physical exams (prostate, testicular). As such, healthcare utilization among men is typically governed by acuity or urgency of illness or injury, need for a specific procedure (e.g., vasectomy), or spousal persuasion. One of the major reasons that young women visit a physician is for family planning. Traditionally, family planning has focused on providing contraception to women as there are numerous reversible options available. This burden may be shifting to men, however, as international surveys have highlighted that men are interested in male contraceptive options, and there has been an increase in clinical research to this end [9]. This may be a potential new driver for men to seek physician care.

Contemporary men's health aims to shift the paradigm to preventative men's health care by emphasizing the importance of well visits, wellness checks, and men's health maintenance. Insurance incentives are one way this paradigm shift may be taking place. Through the Affordable Care Act from 2010 to 2015, for instance, people gaining coverage were more likely to be male (10.3 million or 54%). Additionally, the majority of people gaining coverage were in the 19–34 age group (8.7 million or 45%) [10]. With these incentives and potential drivers in place, clinics specific to men's health have emerged.

1.4 Men's Health Centers

There has been an emergence of medical clinics that have focused on ED and low testosterone ("low T") and branded themselves as "men's health centers." These centers have embraced the men's health platform and have largely been cash-based, taking advantage of the profitability surrounding ED and low T. Most of these centers are not staffed by healthcare professionals with academic training in male endocrinology, sexual medicine, or preventative medicine, and are built on the basis of optimizing men's health via testosterone, supplements, and intra-cavernosal injections [11].

Treatments for low testosterone have been gaining attractiveness since the early 2000s, heavily influenced by direct-to-consumer marketing. From 2001 to 2011, testosterone use in the United States tripled, and consequently, hundreds of testosterone clinics emerged. Rather than offering a traditional medical office visit comprised of history-taking, physical exam, and appropriate lab and imaging studies, these clinics offer memberships with frequent testosterone injections and lab monitoring. Likely as a result, total testosterone sales increased 12-fold globally, rising from $150 million in 2000 to $1.8 billion in 2011 [11]. Additionally, total testosterone use among men over 30 increased from 0.52% in 2002 to 3.20% in 2013. These for-profit low T clinics constitute the original iteration of men's health centers, providing patients with various forms of testosterone replacement therapy, often without a clear indication. These clinics, however, lack the follow-up that is required in patients receiving testosterone therapy and the detailed evaluation necessary for these patients regarding factors such as prostate cancer risk and fertility implications [11].

Over the last decade, men's health clinics have evolved beyond merely testosterone and ED to include a variety of issues and disciplines, including urologic diseases, nutrition, sports medicine, mental health, sleep medicine, cardiology, and dermatology. Academic centers, which have multidisciplinary teams equipped to address a wide variety of men's health issues, began establishing men's health clinics of their own in response. These academic centers now provide a comprehensive approach to men's health, with physicians managing sexual, endocrine, surgical, physical performance, and psychological issues. Fellowship training programs in men's health have emerged in various academic centers in response to the growing attention toward the subject, with the number of programs growing from 8 to 19 within the last decade [11]. With the growing attention toward men's health and the expanding training programs to facilitate experts in the field there has been a heightened interest in male urologic health, especially with the advent of new treatment options for hypogonadism, Peyronie's disease, and ED.

1.5 Men's Health Advocacy

The general interest in men's health was cast into the international spotlight by the "Movember" movement. Established in 2006 as a global charity, the Movember Foundation has become an annual event characterized by the growing of mustaches during the month of November to raise awareness of and funds to deliver innovative research for men's health issues such as prostate cancer, testicular cancer, mental health, and suicide prevention. The foundation also launched the Global Action Plan Prostate Cancer Active Surveillance initiative, creating the largest worldwide collaboration integrating patient data from men with prostate cancer on active surveillance. Similar to the "Pinktober" campaign focused on breast cancer that exploits pink ribbons as a strong visual tag, Movember exploits mustaches as a visual tag to maximize online visibility and to associate the movement specifically with improving men's health. This similarity between the two movements has caused some to question whether Movember is the "pink ribbon for men." The Movember Foundation has been able to raise over $900 million for men's health over the last 16 years [12].

1.6 Men's Health and Urology

Many of the reasons men seek healthcare are related to sexual function or reproductive health, often making urologists the first doctor a patient will see in many years. This puts urologists in an important position to quarterback men's health initiatives and to establish the patient–physician relationship that is essential for the patient to return to the physician's office. In fact, there has been evolving synergistic work between primary care physicians and urologists regarding men's health over the last two decades, as they began to recognize and embrace the relationship between the two fields. Primary care physicians interested in men's health are adept at medically managing a variety of men's health conditions such as BPH, hypogonadism, and ED as well as the comorbidities that can affect these. Urologists are often consulted for advanced medical and surgical management. There have been significant advances in many arenas over the last 20 years in men's urologic health, including prostate cancer, testicular pathology, infertility, and prosthetics.

1.6.1 Prostate Cancer

Prostate cancer is the most commonly diagnosed solid-organ malignancy in men in the USA and the second most common worldwide. Within the last 20 years, extensive research in the field of prostate cancer has resulted in important discoveries and modifications that have influenced our understanding of the disease and its management. Historically, most patients with low-risk prostate cancer were treated with either radical prostatectomy or radiotherapy-based treatment. However, conservative management of low-risk prostate cancer with active surveillance has become one of the most common management approaches.

There have been several advancements made for patients requiring definitive management of their prostate cancer. The last two decades has seen the advent of robot-assisted laparoscopic radical prostatectomy become the most commonly utilized surgical approach for prostate cancer. From 2004 to 2010, the number of patients treated with robotic radical prostatectomy versus open increased from 8% to 67%, a trend that continues to increase and evolve [13]. Prostate radiotherapy (RT) techniques have also experienced improvement in delivery, efficacy, safety, and efficiency. Techniques such as three-dimensional conformal RT, intensity-modulated RT, stereotactic body RT, robotic RT, high-dose-rate brachytherapy, and hypofractionation, to name a few, are revolutionizing the field [14,15]. In nearly every facet of prostate cancer management, tremendous progress has been made and continues to be made with promising techniques on the horizon.

1.6.2 Chronic Testicular Pain

Chronic testicular pain has been a challenging condition for both primary care providers and urologists to address. The condition may occur from previous scrotal surgery, infection, trauma, referred pain, or may be idiopathic. However, the etiology and pathophysiology of testicular pain have remained poorly understood since the term "orchialgia" was defined in the 1970s, contributing to the difficulty in treatment. More recently it was found that Wallerian degeneration of the autonomic nerves that travel along the spermatic cord may play a role in chronic testicular pain [16].

It is important to initially obtain a comprehensive history and physical exam and rule out underlying medical and anatomic causes such as tumors, intermittent torsion, active infection, and varicocele [17]. First-line therapy for chronic testicular pain is focused on conservative and medical management such as analgesics, anti-inflammatory agents, antibiotics, physical therapy, and avoidance of activities that evoke pain. When conservative management fails, surgical options are available depending on the cause of the testicular pain. Over the past two decades studies have demonstrated that a vasovasostomy is effective in the treatment of postvasectomy pain syndrome. When pain is diffuse involving the testicle or epididymis, microsurgical spermatic cord denervation (MSCD) offers a minimally invasive option with minimal morbidity and success rates of 70–80%. Surgical procedures such as orchiectomy and epididymectomy have been historically described as options for treating chronic testicular pain; however, they have variable success rates and are often considered to be a last resort. Though introduced in the 1970s, the technique of MSCD has been continuously developed and refined over the last 20 years and has become a primary surgical intervention for this patient population [17–20].

Though MSCD has gained much popularity, approximately 12–16% of patients will have persistent pain after denervation. In these patients, ultrasound guided targeted micro-cryoablation of the ilioinguinal and genitofemoral nerve fibers, which has been developed within the last 10 years, has proven effective. Similar to cryoablation, pulsed radiofrequency ablation of the cord has been recently developed for this patient population and is another potential treatment option [21].

1.6.3 Erectile Dysfunction

1.6.3.1 Phosphodiesterase Type 5 Inhibitors

Viagra (sildenafil) revolutionized the field of sexual medicine after its introduction to the market as the first oral treatment for ED. Following approval from the US Food and Drug Administration (FDA) for the treatment of ED in March 1998, the "blue pill" made its first appearance in pop culture on the cover of *TIME* magazine in May 1998 and has since had a tremendous impact on men's health. In fact, just 7 years following its market launch, more than 750,000 physicians had prescribed sildenafil to more than 23 million men [22]. Prior to its use, men had the option of testosterone optimization, vacuum erection devices, injection therapies, or surgery. The ability to use an oral medication for ED quickly made sildenafil and other phosphodiesterase type 5 (PDE5) inhibitors, such as tadalafil, vardenafil, and avanafil the first-line treatments of choice for ED.

1.6.3.2 Intracavernosal Injection Therapy

In the 25–50% of patients who do not respond to noninvasive therapies or for those whom PDE5 inhibitors are contraindicated, alternative therapies such as intracavernosal injection (ICI) therapy may be considered. The most commonly used and studied ICI agents currently include prostaglandin-E1 (alprostadil), papaverine, phentolamine, and combination therapy [23]. Various urological bodies have issued guidelines on the management of ED over the past 20 years, many of them recommending ICI therapy as a second-line treatment option for patients who do not respond to PDE5 inhibitors. However, some bodies, such as the American Urological Association (AUA), have come to recommend that male patients should be offered information on all treatment modalities prior to selecting a treatment option. Additionally, within the last 5 years, the AUA and the European Association of Urology (EAU) have produced guidelines advising combination therapy, such as Trimix (alprostadil, papaverine, and phentolamine), as a better alternative to monotherapy [24,25].

1.6.3.3 Prosthetics

The field of prosthetic urology has made significant strides in the past 20 years. Malleable devices and inflatable penile prostheses (IPP) are the currently available penile implants.

Infection rates have been dramatically reduced to 1–2% with the introduction of antibiotic-coated prosthetics, either inhibizone (AMS) or an antibiotic of choice (Coloplast) to adhere to the hydrophilic coating. There have also been improvements in components of the IPP by introduction of the one-touch release button in the pump, more compact and concealable reservoirs, no-crimp tubing, and the introduction of valves that prevent auto-inflation and lockout. The evolution of IPP has continued over the last 10 years with various technologies in development, including mechanized cylinder inflation via battery-operated pumps to eliminate problems associated with manual manipulation of the scrotal pump, and more compact devices to eliminate the need for tubing and connections, leading to lower infection rates and mechanical failures [26]. Battery-operated and heat-activated prostheses are currently undergoing research and development and are on the horizon for prosthetic urology.

1.6.3.4 Future of ED Treatment

Regenerative medicine therapies are being explored in the men's health practice as a way to restore erectile function. Low-intensity extracorporeal shock wave therapy, a technology introduced to medicine in 1978, is another noninvasive treatment that has continued to be developed, and in the last 10 years has proven to have positive effects on erectile function when applied to the penile shaft of men who responded to pharmacotherapy [27,28]. Platelet-rich plasma contains a high concentration of growth factors such as vascular endothelial growth factor, platelet-derived growth factor, and insulin growth factor [29]. Early clinical trials have suggested a small but clinically relevant improvement in ED through the endothelial nitric oxide synthase pathway [30,31]. Mesenchymal stem cells possess regenerative abilities and promote cell growth and survival through the release of a variety of cytokines [32]. Clinical trials have demonstrated safety and minor improvement in erectile function after the injection of stem cells [33]. Other techniques such as wrapping the neurovascular bundle with dehydrated amnion/chorion membrane during radical prostatectomy have emerged to help improve nerve recovery as these grafts are full of growth factors and cytokines [34]. Despite having sound translational evidence behind these therapies, there is still a paucity of data from human studies and further trials need to be completed before their routine clinical use can be recommended.

1.6.4 Fertility

Approximately 15% of couples fail to conceive after one year of trying, and male factor infertility accounts for about half of these cases. In recent years, increasing environmental pollution and psychological stresses have resulted in a decline in sperm counts worldwide [35]. Etiologic factors in male infertility include congenital, acquired, and idiopathic causes.

1.6.4.1 Semen Analysis

As modern statistical analysis has been utilized to examine the metrics of the parameters of the semen analysis over the last two decades, it has become clear that the semen analysis should be used as a part of, not as a complete male evaluation. The World Health Organization updated criteria in 2010 to help delineate a "normal" semen analysis. With the evolution of computers and the development of computer-assisted semen analysis equipment, machines have been able to measure standard semen parameters. Within the last decade, newer assays have been developed including testing for reactive oxygen species and sperm DNA fragmentation. These assays are still being studied and continue to undergo refinement but may prove to be informative in individual cases.

1.6.4.2 In Vitro Fertilization (IVF)

The first IVF birth in 1978 opened the door for the utilization of advanced reproductive technologies (ART) worldwide. One of the most important advances since 1978 in the trajectory of IVF was the ability to insert a single sperm into an ovum and achieve a live birth. This technique, known as intracytoplasmic sperm injection (ICSI), made biological parenthood possible when only a few sperm are available in the ejaculate or retrieved from the testis. The use of ICSI worldwide has steadily grown, representing 67% of all ART cases performed in 60 countries, according to the International Committee Monitoring Assisted Reproductive Technologies for 2008–2010, and revolutionized the treatment of infertility since the first ICSI report in 1992 [36,37]. Currently, ICSI is the preferred insemination protocol, with many centers using it in >90% of their insemination cycles [38].

First described in 1998, microdissection testicular sperm extraction (microTESE) has transformed sperm extraction in men with azoospermia and is useful when used in conjunction with ICSI [39]. In the past two years, microTESE has been reported to yield up to a 90% sperm retrieval rate from dilated seminiferous tubules [40]. The development of microTESE used in conjunction with ICSI has given many men with nonobstructive azoospermia the hope of biological parenthood. However, current methods of sperm retrieval via microTESE specimens are labor-intensive, inefficient, and expensive, so there is strong interest in improving the process. Novel sorting methods have therefore been developed over the last decade and continue to be cultivated. These methods include microfluidics, magnetic-activated cell sorting, and fluorescence-activated cell sorting [41]. In the last 20 years, studies on carriers and single-sperm freezing methods have tremendously improved the recovery and activity rates of sperm after cryopreservation, and there is large developmental potential of these procedures [35].

1.6.4.3 Microsurgical Advances

Since the microsurgical subinguinal approach to varicocelectomy was described in 1985, the technique has exploded worldwide and has resulted in excellent outcomes with lower complication rates than nonmicrosurgical approaches [38]. In the past five years, improved outcomes for both intrauterine insemination and IVF have been shown

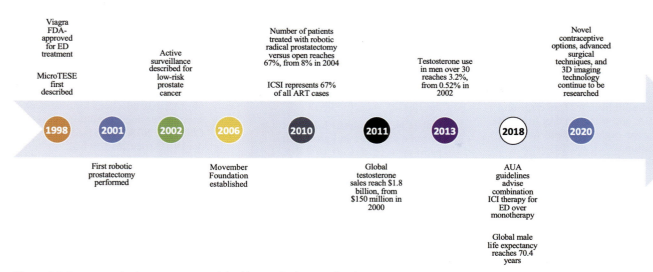

Figure 1.1 Progress and achievements in men's health over the last two decades

in men who first undergo microsurgical varicocelectomy. In fact, recent studies illustrate that both men with low sperm counts and those requiring TESE do indeed benefit from microsurgical varicocele repair even in instances when ART is required [42].

Microsurgical techniques have also been applied to men with obstructive azoospermia, with the first reported microsurgical vasectomy reversal using vasovasostomy in the 1970s [43]. As vasectomy reversal remains the standard of care for men desiring fertility after sterilization, the technique has been constantly refined throughout the past two decades. Currently, vasectomy reversal results in return of sperm to the ejaculate in 85–99% of men, with pregnancy rates from 40% to 80%, depending on time since vasectomy and female age. Additionally, with the constant advancement of technology, techniques such as robotic vasectomy reversal and video microsurgery are emerging. Though the cost-effectiveness of these novel techniques can be debated, literature within the last 20 years has shown that, compared to going directly to IVF/ICSI, vasectomy reversal is significantly more cost-effective than IVF/ICSI in sterilized males by a significant margin [44]. This phenomenon may also be due in part to the increasing accessibility of vasectomies, as five states have passed laws within the last 10 years that require state-regulated health insurance plans to also cover vasectomies at no additional cost to the patient.

1.7 Conclusion

The past 20 years have seen major innovations and refinements with men's health. The next 20 years will likely prove to be even more fruitful for the discipline. Things on the horizon include novel contraceptive options, advanced surgical technologies, incorporation of novel three-dimensional imaging capture in various urologic settings, and the continued advancement of men's health as a whole (Figure 1.1).

References

1. Griffith DM. Biopsychosocial approaches to men's health disparities research and policy. *Behav Med*. 2016;42(3):211–215. doi:10.1080/08964289.2016.1194158.
2. The World Bank. Life expectancy at birth, male (years). 2019. https://data.worldbank.org/indicator/SP.DYN.LE00.MA.IN. Accessed October 25, 2022.
3. Mortality GBD, Causes of Death Collaboration. Global, regional, and national age-sex specific all-cause and cause-specific mortality for 240 causes of death, 1990–2013: a systematic analysis for the Global Burden of Disease Study 2013. *Lancet*. 2015;385 (9963):117–171. doi:10.1016/S0140-6736(14)61682-2.
4. Vaidya V, Partha G, Karmakar M. Gender differences in utilization of preventive care services in the United States. *J Womens Health (Larchmt)*. 2012;21(2):140–145. doi:10.1089/jwh.2011.2876.
5. Kannel WB, Hjortland MC, McNamara PM, Gordon T. Menopause and risk of cardiovascular disease: the Framingham study. *Ann Intern Med*. 1976;85 (4):447–452. doi:10.7326/0003-4819-85-4-447.
6. Vitale C, Fini M, Speziale G, Chierchia S. Gender differences in the cardiovascular effects of sex hormones. *Fundam Clin Pharmacol*. 2010;24 (6):675–685. doi:10.1111/j.1472-8206.2010.00817.x.
7. Yahia N, Wang D, Rapley M, Dey R. Assessment of weight status, dietary habits and beliefs, physical activity, and nutritional knowledge among university students. *Perspect Public Health*. 2016;136(4):231–244. doi:10.1177/1757913915609945.
8. Koopmans GT, Lamers LM. Gender and health care utilization: the role of mental distress and help-seeking propensity. *Soc Sci Med*. 2007;64 (6):1216–1230. doi:10.1016/j.socscimed.2006.11.018.

9. Roth MY, Amory JK. Beyond the condom: frontiers in male contraception. *Semin Reprod Med.* 2016;34(3):183–190. doi:10.1055/s-0036-1571435.

10. Garrett B, Gangopadhyaya A. Who gained health insurance coverage under the ACA, and where do they live? 2016. www.urban.org/sites/default/files/publication/86761/2001041-who-gained-health-insurance-coverage-under-the-aca-and-where-do-they-live.pdf. Accessed October 19, 2022.

11. Houman JJ, Eleswarapu SV, Mills JN. Current and future trends in men's health clinics. *Transl Androl Urol.* 2020;9(Suppl 2):S116–S122. doi:10.21037/tau.2019.08.33.

12. Cacciamani GE, Stern MC, Medina LG, Gill K, Sotelo R, Gill IS. Cancer awareness crusades-pink ribbons and growing moustaches. *Lancet Oncol.* 2019;20(11):1491–1492. doi:10.1016/S1470-2045(19)30639-4.

13. Lowrance WT, Eastham JA, Savage C, et al. Contemporary open and robotic radical prostatectomy practice patterns among urologists in the United States. *J Urol.* 2012;187(6):2087–2092. doi:10.1016/j.juro.2012.01.061.

14. Catton CN, Lukka H, Martin J. Prostate cancer radiotherapy: an evolving paradigm. *J Clin Oncol.* 2018;36(29):2909–2913. doi:10.1200/JCO.2018.79.3257.

15. Podder TK, Fredman ET, Ellis RJ. Advances in radiotherapy for prostate cancer treatment. *Adv Exp Med Biol.* 2018;1096:31–47. doi:10.1007/978-3-319-99286-0_2.

16. Tan WP, Levine LA. What can we do for chronic scrotal content pain? *World J Mens Health.* 2017;35(3):146–155. doi:10.5534/wjmh.17047.

17. Calixte N, Tojuola B, Kartal I, et al. Targeted robotic assisted microsurgical denervation of the spermatic cord for the treatment of chronic orchialgia or groin pain: a single center, large series review. *J Urol.* 2018;199(4):1015–1022. doi:10.1016/j.juro.2017.10.030.

18. Levine LA. Microsurgical denervation of the spermatic cord. *J Sex Med.* 2008;5(3):526–529. doi:10.1111/j.1743-6109.2007.00762.x.

19. Levine LA, Matkov TG, Lubenow TR. Microsurgical denervation of the spermatic cord: a surgical alternative in the treatment of chronic orchialgia. *J Urol.* 1996;155(3):1005–1007. doi:10.1016/s0022-5347(01)66369-9.

20. Tatem A, Kovac JR. Chronic scrotal pain and microsurgical spermatic cord denervation: tricks of the trade. *Transl Androl Urol.* 2017;6(Suppl 1):S30–S36. doi:10.21037/tau.2017.05.17.

21. Calixte N, Brahmbhatt J, Parekattil S. Chronic testicular and groin pain: pathway to relief. *Curr Urol Rep.* 2017;18(10):83. doi:10.1007/s11934-017-0722-7.

22. Martin AL, Huelin R, Wilson D, Foster TS, Mould JF. A systematic review assessing the economic impact of sildenafil citrate (Viagra) in the treatment of erectile dysfunction. *J Sex Med.* 2013;10(5):1389–1400. doi:10.1111/jsm.12068.

23. Duncan C, Omran GJ, Teh J, Davis NF, Bolton DM, Lawrentschuk N. Erectile dysfunction: a global review of intracavernosal injectables. *World J Urol.* 2019;37(6):1007–1014. doi:10.1007/s00345-019-02727-5.

24. Burnett AL, Nehra A, Breau RH, et al. Erectile dysfunction: AUA guideline. *J Urol.* 2018;200(3):633–641. doi:10.1016/j.juro.2018.05.004.

25. Wespes E, Amar E, Hatzichristou D, et al. EAU guidelines on erectile dysfunction: an update. *Eur Urol.* 2006;49(5):806–815. doi:10.1016/j.eururo.2006.01.028.

26. Gurtner K, Saltzman A, Hebert K, Laborde E. Erectile dysfunction: a review of historical treatments with a focus on the development of the inflatable penile prosthesis. *Am J Mens Health.* 2017;11(3):479–486. doi:10.1177/1557988315596566.

27. Vardi Y, Appel B, Kilchevsky A, Gruenwald I. Does low intensity extracorporeal shock wave therapy have a physiological effect on erectile function? Short-term results of a randomized, double-blind, sham controlled study. *J Urol.* 2012;187(5):1769–1775. doi:10.1016/j.juro.2011.12.117.

28. Fojecki GL, Tiessen S, Osther PJ. Extracorporeal shock wave therapy (ESWT) in urology: a systematic review of outcome in Peyronie's disease, erectile dysfunction and chronic pelvic pain. *World J Urol.* 2017;35(1):1–9. doi:10.1007/s00345-016-1834-2.

29. Epifanova MV, Gvasalia BR, Durashov MA, Artemenko SA. Platelet-rich plasma therapy for male sexual dysfunction: myth or reality? *Sex Med Rev.* 2020;8(1):106–113. doi:10.1016/j.sxmr.2019.02.002.

30. Matz EL, Pearlman AM, Terlecki RP. Safety and feasibility of platelet rich fibrin matrix injections for treatment of common urologic conditions. *Investig Clin Urol.* 2018;59(1):61–65. doi:10.4111/icu.2018.59.1.61.

31. Musicki B, Palese MA, Crone JK, Burnett AL. Phosphorylated endothelial nitric oxide synthase mediates vascular endothelial growth factor-induced penile erection. *Biol Reprod.* 2004;70(2):282–289. doi:10.1095/biolreprod.103.021113.

32. Caplan AI, Correa D. The MSC: an injury drugstore. *Cell Stem Cell.* 2011;9(1):11–15. doi:10.1016/j.stem.2011.06.008.

33. Bahk JY, Jung JH, Han H, Min SK, Lee YS. Treatment of diabetic impotence with umbilical cord blood stem cell intracavernosal transplant: preliminary report of 7 cases. *Exp Clin Transplant.* 2010;8(2):150–160.

34. Patel VR, Samavedi S, Bates AS, et al. Dehydrated human amnion/chorion membrane allograft nerve wrap around the prostatic neurovascular bundle accelerates early return to continence and potency following robot-assisted radical prostatectomy: propensity score-matched analysis. *Eur Urol.* 2015;67(6):977–980. doi:10.1016/j.eururo.2015.01.012.

35. Liu S, Li F. Cryopreservation of single-sperm: where are we today? *Reprod Biol Endocrinol.* 2020;18(1):41. doi:10.1186/s12958-020-00607-x.

36. Dyer S, Chambers GM, de Mouzon J, et al. International Committee for Monitoring Assisted Reproductive Technologies world report: Assisted Reproductive Technology 2008, 2009 and 2010. *Hum Reprod.* 2016;31(7):1588–1609. doi:10.1093/humrep/dew082.

37. Palermo G, Joris H, Devroey P, Van Steirteghem AC. Pregnancies after intracytoplasmic injection of single spermatozoon into an oocyte. *Lancet.* 1992;340(8810):17–18. doi:10.1016/0140-6736(92)92425-f.

38. Niederberger C, Pellicer A, Cohen J, et al. Forty years of IVF. *Fertil Steril.* 2018;110(2):185–324 e5. doi:10.1016/j.fertnstert.2018.06.005.

39. Schlegel PN, Li PS. Microdissection TESE: sperm retrieval in non-obstructive azoospermia. *Hum Reprod Update*. 1998;4(4):439. doi:10.1093/humupd/4.4.439.

40. Caroppo E, Colpi EM, Gazzano G, et al. The seminiferous tubule caliber pattern as evaluated at high magnification during microdissection testicular sperm extraction predicts sperm retrieval in patients with non-obstructive azoospermia. *Andrology*. 2019;7(1):8–14. doi:10.1111/andr.12548.

41. Mangum CL, Patel DP, Jafek AR, et al. Towards a better testicular sperm extraction: novel sperm sorting technologies for non-motile sperm extracted by microdissection TESE. *Transl Androl Urol*. 2020;9(Suppl 2):S206–S214. doi:10.21037/tau.2019.08.36.

42. Kirby EW, Wiener LE, Rajanahally S, Crowell K, Coward RM. Undergoing varicocele repair before assisted reproduction improves pregnancy rate and live birth rate in azoospermic and oligospermic men with a varicocele: a systematic review and meta-analysis. *Fertil Steril*. 2016;106(6):1338–1343. doi:10.1016/j.fertnstert.2016.07.1093.

43. Silber SJ. Microscopic technique for reversal of vasectomy. *Surg Gynecol Obstet*. 1976;143(4):631.

44. Lee R, Li PS, Goldstein M, Tanrikut C, Schattman G, Schlegel PN. A decision analysis of treatments for obstructive azoospermia. *Hum Reprod*. 2008;23(9):2043–2049. doi:10.1093/humrep/den200.

Section 1　An Introduction to Men's Health Care

Chapter 2: The Business Landscape of Men's Health

James M. Weinberger and Jesse N. Mills

2.1 Introduction

Over the last two decades, the men's health space has grown exponentially; the International Society of Sexual Medicine now boasts over 2,000 members from 89 countries. Further, the number of fellowships available for urologists to specialize in andrology, infertility, and sexual dysfunction has more than doubled in the last decade alone [1]. The contemporary story of the men's health field is entrenched in the gender health gap; the global life expectancy is 5.1 years longer for women than men [2]. This finding from the Global Burden of Disease study confirmed a well-documented gender gap in mortality. Beyond life expectancy, studies continue to demonstrate that men suffer from worse health-related quality of life compared to age-matched females [3]. This discrepancy appears to be a product of both biology and behavior. Men have higher rates of cardiovascular disease (CVD) risk factors such as hypertension, hypercholesterolemia, and diabetes [3]. They also use more alcohol and tobacco, consume less heart-healthy diets, and practice riskier behavior [4,5]. The result of premature mortality and morbidity for men costs $479 billion annually to the United States economy alone [5].

Given that many risk factors responsible for the gender mortality gap are modifiable and related to diet and lifestyle choices, the burden of premature male morbidity signifies a failure of healthcare delivery and policy. Studies show that men are less likely to see a primary care physician, obtain recommended screening exams, and be aware of disease-related symptoms [1,5]. The inroad to quell this underutilization and aversion to screening came with uncovering the link between erectile dysfunction (ED) in young men and an increased risk of coronary events [6]. In addition, studies associating infertility and metabolic syndrome provided another opportunity for physicians to screen and intervene on younger patients [3]. As such, male sexual and reproductive health represents a touchpoint for promoting a global men's health assessment. Further, given the complex nature of screening for the most common male cancer, prostate cancer, urologists are uniquely equipped to improve male health outcomes. It is this backdrop that solidified urologists as the true stewards of men's health [4]. This trend is evident in the eruption of formal Men's Health Centers, now present in close to half of major hospitals in the United States, up from only one-third in 2014 [4].

Men's health has expanded not only as a discipline, but as an industry. Direct-to-consumer marketing catapulted annual testosterone sales in the USA from a stagnant $18 million in 1988 to more than $2 billion in 2013 [7]. The trend is mirrored in global markets, but the US market predominates, accounting for more than 80% of global testosterone sales in 2016 [8]. The demand for prescriptions targeting ED has similarly increased. In 2018, after sildenafil and tadalafil became generic, ED medications accounted for 0.024% of all prescriptions in the USA [9]. Centers for Medicare & Medicaid Services data indicate that phosphodiesterase type 5 inhibitor (PDE5i) prescriptions were written for 149,582 beneficiaries in 2017 alone, with an aggregate cost of well over $500 million [10]. Both physical men's clinics as well as web-based telemedicine companies have moved aggressively to meet consumer demand. Given the vast disparities in practice standards and patterns, array of covered versus out-of-pocket conditions, and role of adjunct streams of revenue, the business considerations surrounding men's health are complex. The purpose of this chapter is to outline the competitive landscape of men's health.

2.2 Hypogonadism

Low testosterone levels are characteristic of classical hypogonadism and can result because of a disruption of the hypothalamic-pituitary-gonadal axis or due to a primary testicular problem [11]. The variance across clinical settings that treat hypogonadism reflects the evolution of practice patterns. Entrepreneurial providers in the early 2000s recognized the increasing swell in demand for testosterone testing and treatment and opened freestanding men's health clinics. These clinics leveraged the influence of direct-to-consumer (DTC) marketing to portray testosterone therapy as a solution for the effects of aging [11]. As a result, the use of testosterone in the USA more than tripled from 2001 to 2011, often in men without a clear indication for treatment [12,13]. Globally, testosterone sales increased from $150 million in 2000 to $1.8 billion in 2011. The growth of the hypogonadism market segment created a dynamic unique to men's health that perpetuates today; a substantial proportion of testosterone prescribers operate in nontraditional medical settings. These freestanding centers are infrequently staffed by urologists, endocrinologists, or cardiologists [1].

Some of these "low T" for-profit clinics offer a subscription model. Membership includes office visits, labs work, and testosterone injections paid upfront [1]. These membership plans often include multiple months of treatment regardless of treatment response and without rigorous monitoring. These monetization centers forego aspects of the traditional medical visit such as obtaining a medical history, performing a physical exam, and ordering indicated labs and imaging [13]. This structure led to notably inappropriate prescribing patterns; in two studies of collectively more than 11 million men, the rate of initiation of testosterone without obtaining of baseline testosterone levels was remarkably high, ranging from 25.28% [12] to 40.2% [11]. Further, Layton et al. compared testosterone prescribing patterns in the United Kingdom and the USA from 2000 to 2011. Across a large population-based study, the authors found that only 10% of men with low testosterone levels were initiated on therapy in the UK, as compared to ~40% in the USA. Further, 4–9% of US patients with normal or high levels were initiated on testosterone, as compared to <1% in the UK [11].

This growth trend was curbed only by a US Food and Drug Administration (FDA) safety communication in 2014 [12]. Buoyed by two studies that reported an association between testosterone use and an increased risk of myocardial infarction and stroke, the FDA explicitly asserted that prescription testosterone is only indicated for men who have low testosterone due to certain medical conditions and not for men with low testosterone secondary to aging alone [14]. The 2014 communication resulted in a dramatic change in practice patterns; between 2013 and 2016, there was a 62% relative decline in new testosterone prescriptions and, similarly, a 48% relative decrease in established users [12]. Studies since the FDA communication have broadened the indications for prescription testosterone and informed the current American Urological Association (AUA) guidelines. In fact, due to mixed evidence, it cannot be stated whether exogenous testosterone use increases or decreases the risk of myocardial infarction or stroke [15]. Buoyed by the traditional medical community's apprehension to prescribe testosterone, DTC testosterone clinics flourish even more.

The AUA guideline statement on testosterone prescribing indicates that the diagnosis of hypogonadism, by definition, requires the clinical signs and symptoms of low testosterone as well as repeated morning measurements confirming low testosterone levels [15]. Despite the FDA communication, guideline-discordant prescribing persists. In many cases, low-T centers relinquish one, if not both components of the guideline, prescribing to patients regardless of symptoms and without repeated morning measurements [11,16,17]. As evidenced by studies of US insurance claims data, even fewer patients received a PSA test to rule out prostate cancer, a contraindication to testosterone therapy, prior to initiation of therapy [16,17]. A study of Veterans Health Administration prescribing practices demonstrated that over a four-year study period, only 3.1% of men receiving testosterone supplementation received a full guideline-compliant workup including two morning testosterone levels, LH and/or FSH, PSA, and hematocrit [15,17]. Further, studies demonstrate that a not insignificant proportion of testosterone prescriptions are for inappropriate indications such as infertility [11,16,17]. This likely represents evidence of a discrepancy in quality of care between factory-line low-T centers and urology clinics.

Despite the FDA's 2014 communication, entire industries within health care have been built around treating natural aging. Men will continue to seek elective treatment for age-related effects of low testosterone and, as a result, low-T centers continue to monetize out-of-pocket testosterone treatment [1]. Given that a market to treat aging will perpetuate, men would benefit from guideline-driven prescribing and monitoring patterns found in practices staffed by urologists and endocrinologists.

This awareness of the potential dangers associated with inappropriate testosterone prescribing and monitoring coincided with a more systems-based, global methodology to men's health. A layered approach to a men's health workup now involves consideration of urologic, cardiologic, psychologic, and endocrine needs, among others [1]. This multidisciplinary approach is well-suited for academic and well-integrated managed-care centers. This more comprehensive method provides the opportunity to screen for comorbidities and engage in preventative medicine. Reimbursement in this model, however, is more complex. Cash-based low-T centers are able to leverage economies of scale and efficiencies in delivery of care that academic and managed-care settings cannot; properly tailoring workup and treatment regimens and coordinating between multiple specialties does not lend itself to leveraging economies of scale. As a result, these holistic men's health clinics benefit from the infrastructure of a health system to capture the downstream revenue associated with longitudinal care of a patient. For example, if an academic medical center has a men's clinic, it can market effectively to a population that traditionally does not seek medical attention routinely. Smart marketing using the carrot of sexual medicine and health optimization can lead to patients who wouldn't ordinarily get screened for prostate or colon cancer. It therefore is no surprise that many academic centers and Large Urology Group Practices (LUGPA) have created men's centers. The profit lies not in testosterone prescriptions but in associated and otherwise not captured revenue these men provide.

Another advantage of more well-rounded practices taking the helm of men's health is patients get an unbiased discussion on what testosterone formulation is right for them. Direct-to-consumer testosterone clinics rely on the exorbitant markup of generic testosterone injections to drive their profits. If a center's business model does not depend on marking up the product, a patient and physician can choose what delivery mechanism is right.

2.3 Erectile Dysfunction

ED was once thought to be exclusively a disease of the aging man; studies now demonstrate a nontrivial prevalence of ED in men younger than 40 years old (22%) [18,19]. The pathogenesis of ED includes atherosclerosis with associated oxidative stress and endothelial damage; deficient endothelial-mediated vasodilation is characteristic of both ED and coronary artery disease (CAD) [20]. In fact, multiple studies reveal that ED is an independent predictor of future cardiovascular events [20]. In a meta-analysis of prospective trials spanning over 36,000 patients, ED independently increased the risk of CVD by 48%, stroke by 35%, and all-cause mortality by 19% [21]. Moreover, studies determined that ED precedes the development of clinically significant CAD by approximately five years [20]. This predictable timeline underlines the gravity of implementing formal men's health screening in the setting of ED diagnosis and treatment.

Beyond its central role in funneling younger patients into a formal men's health screening program, diagnosing and treating ED and its associated conditions represents a business opportunity for urologists. The global market for pharmaceuticals for ED is projected to be $6.29 billion by 2024 with a 6.3% compound annual growth rate (CAGR) [22]. The market for ED devices, which generally includes penile prostheses, implants, and vacuum devices, is similarly anticipated to grow to over $645 million by 2023 [23].

The opportunity this market segment provides is not new; historically, the track record of for-profit men's clinics is evidence of the financial benefits available to urologists and other healthcare providers. These cash-based clinics originated as "low-T" prescribers but have expanded to address ED as well. These clinics often do not offer the full range of potential treatment options and are driven instead by financial incentives [1]. For example, platelet-rich plasma (PRP) is an autologous blood plasma with growth factors promoting angiogenic, vasculogenic, and regenerative effects. These properties theoretically stimulate blood flow and regulate vascular smooth muscle, accounting for its numerous applications across multiple specialties in medicine [18]. The theoretical application bolstered the advent of the Priapus shot or "P-Shot." This DTC product claims literal regrowth of tissue and vessels leading to rejuvenation of erections [24]. Further, marketing materials claim improvements in penile length, girth, and firmness. These claims have little standing in the literature; no study exists comparing PRP to a placebo arm or to the standard of care, PDE5i [18]. As a result, the AUA has concluded that there is no scientific evidence-based risk-benefit profile for the use of PRP [25]. Both the AUA and Sexual Medicine Society of North America (SMSNA) statements specify that PRP is experimental and only appropriate in the setting of a clinical trial [24–26]. Nonetheless, sales of PRP for ED continue to grow.

For-profit clinics have also leveraged the inelastic demand for ED treatment to create huge industries behind Low intensity Shock Wave Therapy (LiSWT) and intracavernous stem cell therapy. Given the lack of clinical data for treating ED, stem cell treatments are entirely out-of-pocket, and yet, patient willingness to pay supports prices ranging from $2,000 to $20,000 [27]. Further, despite the SMSNA's position statement deeming LiWST for ED as experimental, the current market demonstrates that there exists a model for implementing this into practice [26]. These practices are built on active marketing that leverages public interest. These for-profit clinics employ an effective fiscal model but are not optimized for patient care; they are often not staffed by a urologist, which has concerning implications for the management of complications, and further, they rarely address preventative medicine, lifestyle modifications, and health screening [1].

Other practice settings allow for alternative financial angles and synergies. For example, LUGPAs are frequently dispensing PDE5is directly. This obviates the hassle of prior authorization. Moreover, it lowers the cost to the patient and increases margins for the LUGPA itself. The patient may benefit fiscally, but the practice, unless carefully self-policed, raises ethical concerns. In fact, Boston Medical Group, an international center offering proprietary personalized treatment for ED, premature ejaculation, and low T, was at the center of a legal controversy when it was discovered that physician bonuses were tied to prescriptions written for injections. Further, in parallel to LUGPAs dispensing medications, the Boston Medical Group pharmacy that prepared injections was found to be owned by the founder's wife [28]. The financial appeal of vertical integration by a practice group is enticing but must be structured as to not influence or compromise ethical prescribing patterns.

The academic setting may be best positioned to leverage the synergies of vertical integration. The health system can capitalize on a multidisciplinary approach in which an ED consult can prompt a thorough men's health workup involving urologists, endocrinologists, cardiologists, and nutritionists. Ultimately, the academic center will collect the downstream revenue from prescriptions, long-term screening, and hospitalizations. The managed care setting is similarly optimized to provide a more holistic approach to the ED and men's health visit. In fact, managed care or accountable care organizations (ACOs) are incentivized to champion prevention-based management consistent with the recent evolution toward a comprehensive, multidisciplinary approach to men's health clinics.

The influx and success of DTC companies demonstrates a market inefficiency unaddressed by traditional for-profit clinics and urology offices. Studies suggest that only half of men with ED will actively seek consultation [1]. These online platforms remove the social stigma associated with an office visit for ED that prevents many young men from seeking care. Further, they eliminate obvious access to care issues and fulfill a need for instant gratification and convenience. As a result, these market disrupters have quickly gained market share; Hims is projected for $250 million in annual subscription revenue with 60% gross margins and a 50% retention rate over 18 months [29]. The two largest DTC platforms for ED prescribing, Hims and Ro, have valuations of $1 billion and $500 million, respectively [19]. These platforms have exposed a gap in the care of traditional providers, delivering value to customers through a more comfortable and expedient patient experience. However, there are growing concerns from the medical community that these companies are leveraging a more lax regulatory environment and that the patient intake process for these online platforms does not adhere to guideline-based recommendations for the workup of ED. Specifically, physical examination, laboratory evaluation, and counseling on both risk factors and prevention are often circumvented [1,19]. One study of a large cohort of young men presenting to an academic center for workup of ED found a significant rate of comorbid pathology on workup; 20% of the cohort was discovered to have diabetes or prediabetes. Further, 54% had dyslipidemia, 15% had obesity, and 20% had low testosterone [19]. The DTC platforms omit the guideline-based workup and therefore relinquish the opportunity to intervene on metabolic risk factors that portend significant health consequences. Moreover, the online DTC platforms often dispense through a subscription format with no reevaluation. Ultimately, the DTC prescription platform foregoes the opportunity to discover comorbidities and to counsel patients on risk factors, preventative lifestyle modifications, weight loss, and fertility [19]. However, this successful platform should serve as a wakeup call to traditional medical practices that the market is there and the opportunity to positively intervene in the health of men and drive practice revenues is golden.

The market disrupters uncovered an unmet need for more discrete and accessible workup and treatment of ED but lack the infrastructure to become the initial touch-point for a formal men's health evaluation. The rapid ascension of DTC companies to high valuations further validates the niche discovered by early for-profit clinics that identified ED treatment as a sector with significant demand. In response to the success of Hims and Ro, academic and community physicians must incorporate telemedicine into their practice patterns; models for this are evolving but may include having remote patients follow up with a local primary physician for screening and labs. Ultimately, providers will be able to win back market share based on practice pattern differentiation, combining access and convenience with guideline-based practice that evaluates patients comprehensively. Leveraging young men's desire to seek treatment for ED in order to formally provide a men's health evaluation represents a unique opportunity to close the gender life gap.

2.4 Peyronie's Disease

Peyronie's disease (PD) is characterized by fibrosis of the tunica albuginea, often causing deformity, pain, and ED. The disease process can cause significant distress for patients and, therefore, the willingness to pursue novel treatment methods is high. In 2013, the FDA approved the use of injectable collagenase clostridium histolyticum (CCH) for destruction of Peyronie's plaques. With the support of the AUA practice guidelines, a robust market has developed for CCH treatment [30]. The recommended course includes eight injections at a cost of approximately $3,000 per injection. In 2017, over 180,000 Medicare beneficiaries received Santyl or Xiaflex injections, with an aggregate cost surpassing $150 million [10]. Surgical correction, including plication, plaque excision and graft, and tunical lengthening, remains the gold standard for curvature correction but risks penile shortening and ED [31]. In patients with significant concomitant ED, simultaneous penile prosthesis with intraoperative modeling is indicated. In comparison to a course of CCH, a prosthesis costs more than double at $55,000 [32]. The typical reimbursement structure splits the cost of treatment 80/20 between insurance and the patient, respectively.

Demand for PD treatment is inelastic and therefore patient willingness to pay for out-of-pocket treatment modalities with unclear outcomes data is high. Studies examining PRP in the treatment of PD advocate for its use mechanistically as an adjunct to CCH; while CCH is effective in breaking down plaque, PRP facilitates tissue regeneration [18]. The data for its effectiveness, however, remain lacking. No Level 1 evidence supports its use in PD. Only one trial exists with a placebo arm; this preclinical study of rats found that injections of PRP in fact cause fibrosis and can even be used to model the disease process [33]. Nonetheless, PRP injections are being paid for out-of-pocket at a rate of $1,500–$3,000 per injection [24]. Further, the industry is largely unregulated after it earned the distinction of "minimal manipulation of tissue." As a result, the regulatory restrictions are more lax, resulting in unpredictable variability in PRP formulations between offices [24].

Despite the lack of evidence, some men's health providers continue to offer PRP for PD. Moreover, given the lenient regulatory environment, providers are not held to a protocol for treatment, including confirmation of the appropriate qualitative and quantitative composition of growth factors and platelets in PRP [18]. This has created an opportunity for certain providers to scale a lower-cost production of PRP, with a funnel of customers via DTC marketing. In similar fashion, some men's health providers have capitalized on the distress PD causes by offering other data-agnostic treatments such as extracorporeal LiSWT for a significant financial cost. While the evidence supports the use of shockwave therapy as second-line therapy for refractory penile pain in the setting of PD, the European Association of Urology guidelines explicitly state that LiSWT should not be used for penile curvature correction or plaque reduction [31,34]. Nonetheless, DTC advertising has created a market that supports treatment courses ranging from $3,000 to $6,000 [35]. This theme is pervasive across the disease processes central to men's health: Inelastic demand, in conjunction with platforms enabling direct marketing, create a market for expensive, out-of-pocket treatments that are buoyed only by a theoretical mechanism for clinical improvement. While these novel technologies may show anecdotal promise, one would be remiss to build a sustainable business plan around LiSWT or PRP for treatment of PD without better clinical trials. As more data become available, we may in fact find effective protocols and injectable biologics that will change the marketplace.

2.5 Infertility

Infertility is the inability to initiate a pregnancy after one year of unprotected vaginal intercourse. Despite certain historical narratives, infertility is a condition of both men and women; approximately half of infertility cases involve the male partner. In fact, national surveys demonstrate that 9.4% of men aged 15–44 have clinical infertility [36]. The global market size for male infertility was valued at $3.5 billion in 2019 with a notable projected CAGR of 4.7% over the next five years. Multiple factors contribute to this growth trend, including the rising age of would-be parents, delayed pregnancy, increased alcohol consumption, stress, increased BMI, and the frequent use of pesticides [37]. In fact, Levine et al. performed a meta-regression analysis of over 40,000 men from 185 studies and found that in North America, Europe, Australia, and New Zealand, there has been a significant decline in sperm concentration and total sperm count between 1973 and 2011 [38]. The evidence of decline persisted, even controlling for age, method of collection, and abstinence time, among other modulators. The authors found that in Western men unselected for their fertility status, for example screened for military service or college students, the average decline in sperm concentration was 1.4% per year, with the 2011 value of 47.1 million sperm per mL [38]. The notion that the general Western mean sperm count was approaching the 40 million/mL threshold for subfertility in 2011 predicts the accelerated growth seen in the men's infertility market segment.

The underlying driver of the infertility business landscape is insurance coverage, as determined by State policy. Notably, only 15 states mandate that insurance policies cover infertility benefits (Figure 2.1). Moreover, only eight states require the coverage of in vitro fertilization (IVF), suggesting that even fewer states mandate any robust coverage. In fact, the policies of only eight states even mention the male partner [36]. This may account for survey results indicating that despite guideline recommendations from the American Society of Reproductive Medicine (ASRM) that both partners undergo infertility evaluations, approximately one-quarter of men do not receive a fertility workup [36]. Given limited coverage, this gap in access to care is exacerbated by the high costs of infertility workup and treatment; one 2016 study of San Francisco area men demonstrated that 46% of men were limited by cost in selecting treatment and that 47% of men experienced financial strain due to said infertility treatments. Further, 64% of the cohort reported out-of-pocket costs exceeding $15,000 and 16% indicated that they had spent greater than $50,000 [39]. As a result, states in which fertility is not covered foster large-margin cash practices.

In the few states that mandate coverage for infertility, large fertility centers are able to leverage economies of scale due to the significant patient volume. In some cases, IVF centers have begun to extend the fertility umbrella to include men's infertility workup and treatment. These centers have been able to capitalize on customer recruitment via the female partner. Synergies exist for companies that can provide services to both male and female partners. In particular, these centers can lower the fixed costs of sperm and egg banking, and decrease staffing costs by relying on reproductive endocrinologists well-versed in both male and female infertility. Nonetheless, most of the market remains fragmented; due to disparate insurance coverage and regulations, the majority of fertility providers are comprised of small regional clinics, private physician practices, and hospital or university based centers [40].

Beyond clinic-based synergies uncovered by centers offering male and female infertility treatment, health systems implementing a comprehensive men's health approach are able to leverage a lifetime of healthcare utilization. Accumulating data reveal a concerning correlation between poor semen quality and worse somatic health outcomes [36,37]. The connection between male subfertility and long-term morbidity has been linked to diabetes, metabolic disorders, cardiovascular disease, and cancers, all largely independent of socioeconomic status and lifestyle factors [37]. In one study from two academic medical centers, 6% of male infertility evaluations discovered underlying pathology ranging from testicular cancer to cystic fibrosis [41]. The role of a multidisciplinary approach to men's health is again evident as an initial presentation for infertility evaluation can prompt the establishment of longitudinal, comprehensive care for the patient. In traditional fee-for-service models, this facilitates multispecialty clinic visits and continued downstream revenue. For ACO models, the preventative health component is critical. In both cases, the health center and University-based models are uniquely positioned to capitalize on the holistic approach to infertility and men's health.

An emerging presence in the male fertility marketplace is DTC semen analysis and banking start-ups. These online services offer at-home collection of semen for analysis and cryopreservation. The business model is simple and fulfills an underserved need as many areas of the country have no sperm banking. If a man is diagnosed with a malignancy and wants to preserve sperm prior to radiation or chemotherapy, he would need access to a sperm bank. Legacy and Dadi, two of the current market leaders, raised a combined $3.5 million dollars in early seed rounds in 2019 alone [42]. The Legacy kit offers two semen deposits and 10 years of storage for $1,995. These emerging companies are taking advantage of an expanding market, including oncofertility, same-sex couples planning on a future surrogate, trans women prior to gender affirmation surgery, and military men desiring sperm preservation before deployment. The value proposition of access, discretion, and comfort for sperm banking has resonated with both consumers and investors. These DTC companies appear positioned to win a significant proportion of market share going forward.

Summary of male factor infertility coverage in states with laws related to infertility coverage.

State	Male factor evaluation and treatment coverage included in law	Restrictions	Law/code	Year(s) enacted
AR	None		Ark. State. Ann. § 23-85-137, § 23-86-118	1987, 2011
CA	Diagnosis and treatment (medication and surgery) of conditions causing infertility must be offered to employers		Cal. Health & Safety Code § 1374.55, Cal. Insurance Code § 10119.6	1989
CT	Diagnosis and treatment for individuals unable to "produce conception"		Conn. Gen. Stat. § 38a-509, § 38a-536	1989, 2005
HI	None		Hawaii Rev. Stat. § 431:10A-116.5, § 432.1-604	1989, 2003
IL	None		Ill. Rev. Stat. ch. 215, § 5/356m	1991, 1996
LA	None		La. Rev. Stat. Ann. § 22:1036	2001
MD	None		Md. Insurance Code Ann. § 15-810, Md. Health General Code Ann. § 19-701	2000
MA	Diagnosis and treatment of infertility, including sperm procurement, processing, and banking	Correction of elective sterilization; experimental procedures[a]	Mass. Gen. Laws Ann. Ch. 175, § 47H, ch. 176A, § 8K, ch. 176B, § 4J, ch. 176G, § 4; 211 Code of Massachusetts Regulations 37.00	1987, 2010
MT	Undefined "infertility services" as a basic health care service	Only mandated for Health Maintenance Organizations (HMOs)	Mont. Code Ann. § 33-22-1521, § 33-31-102(2)(v), et seq.	1987
NJ	Diagnosis and treatment of infertility	Correction of elective sterilization; cryopreservation; experimental procedures[a]	N.J. Stat. Ann. § 17:48A-7w, § 17:48E-35.22, § 17B:27-46.1x	2001
NY	Semen analysis, testis biopsy, correction of malformation, disease, or dysfunction resulting in infertility	Correction of elective sterilizations; cryopreservation; experimental procedures[a]	N.Y. Insurance Law § 3216 (13), § 3221 (6) and § 4303	1990, 2002, 2011
OH	Diagnostic and exploratory procedures for testicular failure	Only mandated for HMOs	Ohio Rev. Code Ann § 1751.01 (A) (7)	1991
RI	None		R.I. Gen. Laws § 27-18-30, § 27-19-23, § 27-20-20 and § 27-41-33	1989, 2007
TX	None		Tex. Insurance Code Ann. § 1366.001 et seq.	1987, 2003
WV	Undefined "infertility services" as a basic health care service	Only mandated for HMOs	W. Va. Code § 33-25A-2	1995

[a] Not otherwise defined.

Figure 2.1 Summary of male factor infertility coverage in states with laws related to infertility coverage (reprinted from 43, with permission from Elsevier)

2.6 Conclusions

The business landscape of men's health is diverse, due to the spectrum of practice standards, ranging from cosmetic hormone prescribing to fellowship-driven, evidence-based medicine. The disparity has a historical precedent, as early low-T centers were cash-based for-profit clinics. Fundamental to the fiscal success of many providers is the inelastic demand for solutions to aging, ED, and PD, coupled with DTC marketing. This market dynamic has created booming industries for out-of-pocket products that offer theoretical benefit without rigorous science supporting their use. And while infertility practices are data-driven, the field represents a profitable industry. The infertility landscape is ultimately driven by state insurance coverage laws: In the majority of states, given little coverage, large cash-based practices thrive.

Although the out-of-pocket segments of men's health persist, the contemporary story has been defined by the gender health gap; uncovering the link between CAD and ED unveiled a touchpoint for establishing longitudinal and holistic men's health. Identifying the necessity of multidisciplinary care has prompted a boom in men's health centers. University and large hospital systems have the infrastructure to support comprehensive men's health centers and have therefore maximized the downstream revenue associated with prescriptions, long-term screening, and future hospitalizations. Most recently, the paradigm of men's health delivery has been upended; market disrupters like Hims have acquired billion-dollar valuations by leveraging telehealth to deliver value to patients who otherwise might not feel comfortable having an office visit for ED. Private, academic, and managed care practices are recently beginning to embrace telehealth, indicating that they recognize the need to evolve to compete. Ultimately, companies like Hims provide utility to patients through the discrete and convenient treatment of ED but lack the infrastructure to become the initial touchpoint for a formal men's health evaluation. Leveraging young men's desire to seek treatment for ED, PD, or infertility in order to initiate a comprehensive men's health evaluation represents a unique opportunity to close the gender life gap.

References

1. Houman JJ, Eleswarapu SV, Mills JN. Current and future trends in men's health clinics. *Transl Androl Urol.* 2020;9(I):S116–S122.
2. Dicker D, Nguyen G, Abate D, et al. Global, regional, and national age-sex-specific mortality and life expectancy, 1950–2017: a systematic analysis for the Global Burden of Disease Study 2017. *Lancet.* 2018;392(10159):1684–1735.
3. Tharakan T, Bettocchi C, Carvalho J, et al. Male sexual and reproductive health: does the urologist have a role in addressing gender inequality in life expectancy? *Eur Urol Focus.* 2019;6.
4. Landro L. Why men won't go to the doctor, and how to change that. *Wall Street Journal* [Internet]. 2019;1–9. Available from: www.wsj.com/articles/why-men-wont-go-to-the-doctor-and-how-to-change-that-11556590080
5. Baker P, Shand T. Men's health: time for a new approach to policy and practice? *J Glob Health.* 2017;7(1).
6. Inman BA, St Sauver JL, Jacobson DJ, et al. A population-based, longitudinal study of erectile dysfunction and future coronary artery disease. *Obstet Gynecol Surv.* 2009;64(7):459–460.
7. Bhasin S. A perspective on the evolving landscape in male reproductive medicine. *J Clin Endocrinol Metab.* 2016;101(3):827–836.
8. Straftis A, Gray P. Sex, energy, well-being and low testosterone: an exploratory survey of U.S. men's experiences on prescription testosterone. *Int J Environ Res Public Health.* 2019;16.
9. Marsh T. Which states fill the most (and fewest) prescriptions for erectile dysfunction drugs?. GoodRx. 2018. Available from: www.goodrx.com/blog/which-states-fill-most-prescriptions-for-erectile-dysfunction-drugs/
10. Part D Prescriber Data. Centers Medicare Medicaid Serv. 2017. Available from: www.cms.gov/Research-Statistics-Data-and-Systems/Statistics-Trends-and-Reports/Medicare-Provider-Charge-Data/Part-D-Prescriber
11. Layton JB, Li D, Meier CR, et al. Testosterone lab testing and initiation in the United Kingdom and the United States, 2000 to 2011. *J Clin Endocrinol Metab.* 2014;99(3):835–842.
12. Baillargeon J, Kuo YF, Westra JR, Urban RJ, Goodwin JS. Testosterone prescribing in the United States, 2002–2016. *JAMA - J Am Med Assoc.* 2018;320(2):200–202.
13. Handelsman D. Global trends in testosterone prescribing, 2000–2011: expanding the spectrum of prescription drug misuse. *Med J Aust.* 2013;199:548–551.
14. FDA. Drug Safety Communication: FDA cautions about using testosterone products for low testosterone due to aging. 2015.
15. Statements G. AUA Guideline TRT. AUA Clin Guide. 2018;(February).
16. Baillargeon J, Urban RJ, Ottenbacher KJ, Pierson KS, Goodwin JS. Trends in androgen prescribing in the United States, 2001 to 2011. *JAMA Intern Med.* 2013;173(15):1465–1466.
17. Jasuja GK, Bhasin S, Rose AJ. Patterns of testosterone prescription overuse. *Curr Opin Endocrinol Diabetes Obes.* 2017;24(3):240–245.
18. Epifanova MV, Gvasalia BR, Durashov MA, Artemenko SA. Platelet-rich plasma therapy for male sexual dysfunction: myth or reality? *Sex Med Rev.* 2020;8(1):106–113.
19. Shahinyan RH, Amighi A, Carey AN, et al. Direct-to-consumer internet prescription platforms overlook crucial pathology found during traditional office evaluation of young men with erectile dysfunction. *Urology.* 2020;143:165–172.
20. Imprialos K, Koutsampasopoulos K, Manolis A, Doumas M. Erectile dysfunction as a cardiovascular risk factor: time to step up?. *Curr Vasc Pharmacol.* 2021;19(3):301–312.
21. Dong J, Zhang Y, Qin L. Erectile dysfunction and risk of cardiovascular disease: meta-analysis of prospective cohort studies. *J Am Coll Cardiol.* 2011;58(13):1378–1385.
22. Global Erectile Dysfunction Drugs Market Growth 2019–2024. Mark. Study Rep. 2019.
23. Erectile dysfunction devices therapies market to be worth over $645 million by 2023. Arizton Advisory & Intelligence. January 12, 2018. Available from: www.arizton.com/news/press-release/erectile-dysfunction-devices-therapies-market. Accessed November 11, 2022.
24. Carrier S. Platelet rich plasma: what's the evidence for efficacy in ED/PD?. Nashville: 2019. Available from: www.smsna.org/nashville2019/presentations/122.pdf
25. Burnett AL, Nehra A, Breau RH, et al. AUA Guideline ED. AUA Clin Guidel 2018;(April):1–36.
26. Liu JL, Chu KY, Gabrielson AT, et al. Restorative therapies for erectile dysfunction: position statement from the Sexual Medicine Society of North America (SMSNA). *Sex Med.* 2021;9:100343.
27. Allday E. Merchants of hope. SF Chron. 2018. Available from: https://projects.sfchronicle.com/2018/stem-cells/clinics/
28. Zarembo A. Clinic settles lawsuits but still faces scrutiny over erectile dysfunction injections. *Los Angeles Times.* 2011. Available from: www.latimes.com/local/education/la-xpm-2011-apr-07-la-me-boston-medical-20110404-story.html
29. Farr C. How men's health start-ups are turning erectile dysfunction and hair loss treatment into a booming business. CNBC. 2019. Available from: www.cnbc.com/2019/11/17/hims-aims-to-

raise-200-million-as-sales-of-mens-health-products-grow.html

30. Nehra A, Alterowitz R, Culkin DJ, et al. Peyronie's disease: AUA guideline. *J Urol.* 2016;194(3):745–753.
31. Krieger JR, Rizk PJ, Kohn TP, Pastuszak A. Shockwave therapy in the treatment of Peyronie's disease. *Sex Med Rev.* 2019;7(3):499–507.
32. Gomez de Diego E. The therapies of Peyronie's disease are an unclear business in 2019. NewsWire. 2019. Available from: www.newswire.com/news/the-therapies-of-peyronies-disease-are-an-unclear-business-in-2019-20812142
33. Culha M, Erkan E, Cay T, Yucetas U. The effect of platelet-rich plasma on Peyronie's disease in rat model. *Urol Int.* 2019;102(2):218–223.
34. Hatzimouratidis K, Eardley I, Giuliano F, Moncada I, Salonia A. European Association of Urology Guidelines on Penile Curvature. 2015.
35. Hilton L. Shock wave therapy: ED cure or unproven treatment? [Internet]. *Urol. Times.* 2019. Available from: www.urologytimes.com/view/shock-wave-therapy-ed-cure-or-unproven-treatment
36. Dupree JM. Insurance coverage of male infertility: what should the standard be? *Transl Androl Urol.* 2018;7(Suppl 3):S310–S316.
37. De Jonge C, Barratt CLR. The present crisis in male reproductive health: an urgent need for a political, social, and research roadmap. *Andrology.* 2019;7(6):762–768.
38. Levine H, Jørgensen N, Martino-Andrade A, et al. Temporal trends in sperm count: a systematic review and meta-regression analysis. *Hum Reprod Update.* 2017;23(6):646–659.
39. Elliott PA, Hoffman J, Abad-Santos M, Herndon C, Katz PP, Smith JF. Out of pocket costs of male infertility care and associated financial strain. *Urol Pract.* 2016;3(4):256–261.
40. Fertility Clinics & Infertility Services Industry. Res. Mark. 2020. Available from: www.researchandmarkets.com/reports/5028546/fertility-clinics-and-infertility-services?utm_source=dynamic&utm_medium=GNOM&utm_code=z9m4dj&utm_campaign=1392804+-+Insights+into+the+Fertility+Clinics+%26+Infertility+Services+Industry+in+the+US+to+2025+-+Featuring+Allan+Guttmacher+Institute%2C+California+Cryobank+%26+Cryos+International+Among+Others&utm_exec=jamu273gnomd
41. Kolettis P, Sabanegh E. Significant medical pathology discovered during a male infertility evaluation. *J Urol.* 2001;166:178–180.
42. Loizos C. Newly funded Legacy, a sperm testing and freezing service, conveys a message to men: get checked. Yahoo Financ. 2020. Available from: https://finance.yahoo.com/news/legacy-sperm-testing-freezing-just-211742168.html?bcmt=1
43. Dupree JM, Dickey RM, Lipshultz LI. Inequity between male and female coverage in state infertility laws. *Fertil Steril [Internet].* 2016;105(6):1519–1522.

Section 1 An Introduction to Men's Health Care

Chapter 3

Urologic Men's Health, the Internet, and Social Media

Adithya Balasubramanian, Kassandra E. Zaila, James M. Hotaling, and Jesse N. Mills

3.1 Introduction

Men's health has historically drawn little attention from healthcare practitioners and policymakers across the world [1]. It was not until the twentieth century that men's health became a focus for public health officials [1]. Since then, organizations including the World Health Organization have recognized the significant health disparities across genders and acknowledged the growing need to better understand male-related diseases and health-seeking behaviors [1].

In the United States, across all demographics and socioeconomic strata, male life expectancy at birth is five years shorter than female life expectancy [2,3]. Research shows that men in the USA have an increased disease burden owing to higher rates of heart disease, cancer, HIV/AIDS, suicide, and risk-taking behavior [4]. These disparities are heightened given that men exhibit lower rates of health literacy and healthcare utilization. Notably, when men receive care from practitioners, they tend to be less knowledgeable of specific diseases and risk factors [5]. Consequently, men are less likely to report symptoms of disease or illness during a healthcare encounter [6]. The poor health of men adversely impacts the US economy, with male premature death and morbidity costing federal, state, and local governments in excess of $142 billion annually and US employers an excess of $156 billion annually for direct medical payments and lost productivity [7]. These marked consequences have spawned awareness and garnered an increasing interest in addressing men's health issues and improving male health outcomes.

Professor Louis Ignarro's breakthrough discovery in 1984 elucidating the relationship between the nitric oxide pathway and penile erection played a central role in bringing men's health issues to the forefront [8]. Quite literally, men's health became sexy. In 1998, Dr. Ignarro's research led to the development of sildenafil, commercially marketed as Viagra. Viagra revolutionized men's health. For the first time, the media spotlighted and sparked discussions of penile impotence, rebranded to erectile dysfunction (ED) to destigmatize the condition [4]. The surge in media attention later catalyzed discussion of other male-related health issues including heart disease, depression, and prostate cancer.

Public awareness and interest in men's health has intensified via organizations such as the Movember Foundation, a global charity committed to empowering men through education, research, and innovative projects [9]. Furthermore, men's health issues continue to be publicized through campaigns such as the June Men's Health Month and the September National Prostate Cancer Awareness Month. The prominence and success of these campaigns underscore how men's health initiatives raise awareness and acceptance of the importance of developing male-specific care pathways.

Despite historical disinterest in men's health issues, the last two decades have ushered in a new era of men's health. At the forefront of this movement has been the omnipresence of the Internet and the integration of internet-based tools like social media. These platforms have enabled patients to readily acquire medical information, create social networks among peers, remotely consult healthcare practitioners, and independently undertake treatment decisions.

3.2 Internet and Health Care

The rapid expansion of the Internet has allowed widespread connectivity access to over 5 billion users. Initially, the consumer internet was comprised of rudimentary websites that displayed information for passive consumption [10]. Technical bottlenecks such as slow internet speeds led corporations to become gatekeepers of online content. Consequently, users were relegated to passively consuming information with limited opportunities to produce and share content online.

By early 2000, computer science advancements facilitated new avenues for users to interact online. Activities such as blogging, content uploading, and comment posting promoted users to transition from passive consumption toward active contribution [10–12]. This participatory internet enabled networked individuals to collaborate, critique, and share information among digital communities [13]. Search engines and social media platforms were developed during the early 2000s and furthered online engagement. The Pew Research Center estimated that 5% of United States adults employed at least one social media platform in 2005 [14]. By 2017, this adoption skyrocketed to 69% [14]. Data generated from these Pew studies also revealed that adoption gained traction across several age groups including those in the 65 and older demographic. Such findings indicated that internet and social media participation was not solely limited to younger generations.

The participatory web is reshaping all aspects of daily life including how patients interface with healthcare systems. While the traditional patient–physician relationship was defined through interactions within hospitals, the Internet enables patients to obtain medical care outside these confines. Patients are now enabled to seek medical information or directly interface with healthcare practitioners through internet portals. Patients are also able to catalog healthcare experiences from initial diagnosis through recovery. Additionally, online communities empower patients to broadcast personal illness narratives and receive support from various parties. The flow of medical information along with the rise of digital marketplaces enables patients to curate their treatment with limited oversight.

These trends are noteworthy in the context of men's health. Prior studies highlight that men have an underlying hesitation to visit healthcare practitioners [15]. Second, men's urologic health conditions are stigmatized, therefore reducing prospects that men will seek care [16,17]. These obstacles are reinforced by legislative forces such as insurance coverage limitations which often fail to cover such conditions [18,19]. Despite the many benefits afforded by the Internet and social media, concerns are emerging regarding the quality of medical information shared via these platforms. The remainder of this chapter evaluates the online content landscape for hypogonadism, male infertility, ED, and Peyronie's disease (PD).

3.3 Male Infertility

Infertility is defined as the inability of a couple to conceive after regular unprotected intercourse for at least six months [20]. Although a male factor contributes to 50% of infertility cases, cultural ideas surrounding masculinity create psychosocial barriers to seeking care from healthcare practitioners for the condition. Infertile men experience a higher risk of developing sexual dysfunction, major depressive disorder, and sleep-related disturbances as a consequence of preconceived gendered notions of masculinity surrounding virility [20]. These consequences are compounded by the fact that men have lower utilization rates of mental health services. Studies indicate two main barriers faced by infertile men to request support during fertility treatments include: (1) men preferring to support their partners and tending to neglect and repress their own well-being, and (2) men perceiving help-seeking to be traditionally associated with feminine behavior [21]. This gendered response leads to increased online information- and support-seeking compared to traditional physical encounters [22]. The availability and anonymity of online sources creates a "safe space" and allows infertile men to openly expresses themselves on topics traditionally viewed as private or taboo [23].

Couples struggling with infertility increasingly turn online to overcome stigma. Beeder and Samplaski investigated online male infertility discussion boards to identify themes and concerns of infertile men and their partners [24]. Qualitative thematic analysis revealed that discussion forums are employed to share the emotional experience of infertility while fostering social support and community among users. Common topics included treatment modality appraisal, diagnostic testing interpretation, and lifestyle modifications to improve fertility [24]. Notably, two-thirds of discussion board posts in the study were written by female partners. These findings underscore the impact and popularity of online forums for both infertile men and their partners and the importance of incorporating female partners in male infertility evaluation.

Osadchiy et al. analyzed online discussions on male factor infertility on Reddit, a popular social media platform [25]. Interestingly, the majority of posts analyzed were authored by men. Feelings of emasculation and isolation were prominent themes permeating the majority of posts. Notably, the Reddit forum appeared to fill the void of the underutilization of mental health services. Men commonly used Reddit to connect with others facing similar feelings of isolation and to normalize the psychosocial burden they face. The study also found that posts authored by men had higher authenticity scores compared to female authors, thus emphasizing the value of online anonymity. Overall, the Internet and online discussions forums are transforming how patients empathize with one another and cope with the hardships of illness and medical care.

Discussions regarding male infertility are also occurring on Twitter [26]. Balasubramanian et al. analyzed tweets associated with #Maleinfertility and found increasing associated tweets throughout the 2013–2018 study period, suggesting that Twitter is becoming a prominent platform to discuss male infertility. The study highlights that doctors and advocacy organizations across 20+ countries are leading the discussion on Twitter regarding male infertility. Common conversations involved assisted reproductive technologies and featured various diagnostic and treatment modalities. Over two-thirds of #Maleinfertility tweets contained links to external academic sites, medical device pages, and direct-to-consumer (DTC) platforms. The breadth of external links suggests that Twitter may drive web traffic toward health information that encourages alternative pathways of diagnosis and treatment for male infertility.

Internet-based social networking is profoundly altering how health information is obtained as individuals increasingly turn to these resources for information, guidance, and discussion. Despite the benefits of social media, the lack of scrutiny and vetting of online information facilitates the propagation of unregulated and nonevidenced based content [27]. Zaila et al. critically evaluated male infertility content across social media platforms and found that information is widely shared, but highly sensationalized. The study concluded that misleading or inaccurate information is amplified by user engagement and that patients often encounter low-quality articles that overstate implications of animal research and conclusions founded upon limited sample sizes. Healthcare providers must proactively engage with patients on social media to mitigate issues associated with widely disseminated misinformation.

In response to the spread of misinformation online, a recent study investigated the popularity and reach of a health system-sponsored video intervention using YouTube to facilitate sharing reputable, high-quality, and evidenced based men's health content [28]. The study evaluated six videos focused on several men's health topics and featuring a board-certified urologist with fellowship training in andrology. The authors reported over 100,000 lifetime views across all videos and viewers in 47 countries. The study demonstrates that using a health system approach integrated with video streaming services is an effective method to disseminate high-quality information globally with significant popularity and remarkable reach. Healthcare providers should leverage video streaming and social media platforms such as YouTube to augment their practice and improve the online health information.

3.4 Erectile Dysfunction

ED is defined as the inability to maintain an erection that is sufficient for satisfactory sexual performance [29]. Men with ED face significant psychosocial consequences including feelings of inadequacy in sexual performance, partner-related difficulties, and depression. Additionally, there are well-known associations between ED, cardiovascular disease, diabetes mellitus, and metabolic syndromes [29]. ED is a major health problem with worldwide prevalence predictions reaching 322 million cases by 2025 [29]. Despite ED's high prevalence and the availability of established medical interventions including phosphodiesterase-5 (PDE-5) inhibitors, men continue to go untreated and are increasingly seeking alternative avenues to educate themselves and manage this condition [18].

Various studies highlight how the Internet has become a popular source of information for ED. Zhang et al. characterized health-seeking behaviors of Chinese men with ED and found that physicians and the Internet were the most consulted sources of information about ED [30]. Interestingly, the authors found variations in internet utilization between different age groups. Older men utilized the Internet as an initial information source prior to physician consultation, whereas younger men exclusively relied on the Internet for knowledge acquisition and self-treatment.

Baunacke et al. surveyed visitors to a German urology-oriented website providing health information on common urologic topics and found that ED was the second-highest searched topic [31]. Survey respondents indicated that they consulted ED-oriented websites prior to any physician encounter. Baunacke and colleagues also highlighted that given that ED does not require urgent therapy as a result of its insidious nature, patients have adequate time to search information online at their convenience while monitoring their own disease progression. Additionally, the authors postulate that the shame and embarrassment often faced by patients with ED further encourages patients to seek at-home treatments in lieu of care from a medical provider.

Social media creates a unique experience for online users as it does not just purvey information but also provides a platform for user engagement and discussion. Online discussion forums such as Reddit, with over 330 million monthly active users, have become increasingly popularized among men with ED to share personal medical anecdotes, gain advice on evaluation and treatment options, as well as form support networks with other individuals experiencing the same issue [32]. Jiang et al. applied a mixed-methodology approach to investigate content found in online discussions on the Reddit subforum r/ErectileDysfunction [32]. The authors discovered that the most popular self-reported causes of ED among discussants were psychogenic in nature, with individuals openly expressing feelings of depression and suicidality related to their condition. The authors highlighted that young men in particular are more likely to seek information and guidance on ED discussions forums as their first source of information. Online discussion boards are thus providing health-related information and safe spaces for men to have unfiltered and anonymous conversations about their condition.

There are several benefits of online health-seeking behaviors including patient empowerment in better understanding their condition, seeking different treatment modalities, and creating social networks. However, there remain concerns that patients are making unsuitable treatment decisions after reading unreliable information online. Limited studies have evaluated the quality of online health content about ED. A study by Read and Mati appraised 70 websites for their reporting style of causes and treatments for ED, as well as their authorship [33]. Interestingly, they found that the pharmaceutical industry funds a high proportion of websites. The authors also discovered that 77% of all the websites and 90% of the drug company-funded websites emphasized a biological cause of ED and were biased toward medical management while overlooking the psychosocial aspect of ED. Although these conclusions are important to recognize in the discussion of the use of the Internet and men's health, it must be noted that studies critically evaluating online ED content remain scarce.

Although critical content evaluation of ED information online is limited, several studies have investigated online platforms targeted toward ED evaluation and treatment. Telemedicine websites such as forhims.com (Hims) and getroman.com (Ro) have recently gained significant traction and offer DTC ED evaluation and treatment. Fantus et al. examined traffic patterns to ED specific telemedicine platforms and found that these websites are reaching approximately 4 million monthly visits [34]. These websites are offering men a rapid, discreet, and affordable solution to their condition all from the privacy of their own home.

However, recent investigations suggest that these DTC platforms do not adhere to the comprehensive ED evaluation guidelines created by the American Urological Association [35]. Shahinyan et al. assessed the role of urology office visits for young men in the diagnosis and management of ED, as this age group is increasingly targeted by DTC platforms for oral PDE-5 inhibitors and other prescription medications without a formal clinical evaluation. The study showed that office consultations identify young men with comorbid conditions including obesity, dyslipidemia, diabetes, and hypogonadism.

Additionally, a significant proportion of these patients had evidence of subfertility with varicocele or elevated FSH. The authors argue that although these DTC platforms augment conventional pathways to care, they overlook crucial pathology, carry the risk of unnecessary overtreatment with their auto-renewal of medication, and do not provide adequate follow-up or reevaluation. Overall, telemedicine platforms are increasing men's access to health services; however, there remains concern about the limitations of the Internet in providing adequate evidence-based care.

3.5 Hypogonadism

Hypogonadism is a clinical syndrome characterized by low serum testosterone levels and the presence of symptoms such as low libido, fatigue, and sexual dysfunction. Testosterone therapy (TTh) has emerged as a popular treatment for hypogonadism [36]. Although TTh prescriptions have spiked since the early 2000s, studies have repeatedly shown that the treatment is often prescribed without appropriate scrutiny [37].

The Internet has emerged as a first-line option for men to acquire information about testosterone [38]. Ivanov et al. surveyed popular testosterone-related websites from across the USA. Their analysis highlighted that website content was designed to motivate the sale of testosterone-boosting products such as TTh [39]. Website content also centered around elucidating relationships between testosterone products and muscle development. The sites also overviewed how androgens heighten sexual function, stymie aging, and improve well-being.

Content displayed on websites related to testosterone have been critically analyzed by urologists. A Google search–based study evaluated androgen replacement-oriented websites produced by practitioners from major US metropolitan regions [40]. The authors analyzed 75 popular websites based on content creator type, displayed information, and industry affiliations. A majority of these websites were not created by physicians, thereby bringing into question the quality of health information displayed on these domains.

Additionally, only 20% of websites mentioned possible industry relationships or conflicts. Their analysis also showcased that a majority of these websites touted benefits affiliated with starting TTh including heightened libido, cognition, sports performance, and energy. However, fewer than 30% of websites discussed side effects associated with TTh. This disparity sheds light upon potential biases that are prevalent among online resources related to hypogonadism. The importance of physician-curated content was reinforced by the fact that websites produced by specialists were more than twice as likely to detail TTh side effects.

McBride and colleagues scrutinized online patient-centered information related to hypogonadism and TTh [41]. Popular testosterone-oriented websites identified via Google were evaluated based on information quality, readability, and credibility. Analyzed websites were deemed to be of poor quality and overly complex for average patients. Most websites were again developed by nonphysicians, thereby underscoring the lack of physician-produced online information on these topics. Additionally, less than half of studied websites discussed the appropriate management of hypogonadism or TTh-associated risks. The preceding investigations thereby showcase a critical shortage of accurate online information related to hypogonadism and TTh.

The Internet also facilitates the ability to procure testosterone products, such as androgenic anabolic steroids (AAS) without a healthcare practitioner consultation [42]. A survey conducted in 2011 overviewed the content hosted on 30 AAS-oriented websites [43]. Several synthetic, anabolic steroid analogs of testosterone including nandrolone and methandrostenolone were routinely hosted on these sites. Other products such as estrogen blockers, and 5 alpha-reductase inhibitors were also available. Concerningly, the study revealed that adverse effects of products hosted on these sites were sparingly reported, even though reported dosages were several-fold higher than recommended.

McBride and colleagues further analyzed the products and services marketed on AAS websites [44]. They revealed that several synthetic AAS derivatives such as methandienone were available for purchase via these portals. The significance of this distribution of products was magnified by the fact that none of these AAS websites required prescriptions at time of purchase. Moreover, drugs accessible via these portals were manufactured and distributed by unregulated vendors. Of note, AAS websites included in the study also provided supplementation recommendations despite limited evidence-based research to support displayed claims.

Popular online marketplaces routinely broadcasted via social media channels are also employed to distribute testosterone boosting supplements (T-Boosters) which claim to "naturally" improve hypogonadal symptoms [45]. Balasubramanian et al. showcased that T-Boosters are featured on Amazon.com, with a considerable number of affiliated product reviews stating that these nutraceutical products can boost testosterone levels despite limited scientific evidence validating their claims. Given the concerning landscape, the authors rigorously evaluated the T-Booster ingredients as well as affiliated product reviews. Their literature review of product ingredients demonstrated that the few human studies that appraised T-Booster ingredient efficacy displayed no conclusive findings of effectiveness.

Additionally, their analysis of top customer reviews for each product revealed substantial differences between popular and trustworthy reviews. Popular product reviews made assertions that T-Boosters improve libido, energy, and strength. In contrast, trustworthy reviews identified via a proprietary Amazon review analyzing software displayed a considerable reduction in the volume of reviews claiming such improvements. The study underscored how the Internet and social media facilitate the broadcasting of exaggerated product efficacy claims.

3.6 Peyronie's Disease

PD is a superficial fibrosing condition in which aberrant collagen deposition leads to fibrotic scar formation within the penile tunica albuginea [46]. Patients with PD present with curved, often painful erections and other penile deformities that impair penetrative intercourse [46]. The psychosocial effects of PD are considerable given that men with the condition often report shame and poor libido [47–49]. These issues are compounded given that men with PD may hesitate to discuss sexual dysfunction with healthcare practitioners. Hesitancy to discuss PD with physicians heightens a man's depression and anxiety [47–49]. Lastly, although therapies for PD exist, awareness remains low.

Several studies characterize the online resources available to men seeking information about PD. A Mayo Clinic study surveyed over 700 PD patients to understand their health information resource preferences. This analysis revealed that websites were the most popular avenue for patients to obtain information about PD [47]. Surveyed patients indicated that they primarily visited websites produced by hospitals or government agencies. Other internet portals such as forums, blogs, and chat rooms were less popular. These findings highlight that the Internet has emerged as a first-line portal for patients to obtain insight on the condition. Additionally, Bella et al. explored PD-oriented websites and showcased that site content was created by advocacy groups [48]. Their study also revealed that patients employing these sites reported lower rates of stigma and that online content facilitated a deeper understanding of PD etiology and symptomatology.

New social media platforms such as Twitter are being employed to discuss PD. Balasubramanian et al. analyzed PD Twitter discussions [49]. Across the five-year study interval, their investigation revealed statistically significant increases in tweet activity and users. #Peyronies contributors primarily included physicians and advocacy organizations. The study found that hashtags such as #Peyronies, #Menshealth, #Curvedpenis, and #Bentpenis were employed to structure the conversation. The authors also discovered that #Peyronies Twitter discussions were utilized to drive internet traffic to advocacy, academic, commercial, and alternative social media websites. Although this investigation provided insight into the online Twitter discussion for the condition, the authors recognized that further work would be required to understand the potential downstream effects of these discussions on real-world behavior.

3.7 Conclusion

Men increasingly turn to the Internet to learn about various men's health conditions. The healthcare community must recognize and adapt to this emerging landscape given that online portals including websites, social media platforms, and digital marketplaces enable men to self-diagnose and self-treat. Although the Internet allows faster, more convenient access to care, healthcare practitioners and patients alike must be vigilant that the quality and readability of men's health digital content remains circumspect. The established medical community must therefore ensure the accuracy of digital content for patients to educate themselves. The Internet will continue to transform healthcare delivery and physicians should actively shape how this technology can empower men to optimize their health. Failure of the medical establishment to adapt to this new reality will ultimately lead to a defunct traditional business model and reduction in high-quality patient care.

References

1. Hooper GL, Quallich SA. Health seeking in men: a concept analysis. *Urol Nurs*. 2016;36(4):163–172.
2. Arias E, Xu J. United States life tables, 2017. *Natl Vital Stat Rep*. 2019;68 (7):1–66.
3. Balasubramanian A, Zhang CA, Spradling K, Eisenberg ML. The most common reasons for health care provider visits in reproductive aged men differ by race and age stratification. *Urol Pract*. 2020;7(3):194–198.
4. Houman JJ, Eleswarapu SV, Mills JN. Current and future trends in men's health clinics. *Transl Androl Urol*. 2020;9(S2):S116–S22.
5. Baker P, Shand T. Men's health: time for a new approach to policy and practice? *J Glob Health*. 2017;7(1).
6. Marmot M, Allen J, Bell R, Bloomer E, Goldblatt P. WHO European review of social determinants of health and the health divide. *Lancet*. 2012;380 (9846):1011–1029.
7. Brott A, Dougherty A, Williams ST, Matope JH, Fadich A, Taddelle M. The economic burden shouldered by public and private entities as a consequence of health disparities between men and women. *Am J Mens Health*. 2011;5 (6):528–539.
8. Ignarro LJ. Nitric oxide: a unique endogenous signaling molecule in vascular biology. *Biosci Rep*. 1999;19 (2):51–71.
9. Movember Foundation Annual Report 2019. 2019.
10. Murugesan S. Understanding Web 2.0. *IT Prof*. 2007;9(4):34–41.
11. Constantinides E, Fountain SJ. Web 2.0: Conceptual foundations and marketing issues. *J Direct, Data Digit Mark Pract*. 2008;9:231–244.
12. O'Reilly T. What is Web 2.0: design patterns and business models for the next generation of software. oreilly. com. 2005. www.oreilly.com/pub/a/web2/archive/what-is-web-20.html. Accessed October 26, 2022.
13. Cormode G, Krishnamurthy B. Key differences Web 1.0 and Web 2.0. *First Monday*. 2008;13(6). https://firstmonday.org/ojs/index.php/fm/article/view/2125. Available October 26, 2022.
14. Pew Research Center. Social media fact sheet. PewInternet.org 2018.
15. Pinkhasov RM, Wong J, Kashanian J, et al. Are men shortchanged on health? Perspective on health care utilization and health risk behavior in men and women in the United States. *Int J Clin Pract*. 2010;64(4):475–487.
16. Pontin D, Porter T, McDonagh R. Investigating the effect of erectile dysfunction on the lives of men: a qualitative research study. *J Clin Nurs*. 2002;11(2):264–272.
17. Arya ST, Dibb B. The experience of infertility treatment: the male

perspective. *Hum Fertil (Camb).* 2016;19(4):242–248.
18. Frederick LR, Cakir OO, Arora H, Helfand BT, McVary KT. Undertreatment of erectile dysfunction: claims analysis of 6.2 million patients. *J Sex Med.* 2014;11(10):2546–2553.
19. Le B, McAchran S, Paolone D, Gralnek D, Williams D, Bushman W. Assessing the variability in insurance coverage transparency for male sexual health conditions in the United States. *Urology.* 2017;102:126–129.
20. Balasubramanian A, Yu J, Srivatsav A, et al. A review of the evolving landscape between the consumer internet and men's health. *Transl Androl Urol.* 2020;9(S2):S123–S134.
21. Miner SA, Daumler D, Chan P, Gupta A, Lo K, Zelkowitz P. Masculinity, mental health, and desire for social support among male cancer and infertility patients. *Am J Mens Health.* 2019;13(1):155798831882039.
22. Hanna E, Gough B. Searching for help online: an analysis of peer-to-peer posts on a male-only infertility forum. *J Health Psychol.* 2018;23(7):917–928.
23. Hanna E, Gough B. Emoting infertility online: a qualitative analysis of men's forum posts. *Heal An Interduces J Soc Study Heal Illn Med.* 2016;20(4):363–382.
24. Beeder L, Samplaski MK. Analysis of online discussion boards for male infertility. *Andrologia.* 2019;51:e13422. https://doi.org/10.1111/and.13422.
25. Osadchiy V, Mills JN, Eleswarapu SV. Understanding patient anxieties in the social media era: qualitative analysis and natural language processing of an online male infertility community. *J Med Internet Res.* 2020;22(3):e16728.
26. Balasubramanian A, Yu J, Thirumavalavan N, Lipshultz LI, Hotaling JM, Pastuszak AW. Analyzing online Twitter discussion for male infertility via the hashtag #MaleInfertility. *Urol Pract.* 2020;7(1):68–74.
27. Zaila KE, Osadchiy V, Shahinyan RH, Mills JN, Eleswarapu SV. Social media sensationalism in the male infertility space: a mixed methodology analysis. *World J Mens Health.* 2020;38(4):591–598.
28. Zaila K, Osadchiy V, Anderson A, Eleswarapu S, Mills J. MP02–13 popularity and worldwide reach of targeted, evidence-based internet streaming video interventions focused on men's health topics. *J Urol.* 2020;203:e16.
29. Shamloul R, Ghanem H. Erectile dysfunction. *Lancet.* 2013;381(9861):153–165.
30. Zhang K, Yu W, He Z-J, Jin J. Help-seeking behavior for erectile dysfunction: a clinic-based survey in China. *Asian J Androl.* 2014;16(1):131–135.
31. Baunacke M, Groeben C, Borgmann H, Salem J, Kliesch S, Huber J. Andrology on the Internet: most wanted, controversial and often primary source of information for patients. *Andrologia.* 2018;50:e12877. https://doi.org/10.1111/and.12877.
32. Jiang T, Osadchiy V, Mills JN, Eleswarapu SV. Is it all in my head? Self-reported psychogenic erectile dysfunction and depression are common among young men seeking advice on social media. *Urology.* 2020;142:133–140.
33. Read J, Mati E. Erectile dysfunction and the Internet: drug company manipulation of public and professional opinion. *J Sex Marital Ther.* 2013;39(6):541–559.
34. Fantus R, Darves-Bornoz A, Hehemann M, et al. PD28–03 examining online traffic patterns to popular telemedicine websites for evaluation and treatment of erectile dysfunction. *J Urol.* 2020;203:e613.
35. Shahinyan R, Amighi A, Carey A, et al. PD28–05 direct-to-consumer PDE-5 inhibitor telemedicine marketing platforms overlook crucial pathology. *J Urol.* 2020;203:e613–614.
36. Baillargeon J, Urban RJ, Ottenbacher KJ, Pierson KS, Goodwin JS. Trends in androgen prescribing in the United States, 2001 to 2011. *JAMA Intern Med.* 2013;173(15):1465–1466.
37. Jasuja GK, Bhasin S, Rose AJ. Patterns of testosterone prescription overuse. *Curr Opin Endocrinol Diabetes Obes.* 2017;24(3):240–245.
38. Mascarenhas A, Khan S, Sayal R, Knowles S, Gomes T, Moore JE. Factors that may be influencing the rise in prescription testosterone replacement therapy in adult men: a qualitative study. *Aging Male.* 2016;19(2):90–95.
39. Ivanov N, Vuong J, Gray PB. A content analysis of testosterone websites: sex, muscle, and male age-related thematic differences. *Am J Mens Health.* 2018;12(2):388–397.
40. Oberlin DT, Masson P, Brannigan RE. Testosterone replacement therapy and the Internet: an assessment of providers' health-related web site information content. *Urology.* 2015;85(4):814–818.
41. McBride JA, Carson CC, Coward RM. Readability, credibility and quality of patient information for hypogonadism and testosterone replacement therapy on the Internet. *Int J Impot Res.* 2017;29(3):110–114.
42. Pirola I, Cappelli C, Delbarba A, et al. Anabolic steroids purchased on the Internet as a cause of prolonged hypogonadotropic hypogonadism. *Fertil Steril.* 2010;94(6):2331.e1–3.
43. Cordaro FG, Lombardo S, Cosentino M. Selling androgenic anabolic steroids by the pound: identification and analysis of popular websites on the Internet. *Scand J Med Sci Sports.* 2011;21(6):e247–259.
44. McBride JA, Carson CC, Coward RM. The availability and acquisition of illicit anabolic androgenic steroids and testosterone preparations on the Internet. *Am J Mens Health.* 2018;12(5):1352–1357.
45. Balasubramanian A, Thirumavalavan N, Srivatsav A, Yu J, Lipshultz LI, Pastuszak AW. Testosterone imposters: an analysis of popular online testosterone boosting supplements. *J Sex Med.* 2019;16(2):203–312.
46. Pryor JP, Ralph DJ. Clinical presentations of Peyronie's disease. *Int J Impot Res.* 2002;14(5):414–417.
47. Bole R, Ziegelmann M, Avant R, Montgomery B, Kohler T, Trost L. Patient's choice of health information and treatment modality for Peyronie's disease: a long-term assessment. *Int J Impot Res.* 2018;30(5):243–248.
48. Bella AJ, Perelman MA, Brant WO, Lue TF. Peyronie's disease (CME). *J Sex Med.* 2007;4(6):1527–1538.
49. Balasubramanian A, Yu J, Lipshultz LI, Hotaling JM, Pastuszak AW. #Peyronies: an analysis of online Twitter discussion of Peyronie's disease. *Urol Pract.* 2019;7(1):75–81.

Section 2 The Biology of Male Reproduction and Infertility

Chapter 4

Current Understanding of the Physiology and Histology of Human Spermatogenesis

Chiara Capponi and Elena Vicini

4.1 Introduction

Spermatogenesis is a complex process involving the differentiation of spermatogonial stem cells (SSCs) into highly specialized mature male gametes. Even if its efficiency declines with aging, spermatogenesis is a lifetime process, starting at puberty and proceeding until the end of life. It is maintained by the remarkable activity of the SSCs that have the ability to self-renew and to generate cells committed to differentiation. Spermatogenesis takes place inside the seminiferous tubules of the testis: The mitotic germ cells are located at the basal layer of the seminiferous tubules, and as their maturation proceeds, they move from the basal layer up to the lumen of the seminiferous tubules where they are eventually released as mature spermatids. Thus, spermatogenesis requires the coordinate activity of several cell types within the testis. A transcriptomic analysis of several human tissues revealed that the testis expresses the largest fraction of genes among all tissues and organs, with over 80% of all protein-coding genes being expressed in the testis, a testament of the complexity of this organ [1,2]. Most of the testis-enriched genes are related to testis-specific functions and spermatogenesis [3].

4.2 Morpho-functional Arrangement of the Human Testis

The testis is a paired organ specialized for the production of sex hormones and spermatozoa. To carry out these functions, the testis is separated into two morpho-functional distinct compartments, the interstitial compartment, where the steroidogenic Leydig cells produce androgens, and the seminiferous tubules where spermatogenesis occurs (Figure 4.1). In men, the dimensions of the testis are in the range of 4–5 cm in length, 2.5–3 cm in width, and 1.8–2.4 in thickness, whilst the average volume is 18 mL with a range between 12 and 30 mL [4]. The testis is protected by a dense capsule of connective tissue called the tunica albuginea. Several septa of connective tissues extend radially from the capsule into the parenchyma dividing the testis into 250–300 pyramidal lobules each containing 1–4 highly convoluted seminiferous tubules.

4.2.1 The Interstitial Compartment

The interstitial compartment of the testis contains lymphatic and blood vessels, nerve fibers, Leydig cells, and several other cell types, including resident cells, that is, fibroblasts, pericytes, macrophages, and mast cells, and wandering cells, that is, monocytes, and T and NK lymphocytes. Blood-derived nutrients, respiratory gases, and hormones are filtered from vessels into the interstitial fluid that is vital for the avascular seminiferous tubules. Leydig cells are the most prominent cell type in the interstitial compartment, where they can be found isolated or in small clusters, mostly around the blood vessels (Figure 4.1). They can be recognized for their spherical euchromatic nucleus, with a well-visible nuclear envelope, and a prominent nucleolus. The total number of Leydig cells in the human testis is approximately 99×10^6 cells with a range between 47 and 245×10^6 [5]. These cells produce testosterone, the most important sex hormone of the male body, and insulin-like factor 3 (INSL-3), a marker for Leydig cell activity [6].

In humans, Leydig cell development can be divided into three phases (fetal, neonatal, and adult) based on morphological characteristics and a triphasic pattern of hormone release [7]. The first population of Leydig cells appears during fetal life and is responsible for testosterone production between two and four months of gestation. The second generation of Leydig cells develops at two to three months after birth, giving rise to a second peak in testosterone levels (mini-puberty). Finally, just before puberty, the adult population of Leydig cells arise under the regulation of the hypothalamic-pituitary-gonadal axis. Adult Leydig cells derive from differentiation of stem/precursor cells or from regressed neonatal and infantile Leydig cells (reviewed in [7,8]).

In man, the development of mature germ cells from spermatogonia starts at puberty, long after the immune self-tolerance has been established. Spermatogenesis is associated with expression and production of novel antigens that do not belong to those recognized as self-antigens by the immune system. Remarkably, the testis tolerates autoantigenic germ cells as well as allografts and xenografts leading to the conclusion that the testis is an immune-privileged site [9,10]. Several factors contribute to testis immunotolerance and protection of autoantigenic germ cells: the blood–testis barrier formed by Sertoli cells, expression of immunoregulatory and immunosuppressive factors by different somatic cell types, and the molecular makeup of interstitial immune cells (reviewed in [10]).

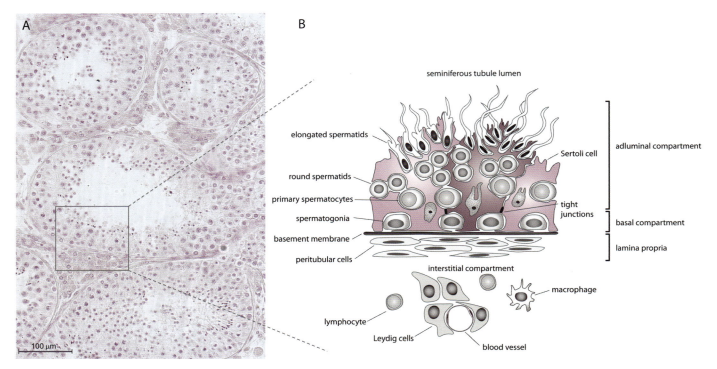

Figure 4.1 Histology of the human testis parenchyma. (A) Formalin-fixed, carmallume-stained testis section from 19-year-old man. (B) Schematic representation of the human seminiferous tubule and the interstitial compartment.

4.2.2 Seminiferous Tubules

The seminiferous tubules consist of the seminiferous epithelium, including germ cells and Sertoli cells, and a supporting lamina propria, comprised of a basement membrane and peritubular cells (Figure 4.1). The diameter of a seminiferous tubule in human is approx. 180–250 μm while its length varies from 40 to 80 cm.

Peritubular cells (PTC), the main cellular components of the lamina propria of seminiferous tubules, are organized into five to seven noncontinuous concentric layers [11], for a total number of approx. 400×10^6 cell per testis [12] (Figure 4.1). Ultrastructural and markers analysis show that PTC in the inner layers show a smooth muscle-like (myoid) phenotype while PTC of the outermost layers are fibroblasts forming the borderline to the interstitial compartment [12,13]. Peritubular myoid cells are contractile cells involved in transport of spermatozoa and testicular fluid in the seminiferous tubules [14]. Moreover, PTC secrete a large array of molecules that could act as paracrine signals for Sertoli, Leydig, or germ cells (reviewed in [15]). Ultrastructural observation indicates that the space among different peritubular cell layers presents a variable amount of extracellular matrix (ECM), mainly collagen fibril network [11]. The amount of the ECM is considerably increased in several pathological conditions and during aging thereby causing a thickening of the lamina propria [12,16]. The thickening of the lamina propria inversely correlates with the quality of spermatogenesis evaluated by the Johnsen's score [17]. It remains to be established whether changes in the lamina propria are the basis for subfertility or infertility or if they are a by-product of other primary causes.

Sertoli cells, the only type of somatic cells in the seminiferous epithelium, play a key function in the initiation and maintenance of spermatogenesis (Figure 4.1). The total number of Sertoli cells in the human testis is approximately 407×10^6 cells with a range between 86 and 665×10^6 [5]. The number of Sertoli cells declines significantly with age and is significantly correlated to the sperm production rate [18]. Sertoli cells are located on the basement membrane and extend up to the lumen of the tubules. The nucleus is large, uniformly euchromatic with a prominent nucleolus, facilitating Sertoli cell identification in histological analysis. The cytoplasm is highly branched with long and thin processes embracing and supporting germ cells during each step of their differentiation. The cytoplasm contains abundant mitochondria, a smooth endoplasmic reticulum, and a well-developed cytoskeleton that is involved in the organization of two remarkable structures, the ectoplasmic specialization and the tubulobulbar complex. These structures, localized between Sertoli and developing spermatids, are responsible for anchoring developing germ and to facilitate their movement across and away from the seminiferous epithelium [19]. Adjacent Sertoli cells are linked by occluding tight junctions forming the blood–testis barrier (BTB). The BTB divides the seminiferous epithelium into a basal compartment containing spermatogonia and preleptotene spermatocytes and an adluminal compartment, containing all the other germ cell types. The transepithelial transport

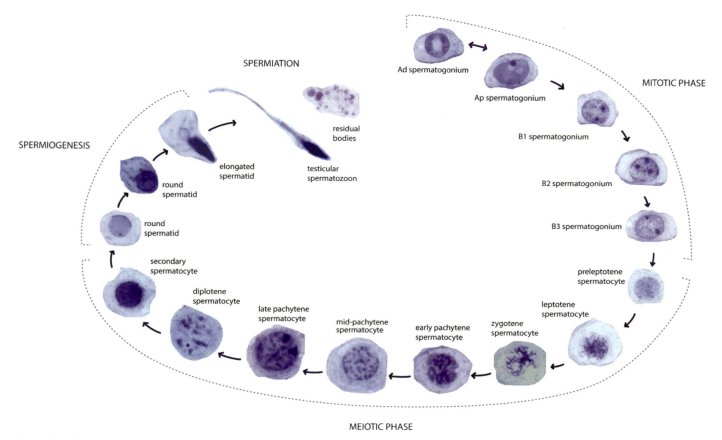

Figure 4.2 The progression of male germ cell differentiation in humans. The arrows indicate the direction of germ cell development. The four phases of spermatogenesis are also shown. The different germ cell types were selected from light microscopy photomicrographs of toluidine blue-stained human testis semi-thin sections.

of ions, water, and micronutrients across the two compartments is mediated by Sertoli cells that are responsible for the formation and secretion of the tubular fluid, a special milieu for the development of the adluminal germ cells [20]. The BTB undergoes cyclical rearrangements to allow the translocation of developing germ cells from the basal to the adluminal compartment. The synchronous passage of large numbers of germ cells requires a stage-specific temporal rearrangement of the BTB and is regulated by hormones, cytokines, and protein phosphorylation [21,22]. Compelling evidence, obtained in animal models, indicates that Sertoli cells represent one key component of the "niche," a specialized microenvironment that regulates spermatogonial stem cell self-renewal and differentiation [23]. Several soluble factors produced by Sertoli cells are critical for spermatogonial stem cell maintenance. This is not surprising, considering that in mammals, spermatogonial stem cells reside on the basement membrane of the seminiferous tubules in close contact to Sertoli cells. In humans, the identity of the spermatogonial stem cells and nature and location of the stem cell niche are areas of intense investigation. At the present, however, our understanding of the contribution of the Sertoli cell to the spermatogonial stem cells niche in human is lagging. Sertoli cells play a key function for the hormonal regulation of spermatogenesis, being the only cells in the seminiferous epithelium that express the cognate receptors for FSH and testosterone. Thus, Sertoli cells convert endocrine signals into paracrine regulation of germ cells at different steps of development [24].

The different types of germ cells of the seminiferous epithelium are typically recognized on morphological characteristics (Figure 4.2). In a mature testis they include dark type A (Ad), pale type A (Ap) and type B spermatogonia, preleptotene, leptotene, zygotene, pachytene, and diplotene spermatocytes, secondary spermatocytes, round and elongating spermatids, and spermatozoa.

4.3 The Unfolding of Germ Cell Development in Humans

Spermatogenesis is a cyclical continuous process that can be schematically divided into four main phases: mitotic phase, meiotic phase, spermiogenesis, and spermiation. In the mitotic phase, diploid spermatogonial stem cells produce cells that go through amplifying divisions, become differentiating spermatogonia, and then form spermatocytes. Spermatocytes enter the lengthy meiotic phase, which includes the critical events of homologous recombination and reduction of chromosomes, ending with the production of haploid round spermatids. During spermiogenesis, round spermatids undergo transformation into mature elongated spermatids. Spermiation is the process by which mature elongated spermatids are released from the Sertoli cell and become testicular spermatozoa.

In all mammals, spermatogonia comprise stem, undifferentiated, and differentiating cell types. They are distributed in a horizontal layer on the basement membrane of the seminiferous epithelium. During their mitotic expansion spermatogonia are arranged as single cells or chains of different lengths interconnected by cytoplasmic bridges generated by incomplete cytokinesis [25]. The distinction between undifferentiated and differentiating spermatogonia, classically based on nuclear morphology, includes important differences in markers expression, apoptotic, and cell cycle regulation [26]. In man, there are three main types of spermatogonia: Ad, Ap, and B [27,28](Figure 4.2). The Ap and Ad spermatogonia are considered undifferentiated spermatogonia and type B as differentiating spermatogonia. Ad and Ap spermatogonia are almost equal in number, while conflicting data are reported for the relative number of B spermatogonia [28,29].

The nuclei of Ad spermatogonia are spherical or ovoid shaped, containing a deeply stained dust-like chromatin with or without a vacuole-like cavity (chromatin rarefaction zone), and with a nucleolus at the nuclear periphery. The nuclei of Ap spermatogonia are ovoid shaped, containing a fine homogenous, and weakly stained chromatin and no vacuoles, with a nucleolus at the nuclear periphery. In primates, Ad spermatogonia are quiescent because they do not or rarely incorporate S phase markers (i.e., 3H-thymidine or BrdU) or express PCNA (a marker for proliferating cells) (reviewed in [30]). Ad and Ap spermatogonia have been indicated as the "reserve stem cells" and the "active stem cells," respectively [31]. In nonhuman primates, the quiescent Ad spermatogonia can be immediately activated upon depletion of the active Ap population, following a cytotoxic treatment with ionizing radiation [32]. At present, the relationship between Ad and Ap spermatogonia has not yet been clarified. In recent years, the classical long-lasting view on the functional arrangement of the spermatogonial compartment in humans, has been challenged by immunostaining and transcriptome data that clearly show the presence of numerous subsets of spermatogonia with high degree of heterogeneity [33,34]. The current model of the stem cell hierarchy in human spermatogenesis with the concomitant presence of two homogenous pools of stem cells, the "reserve" (Ad spermatogonia) and the "active" (Ap spermatogonia), may have to be revised to accommodate new experimental data (see Section 4.4.2).

For recognition of spermatogonia types by light microscopy, in conventional paraffin-embedded testis sections, appropriate preservation of nuclear details is of crucial importance. In formalin-, paraformaldehyde-, and Bouin-fixed testes a reliable morphological distinction between Ad, Ap, and B spermatogonia is not always possible, whereas the Zenkerformal-fixed testis is best suited [27,35]. However, even in well-fixed samples, many spermatogonia show an intermediate nuclear morphology and cannot be unequivocally characterized. Spermatogonia with an intermediate morphology between Ad and Ap spermatogonia have been defined as A-transition (At) or A-unclassified (Aunc) spermatogonia. The rate of spermatogonial recognition can be increased by high-resolution light microscopy, an improved method for the visualization of spermatogonial features requiring glutaraldehyde/osmium fixation, epoxy resin embedding, and semithin sections of testis specimens [36]. A classical method for the analysis of spermatogonial subtypes is the histological analysis of whole mounted seminiferous tubules (Figure 4.3). In this method seminiferous tubules are mechanically untangled from testis biopsies and are left intact for downstream applications [37]. This approach allows the concomitant analysis of nuclear morphology, the topographical arrangements of spermatogonial clones over the basement membrane, and the expression profile of spermatogonial markers [33] (Figure 4.3).

It is generally accepted that Ap give rise to B spermatogonia. The nuclei of B spermatogonia are spherical, characterized by a fine granulated chromatin with some intensively stained chromatin clumps that can be attached to the nuclear envelope that appears well delineated, with one or more centrally located nucleoli (Figure 4.2). It has been recently shown that in man there are three generations of B spermatogonia (B1, B2, and B3 spermatogonia) and not only one as previously supposed [33]. The last generation of B spermatogonia divides to form preleptotene spermatocytes that enter meiosis.

Meiosis (from Greek μείωσις, lessening) is unique to germ cells and involves a single round of DNA replication followed by two consecutive divisions (meiosis I and II) to form haploid germ cells. During meiosis I, the homologous chromosomes – each consisting of two sister chromatids – are segregated (reduction division) while in meiosis II the sister chromatids are segregated by equatorial division.

The critical events of homologous recombination, that is, the formation of DNA double-strand breaks (DSBs) and chromosome synapsis, occur during the prophase of meiosis I [38]. Prophase I is prolonged and can be further subdivided into four stages named leptonema, zygonema, pachynema, and diplonema, each characterized by a particular nuclear morphology that can be readily assessed in toluidine-stained semithin sections (Figure 4.2). Meiosis is a critical step of spermatogenesis because it involves: (a) the formation and repair of DSBs that are essential for homologous recombination but are potentially lethal lesions and (b) the pairing and synapsis of homologous chromosomes including the partial synapsis of X and Y chromosomes with the formation of the XY body. When homologous chromosomes fail to synapse appropriately or meiotic DSBs are not adequately repaired this could lead to transmission of harmful aberrations to the offspring. However, the production of defective spermatozoa is prevented by several meiotic checkpoints, set in place to block or delay

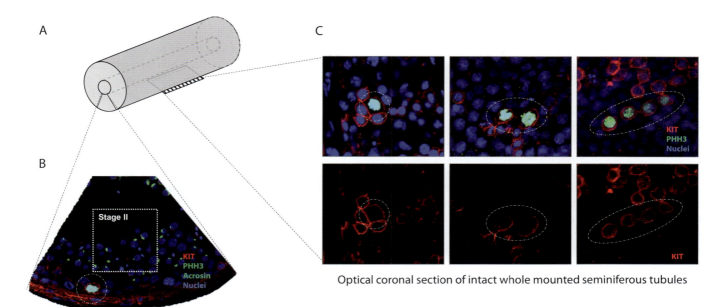

Figure 4.3 Different methodological approaches for the detection of spermatogonia. (A) Schematic drawing of a seminiferous tubule. (B) In conventional testis cross-sections spermatogonia are detected above the basement membrane of the seminiferous tubules. (C) In intact whole mounted tubules, the spermatogonial layer is underneath the peritubular layer and the basement membrane. The whole mounted approach permits the analysis of the topography of spermatogonial clones while in a conventional cross-section it is not possible to establish the clonal size of spermatogonia. Dashed white lines indicate mitotic differentiating spermatogonia detected by co-immunostaining for KIT (marker of B spermatogonia), and PHH3 (marker for mitotic cells) (B, C). Anti-acrosin (green) staining decorates the acrosome of round spermatids (B).

prophase I progression in the presence of cellular defects or DNA lesions [39]. Consequently, aberrant spermatocytes are removed leading to partial or complete meiotic arrest, which is diagnosed in 10–20% of man with nonobstructive azoospermia [40]. A meiotic arrest can be caused by known genetic aberrations or unknown factors including gene mutations and noxious agents. While the list of validated causative mutations for meiotic arrest has recently lengthened [41–43], fewer studies have addressed the general mechanism for meiotic arrest in man. Jan and colleagues recently unveiled two distinct mechanisms of meiotic arrest occurring during prophase I in man [44]. By histological analysis of testis biopsies obtained from 14 patients with complete meiotic arrest, two types of meiotic arrest were found. The first type displays severe asynapsis of homologous chromosomes and disturbed XY-body formation, while the second type displays normal chromosome synapsis, normal XY-body morphology, and meiotic crossover formation. Comparative transcriptome analysis of isolated single spermatocytes revealed that in the first type of meiotic arrest the underlying problem is the chromatin structure and organization while the second type of meiotic arrest is characterized by downregulation of genes involved in RNA processing and cell cycle progression.

An emerging aspect of male germ cell biology is the importance of the higher-order chromosome positioning for basic genome functions, including gene expression [45]. The analysis of chromatin architecture in germ cells and its interplay with the control of gene expression during spermatogenesis, and particularly at meiosis, may give important clues for a better understanding of male infertility [46,47].

At the end of meiotic division, four haploid spermatids are generated from one spermatocyte. Newly generated spermatids undergo an extensive morphological and functional rearrangement called spermiogenesis. Spermiogenesis represents the final remodeling phase of spermatogenesis transforming round haploid germ cells to highly polarized spermatozoa (Figure 4.2). This phase includes: the development of the acrosome covering the anterior portion of the nucleus; the development of the flagellum at the opposite side of the nucleus; the nuclear condensation and remodeling into its final shape; the packaging of mitochondria around the mid-piece of the sperm tail; and dislocation and removal of the cell cytoplasm. It can be anticipated that failure to correctly execute any of these processes could impact human fertility.

The acrosome is a cap-like structure containing digestive enzymes required for sperm penetration through the corona radiata and the zona pellucida surrounding the oocyte. In mammals the development of the acrosome consists of four distinct phases: Golgi, cap, acrosomal, and maturation [48]. Based on morphological changes of the acrosome detected by periodic acid-Schiff (PAS) staining method, the four phases can be further subdivided in several steps, defined as the steps of spermiogenesis [48]. The steps of spermiogenesis can be used to identify the stages of the cycle of the seminiferous epithelium (see Section 4.4.1).

A critical role for spermatid shaping is played by the manchette, a microtubular and actin-based transient cylindric structure, surrounding the elongating spermatid head and attached to the perinuclear ring. During the elongation of the spermatid head, the perinuclear ring and the manchette move toward the nascent spermatid tail, concomitantly with the expansion of the acrosome on the anterior part of the nucleus [49]. The manchette acts as a platform for the transport of structural proteins of the sperm tail axoneme. Proteins are transported through the manchette by the intra-manchette transport to the base of the sperm tail and then to the developing tail by intra-flagellar transport [50]. When the manchette is absent or abnormal, the sperm head is abnormally shaped and the sperm tail fragile [50].

During spermiogenesis, a unique chromatin remodeling process takes place leading to replacement of core histones with protamines and finally to nuclear condensation. The histone-based nucleosome structure of chromatin in spermatids is progressively disassembled, then replaced with transition proteins (TP1 and TP2) and finally by protamines. Any defects during the histone-to-protamine transition would lead to male infertility [51]. The histone-to-protamine transition is a stepwise process that gradually reduces chromatin accessibility for the transcriptional machinery, resulting in transcriptional silencing. Therefore, relevant mRNA required for the final steps of spermiogenesis must be transcribed earlier, stored, and selectively translated at an appropriate time during spermiogenesis [52].

Protamines constitute the most abundant nucleoproteins in mature sperm. They stabilize and compact the sperm chromatin conferring a more hydrodynamic nucleus best fitted for motility, protecting paternal genome during the transport of sperm through male and female reproductive tracts, and enabling the silencing and reprogramming of the paternal genome. In humans, protamines are encoded by two different genes protamine 1 and 2 (PRM1 and PRM2) and in human sperm the protein level of protamine P1 and protamine P2 are similar (reviewed in [53]). An abnormal P1/P2 ratio in sperm is associated with infertility [54].

4.4 The Kinetics of Human Spermatogenesis
4.4.1 Redefinition of the Cycle of Seminiferous Epithelium

Spermatogenesis is a continuous and highly regulated process both in space and time. In man, approximatively every 16 days, spermatogonial stem cells produce a new generation of differentiating spermatogonia, that develop and complete the process of differentiation to spermatozoa in approximatively 74 days [55]. While maturing, the descendants of the spermatogonia move from the basal to the adluminal compartment and then to the lumen, where they are released as spermatozoa. In the meantime, at 16-day intervals, before the first generation reaches the lumen, a successive generation of differentiating spermatogonia is produced. Therefore, in each area of the seminiferous epithelium more generations of germ cells are concomitantly present. Remarkably, germ cells of different generations are not randomly associated to one another but develop in synchrony forming stereotypical germ cell associations. During the 16-day interval, in between successive generation of differentiating spermatogonia, each area of the seminiferous epithelium shows all the germ cell associations, following each other in time, and then returns to the first one. This is called the cycle of the seminiferous epithelium and the germ cell associations are called stages [56]. In each stage, types of germ cells are always the same. It follows that it is possible to determine the specific stage of the seminiferous epithelium by evaluating the developmental steps of one generation of germ cells, using cytological or histological criteria.

In mammals, the stages of the cycle have been largely characterized using the morphological development of the acrosome in spermatids (i.e., steps of spermiogenesis), assessed by PAS staining in conventional paraffin-embedded testis sections. The stages of the cycle have been described in many mammals and often 12 stages can be distinguished, as in the mouse, hamster, and various monkeys. In the human testis, however, the PAS staining method does not allow clear characterization of acrosome development. Consequently, the germ cell associations are recognized by combining the morphology of the spermatid's nucleus and the presence of other relevant germ cell types. Spermatids are morphologically divided in six types (Sa, Sb1, Sb2, Sc, Sd1, and Sd2) and the epithelial cycle is divided in six germ cell associations [57]. The relative duration of each stage can be estimated by the frequency of their presence in sections of the seminiferous tubules. Since, in man the epithelial cycle last around 16 days, the histological frequency of each stage can be translated in duration of each stage. Individual germ cell associations encompass less than one to around five days [27,28,36].

There are important differences in the histological arrangement of germ cell associations between man and other mammalian species. In man, a stage occupies only a small patchy area of tubule basement membrane as opposed to a full cross-section in most other mammals. Therefore, in man, more than one stage can be found in a cross-section. Sometimes, the boundary between different stages is not clearly delineated forming a heterogeneously mixed germ cell association. Moreover, in some cross-sections, a germ cell association may lack one or two generations of germ cells and is defined as an incomplete germ cell association.

In the six-stage classification of the epithelial cycle, the long duration of the stages and their reduced number compared to other mammals has hampered detailed studies on germ cell development. More recently, the acrosomal development in

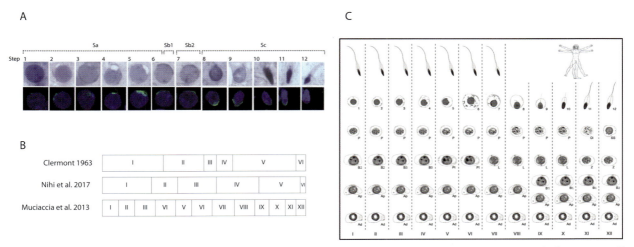

Figure 4.4 Comparison between the subdivision of the cycle of the human seminiferous epithelium in 6 and 12 stages. (A) The first 12 steps of human spermatid development based on immunodetection of acrosine (green) in the acrosome (below) and the corresponding morphology of spermatids in semi-thin sections (above). The dashed lines indicate the relative alignment of spermatids in 6-step versus 12-step classifications. Acrosin cannot be detected in Sd1 and Sd2 spermatids. (B) Schematic comparison between the stage frequencies in the two classifications. (C) Schematic diagram of the human seminiferous epithelium showing the cell types present in each of its 12 epithelial stages. Ap – A-pale spermatogonium; Ad – A-dark spermatogonium; B1, B2, B3 – B spermatogonia; pL – preleptotene spermatocytes; L – leptotene spermatocytes; Z – zygotene spermatocytes; eP – early pachytene spermatocytes; mP – mid pachytene spermatocytes; lP – late pachytene spermatocytes; D – diplotene spermatocytes; SS – secondary spermatocytes; 1 to 12, first 12 steps in the development of spermatids.

man has been described by immunohistochemical (IHC) detection of acrosin, an acrosomal protein, allowing the identification of 12 different steps of spermiogenesis [35]. The 12 steps of acrosome development can be identified also by immunofluorescence (IF) detection of acrosin (Figure 4.4A). Figure 4.4A also shows the relative alignment of spermatids development in 6-step versus 12-step classifications. Importantly, in both IHC and IF methodology, the last step recognizable by acrosin staining is step 12, which corresponds to Sc spermatids in the 6-steps classification. Acrosin cannot be detected in Sd1 and Sd2 spermatids.

Taking advantage of the more detailed description of the developing acrosome, a novel classification of the stages of human spermatogenesis has been proposed. By analyzing germ cell types and germ cell associations in acrosin-stained samples, 12 epithelial stages were detected. The frequency of stages in seven individuals (from 19 to 75 years) with normal spermatogenesis was estimated and their time span calculated based on the 16 days of one seminiferous cycle. Interestingly, the relative duration of each stage did not significantly vary with age and with the genetic variability of the individuals. Most of the stages last from 30 to 40 hours and only two stages (stage XI and XII) are shorter than 24 hours, showing that their duration does not differ more than about a factor of two [35]. IHC detection of acrosin can be achieved in formalin-, Bouin-, Cleland-, and Davidson-fixed testis biopsies. There are limitations to the identification of stages using the novel classification. Acrosin must be detected by IHC or IF, a methodology that may not be readily available in clinical practice. Moreover, in humans a stage occupies a small area of the tubule and in such an area spermatids at the same step of development may be very few, making identification of the stage difficult. In any case, the 12-stage classification will prove valuable in andrology to study spermatogenesis impairments and, importantly, it gives an accurate timing of the molecular and cellular events regulating germ cell progression. This is well evident when the frequency of stages in the two subdivisions are directly compared. Stage I, II, and V of the old classification are further subdivided respectively into three, two, and four stages in the novel classification (Figure 4.4B). The germ cell types present in each of the 12 stages of the epithelial cycle in humans are shown in Figure 4.4C. Most of our current knowledge about spermatogenesis has been obtained in monkeys and rodents, whose epithelial cycle is divided in 12 stages. Therefore, the novel classification allows a more direct comparison between data obtained in animal models and humans.

4.4.2 Current Knowledge on the Spermatogonial Compartment in Humans

In mammals, the undifferentiated spermatogonial subtypes are classically recognized by their nuclear morphology. However, when spermatogonia are stratified by marker expression, a striking level of heterogeneity is promptly observed, reflecting a complex regulation of the kinetics of the spermatogonial compartment in mammals [23,30]. A large body of evidence shows that human undifferentiated spermatogonia are not an exception, being highly heterogeneous in term of gene expression. The analysis of the transcriptional profile of single spermatogonia by the single-cell RNA sequencing (scRNAseq) technology showed that the human spermatogonia can be further subdivided into several cell clusters, from three up to ten cell clusters as reported in different studies [58]. Remarkably, there is not a specific transcriptional profile associated with the classic nuclear morphology of Ad and Ap spermatogonia [59,60]. Taken together, these data clearly show that different spermatogonial subsets coexist within the Ad and Ap spermatogonial populations.

To describe the kinetics of spermatogonial expansion in humans, several basic questions need to be addressed, such as the proliferation pattern of the different spermatogonial subtypes, the number of cells in individual chains (clonal size), the stage at which spermatogonial subtypes undergo S-phase and mitosis, etc. A detailed description of the kinetics of spermatogonial expansion is required for the understanding of the basic regulatory molecular mechanisms regulating the mitotic compartment, both in normal and pathological conditions. In the six-stage classification, two spermatogonial mitotic peaks are described at stage II and V [29]. Given the length of these stages, however, the mitotic peaks could include multiple proliferative events. Moreover, conflicting data have been reported about when B spermatogonia are first formed during the cycle (reviewed in [61]). Di Persio and colleagues recently reassessed the expansion of the spermatogonial clones, within the frame of the novel classification of the cycle in 12 stages. In this study, spermatogonial types were recognized based on marker expression and not by nuclear morphology. MAGEA4 was employed as a marker for all spermatogonia; UCHL1, UTF1, and GFRA1 as markers for the undifferentiated spermatogonia (Ad and Ap spermatogonia); and KIT as a marker for differentiating spermatogonia (B spermatogonia). In this study the classical distinction between Ad and Ap was abandoned and undifferentiated spermatogonia were collectively defined as Ap-d. Using different combinations of markers, a high degree of molecular heterogeneity was evident, and four spermatogonial cell subsets were distinguished. The analysis of the proliferative activity (Ki67-index) indicated that the great majority (around 95%) of Ap-d spermatogonia are quiescent. The clonal expansion of the Ap-d was assessed in wholemount seminiferous tubules by looking at PHH3-positive, mitotic Ap-d. The analysis of the topographical arrangement of mitotic spermatogonia showed that mitotic Ap-d are extremely rare, mostly formed by single cells and some pairs, while chains of mitotic Ap-d were never observed. This indicates that in humans most if not all Ap-d spermatogonia are single cells. The analysis of mitotic Ap-d in testis cross-sections indicates that Ap-d proliferate throughout the cycle, but the number of mitotic Ap-d are significantly higher at stage IX. It was suggested that, among the four spermatogonial subsets identified by marker analysis, the SSCs reside in the subset of GFRA1^{high}/UTF1^{neg}. However, other studies suggest that GFRA1 is also expressed by more advanced subsets of spermatogonia, and that more primitive spermatogonia are GFRA1^{low}/UTF1^{high} [62,63]. This discrepancy could be due to different stability of mRNA and encoded proteins from each gene. The analysis of mitotic KIT+ B spermatogonia showed three peaks of mitotic cells at stage IX, II/III, and V/VI indicating the presence of three generations of B spermatogonia (B1, B2, and B3 spermatogonia) and not one as previously suggested by Clermont [29]. When B1 spermatogonia are single cells and probably some paired cells, after three divisions the number of cells of a clone of preleptotene spermatocytes entering meiosis is 8–16 cells. Surprisingly, almost half of B spermatogonia are not actively in cell cycle, as judged by their Ki67 index. This is in contrast with other mammalian species: In rodents, there are six generations of differentiating spermatogonia that are always in cell cycle. The reason underlying the downregulation of B spermatogonia proliferation in humans deserves further investigation.

To guarantee the constant production of mature germ cells, once during each epithelial, new B1 spermatogonia should be derived by differentiation of Ap-d and meanwhile the rest of the Ap-d should proliferate to replace the Ap-d lost to differentiation. Based on the relative proportion of Ap-d and B spermatogonia and the percentage of Ap-d spermatogonia actively in cell cycle, it was suggested that at a population level a single Ap-d divides approximately only once every three epithelial cycles (i.e., once every one-and-a-half months) with the majority Ad-p being out of the cycle for protracted periods of time. Moreover, only a small proportion of the Ad-p can be recruited into the differentiation pathway, during each epithelial cycle [33]. Apparently, human undifferentiated spermatogonia including SSCs are almost all quiescent cells, as also shown by scRNAseq studies on human spermatogonia [34]. The low rate of SSCs proliferation may be protective for the risk of de-novo germline mutations or susceptibility to cytotoxic events [64]. The low rate of cell division of SSCs may not be the only mechanism set in place to minimize germline mutations rate in humans. Recently, it has been suggested that the observed widespread transcription during spermatogenesis systematically reduces germline mutations by a mechanism of transcriptional-coupled repair (TCR) [65]. The TCR is the fast and preferential repair of mutations in the transcribed strand of an active gene, performed by the nucleotide excision repair (NER) or the base excision repair (BER) pathways. Interestingly, in TCR the transcribed strand is preferentially repaired while the nontranscribed strand of the same gene is repaired at a rate comparable to that in nontranscribed regions. Therefore, highly expressed genes have a low chance to accumulate deleterious mutations compared to nontranscribed genes [66]. According to the "transcriptional scanning" hypothesis, the widespread germ cell transcription facilitates germline DNA repair and could modulate gene evolution rate [65].

In the last few years, several scRNAseq studies have shed light on the heterogeneity of different spermatogonial cell types (reviewed in [58]). The scRNAseq technology can measure the expression level of thousands of genes at single cell level and allows: (a) the definition of cell clusters based on their transcriptome profile; (b) the identification of specific markers (differential-expressed genes) for a given cell cluster for both germ and somatic cells; and (c) the alignments of cell clusters according to their developmental trajectory. Sohni and colleagues have recently analyzed the transcriptome profile of neonatal and human testis. Four different cell clusters of human

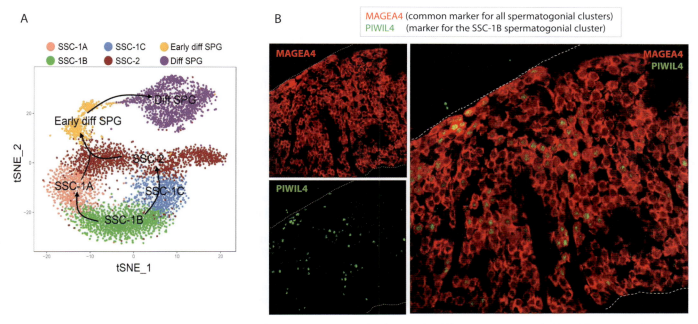

Figure 4.5 Identification of human spermatogonial subsets by scRNAseq. (A) tSNE plot showing the different spermatogonial subsets. The arrows indicate the putative developmental trajectories of germ cells from the SSC-1B subset (see text). Reproduced with permission from [36]. (B) Immunofluorescence analysis of intact seminiferous tubules co-immunostained for the indicated spermatogonial markers. Dashed lines outline the seminiferous tubules.

spermatogonia were identified in the adult testis, defined as SSC-1, SSC-2, early differentiating SPG, and differentiating SPG. Based on marker analysis, the first two subsets comprise undifferentiated spermatogonia that should therefore include classical Ap-d spermatogonia, while the last two include B spermatogonia. The cell cycle gene expression profile of cells in SSC-1 and SSC-2 suggest that they are not proliferating or undergo slow proliferation, in line with previous results [34]. SSC-1 could be further subdivided into three subclusters, SSC-1A, SSC1-B, and SSC-1C (Figure 4.5A). The pseudotime trajectory analysis, which aligns the developmental order of cells based on transcriptome changes, indicated that cells in the SSC-1B subset are the least developmentally advanced and might be the most enriched in SSCs. Pseudotime analysis also indicated that the differentiation pathway from SSC-1B to early differentiating spermatogonia is not linear: SSC-1B could convert into either SSC-1A or SSC-1C before becoming early differentiating spermatogonia. At present it remains to establish whether the different clusters represent successive generations of spermatogonia or different cellular states whose transcriptional profile varies in relation to their cell cycle, to the microenvironment or to the stage of the epithelial cycle. Even though single-cell transcriptome analysis enables the identification of rare cell populations or identifies small differences between similar cell types, the dissociation of cells eliminates the spatial information required to map their relative localization in situ. The next challenge will be the histological identification and the morphological and functional description of each of the undifferentiated spermatogonial subsets pinpointed by scRNAseq (Figure 4.5B). The understanding of human spermatogonial biology has important implications for the study of male infertility, male contraception, and human genetics.

4.5 Transcriptome Analysis of the Testis at Single-Cell Level: Clarifying the Blueprint of Human Spermatogenesis in Normal and Pathological Conditions

In the last few years, the increased accessibility to the scRNAseq technology has stimulated several studies on human testis (reviewed in [58]). Human spermatogenesis is mediated by a highly orchestrated cellular crosstalk between somatic and germ cells, and scRNAseq studies offer the possibility to explore this crosstalk at an unprecedent resolution. Comparative studies in mice and nonhuman primates give important clues as to the nature of the spermatogonial stem cell niche, a specialized microenvironment tailored to regulate SSCs quiescence, self-renewal, survival, and differentiation [60]. Elucidating how the crosstalk between somatic cells and germline is established, maintained, and altered in pathological conditions represents a major challenge.

The transcriptome analysis of dissociated cells from the human testis allowed the identification of the major cell types including germ cell types (spermatogonia, spermatocytes, and spermatids) and the somatic cells of the testis (Sertoli cells, peritubular myoid cells, Leydig cells, macrophages). The datasets obtained in these studies might be used as a reference for the diagnosis of male fertility disorders [67]. Several rare mutations causing nonobstructive azoospermia have recently been identified including NR5A1, DMRT1, FANCA, MEIOB, etc. (reviewed in [68]). To determine the relationship between a causative genetic variant and azoospermia, detailed knowledge of the specific cell types that express the gene in question is needed. Therefore, datasets from normal spermatogenesis might be very informative. Comparison of transcriptomic data from patients with arrested or disturbed spermatogenesis with transcriptomic data from fertile patients could help to elucidate many cases of yet unexplained male infertility.

Acknowledgments:
We are grateful to Dirk G. de Rooij for critical reading of the manuscript and to Elisa Perlas for drawing Figure 4.1B.

References

1. Soumillon M, Necsulea A, Weier M, et al. Cellular source and mechanisms of high transcriptome complexity in the mammalian testis. *Cell Rep.* 2013;3 (6):2179–2190.
2. Uhlen M, Fagerberg L, Hallstrom BM, et al. Proteomics. Tissue-based map of the human proteome. *Science*. 2015;347 (6220):1260419.
3. Pineau C, Hikmet F, Zhang C, et al. Cell type-specific expression of testis elevated genes based on transcriptomics and antibody-based proteomics. *J Proteome Res.* 2019;18(12):4215–4230.
4. Weinbauer G, Luetjens C, Simoni M, Nieschlag E. Physiology of testicular fuction. In: Nieschlag E., Behre HM, Nieschlag S, eds. *Andrology Male Reproductive Health and Dysfunction*. 3rd ed. Springer-Verlag; 2010:11–59.
5. Petersen PM, Seieroe K, Pakkenberg B. The total number of Leydig and Sertoli cells in the testes of men across various age groups: a stereological study. *J Anat.* 2015;226(2):175–179.
6. Ivell R, Agoulnik AI, Anand-Ivell R. Relaxin-like peptides in male reproduction – a human perspective. *Br J Pharmacol.* 2017;174(10):990–1001.
7. Prince FP. The human Leydig cell. In: Payne AH, Hardy MP, eds. *The Leydig Cell in Health and Disease*. Humana Press; 2007:71–89.
8. Chen P, Zirkin BR, Chen H. Stem Leydig cells in the adult testis: characterization, regulation and potential applications. *Endocrine Reviews*. 41(1):22–32.
9. Head JR, Neaves WB, Billingham RE. Immune privilege in the testis. I. Basic parameters of allograft survival. *Transplantation*. 1983;36(4):423–431.
10. Fijak M, Pilatz A, Hedger MP, et al. Infectious, inflammatory and 'autoimmune' male factor infertility: how do rodent models inform clinical practice? *Hum Reprod Update*. 2018;24 (4):416–441.
11. Maekawa M, Kamimura K, Nagano T. Peritubular myoid cells in the testis: their structure and function. *Arch Histol Cytol*. 1996;59(1):1–13.
12. Arenas MI, Bethencourt FR, Fraile B, Paniagua R. Immunocytochemical and quantitative study of the tunica albuginea testis in young and ageing men. *Histochem Cell Biol*. 1997;107 (6):469–477.
13. Davidoff MS, Breucker H, Holstein AF, Seidl K. Cellular architecture of the lamina propria of human seminiferous tubules. *Cell Tissue Res*. 1990;262 (2):253–261.
14. Hargrove JL, MacIndoe JH, Ellis LC. Testicular contractile cells and sperm transport. *Fertil Steril*. 1977;28 (11):1146–1157.
15. Mayerhofer A. Human testicular peritubular cells: more than meets the eye. *Reproduction*. 2013;145(5): R107–R116.
16. Volkmann J, Muller D, Feuerstacke C, et al. Disturbed spermatogenesis associated with thickened lamina propria of seminiferous tubules is not caused by dedifferentiation of myofibroblasts. *Hum Reprod*. 2011;26 (6):1450–1461.
17. Sato Y, Nozawa S, Iwamoto T. Study of spermatogenesis and thickening of lamina propria in the human seminiferous tubules. *Fertil Steril*. 2008;90(4):1310–1312.
18. Johnson L, Zane RS, Petty CS, Neaves WB. Quantification of the human Sertoli cell population: its distribution, relation to germ cell numbers, and age-related decline. *Biol Reprod*. 1984;31 (4):785–795.
19. Franca LR, Hess RA, Dufour JM, Hofmann MC, Griswold MD. The Sertoli cell: one hundred fifty years of beauty and plasticity. *Andrology*. 2016;4 (2):189–212.
20. Setchell BP. The secretion of fluid by the testes of rats, rams and goats with some observations on the effect of age, cryptorchidism and hypophysectomy. *J Reprod Fertil*. 1970;23(1):79–85.
21. Stanton PG. Regulation of the blood-testis barrier. *Semin Cell Dev Biol*. 2016;59:166–173.
22. Mruk DD, Cheng CY. The mammalian blood-testis barrier: its biology and regulation. *Endocr Rev*. 2015;36 (5):564–591.
23. Makela JA, Hobbs RM. Molecular regulation of spermatogonial stem cell renewal and differentiation. *Reproduction*. 2019;158(5):R169–R187.
24. Santi D, Crepieux P, Reiter E, et al. Follicle-stimulating hormone (FSH) action on spermatogenesis: a focus on physiological and therapeutic roles. *J Clin Med*. 2020;9(4):1014.
25. de Rooij DG, Russell LD. All you wanted to know about spermatogonia but were afraid to ask. *J Androl*. 2000;21 (6):776–798.
26. Boitani C, Di PS, Esposito V, Vicini E. Spermatogonial cells: mouse, monkey and man comparison. *Semin Cell Dev Biol*. 2016;59:79–88.
27. Clermont Y. The cycle of the seminiferous epithelium in man. *Am J Anat*. 1963;112:35–51.
28. Rowley MJ, Heller CG. Quantitation of the cells of the seminiferous epithelium of the human testis employing the sertoli cell as a constant. *Z Zellforsch Mikrosk Anat*. 1971;115(4):461–472.
29. Clermont Y. Renewal of spermatogonia in man. *Am J Anat*. 1966;118 (2):509–524.
30. Hermann BP, Sukhwani M, Hansel MC, Orwig KE. Spermatogonial stem cells in higher primates: are there differences from those in rodents? *Reproduction*. 2010;139(3):479–493.
31. Clermont Y. Two classes of spermatogonial stem cells in the monkey (*Cercopithecus aethiops*). *Am J Anat*. 1969;126(1):57–71.
32. van Alphen MM, de Rooij DG. Depletion of the seminiferous

33. Di Persio S, Saracino R, Fera S, et al. Spermatogonial kinetics in humans. *Development.* 2017;144(19):3430–3439.

34. Sohni A, Tan K, Song HW, et al. The neonatal and adult human testis defined at the single-cell level. *Cell Rep.* 2019;26(6):1501–1517.

35. Muciaccia B, Boitani C, Berloco BP, et al. Novel stage classification of human spermatogenesis based on acrosome development. *Biol Reprod.* 2013;89(3):60.

36. Nihi F, Gomes MLM, Carvalho FAR, et al. Revisiting the human seminiferous epithelium cycle. *Hum Reprod.* 2017;32(6):1170–1182.

37. Clermont Y, Bustos-Obregon E. Re-examination of spermatogonial renewal in the rat by means of seminiferous tubules mounted "in toto." *Am J Anat.* 1968;122(2):237–247.

38. Bolcun-Filas E, Handel MA. Meiosis: the chromosomal foundation of reproduction. *Biol Reprod.* 2018;99(1):112–126.

39. Barchi M, Mahadevaiah S, Di GM, et al. Surveillance of different recombination defects in mouse spermatocytes yields distinct responses despite elimination at an identical developmental stage. *Mol Cell Biol.* 2005;25(16):7203–7215.

40. Tsai MC, Cheng YS, Lin TY, Yang WH, Lin YM. Clinical characteristics and reproductive outcomes in infertile men with testicular early and late maturation arrest. *Urology.* 2012;80(4):826–832.

41. Gershoni M, Hauser R, Barda S, et al. A new MEIOB mutation is a recurrent cause for azoospermia and testicular meiotic arrest. *Hum Reprod.* 2019;34(4):666–671.

42. Wyrwoll MJ, Temel SG, Nagirnaja L, et al. Bi-allelic mutations in M1AP are a frequent cause of meiotic arrest and severely impaired spermatogenesis leading to male infertility. *Am J Hum Genet.* 2020;107(2):342–351.

43. Riera-Escamilla A, Enguita-Marruedo A, Moreno-Mendoza D, et al. Sequencing of a 'mouse azoospermia' gene panel in azoospermic men: identification of RNF212 and STAG3 mutations as novel genetic causes of meiotic arrest. *Hum Reprod.* 2019;34(6):978–988.

44. Jan SZ, Jongejan A, Korver CM, et al. Distinct prophase arrest mechanisms in human male meiosis. *Development.* 2018;145(16).

45. Sarrate Z, Sole M, Vidal F, Anton E, Blanco J. Chromosome positioning and male infertility: it comes with the territory. *J Assist Reprod Genet.* 2018;35(11):1929–1938.

46. Wang Y, Wang H, Zhang Y, et al. Reprogramming of meiotic chromatin architecture during spermatogenesis. *Mol Cell.* 2019;73(3):547–561.

47. Vara C, Paytuvi-Gallart A, Cuartero Y, et al. Three-dimensional genomic structure and cohesin occupancy correlate with transcriptional activity during spermatogenesis. *Cell Rep.* 2019;28(2):352–367.

48. Clermont Y, Leblond CP. Spermiogenesis of man, monkey, ram and other mammals as shown by the periodic acid-Schiff technique. *Am J Anat.* 1955;96(2):229–253.

49. Lehti MS, Sironen A. Formation and function of the manchette and flagellum during spermatogenesis. *Reproduction.* 2016;151(4):R43–R54.

50. Pleuger C, Lehti MS, Dunleavy JE, Fietz D, O'Bryan MK. Haploid male germ cells-the Grand Central Station of protein transport. *Hum Reprod Update.* 2020;26(4):474–500.

51. Bao J, Bedford MT. Epigenetic regulation of the histone-to-protamine transition during spermiogenesis. *Reproduction.* 2016;151(5):R55–R70.

52. Monesi V. Ribonucleic acid synthesis during mitosis and meiosis in the mouse testis. *J Cell Biol.* 1964;22:521–532.

53. Oliva R. Protamines and male infertility. *Hum Reprod Update.* 2006;12(4):417–435.

54. Carrell DT, Emery BR, Hammoud S. Altered protamine expression and diminished spermatogenesis: what is the link? *Hum Reprod Update.* 2007;13(3):313–327.

55. Heller CG, Clermont Y. Spermatogenesis in man: an estimate of its duration. *Science.* 1963;140(3563):184–186.

56. Russell LD, Ettlin RA, Hikim APS, Clegg ED. Histological and histopathological evaluation of the testis. *J Androl.* 1993;17(6):615–627.

57. Heller CH, Clermont Y. Kinetics of the germinal epithelium in man. *Recent Prog Horm Res.* 1964;20:545–575.

58. Suzuki S, Diaz VD, Hermann BP. What has single-cell RNA-seq taught us about mammalian spermatogenesis? *Biol Reprod.* 2019;101(3):617–634.

59. Jan SZ, Vormer TL, Jongejan A, et al. Unraveling transcriptome dynamics in human spermatogenesis. *Development.* 2017;144(20):3659–3673.

60. Shami AN, Zheng X, Munyoki SK, et al. Single-cell RNA sequencing of human, macaque, and mouse testes uncovers conserved and divergent features of mammalian spermatogenesis. *Dev Cell.* 2020;54(4):529–547.

61. Amann RP. The cycle of the seminiferous epithelium in humans: a need to revisit? *J Androl.* 2008;29(5):469–487.

62. Guo J, Grow EJ, Mlcochova H, et al. The adult human testis transcriptional cell atlas. *Cell Res.* 2018;28(12):1141–1157.

63. Hermann BP, Cheng K, Singh A, et al. The mammalian spermatogenesis single-cell transcriptome, from spermatogonial stem cells to spermatids. *Cell Rep.* 2018;25(6):1650–1667.

64. Goldmann JM, Veltman JA, Gilissen C. De novo mutations reflect development and aging of the human germline. *Trends Genet.* 2019;35(11):828–839.

65. Xia B, Yan Y, Baron M, et al. Widespread transcriptional scanning in the testis modulates gene evolution rates. *Cell.* 2020;180(2):248–262.

66. Svejstrup JQ. Mechanisms of transcription-coupled DNA repair. *Nat Rev Mol Cell Biol.* 2002;3(1):21–29.

67. Gille AS, Lapoujade C, Wolf JP, Fouchet P, Barraud-Lange V. Contribution of single-cell transcriptomics to the characterization of human spermatogonial stem cells: toward an application in male fertility regenerative medicine? *Int J Mol Sci.* 2019;20(22):5773.

68. Soraggi S, Riera M, Rajpert-De ME, Schierup MH, Almstrup K. Evaluating genetic causes of azoospermia: what can we learn from a complex cellular structure and single-cell transcriptomics of the human testis? *Hum Genet.* 2021;140(1):183–201.

Section 2: The Biology of Male Reproduction and Infertility

Chapter 5: Male Reproductive Endocrinology

Christos Tsametis, George Kanakis, and Dimitrios G. Goulis

Abbreviations

17β-HSD$_3$	17β-hydroxysteroid dehydrogenase type 3
17OHP	17(OH)-progesterone
3β-HSD$_2$	3β-hydroxysteroid dehydrogenase type 2
Δ$_4$-A	Δ4-androstenedione
aa	amino acid
AC	adenylyl cyclase
AgRP	agouti-related peptide
AMH	anti-Müllerian hormone
AR	androgen receptor
ARE	androgens response elements
cAMP	cyclic adenosine monophosphate
CART	cocaine- and amphetamine-regulated transcript
CNS	central nervous system
CREB	cAMP response element-binding protein
CRH	corticotropin-releasing hormone
DBP	DNA-binding domain
DHEA	dehydroepiandrosterone
DHT	dihydrotestosterone
E$_1$	estrone
E$_2$	estradiol
ECND	extracellular N-terminal domain
ERα	estrogen receptor-alpha
ERK$_{1/2}$	extracellular-regulated kinase $_{1/2}$
FGFR1	fibroblast growth factor receptor-1
FSH	follicle-stimulating hormone
FSHβ	follicle-stimulating hormone β-subunit
GABA	gamma-aminobutyric acid
GAP	GnRH-associated peptide
GnIH	gonadotropin-inhibitory hormone
GnRH	gonadotropin-releasing hormone
GnRHR	GnRH receptor
GPR54	G–protein-coupled receptor 54
GR	glucocorticoid receptor
GRK	GPCR kinases
hCG	human chorionic gonadotropin
HH	hypogonodatrophic hypogonadism
HPA	hypothalamic-pituitary-adrenal
HPG	hypothalamic-pituitary-gonadal
HPT	hypothalamic-pituitary-testicular
IGF-1	insulin-like growth factor 1
Inh-A	Inhibin A
Inh-B	Inhibin B
INSL3	insulin-like factor 3
IP3	inositol-trisphosphate
LBD	ligand-binding domain
LepR	leptin receptor
LH	luteinizing hormone
LH-RH	luteinizing hormone-releasing hormone
LHβ	luteinizing hormone β-subunit
LIF	leukemia inhibitory factor
LRP	LDL receptor-related protein
MAPK	mitogen-activated protein kinase
miRNA	microRNAs
MPS	male reproductive system
NEFL	nasal embryonic LHRH factor
NPY	neuropeptide Y
PIP	phosphatidylinositol 4,5-trisphosphate
PKA	protein kinase A
PKC	protein kinase C
POA	preoptic area
POMC	proopiomelanocortin
PR	progesterone receptor
PROK2	prokineticin 2
PSA-NCAM	polysialic acid form of neural adhesion molecule
RFRP	RFamide-related peptide
RFRP-3	RFamide-related peptide-3
SHBG	sex hormone-binding globulin
Shp2	phosphotyrosine phosphatase
SRC	steroid receptor coactivator
STAR	steroidogenic acute regulatory protein
T	testosterone
TGF-β	transforming growth factor-β
TSH	thyroid-stimulating hormone
TSPO	translocator protein
VDAC1	voltage-dependent anion channel 1
VIP	vasoactive intestinal peptide

5.1 Physiology of the Hypothalamic-Pituitary-Testicular Axis

5.1.1 Introduction

The male reproductive system (MRS) has three main functions: synthesis and secretion of male sex steroids (androgens), production of male gametes (spermatozoa), and transport of sperm into the female genital tract. The development, maturation, and normal function of the MRS are mainly under the control of the hypothalamic-pituitary-testicular (HPT) axis, which constitutes the hormonal component of an interplaying and intercommunicating neuronal and endocrine system. The axis is anatomically and functionally organized at three levels: The hypothalamic level consists of two different neuronal populations that produce gonadotropin-releasing hormone (GnRH) and the neuropeptide kisspeptin, the latter being the principal secretagogue for the former. At the pituitary level, a group of cells called gonadotrophs synthesize and secrete follicle-stimulating hormone (FSH) and luteinizing hormone (LH), collectively known as gonadotropins, under the stimulatory effect of GnRH. At the testicular level, Leydig cells following stimulation by LH, produce mainly androgens, testosterone (T) being the most important; Sertoli cells, under the action of FSH, promote and support spermatogenesis and produce numerous biologically active molecules. The homeostasis of the HPT axis is maintained through a negative feedback regulatory loop. Testicular hormones produced in response to gonadotropins enter the systemic circulation and feed back on both hypothalamic and pituitary levels, suppressing the secretion of their stimulators. Moreover, locally produced substances at each level of the HPT axis, acting in a paracrine or autocrine way, contribute to the regulation of the axis, as well as neuronal, metabolic, inflammatory, and environmental signals.

5.1.2 Hypothalamus: The GnRH and Kisspeptin Networks

5.1.2.1 Structure and Synthesis of GnRH

The idea that the central nervous system (CNS) controls the pituitary-gonadal axis was first documented by a medical student in Cambridge, Geoffrey Harris, in 1937 [1]. Several years later, two different groups, led by Andrew Schally and Roger Guillemin, isolated an hypothalamic substance from porcine and ovine brain, respectively, that regulates the production of gonadotropins [2,3]. The active molecule was a decapeptide, formerly known as luteinizing hormone-releasing hormone (LH-RH), but now widely referred to as GnRH, to reflect its dual stimulatory effect on the secretion of both gonadotropins [4]. Different forms of GnRH, according to amino acid (aa) sequence, localization, and embryonic origin, have been found among vertebrates. At least 20 primary structures have been identified across species, reflecting the early development of the GnRH system in the evolutionary process. The structure of GnRH was first described in mammals and is designated GnRH-I (pGlu-His-Trp-Ser-Tyr-Gly-Leu-Arg-Pro-GlyNH$_2$). Subsequently, a structurally different vertebral GnRH subtype was isolated from chicken hypothalamus and is referred to as GnRH-II (pGlu-His-Trp-Ser-His-Gly-Trp-Tyr-Pro-Gly-NH$_2$). A third type has been identified in the telencephalon of teleost fish (GnRH-III) [5,6].

In humans, two subtypes of GnRH have been identified: GnRH-I and -II. The former is the principal regulator of gonadotropin synthesis and secretion and is produced by neurosecretory cells (GnRH neurons) located in the mediobasal hypothalamus. GnRH-I has also been found in tissues outside the brain (placenta, immune system, gonads, endocrine tumors), where its physiological role is not yet fully elucidated [7]. GnRH-II is produced by neurons located in the midbrain region, where it functions mainly as a neurotransmitter, rather than a pituitary-releasing hormone. However, there is evidence that GnRH-II can also stimulate gonadotropin release in vivo by binding to the same receptor as GnRH-I [8,9]. GnRH-I is encoded by a gene (*GnRH1*) located on chromosome 8p11.2-p21, whereas a different gene (*GnRH2*), mapped to chromosome 20p13, encodes GnRH-II [8,10]. GnRH-I is produced by successive cleavage steps from a larger 92-aa precursor peptide, the preproGnRH. This prohormone consists of a 23-aa signal peptide, the functional GnRH decapeptide, an amidation/proteolytic processing signal (Gly-Lys-Arg) and the 56-aa GnRH-associated peptide (GAP). PreproGnRH is processed in the rough endoplasmic reticulum and the Golgi apparatus and transported along the axons of GnRH neurons to the median eminence. Mature GnRH is a single decapeptide chain that is cyclized at the N-terminus and amidated at the C-terminus. As a result of a ß-II type bend involving the central Tyr-Gly-Leu-Arg residues, the mature molecule assumes a folded conformation bringing in close proximity the N- and C-termini [5]. The development of GnRH analogs has provided information regarding the relative role of each section of the decapeptide chain. Aa in position 6–10 are important for binding to the receptor; positions 1–3 are involved in biological activity, whereas positions 5–6 and 9–10 are related to enzymatic degradation [11].

5.1.2.2 Neuroanatomy and Embryology of GnRH Neurons

In humans, the cell bodies of GnRH neurons are located in the medial preoptic area (POA) and the infundibular hypothalamic nucleus (the human analog of the arcuate nucleus). It is estimated that 1,000–1,500 GnRH neurons exist in the adult human hypothalamus [5]. A typical GnRH neuron has two dendritic projections which extend a distance of 2–3 mm from their cell body [12]. Their axons end up in the median eminence where GnRH is secreted into the fenestrated capillaries of the hypophyseal portal system to reach the anterior pituitary and stimulate the activity of the gonadotrophs [13]. A unique characteristic of GnRH-producing neuronal population is the fact that during embryological development, they originate outside the CNS, specifically in the medial olfactory placode and then migrate across the nasal septum, together with vomeronasal axons and enter into the forebrain with the nervus terminalis, arching into the septal-preoptic area and hypothalamus [14].

The migratory process is regulated by numerous factors, including adhesion molecules, such as anosmin-1 (the product of *KAL1* gene), the polysialic acid form of neural adhesion molecule (PSA-NCAM) and cell surface glycoconjugate. Other molecules involved in the regulation of GnRH neuronal migration are gamma-aminobutyric acid (GABA), cholecystokinin, neuropillins, leukemia inhibitory factor (LIF), fibroblast growth factor receptor-1 (FGFR1) and its ligand FGF8, prokineticin-2 (PROK2), transcription factors (Ebf2), ephrins, and nasal embryonic LHRH factor (NELF) [7]. Some factors play an important role in specific steps of the migratory process. Semaphorins, plexins, and reelin seem to guide GnRH neurons toward the forebrain, whereas hepatocyte growth factor (HGF), Axl, Tyro3, and chemokine attractants provide guidance as the GnRH neurons migrate through the cribriform plate to the hypothalamus [7,15]. The embryonic migration of GnRH neurons is of paramount importance for the normal functioning of the HPT axis. Disruption of the migratory process at any stage results in hypogonadotropic hypogonadism associated with anosmia/hyposmia (Kallmann syndrome) or not [15].

5.1.2.3 Secretion of GnRH

There are two modes of GnRH secretion: pulsatile and surge mode. The surge mode appears only in females during the preovulatory phase of the menstrual cycle. The pulsatile mode is characterized by the release of GnRH into the portal circulation in discrete, random but regular bursts (pulses) with undetectable GnRH concentrations during the inter-pulse interval [16,17]. The pulsatile fashion of GnRH secretion was first demonstrated in ovariectomized rhesus monkeys and confirmed subsequently in humans using serial blood sampling during pituitary surgery [18,19]. In adult males, GnRH pulses occur approximately every 90–120 minutes. GnRH has a very short half-life (<10 min) and is mainly degraded in the pituitary gland immediately after secretion by several peptidase systems [11].

The pulsatility of GnRH secretion is a prerequisite for its stimulatory effect on gonadotropin release and, consequently, for normal sexual and reproductive function. This was documented in rhesus monkeys, whose endogenous GnRH secretion was abolished by hypothalamic radio-frequency. Pulsatile administration of GnRH restored gonadotropin secretion in these animals, whereas continuous GnRH produced only a transient response. Switching from continuous to pulsatile GnRH administration reinstituted gonadotropin secretion [20]. The suppression of gonadotropin secretion following continuous exposure to GnRH is caused by the downregulation of pituitary GnRH receptors, a phenomenon known as desensitization. It is the basis for the development and clinical use of GnRH analogs exerting agonistic activity in cases where suppression of the HPT axis is required (prostate cancer, premature puberty) [21].

The mechanisms underlying GnRH pulsatility remain still unclear. GnRH neurons can coordinate their activity [22] and show intrinsic electric pulsatility, at least in vitro [16,23]. There is evidence that LH secretion, a surrogate marker of GnRH release, is correlated with episodic multi-unit electrical activity in the medial-basal hypothalamus, indicating that the "GnRH pulse generator" is probably located there [24]. Functionally, the GnRH pulse generator seems to result from a complex interplay between the intrinsic pulsatility of GnRH neurons and the effect of other neuronal networks such as those expressing norepinephrine, dopamine, serotonin, glutamate, GABA, galanin, and neuropeptide Y (NPY) [7]. The kisspeptin-neurokinin B-dynorphin system may also have a pivotal role in regulating GnRH pulsatility [25].

The GnRH pulse generator starts its activity after completing the embryonal migration of GnRH neurons [3,7]. In infancy, GnRH and consequently LH pulsatile secretion is increased (often termed mini-puberty), resulting in activation of gonadal steroidogenesis usually between the third and sixth postnatal month and then becomes quiescent until puberty sets in [26]. This prepubertal suppression of the HPT axis has been shown to occur in agonadal humans [27] and primates [28], suggesting that hypothalamo-hypophyseal factors play the dominant role in this process. The onset of pubertal maturation is characterized by a steady increase in GnRH and LH pulse frequency [29].

5.1.2.4 Regulation of GnRH Secretion: The Kisspeptin-Neurokinin B-Dynorphin System

The discovery of kisspeptins revolutionized the field of neuroendocrine control of reproduction by providing the intermediary mechanism by which neuroendocrine, metabolic, and environmental inputs influence GnRH secretion and the function of the HPT axis. Kisspeptins are neuropeptides encoded by the *KISS1* gene, which was first discovered in Hershey in 1996 as a suppressor of metastasis in malignant melanoma [30]. It was named after the famous "Hershey's Kisses" chocolates, and the inclusion of SS was indicative of "suppressive sequence." The *KISS1* gene is localized to chromosome 1q32 and produces a 145-aa precursor peptide, which is cleaved down to a 54-aa peptide (kisspeptin-54). This peptide can be further cleaved to 14 (kp-14), 13 (kp-13), and 10-aa peptides (kp-10), all sharing the C-terminal sequence of Arg-Phe-NH2 and collectively known as human kisspeptins [31,32]. In 2001, the orphan G–protein-coupled receptor-54 (GPR54) was identified as the receptor for kisspeptins and is currently named KISS1R [33]. It is a 398-aa protein with seven transmembrane domains and is encoded by the *KISS1R* gene, which maps to human chromosome 19p13.3 [32]. Binding of KISS1R to its ligand activates phospholipase C and uses inositol triphosphate and diacylglycerol as intracellular messengers leading to the intracellular release of calcium and activation of protein kinase C [34].

In humans, two populations of kisspeptin-producing neurons are identified: one in the infundibular nucleus and a second, smaller one, in the rostral POA [35]. The axons of kisspeptin neurons create dense plexuses in the human infundibular stalk, where the secretion of GnRH takes place. At this level, axo-somatic, axodendritic, and axo-axonal synaptic contacts exist between kisspeptin and GnRH neurons, providing the neuroanatomical basis for the interaction between these two networks [35,36]. Moreover, GnRH neurons express KISS1R, indicating a direct effect of kisspeptin on GnRH secretion [37]. Three-quarters of kisspeptin-immunoreactive cells in the human infundibular nucleus of the hypothalamus coexpress neurokinin B and dynorphin. These neurons are known by the acronym KNDy [38]. However, neurokinin B and dynorphin are absent from kisspeptin neurons in the hypothalamic POA indicating differences in these two populations [39]. Neurokinins (A and B) belong to the tachykinin family of peptides and act through G-protein coupled receptors (TACR1, TACR2, and TACR3). Neurokinin B predominantly activates TACR3 [40]. Dynorphin is an endogenous opioid that exerts its biological action by binding to the kappa opioid receptor [41].

KNDy neurons act synergistically in order to induce pulsatile GnRH secretion by modifying the activity of other KNDy cells. This is supported by the expression of TACR3 and kappa-opioid peptide receptors but not KISS1R (which are expressed mainly on GnRH neurons) on KNDy neurons, thus creating autocrine and paracrine regulatory loops. Moreover, the existence of gap junctions between KNDy neurons and between neurons and glia further facilitates the synchronized activity of KNDy cells [38,42,43].

Kisspeptin stimulates GnRH secretion and it is the most potent GnRH secretagogue [44]. Kisspeptin signals directly to GnRH neurons through the activation of KISS1R [37]. Animal and human studies have shown the indirect stimulatory effect of kisspeptin on FSH and LH secretion, although it is more intense and consistent on the latter [7]. However, there is also evidence for a direct role of kisspeptin in stimulating gonadotropin secretion, although this direct effect remains debatable [41,45]. Kisspeptin signaling seems to be sexually dimorphic. In men, kisspeptin potently stimulates GnRH, and in turn, LH secretion, but in females, the response is variable and dependent on the phase of the menstrual cycle [39]. Moreover, the number of kisspeptin neurons in infundibular nuclei and POA is more in women than men. These sex differences appear early in perinatal development, probably due to the effects of sex steroids and likely reflect different roles of the kisspeptin signaling system in regulating reproductive function between both sexes [41].

Neurokinin B stimulates KNDy neurons to secrete kisspeptin, leading to GnRH release [46]. In contrast, dynorphin exerts an inhibitory effect on KNDy activity and, consequently, on GnRH secretion. KNDy neurons through the stimulatory effects of kisspeptin and neurokinin and the suppressive action of dynorphin coordinate pulsatile GnRH secretion [41].

The KNDy signaling system plays a pivotal role in normal puberty. Hypothalamic expression of *KISS1* and *KISS1R* increases during puberty as well as the percentage of GnRH neurons, which are responsive to kisspeptin [47]. In humans, the significant role of the KNDy system in regulating the reproductive axis became apparent from patients with pubertal disorders. Inactivating mutations in *KISS1R* have been described in patients with hypogonadotrophic hypogonadism (HH) presenting with pubertal delay [48]. Missense mutations in *TAC3* (which encodes neurokinin B) and *TAC3R* also resulted in HH and delayed puberty [49]. On the other hand, activating mutations in *KISS1R* and *KISS1* have been demonstrated in children with central precocious puberty [50,51].

Moreover, the KNDy neuronal network may act as an intermediary in the regulation of GnRH secretion by other hormonal, metabolic, and stress signals. KNDy neurons express receptors for estrogens (ERα), progesterone (PR), androgens (AR), glucocorticoids (GR), prolactin, and leptin (LepR), whereas many of them (ERα, PR, AR, LepR) are not expressed on GnRH neurons [41]. Apart from its significant contribution to the regulation of GnRH secretion, kisspeptin signaling may have other roles such as the regulation of sexual and social behavior, emotional brain processing, mood, metabolism, body composition, and cardiac function [52–54].

5.1.2.5 Regulation of GnRH Secretion: Sex Steroids, Metabolic Signals and Other Factors

Sex Steroids

The GnRH pulse generator is under the tonic inhibition of peripheral sex steroids. In men, testosterone (T) comprises the most important hormonal regulator of GnRH secretion. T decreases GnRH secretion by reducing its pulse frequency and may act as such or after conversion to DHT or estradiol [11]. Expression of AR on GnRH neurons has been difficult to identify, and it seems that the negative feedback of T on GnRH secretion is mediated through KNDy signaling neurons, which express AR [41]. T reduces Kiss1 and augments dynorphin mRNA expression in KNDy neurons, through activation of ER and AR, leading to suppression of kisspeptin neuronal firing and, consequently, reduction of GnRH secretion [41,55,56]. At least part of the inhibitory effect of T may be realized through aromatization to estradiol. This is supported by studies showing that T-induced suppression of Kiss1 mRNA in the arcuate nucleus is similar to that produced by estradiol but more than that produced by DHT, a nonaromatizable androgen [57].

Estrogens exert both negative and positive effects on GnRH secretion. The positive feedback action is evident only in females during the late follicular phase of the menstrual cycle and induces the preovulatory GnRH and LH surge [41]. As mentioned before, ERα has been identified in KNDy neurons but not in GnRH ones and this fact implies that the estrogen negative feedback on GnRH secretion is mediated by KNDy neurons, which are located in the infundibular nucleus in humans and the arcuate nucleus in other mammals [39,42].

Estrogens decrease kisspeptin and neurokinin B release from KNDy cells, leading to diminished GnRH production [39]. Data from healthy men and men with HH or aromatase deficiency have shown that circulating rather than locally produced estrogens play the dominant role in the regulation of GnRH and gonadotropin secretion [58,59]. Progesterone also reduces GnRH and LH pulse frequency by inducing dynorphin release, which suppresses KNDy activity [60].

Metabolic Signals

It is well known that reproductive function and energy balance are closely related. States of negative energy balance, as well as metabolic disorders such as diabetes and obesity, have a negative impact on reproductive function both in males and females [61,62]. One of the most important metabolic cues regulating GnRH secretion is leptin. Leptin is a peptide encoded by the *ob (lep)* gene and secreted mainly from white adipose tissue. Its main function is to reduce food intake and increase energy expenditure [63]. Leptin stimulates GnRH secretion and, in turn, increases LH pulsatility, but this effect is indirect because GnRH neurons do not express LepR [64]. In contrast, at least 40% of kisspeptin neurons located in arcuate nucleus express LepR and respond to leptin by increasing kisspeptin release, indicating that the KNDy network mediates the effect of leptin on GnRH secretion [65]. However, there is evidence that the mechanism by which leptin regulates reproductive function may be more complex, involving stimulation of anorexigenic proopiomelanocortin (POMC) and cocaine- and amphetamine-regulated transcript (CART) expressing neurons and inhibition of orexigenic agouti-related peptide (AgRP) and NPY neurons [64,66]. The clinical significance of the regulatory role of leptin in the HPT axis is supported by evidence showing that men with mutations in leptin or LepR present with hypogonadism [67].

Apart from leptin, other metabolic signals such as insulin and insulin-like growth factor-1 (IGF-1) stimulate GnRH production by inducing *GnRH1* expression through the activation of mitogen-activated protein kinase (MAPK) pathway and early growth response-1 (Egr-1) [68,69]. On the contrary, ghrelin, an orexigenic peptide secreted by the stomach at the fasting state, decreases the firing rate of GnRH neurons in an estrogen- and endocannabinoid-dependent manner [70].

Other Factors

Physical and psychological stress is associated with suppression of the reproductive axis both in men and women, likely due to activation of the hypothalamic-pituitary-adrenal (HPA) axis [41]. Glucocorticoids decrease GnRH pulse frequency and this effect is probably modulated by sex steroids and kisspeptin signaling [71,72]. Moreover, there is evidence that upstream factors in the HPA axis, such as corticotropin-releasing hormone (CRH), may play an intermediary role in suppressing GnRH activity during stress [41]. Prolactin also inhibits GnRH pulse frequency through several putative mechanisms involving a direct suppressive effect on GnRH neurons, inhibition of kisspeptin signaling, or modulating the activity of GABA, NPY, β-endorphin, and dopamine secreting cells [41]. A neuropeptide called gonadotropin-inhibitory hormone (GnIH), first described in birds and its mammalian analog, RFamide-related peptide-3 (RFRP-3), is another inhibitor of kisspeptin and GnRH neuronal activity [73,74]. Other inhibitory signals include opioids, inflammatory cues such as interleukin-1, dopaminergic and serotoninergic systems, melatonin, and nitric oxide. On the contrary, the noradrenergic system, vasoactive intestinal peptide (VIP), glutamate, and GABA exert a stimulatory effect on GnRH secretion [7,11,41].

5.1.2.6 Actions of GnRH

GnRH reaches anterior pituitary via the hypophyseal portal system and binds to its receptor on gonadotrophs to stimulate synthesis and release of gonadotropins. GnRH receptor (GnRHR) is a 328-aa peptide belonging to the GPCR superfamily characterized by a seven-transmembrane domain structure. A characteristic feature of mammalian GnRHR is the absence of the cytoplasmic C-terminal tail, which is present in nonmammalian species [75]. In humans, the gene encoding GnRHR maps on chromosome 4q21.2 and possesses some unique features such as the location of the transcription start sites and the presence of TATA boxes [76].

Binding of GnRH to its receptor leads to the formation of a hormone-receptor complex, which can interact with multiple G proteins. In gonadotrophs, however, the main pathway involves coupling with Gq/11 [77] proteins leading to activation of phospholipase C, which promotes the formation of diacylglycerols and inositol-trisphosphate (IP3), resulting in the activation of several protein kinase C (PKC) isoforms and the mobilization of intracellular calcium, respectively. Increased calcium entry causes the release of FSH and LH via exocytosis. In addition, PKC activates the MAPK pathway, which plays an important role in inducing gonadotropin gene transcription [78]. Alternatively, the GnRH hormone-receptor complex can interact with Gs protein, which activates adenylyl cyclase (AC), producing a rise in cyclic adenosine monophosphate (cAMP) concentrations leading finally to the activation of protein kinase A (PKA) and cAMP response element-binding protein (CREB) [79]. Upon completing its biological action, the hormone-receptor complex is internalized by endocytosis and undergoes degradation in lysosomes [11].

GnRH is the sole releasing factor for both FSH and LH, but its effects on each one is not the same. Human and animal studies demonstrated that FSH secretion is more irregular than LH. Possible reasons include differences in the stimulatory action of GnRH, storage of FSH and LH in separate granules, diverse response times to GnRH, the existence of different gonadotroph subpopulations, and constitutive, in addition to pulsatile, secretion of FSH but not of LH [41]. Studies have shown that 93% of GnRH pulses are associated with FSH pulses, while each secretory burst of GnRH is followed by an LH pulse [80]. Moreover, GnRH pulse frequency differentially regulates gonadotropin subunit gene transcription. Increased pulse rates preferentially promote α-subunit and LHβ synthesis and secretion, whereas slow GnRH pulse rates increase FSHβ gene transcription [81].

GnRH regulates the expression of its receptors, an effect that depends on the secretory pattern and the released quantity of the neuropeptide [11]. When the pituitary is not stimulated by GnRH for a period of time, the number of GnRHR declines, but is restored after subsequent exposure of gonadotrophs to GnRH. This phenomenon is referred to as upregulation or self-priming and differs among species. The upregulation of GnRHR is differentially modulated by varying GnRH pulse rates [82]. In contrast, continuous exposure of pituitary to GnRH causes an initial rise in response followed by downregulation of the receptors and, eventually, inhibition of gonadotropin synthesis and secretion, an effect known as desensitization [7,11]. The underlying mechanism of desensitization is not clarified yet, but there is evidence that it may be due to postreceptor events such as downregulation of IP3 receptors or desensitization of calcium mobilization in gonadotrophs [83]. Apart from GnRH itself, the expression of GnRHR in the pituitary is also stimulated by activin but suppressed by estradiol, progesterone, and follistatin [7]. A second type of GnRHR (GnRHR type II) has been described in vertebrates, but the gene encoding this receptor has been disrupted or deleted in many mammalian species, including humans.

5.1.3 Pituitary: The Gonadotropins
5.1.3.1 Structure and Synthesis of Gonadotropins

FSH and LH are heterodimeric glycoproteins belonging to the same hormone family with human chorionic gonadotropin (hCG) and thyroid-stimulating hormone (TSH). They consist of two peptide chains, α and β, noncovalently attached to each other. The α-subunit, encoded by a gene on chromosome 6q12.21, contains 92 aa and is common to all members of the glycoprotein hormone family, while β-subunit differs in each hormone and confers specificity of action. The FSH β-subunit (FSHβ) consists of 111 aa and is encoded by a gene localized on chromosome 11p13 whereas LH's β-subunit (LHβ) contains 120 aa and the coding gene is mapped on chromosome 19q13.32. LHβ and βhCG are structurally very similar and the two hormones act by binding to the same receptor [11].

The synthesis of α- and β-subunits in pituitary gonadotrophs is calcium-dependent and requires activation of PKC and the MAPK-signaling pathway [84]. Translation of the relevant RNAs results in precursor peptides containing the original subunit sequence preceded by a signal aa chain. The precursor α- and β-peptides undergo cleavage of the signal peptide and N-glycosylation in the endoplasmic reticulum resulting in the formation of immature α/β heterodimers. In the Golgi apparatus, the glycosylation is completed, and the heterodimers acquire their final conformation. FSH and LH are stored in separate granules before secretion takes place [7].

Glycosylation of gonadotropins refers to oligosaccharide structures N-linked to asparagine (Asn) residues. These carbohydrate moieties are usually branched and contain simple sugars (mannose, galactose), aminosugars (N-acetyl-glycosamine, galactosamine), and sialic acid (FSH) or sulfate (LH) residues. The extend and type of glycosylation, which is different between the two gonadotropins, influence their secretion, biological activity, and rate of degradation. Glycosylation is not important for receptor binding but is crucial for receptor activation. FSH contains four glycosylation sites (α-subunit at positions 52 and 78, β-subunit at positions 7 and 24) but LH only three (α-subunit at positions 52 and 78, β-subunit at position 30). Glycosylation at position 52 of α-subunit is necessary for biological function, while isoforms of gonadotropins without glycosylation cannot be secreted and function as competitive antagonists of the wild type. LH is rich in N-acetyl-glucosamine sulfate and therefore is quickly removed from circulation resulting in a short half-life of 25 minutes. In contrast, FSH is predominantly sialylated, which protects immediate liver metabolism, resulting in a longer half-life of about two hours [11].

5.1.3.2 Secretion of Gonadotropins

FSH and LH are secreted by gonadotrophs in a pulsatile manner following the corresponding secretory bursts of GnRH. However, a fraction of synthesized hormones is not stored in granules and is constitutively secreted. The latter mode has been described only for FSH [41]. This bimodal pattern of secretion in conjunction with its long half-life may explain why FSH concentration in systemic circulation seems to fluctuate less than LH. As mentioned before, the same GnRH stimulus can cause preferential secretion of one gonadotropin over the other, depending on the GnRH pulse frequency.

The gonadotropins are detectable in the pituitary of embryos as early as the 9th week of gestation and become measurable in systemic circulation not until the 12th–14th gestational week. The concentration of gonadotropins in the fetus reaches a maximum level at mid-gestation and declines after that until they become suppressed at term, probably due to the progressive inhibition of fetal HPT axis by the gradual rise in the production of placental steroids toward birth. Male fetuses produce fewer gonadotropins than females and have higher LH concentrations than FSH, while the opposite occurs in females [85].

In male infants, a few minutes after birth, the concentration of LH increases by 10-fold and this rise lasts for ~12 hours. Due to the gradual decline in the levels of placentally produced sex steroids after birth and the lack of their inhibitory effect, the GnRH pulse generator is reactivated, leading to a rise in gonadotropin production between postnatal days 6 and 10. In infant boys, serum LH concentration enters the pubertal range by 1 week of age, peaks during the 2nd and 10th postnatal week and declines subsequently to prepubertal levels by 4–6 months of age. Serum FSH concentration, which is lower than LH in male infants compared to females, reaches a maximum level between 1 week and 3 months and decreases to prepubertal range within 4 months of age. This re-activation of the HPT axis during the neonatal period of life is known as mini-puberty and has been linked to a variety of developmental processes such as penile and testicular growth and differentiation and proliferation of germ cells [85]. During childhood, the GnRH pulse generator remains dormant and the secretion of gonadotropins very low until the onset of puberty, when the GnRH pulse frequency steadily increases, leading to increased rates and amplitude of LH and FSH pulses. This augmentation of gonadotropin secretion is first detected at night, during sleep, and gradually extends during the day [11].

5.1.3.3 Regulation of Gonadotropin Secretion

The main stimulus for the production of gonadotropins is GnRH-I. In contrast, the principal inhibitors of gonadotropin secretion are the sex steroids and a testicular peptide, inhibin B (Inh-B), via a negative feedback mechanism. The regulatory process also involves the paracrine/autocrine actions of other pituitary-derived peptides such as activin and follistatin and the effect of the hypothalamic neuropeptide GnIH/RFRP-3 [86].

The Role of Sex Steroids

T is the main inhibitor of LH secretion in men. T may act as such or after its conversion to DHT by 5α-reductase or E_2 by aromatase. Both metabolic pathways are important for mediating T's negative feedback effect. Available data show that the administration of nonaromatizable androgen (dihydrotestosterone – DHT) suppresses LH secretion and, on the other hand, LH is increased in men with aromatase deficiency, resistance to estrogens, or treated with aromatase inhibitors. T suppresses LH secretion by acting both indirectly at the hypothalamic level and directly on gonadotrophs. At the hypothalamus, T reduces GnRH pulse frequency, probably through an opioid-induced inhibition of KNDy neurons, leading to reduced LH pulse rate. At the pituitary level, T acts on gonadotrophs to reduce LH release, an effect that requires aromatization to estradiol (E_2), which is not necessary for the hypothalamic effect [87,88]. T, through aromatization to E_2, acts on gonadotrophs and inhibits FSH secretion as well [88]. However, in normal men, T seems to be less important than E_2 and inhibin in the control of FSH [89].

Estrogens are secreted by testes, after the conversion of testicular androgens, such as T and androstenedione to E_2 and estrone (E_1), respectively, by aromatase, an enzyme expressed mainly in Sertoli cells. However, aromatase has also been detected in other tissues such as the adipose tissue, muscles, CNS, liver, mammary gland, endothelium, skin, and parietal cells of the stomach. The main source of estrogens in men is the aromatization of circulating androgens in peripheral tissues [90]. Estrogens suppress the secretion of both LH and FSH by acting on the hypothalamus and pituitary. At the hypothalamic level, estrogens reduce the frequency of GnRH pulse generator, by suppressing the KNDy neurons that express the relevant receptor (ERα), whereas in the pituitary, they reduce the responsiveness of the gonadotrophs to GnRH stimuli by suppressing the expression of *GnRHR* [7]. The result of estrogen negative feedback is a reduction in the mean serum concentration of FSH and LH, and decreased frequency and amplitude of LH pulses [90].

The Role of Inhibin, Activins, and Follistatin

During the last three decades, much evidence has emerged, showing that sex steroids are not the only testicular products exerting a negative feedback effect on gonadotropin secretion. This is manifested in subfertile men with disturbed spermatogenesis, in whom serum FSH concentration is elevated despite normal LH and T concentrations. It was assumed that a hormonal product of the testes conveys to the hypothalamo-pituitary control system information related to the efficiency of spermatogenesis. This hormone is now known as inhibin and comprises the major regulator of FSH secretion in men [91].

Inhibin is a dimeric glycoprotein, belonging to the transforming growth factor-β (TGF-β) superfamily and consists of two disulfide-linked peptide chains, α and β. Subunit β exists in two isoforms, βA and βB, giving rise to two forms of inhibin: inhibin A (α/βA) and B (α/βB). Inh-B is the main circulating and physiologically relevant form of inhibin in men. It is produced, under the stimulation of FSH, by Sertoli cells in prepubertal testis, but in adults, its secretion requires the synergistic contribution of both Sertoli and germ cells. In adult males, serum Inh-B concentration is inversely correlated with serum FSH and positively associated with Sertoli cell number, sperm concentration and total count, and testicular volume [92]. Inhibin B (Inh-B), via systemic circulation, reaches pituitary gonadotrophs and inhibits FSH secretion exclusively. Specifically, it downregulates the expression of FSHβ mRNA and FSH protein, by blocking the activin-induced stimulation of transcription. Inh-B and activins compete for binding to the same receptor (type II activin receptor). Inhibin β subunit binds to a single type II activin receptor while α subunit binds to a membrane proteoglycan, called betaglycan or type III TGF-β receptor, thus creating an inactive inhibin-receptor complex. This complex cannot induce signal transduction and by sequestering type II receptors blocks activin signaling [93].

Activins, which also belong to the TGF-β superfamily, are dimeric proteins consisting of two β subunits, the same as inhibin. Three forms of activins exist: A (βA/βA), B (βB/βB), and AB (βA/βB). Two more β-subunits have been described (βC, βE) but their function is yet unknown. Activins are produced by the gonadotrophs and can bind to two type I (ActRIB [ALK-4] and ActRIC [ALK-7]) and two type II activin receptors (ActRII and ActRIIB) creating an active hexameric complex that signals intracellularly through mainly Smad proteins [7,93]. The production of pituitary activin B is controlled by GnRH pulse frequency [94]. Activins function in a paracrine/autocrine manner to enhance the expression of

GnRH receptors on gonadotrophs, thereby increasing the responsiveness of the pituitary to GnRH. Pituitary-derived activin B stimulates GnRH-induced FSH synthesis and release, while activin-A stimulates GnRH-induced LH production. The latter effect is inhibited by T [93]. Activins are also produced in testes by Sertoli, Leydig, and peritubular myoid cells. However, the absence of a reduction in activin A serum levels after castration precludes a major role of this peptide in the negative feedback control of gonadotropin secretion. Instead, testicular-derived activins may exert many local actions such as stimulation of spermatogonial mitosis and Sertoli cell proliferation during testis development [86].

Follistatin is a monomeric glycoprotein rich in cysteine, structurally different from inhibins and activins. It exists in three isoforms, designated Fst288, Fst303, and Fst315, which are products of alternative splicing of a single follistatin gene (*Fst*). Fst315 is the main circulating form of follistatin, whereas Fst288 and Fst303 are bound to cell-surface heparan sulfate proteoglycans, indicating different physiological roles for the three isoforms. Follistatins act as functional antagonists of activins. In particular, two follistatin molecules bind irreversibly to dimeric activin and inhibit its interaction with type I and II receptors. The activin-Fst288 complex is then internalized and degraded in lysosomes. Follistatins bind both activin A and B but have a higher affinity for the former. Fst288 binds to activins with higher affinity than Fst303 [93]. They are generally coexpressed with activins and the highest level of expression has been demonstrated in the pituitary and gonadal tissues. At the pituitary level, follistatin mRNA has been found in different pituitary cell types, including gonadotrophs and folliculo-stelate cells. Locally produced follistatin blocks activin-induced FSH secretion and upregulation of GnRHR expression on gonadotrophs [7,86,93]. Moreover, FSH stimulates the pituitary production of follistatin, which in turn inhibits activin-mediated FSH release, thus creating a negative feedback autocrine/paracrine loop [95]. At the testicular level, follistatin is produced by Sertoli cells, spermatogonia, primary spermatocytes, and round spermatids. However, castration does not result in a decrease in follistatin-circulating concentration, suggesting that testes are not the major source of circulating follistatin [86]. In addition, it seems that testicular-derived follistatin does not feed back on the pituitary but instead acts locally in a paracrine manner to regulate spermatogenesis and Sertoli cell proliferation according to animal studies [93].

In conclusion, the activin-inhibin B-follistatin system plays an important role in the regulation of mainly FSH secretion. Activin functions in a paracrine/autocrine way to stimulate GnRH-induced FSH production, whereas testicular inhibin B acting via a negative feedback mechanism and pituitary-derived follistatin acting in a paracrine/autocrine manner, block activin's effect on FSH release. The fact that GnRH, T, and E_2 can modulate the expression of α, βA, βB, and follistatin mRNA expression in the pituitary [86] indicates the existence of a complex interplay among the major regulators of gonadotropin secretion.

The Role of GnIH/RFRP

In 2000, a neuropeptide was isolated from the Japanese quail's hypothalamus capable of suppressing gonadotropin secretion [96]. This dodecapeptide (Ser-Ile-Lys-Pro-Ser-Ala-Tyr-Leu-Pro-Leu-Arg-Phe-NH2 or SIKPSAYLPLRFamide), which was named gonadotropin-inhibitory hormone (GnIH) after its inhibitory effect on gonadotropins, belongs to the RFamide-related peptides (RFRP) family that is characterized by the presence of a common C-terminal Leu-Pro-X-Arg-Phe-NH2 (X = Leu or Gln) sequence. Peptides with GnIH action have been identified in the CNS of mammals, amphibians, fish, and also in humans [97,98]. Two human GnIH homologs have been identified and are referred to as RFRP-1 and RFRP-3 [98]. Although RFRP-1 rather than RFRP-3 resembles structurally avian GnIH, functional studies have shown that RFRP-3 is most likely the main regulator of gonadotropin secretion in mammalian species [99]. These neuropeptides act through a G-protein coupled receptor designated GPR147 (neuropeptide FF receptor 1 [NPFF1R] or OT7T022) [99,100]. In humans, the cell bodies of GnIH/RFRP neurons have been localized in the dorsomedial hypothalamus and their axon terminal-like structures have been observed in the preoptic and infundibulum area close to GnRH and kisspeptin neurons and the neurosecretory area of the median eminence. These neuroanatomical correlations indicate a role for GnIH in the regulation of the reproductive axis at both the hypothalamic and pituitary levels. In support of this notion, the expression of the cognate receptor (GPR147) has been demonstrated in both the hypothalamic nuclei and gonadotrophs [98].

Studies, predominantly in animals, have shown that GnIH/RFRP-3 acts on gonadotrophs to inhibit GnRH-induced gonadotropin synthesis and release. The inhibitory effect is more prominent for LH than FSH. The intracellular mechanism, by which GnIH/RFRP-3 reduces GnRH-induced gonadotropin secretion, is probably interference with the adenylate cyclase/cAMP/PKA-dependent ERK pathway of GnRH signaling and inhibition of intracellular calcium mobilization [99,101]. Apart from the direct action on the pituitary responsiveness to GnRH, GnIH/RFRP-3 may also modulate gonadotropin secretion indirectly by affecting GnRH and kisspeptin neuronal activity. Animal studies (rodents, ewes, cattle, gilt, mares) have produced inconsistent results regarding the action of RFRP-3 on GnRH and kisspeptin neurons, showing either an inhibitory (most of them), a neutral, or even a stimulatory effect. It seems that the impact of GnIH on upstream regulators of gonadotropin secretion depends on many factors, including animal species, gender, age, estrogen level, and photoperiod [99]. In humans, the role of GnIH in the neuroendocrine regulation of reproduction is far from being elucidated. The only study published so far has shown that exogenously administered GnIH/RFRP-3 modestly suppressed LH secretion in postmenopausal women but failed to prevent the increase in LH, induced by the concurrent administration of kisspeptin-10 in normal men [102].

5.1.3.4 Actions of Gonadotropins

The gonadotropins reach testes via the systemic circulation, where they exert their biological actions by binding to hormone-specific receptors. FSH receptor (FSHR) binds only the cognate hormone, whereas LH receptor (LHR/LHCGR) is activated by LH and hCG. The genes encoding FSHR and LHCGR map on chromosome 2 and consist of 10 and 11 exons, respectively [11]. The gonadotropin receptors belong to the rhodopsin-like class of GPCR and display the characteristic seven-transmembrane domain architecture. A unique feature of these receptors is the very large extracellular N-terminal domain (ECND), which contains a cysteine-rich section followed by several leucine-rich repeats [103]. The latter area of the extracellular domain creates a curved solenoid structure, the inner surface of which comprises the binding site of the gonadotropin. Upon binding, the gonadotropin molecule interacts with a sulfated tyrosine residue in a region of the ECND proximal to the extracellular loops of the transmembrane domain, known as the "hinge region," leading to receptor activation [104]. Another phenomenon shared by FSHR and LHCGR is agonist-induced desensitization, which takes place a few minutes after exposure to their ligand and is mediated by the phosphorylation of their intracellular domain by GPCR kinases (GRK) and subsequent internalization through the recruitment of β-arrestins. Desensitization of the receptors serves as a local safety valve to prevent untamed stimulation of target cells.

LH Actions

The target of LH action in testes is the Leydig cell, which express the relevant receptor (LHCGR). In addition to testes, LHCGR has also been identified in adrenals, seminal vesicles, prostate, and certain brain regions. However, the physiologic role of LH in these extragonadal tissues in men is not yet known [105]. On the contrary, the main actions of LH in testes are documented and include:

- differentiation of Leydig cells during puberty when the adult-type Leydig cell population arises from mesenchymal stem cells [106]; and
- stimulation of synthesis and secretion of androgens, especially testosterone, a process called steroidogenesis.

Regarding the latter effect, the regulatory role of LH is double: (a) translocation of cholesterol from lipid droplets and/or plasma membrane into the inner membrane of mitochondria, which is the rate-limiting step in steroidogenesis (acute regulation) and (b) maintenance of optimal levels of the enzymes involved in steroidogenesis (trophic regulation) [107,108]. T, under the stimulus of LH, is secreted by Leydig cells into the systemic circulation and reaches all its target tissues where the hormone exerts its androgenic/sexual, anabolic, and feedback regulatory actions. Moreover, the LH-driven production of T raises its intratesticular concentration 60–100 times higher than that in the bloodstream, which is necessary for the paracrine stimulatory effect of T on spermatogenesis [11].

The study of human male phenotypes associated with mutations in *LHβ* or *LHCGR* genes has provided evidence supporting the importance of LH action in male reproductive physiology. Inactivating mutations in *LHβ* result in hypogonadotropic hypogonadism with delayed puberty, eunuchoid proportions, and defective spermatogenesis, ranging from complete arrest to hypospermatogenesis depending on the functional severity of the mutation and infertility but not genital ambiguity. On the contrary, loss-of-function mutations in *LHCGR* in genetic males were associated with 46XY disorders of sexual differentiation (male pseudohermaphroditism) phenotypically ranging from the complete feminization of external genitalia to less severe abnormalities such as micropenis and/or hypospadias or infertility without ambiguity. The milder phenotypes associated with *LHβ* mutations compared with those resulting from *LHCGR* mutations are likely due to activation of fetal Leydig cell proliferation, differentiation, and T production by placental hCG during the crucial first trimester of gestation [105]. On the other hand, gain-of-function mutations in *LHCGR* result in precocious puberty in males, whereas severe somatic activating *LHCGR* mutations have been associated with Leydig-cell tumors.

The actions of LH are mediated by intracellular signaling pathways, among which AC/cAMP/PKA-dependent cascade plays the dominant role. LHCGR activation leads to dissociation of Ga_s protein from βγ dimer, activation of AC, increased production of cAMP, and activation of PKA, which phosphorylates the transcription factor CREB. The latter binds to relevant DNA sequences and upregulates the transcription of genes encoding proteins and enzymes involved in steroidogenesis. Moreover, cAMP signaling through PKA is very important for the acute effect of LH as it stimulates the translocation of cholesterol to the outer mitochondrial membrane and then its transport into the inner membrane via the activation (phosphorylation) by PKA of the steroidogenic acute regulatory protein (STAR). STAR is essential for steroidogenesis as it interacts with other proteins, such as translocator protein (TSPO) and voltage-dependent anion channel-1 (VDAC1), to form a complex, known as transduceosome, which is responsible for cholesterol import into mitochondria [107]. Transduction of LH signal may also involve other pathways such as increased calcium mobilization through the Ga_q/phospholipase C/inositol triphosphate (IP_3) cascade, stimulation of the extracellular-regulated kinase $_{1/2}$ ($ERK_{1/2}$) signaling, and activation of AKT (protein kinase B) via the $G_{βγ}$ dimer/phosphatidylinositol 4,5-trisphosphate (PIP_3) route [109]. In addition, LH stimulation increases arachidonic acid release in Leydig cells through the coupling of the LHCGR with G_i protein and activation of phospholipase A2. The released arachidonic acid produces metabolites, via the action of cyclooxygenases, that influence steroidogenesis by modulating STAR protein expression [108].

FSH Actions

The principal function of FSH in males is to promote spermatogenesis, which is realized indirectly through its effect on

Sertoli cells, the only testicular cells documented to express FSHR. In humans, FSHR appears on Sertoli cells during the second half of gestation but become activated after the onset of FSH secretion in the neonate [110]. FSHR is also expressed on monocytes, adipocytes, and bones, but the physiology of FSH signaling in these tissues has not been clarified yet. However, animal studies have shown that FSH contributes to fat accumulation and possibly regulates bone mass [105].

On the other hand, the reproductive effects of FSH have been studied more extensively, although the exact role of this gonadotropin in male gametogenesis is not fully elucidated. The main actions of FSH include:

- Induction of Sertoli cell proliferation during the neonatal and pubertal stages of life. This proliferative effect occurs due to the upregulation of genes involved in DNA replication and cell cycle progression, such as cyclin D1 and D2. FSH is the main determinant of the final adult population of Sertoli cells, which in turn defines the adult total sperm output and testicular volume, given the fact that each Sertoli cell can support structurally and functionally only a specific number of germ cells (~10 in humans) [11].
- Stimulation of Sertoli cells to produce regulatory molecules and nutrients, necessary for spermatogenesis, such as retinoic acid, lactate, type 2 plasminogen-activator, and substances related to fatty acid metabolism and mitochondrial biogenesis [110].
- Production of anti-apoptotic survival factors. FSH acts as a survival factor rather than a mitogen, supporting the germ cell population up to the stage of pachytene spermatocytes [111].
- Production of adhesion molecules and organization of tight junctions and ectoplasmic specializations [110,111]. FSH, in concert with T, upregulates genes involved in the structure and function of the blood–testis barrier [110].
- Induction of spermiation (the release of mature elongated spermatids into the tubular lumen), in synergy with T [111].
- Upregulation of anti-Müllerian hormone (AMH) gene transcription in Sertoli cells, in the absence of androgen signaling [112].
- Stimulation of Inh-B production. In particular, FSH stimulates the production of the α-subunit from Sertoli cells [113].

Regarding the regulation of spermatogenesis, the available data converge to the fact that FSH acts in synergy with LH-driven intratesticular T to achieve a qualitatively and quantitatively normal sperm production. The major contributions of FSH are the regulation of Sertoli cell population and the support of premeiotic germ cells as a survival factor. Mutations in *FSHβ* and *FSHR* genes have been described in humans and the associated phenotypes support the importance of FSH for normal spermatogenesis. In particular, all men bearing inactivating mutations in *FSHR* were subfertile with reduced testicular volumes but not azoospermic, whereas all men with inactivating mutations in *FSHβ* were azoospermic. On the other hand, evidence from animal and human studies indicates that the role of FSH is not indispensable for spermatogenesis. An example comes from studies in gonadotropin-suppressed men where the administration of β-hCG achieved the desirable intratesticular T concentration and restored almost normal spermatogenesis in the absence of FSH action [114].

The biological effects of FSH are mediated through a network of intracellular signaling pathways. Apart from coupling to $G\alpha_s$ protein and activation of the AC/cAMP/PKA/CREB cascade, FSHR may also interact with $G\alpha_i$ protein, associated with the FSH-induced postnatal proliferation of Sertoli cells, via the ERK/MAPK-dependent signal transduction route. Moreover, FSH can stimulate the PIP3/AKT pathway and it seems that ERK and AKT signaling systems are oppositely regulated by FSH during postnatal Sertoli cell development. This dual regulation is most likely mediated by the tyrosine kinase receptor phosphatase Src homology 2-containing phosphotyrosine phosphatase (Shp2), given the fact that absent Shp2 activity, as is the case in Shp2 knock-out mice, leads to infertility. B-arrestins may also play a role in FSH signaling by inducing ERK activation associated with the internalization of the ligand-bound FSHR complex. This β-arrestin-induced ERK activation is more sustained than the transient one produced by the Gs pathway. Finally, data from rat models indicate that another intracellular mechanism mediating the FSH signal could regulate micro RNAs (miRNA) turnover [110].

5.2 Testicular Function

The testis is the principal male reproductive organ, which has a dual role: the production of the male gametes (spermatozoa), a process called spermatogenesis, and the synthesis and secretion of the male sex hormones (androgens), which is referred to as steroidogenesis [115]. These functions take place into two different histological compartments of the testis: the interstitial compartment, which is responsible for steroidogenesis, and the tubular compartment, which carries out spermatogenesis [116]. However, this division is grossly due to educational reasons, since the two compartments are one adjacent to the other and a substantial functional interplay exists between them.

5.2.1 Leydig Cell Function

The interstitial compartment represents 12–15% of the total testicular volume and contains the Leydig cells, immune cells such as macrophages and lymphocytes, blood and lymph vessels, nerves, fibroblasts, and loose connective tissue [117]. Leydig cells are capable of producing steroid hormones, among which the major product is T, the principal male hormone that plays a crucial role in every aspect and stage of a man's life, including sexual differentiation, sexual maturation, and reproductive health, as well as in the general health and quality of life of men [118].

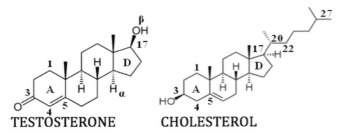

Figure 5.1 Testosterone (C19 steroid) and its precursor cholesterol (C27 steroid). This figure depicts the cycloperhydropentano-phenanthrene structure common to all steroid compounds and explains the basic steroid nomenclature. The numbers indicate the carbon atoms that are more relevant for steroid metabolism. Capital letters (A–D) correspond to the three cyclohexane and fourth (D) cyclopentane rings, according to standard convention. Attached groups and hydrogens are labeled as α or β according to their cis- or trans-configuration. Another important site is the double bond at C5. The steroid is classified as "Δ_4- or Δ_5-compound," whether the double bond resides between C4 and C5 or C5 and C6, respectively.

The synthesis of testosterone takes place in the endoplasmic reticulum and mitochondria of Leydig cells. The initial substrate is cholesterol, a C27-steroid, which may be synthesized de novo from acetate within the Leydig cell or derived from hydrolysis of cholesterol esters or circulating cholesterol and subsequently, through a sequence of enzymatic driven reactions, is converted to testosterone (C19-steroid) [119] (Figure 5.1).

1. The biosynthetic pathway starts with the transfer of cholesterol from the outer to the inner mitochondrial membrane, which is performed by StAR [120].
2. The translocation of cholesterol in the mitochondria is followed by a first side-chain cleavage of cholesterol at C20–C22, catalyzed by Cytochrome P450 isoenzyme 11a1 (P450scc), which results in the conversion of cholesterol to pregnenolone [121]. This is the first and essential step of the synthesis of all steroid hormones, since mutations of the CYP11A1 gene result in severe combined gonadal and adrenal deficiency [122].
3. Once pregnenolone is formatted, steroidogenesis may follow two different pathways. In the first, classical (Δ_5-pathway), pregnenolone undergoes hydroxylation coupled with a second side-chain cleavage, which leads successively to 17(OH)-pregnenolone and dehydroepiandrosterone (DHEA). These reactions take place in the endoplasmic reticulum and are catalyzed by a single enzyme, P450c17, which possesses both 17-alpha-hydroxylase and 17,20-lyase activities [123]. In the second, alternative pathway (Δ_4-), pregnenolone is converted to progesterone by 3β-hydroxysteroid dehydrogenase type 2 (3β-HSD$_2$) [124]. Subsequently, progesterone undergoes hydroxylation and side-chain cleavage by P450c17, leading to the successive production of 17(OH)-progesterone (17OHP) and Δ_4-androstenedione (Δ_4-A). The activity of the P450c17 enzyme exceeds that of 3β-HSD$_2$, while it is nearly 50 times more efficient in converting 17α-hydroxypregnenolone to DHEA than 17OHP to Δ_4-A. Consequently, the predominant biosynthetic pathway in the human testis is the Δ_5-pathway [125].
4. The final steps of the Δ_5-pathway comprise the conversion of DHEA by 17β-hydroxysteroid dehydrogenase type 3 (17β-HSD$_3$) to Δ_5-androstenediol, which in turn is further reduced by 3β-HSD$_2$ to T. Various types of human 17β-HSD exist with tissue-specific expression. 17β-HSD$_3$ is encountered almost exclusively in the testis and is considered the principal androgenic isoform of the enzyme [126]. Accordingly, in the Δ_4- pathway, Δ_4-A is converted to T by 17β-HSD$_3$. As a result of the superior efficiency of P450C17 over 3β-HSD$_2$ in Leydig cells, several intermediate products of the Δ_5-biosynthetic pathway are released in the circulation along with T. The pathways of steroidogenesis are summarized in Figure 5.2.

Each day, 5–7 mg of T is secreted by the testes. The synthesis and secretion of T are under the control of the LH [117]. Although the enzymatic rate-limiting step of steroidogenesis is the conversion of cholesterol to pregnenolone by P450scc, actually the rate is determined by the adequacy of the substrate (e.g., cholesterol) in the inner mitochondrial membrane, which is regulated by StAR protein [127]. LH acts on the corresponding G protein-coupled receptor on the membrane of Leydig cells, which, through a cascade of intracellular pathways, induce StAR activity. Accordingly, T is secreted episodically and shows a diurnal variation, which vaguely follows the fluctuations of LH [128]. Besides, T concentrations show a circadian variation, peaking in the early morning. Thus, T values obtained at 16:00 are 20–25% lower compared to those received at 08:00 [129].

Conversely, LH secretion is regulated by the negative feedback that T exerts on the hypothalamus, reducing the frequency of the hypothalamic pulse generator and the corresponding LH pulse frequency, the net effect of which is the reduction of LH activity on the testis [115]. T is also shown to directly inhibit LH secretion at the pituitary level by reducing pituitary responsiveness to GnRH [130]. Some of these effects could be indirect and mediated by the local aromatization of T to estradiol [131]. This feedback loop allows the fine regulation of the hypothalamic-pituitary-gonadal (HPG) axis.

Leydig cells also secrete insulin-like factor 3 (INSL3), a peptide hormone of the relaxin-insulin superfamily. It acts by binding on a membrane-bound G-coupled receptor (LGR8) and has been demonstrated to play an important role in transabdominal testicular descent during fetal life [132]. The secretion of INSL3 is constitutive, lacking a direct acute regulation by the HPG axis, and thus represents a reliable marker of the number and differentiation status of the Leydig cells. As such, in men with anorchia or bilateral orchiectomy, INSL3 is undetectable [133]. Interestingly, men who have undergone unilateral orchiectomy have INSL3 concentration intermediate

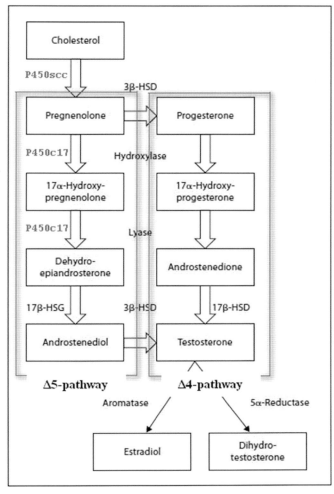

Figure 5.2 Overview of steroidogenesis and testosterone conversion to its active metabolites. The Δ5-pathway is the predominant in the human testis. P450scc is the rate-limiting step of steroidogenesis, while the action of P450c17 is the key branch point for the biosynthesis of androgens. The abundance of 17βHSD3 in Leydig cells directs steroidogenesis to the formation of T.
Notes: P450scc: side-chain cleavage enzyme; P450c17: 17α-hydroxylase/17,20-lyase; 3β-HSD: 3β-hydroxysteroid dehydrogenase/Δ5→Δ4 isomerase; 17β-HSD: 17β-hydroxysteroid dehydrogenase.

spermatogenesis: glycoprotein hormones (Inh-B, AMH), proteins (androgen-binding protein), steroids (E$_2$), cytokines, growth factors, opioids, and prostaglandins [116].

Inhibins are glycoprotein hormones, which belong to the TGF-β superfamily and form heterodimers that consist of two subunits connected one to another by a disulfide bridge. The combination of an α-subunit with a βA-subunit result in Inh-A, whereas the combination with a βB-subunit result in Inh-B [135]. Among inhibins, Inh-B is of clinical importance, as it is the main physiologic negative feedback regulator of FSH secretion [136]. Moreover, it reflects the proliferation rate of spermatogonia and their interaction with Sertoli cells, serving as a marker of the integrity of the germinal epithelium [137]. The levels of Inh-B show a circadian variation, with the highest values observed early in the morning, and act by binding to a heteromeric complex composed of one type III TGF-β receptor and a type IIB activin receptor.

AMH is also a glycoprotein of the TGF-β family, which similarly to INH-B binds to a heteromeric complex of transmembrane serine/threonine kinase receptors. In the male fetus, AMH evokes the regression of Müllerian ducts preventing thus the development of female accessory sex organs [138]. AMH is believed to be the earliest Sertoli cell hormone secretion during fetal life and its secretion follows a continuous pattern. AMH is a marker of immature Sertoli cell function and is used in suspected anorchia to confirm or exclude the presence of testicular tissue [132].

5.2.3 Testosterone Transport

Leydig cells produce and release T under the stimulation of LH initially in the testicular vasculature, which results in approximately 60–100 times higher intratesticular T concentration than that in the systemic circulation [139]. In normal men, only 2% of total T circulates unbound (free T) in plasma, while 44% is bound to sex hormone-binding globulin (SHBG) and 54% loosely bound to albumin. According to the "free hormone hypothesis," the actions of T are mediated through free T, which can enter cells by passive diffusion [140]. SHBG is a specific transporter of sex steroids through the bloodstream with a substantially high affinity to T (1.6×10^{-1} mol/l), which hampers dissociation and availability of T to target tissues. Albumin has about 1,000-fold lower affinity for T binding than SHBG (1.0×10^{-1} mol/l), however, due to its high concentration its binding capacity is high enough to bind more than half of plasma T. On the other hand, this looser bond between T and albumin allows dissociation of T at the capillary level and renders albumin-bound T available for tissue uptake. The sum of albumin-bound with the freeT fraction equates the bioavailable T [141]. Nevertheless, the amounts of bioavailable T measured with the ammonium sulfate precipitation and concanavalin A methods do not equal the sum of albumin-bound and freeT, suggesting that there are also other fractions of T playing a distinct role in total T activity [142]. Recent data suggest that additional proteins such as cortisol-binding

between normal and those with bilateral orchiectomy, despite having normal T, indicating the superiority of INSL3 over T as a marker of Leydig cell number. Accordingly, INSL3 concentration increases during puberty, following Leydig cell proliferation and differentiation, reach a steady state during adulthood, and decline with aging [134].

5.2.2 Sertoli Cell Endocrine Function

Sertoli cells are the main somatic cells of the tubular compartment of the testis, which maintain the proliferation and maturation of germ cells into mature spermatozoa, including their nutritional support, topographical and functional coordination, the formation of the blood–testis barrier, and the synthesis and secretion of several factors that regulate

Table 5.1 Conditions associated with increased or decreased SHBG concentrations

Increased SHBG concentrations	Decreased SHBG concentrations
Aging	Obesity
HIV disease	Diabetes mellitus
Hyperthyroidism	Hypothyroidism
Cirrhosis and hepatitis	Nephrotic syndrome
Use of some anticonvulsants	Acromegaly
Use of estrogens	Use of glucocorticoids, some progestins, and androgenic steroids
Polymorphisms in the SHBG gene	Polymorphisms in the SHBG gene

Notes: HIV: human immunodeficiency virus; SHBG: sex hormone-binding protein.

globulin and orosomucoid take part in T transport, whereas the "free hormone hypothesis," according to which SHBG-bound T should be considered inactive, is largely debated [143].

SHBG is a homodimeric β-globulin produced by hepatocytes in the liver, while a homolog of SHBG is produced by Sertoli cells (androgen binding protein), contributing to the high intratesticular T concentration that is crucial for spermatogenesis [144]. The concentration of sex steroids has a profound impact on SHBG biosynthesis. A preponderance of androgen steroids diminishes serum SHBG concentration, whereas estrogens increase SHBG. Consequently, the levels of SHBG in adult men are about one-third to one-half that in women, while senescence and hypogonadism are associated with elevation of SHBG. Several other conditions, such as androgen administration, obesity, and hypothyroidism, may decrease SHBG, while estrogen administration and hyperthyroidism may increase SHBG. Nevertheless, recent data show that interindividual differences in plasma SHBG levels are largely inherited [145]. Conditions associated with altered SHBG concentrations are summarized in Table 5.1. Normally, such alterations of SHBG have no biological impact on normal men because they are counteracted by equivalent modifications of the HPG axis [115]. However, they should be considered when evaluating T values, particularly if they lie near the lower limit of the adult male range. In such a case, free T should be measured or calculated using approved equations [146,147].

5.2.4 Testosterone Metabolism

The physiological actions of T are the result of T itself plus the actions of its active metabolites, E_2 and dihydrotestosterone (DHT) [148].

The conversion of T to DHT is catalyzed by the enzyme 5-alpha-reductase (SRD5A) and takes place mainly locally at the androgen target tissues. SRD5A exists as two distinct isoenzymes: SRD5A1 and SRD5A2 [149]. SRD5A1 is expressed in the liver and the skin, except the genital area, while SRD5A2 is expressed in the male urogenital tract, genital skin, and liver. Normally, 6–8% of circulating T is converted to DHT, resulting in a ratio of plasma T to DHT of approximately 10–15:1. Disorders in the function of SRD5A result in a distinct feminizing phenotype and may be identified by derangement of this ratio (>20:1) [150]. Both T and DHT exert their effects by binding to the same AR, with DHT being more potent (2.5- to 4-fold) due to its higher affinity to the receptor [151,152].

A smaller proportion of T (<1%) is metabolized to E_2, which also takes place predominantly (85%) in the periphery (adipose tissue and, to a lesser extent the brain, bone, breast, liver, and blood vessels), with the remainder in the testes. This reaction includes the aromatization of the A-ring of T and is catalyzed by the enzyme aromatase (CYP19A1), present in the endoplasmic reticulum [153]. The activity of aromatase is increased by LH and the actions of E_2 can be independent, complementary, or even opposing to those of T as it is observed at the bone, the hypothalamus, and the breast, respectively [148].

Since Leydig cells cannot store T, they are forced to synthesize T continuously. In order to maintain a steady state of androgen concentrations, the remainder of testosterone that is not protein-bound or metabolized to its active compounds is catabolized in the liver and the peripheral tissues [119]. Metabolism of T in the liver comprises two phases. The major target sites of Phase 1 hepatic T degradation are C-3, C-5, and C-17 and the corresponding enzymes involved are 3α- and 3β-hydroxysteroid dehydrogenases, 5α- and 5β-steroid reductases, and 17β-hydroxysteroid dehydrogenase respectively. The action of these enzymes leads successively through the formation of 3α-diol (3α,5α-androstanediol) to androsterone (3-hydroxy-5-androstane-17-one) and etiocholanolone (3-hydroxy-5-androstane-17-one), the most abundant urinary androgen metabolites [148]. During Phase 2, these compounds undergo glucuronidation and, to a lesser degree, sulfation in the liver to form more hydrophilic conjugates that can be excreted in urine and bile [154].

5.2.5 Testosterone Actions

The principal biological actions of T depending on the different stages of the lifespan of a man include the following [155]:
- induction of the fetal male phenotype during embryogenesis
- induction of secondary sexual characteristics at puberty and maintenance during adulthood
- initiation and maintenance of spermatogenesis
- regulation of gonadotropin secretion by the hypothalamic-pituitary unit
- maintenance of normal sexual function
- enhancement of muscle and bone mass and reduction of fat mass

- closure of long-bone epiphyses resulting in cessation of growth at puberty
- stimulation of erythropoiesis

Both T and DHT exert their effects by binding to the same androgen receptor (AR), a nuclear receptor, and a member of the steroid hormone receptor family that acts as a transcription factor (classical pathway) [156]. According to current knowledge, AR resides in the cytoplasm of the cells bound to heat shock proteins, such as hsp90, which maintain its inactive state. Binding of the ligand to the receptor evokes a conformational change that causes dissociation of the receptor from heat shock proteins, a modification that facilitates the translocation of the AR into the cell nucleus. Thereafter, the hormone-receptor complex forms a homodimer with a second hormone-AR receptor molecule, which can interact with specific DNA response elements for androgens (AREs), located adjacent to the relevant target genes, regulating their transcription [157].

The human AR gene is located on the long arm of the X chromosome (Xq11–12). The receptor molecule has a modular structure and can be divided into functional domains: (a) the ligand-binding domain (LBD) and (b) the DNA-binding domain (DBD), which are located at the C-terminal; (c) the hinge region, a flexible region that connects the DBD with the LBD; and (d) the N-terminal domain, which is responsible for most of the transcriptional activity of the AR [158]. This domain also contains three homopolymeric repeat regions, among which the glutamine-repeat region is of clinical importance since it correlates with the AR sensitivity. The length of this region averages 20 amino acids and is encoded by an equal number of trinucleotide CAG repeats in the first exon of the AR gene; the number of repeats (CAG)n normally varies from 11 to 35. It has been demonstrated that fewer repeats lead to increased AR affinity to circulating androgens, whereas more repeats lead to decreased receptor affinity [159].

Apart from the classical actions of T, which require binding to the AR and subsequent gene transcription, which may take hours to days to take place, it has been apparent that there are also androgen actions that may occur within minutes or even seconds such as the vasodilatory effects of T, which involve a rapid rise of intracellular calcium concentration (nonclassical or rapid actions) [160]. Similar actions have also been described in other tissues and cell types such as Sertoli cells, the brain, muscle, prostate, and immune cells [161]. Second messenger pathways have been implicated, such as the interaction of the AR with the tyrosine kinase c-SRC (steroid receptor coactivator), which does not require gene transcription [162], while in vitro studies have shown that T may interact with membrane-bound proteins. As such, megalin, a member of the LDL receptor-related protein (LRP) family, has been shown to facilitate endocytosis and cellular uptake of SHBG-bound T [163].

5.2.6 Testicular Function at the Different Phases of the Lifespan

Hormonal secretion from the testes is not steady throughout a man's lifespan, since it depends on the various stages of testicular ontogenesis and maturation. This becomes profound in disorders of gonadal function, which result in markedly different phenotypes according to the age of the insult [118].

T production is evident during fetal life, already by the seventh week of gestation. T concentrations increase during the first trimester, driven by the surge of chorionic gonadotropin and reach almost adult levels maintained throughout the second trimester. T levels fall afterward so that at the time of birth they reach a nadir similar to that of females [164]. Soon after birth, serum T rises and remains elevated until mid-infancy (six months of age) due to a temporary activation of the GnRH pulse generator. This phenomenon is also known as

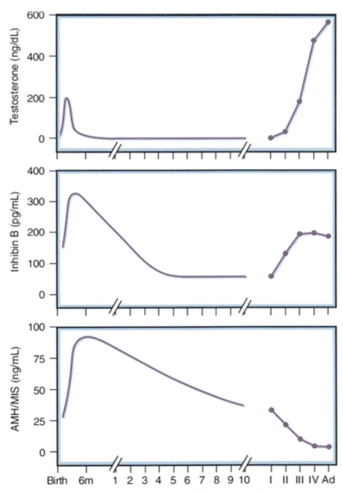

Figure 5.3 Concentrations of T, Inh-B, and AMH during lifetime
Notes: AMH/MIS: Anti-Müllerian hormone; Inh-B: inhibin B; T: testosterone.

"mini puberty" and usually ceases by the first year of age [165], while T levels return to a nadir during childhood (juvenile pause) and until the early pubertal phase when they rise again and gradually reach adult levels by the end of puberty [300–1,000 ng/dL (10.4–34.7 nmol/L)] [166]. T levels remain constant during adulthood, until the fifth decade when cross-sectional and longitudinal studies have shown that they begin to decline at an annual rate of 0.5–2% or 3.2 ng/dL [167].

Inh-B concentrations also rise during the neonatal period when they reach concentrations exceeding normal adults and decrease to a nadir from three to nine years of age [117]. In prepubertal children and at the initial stages of puberty, Inh-B gradually increases and shows a positive correlation with FSH concentrations as Sertoli cells proliferate in an FSH-dependent manner. At mid-puberty, when Sertoli cells become mature and start to interact with the germ cells, Inh-B–mediated negative feedback on FSH becomes activated and Inh-B concentrations reach a plateau that remains steady during adult life [168].

AMH is an early product of Sertoli cell function during fetal life and is present in cord blood at birth [132]. Thereafter, its concentration rises rapidly until mid-infancy, following the gonadotropin surge of "mini puberty" and the FSH-driven proliferation of Sertoli cells. During childhood, AMH declines slowly, falling further in puberty to reach low adult levels. AMH is believed to be blunted during puberty by increased testosterone secretion due to Sertoli cell maturation, which is characterized by enhancement of the AR expression [169]. The fluctuations of testicular hormonal secretion from birth to adulthood are illustrated in Figure 5.3.

References

1. Fink G. 60 years of neuroendocrinology: memoir: Harris' neuroendocrine revolution: of portal vessels and self-priming. *J Endocrinol*. 2015;226:T13–T24.
2. Schally AV, Arimura A, Kastin AJ, et al. Gonadotropin-releasing hormone: one polypeptide regulates secretion of luteinizing and follicle-stimulating hormones. *Science*. 1971;173:1036–1038.
3. Plant TM. 60 years of neuroendocrinology: the hypothalamo-pituitary-gonadal axis. *J Endocrinol*. 2015;226:T41–T54.
4. Schally AV. Use of GnRH in preference to LH-RH terminology in scientific papers. *Hum Reprod*. 2000;15:2059–2061.
5. Millar RP. GnRHs and GnRH receptors. *Anim Reprod Sci*. 2005;88:5–28.
6. Okubo K, Nagahama Y. Structural and functional evolution of gonadotropin-releasing hormone in vertebrates. *Acta Physiol (Oxf)*. 2008;193:3–15.
7. Kaprara A, Huhtaniemi IT. The hypothalamus-pituitary-gonad axis: tales of mice and men. *Metabolism*. 2018;86:3–17.
8. White RB, Eisen JA, Kasten TL, Fernald RD. Second form of gonadotropin-releasing hormone in humans. *Proc Natl Acad Sci USA*. 1998;95:305–309.
9. Densmore VS, Urbanski HF. Relative effect of gonadotropin releasing hormone (GnRH)-I and GnRH-II on gonadotropin release. *J Clin Endocrinol Metab*. 2003;88:2126–2134.
10. Lee VH, Lee LT, Chow BK. Gonadotropin-releasing hormone: regulation of the GnRH gene. *FEBS J*. 2008;275:5458–5478.
11. Weinbauer GF, Luetjens CM, Simoni M, Nieschlag E. Physiology of testicular function. In: Nieschlag E, Behre HM, Nieschlag S, eds. *Andrology: Male Reproductive Health and Disfunction*. 3rd ed. Springer-Verlag; 2010:11–59.
12. Herbison AE. Physiology of the adult gonadotropin-releasing hormone neuronal network. In: Plant TM, Zeleznik AJ, eds. *Knobil and Neill's Physiology of Reproduction*. 5th ed. Elsevier Inc.; 2015:399–467.
13. Clifton DKS. Neuroendocrinology of reproduction. In: Strauss JF, Barberi RL, eds. *Yen & Jaffe's Reproductive Endocrinology*. Elsevier; 2009: Ch. 1.
14. Schwanzel-Fukuda M, Pfaff DW. Origin of luteinizing hormone-releasing hormone neurons. *Nature*. 1989;338:161–164.
15. Wierman ME, Kiseljak-Vassiliades K, Tobet S. Gonadotropin-releasing hormone (GnRH) neuron migration: initiation, maintenance and cessation as critical steps to ensure normal reproductive function. *Front Neuroendocrinol*. 2011;32:43–52.
16. Maeda K, Ohkura S, Uenoyama Y, et al. Neurobiological mechanisms underlying GnRH pulse generation by the hypothalamus. *Brain Res*. 2010;1364:103–115.
17. Moenter SM, DeFazio AR, Pitts GR, Nunemaker CS. Mechanisms underlying episodic gonadotropin-releasing hormone secretion. *Front Neuroendocrinol*. 2003;24:79–93.
18. Carmel PW, Araki S, Ferin M. Pituitary stalk portal blood collection in rhesus monkeys: evidence for pulsatile release of gonadotropin-releasing hormone (GnRH). *Endocrinology*. 1976;99:243–248.
19. Antunes JL, Carmel PW, Housepian EM, Ferin M. Luteinizing hormone-releasing hormone in human pituitary blood. *J Neurosurg*. 1978;49:382–386.
20. Belchetz PE, Plant TM, Nakai Y, Keogh EJ, Knobil E. Hypophysial responses to continuous and intermittent delivery of hypothalamic gonadotropin-releasing hormone. *Science*. 1978;202:631–633.
21. Blumenfeld Z. Investigational and experimental GnRH analogs and associated neurotransmitters. *Expert Opin Investig Drugs*. 2017;26:661–667.
22. Moenter SM, DeFazio AR, Pitts GR, Nunemaker CS. Mechanisms underlying episodic gonadotropin-releasing hormone secretion. *Front Neuroendocrinol*. 2003;24:79–93.
23. Martinez de la Escalera G, Choi AL, Weiner RI. Generation and synchronization of gonadotropin-releasing hormone (GnRH) pulses: intrinsic properties of the GT1-1 GnRH neuronal cell line. *Proc Natl Acad Sci USA*. 1992;89:1852–1855.
24. Wilson RC, Kesner JS, Kaufman JM, Uemura T, Akema T, Knobil E. Central electrophysiologic correlates of pulsatile luteinizing hormone secretion in the rhesus monkey. *Neuroendocrinology*. 1984;39:256–260.
25. Ezzat A, Pereira A, Clarke IJ. Kisspeptin is a component of the pulse generator for GnRH secretion in female sheep but

26. Waldhauser F, Weissenbacher G, Frisch H, Pollak A. Pulsatile secretion of gonadotropins in early infancy. *Eur J Pediatr*. 1981;137:71–74.

27. Conte FA, Grumbach MM, Kaplan SL, Reiter EO. Correlation of luteinizing hormone-releasing factor-induced luteinizing hormone and follicle-stimulating hormone release from infancy to 19 years with the changing pattern of gonadotropin secretion in agonadal patients: relation to the restraint of puberty. *J Clin Endocrinol Metab*. 1980;50:163–168.

28. Pohl CR, deRidder CM, Plant TM. Gonadal and nongonadal mechanisms contribute to the prepubertal hiatus in gonadotropin secretion in the female rhesus monkey (*Macaca mulatta*). *J Clin Endocrinol Metab*. 1995;80:2094–2101.

29. Boyar R, Finkelstein J, Roffwarg H, Kapen S, Weitzman E, Hellman L. Synchronization of augmented luteinizing hormone secretion with sleep during puberty. *N Engl J Med*. 1972;287:582–586.

30. Lee JH, Miele ME, Hicks DJ, et al. KiSS-1, a novel human malignant melanoma metastasis-suppressor gene. *J Natl Cancer Inst*. 1996;88:1731–1737.

31. West A, Vojta PJ, Welch DR, Weissman BE. Chromosome localization and genomic structure of the KiSS-1 metastasis suppressor gene (KISS1). *Genomics*. 1998;54:145–148.

32. Pasquier J, Kamech N, Lafont AG, Vaudry H, Rousseau K, Dufour S. Molecular evolution of GPCRs: kisspeptin/kisspeptin receptors. *J Mol Endocrinol*. 2014;52:T101–T117.

33. Ohtaki T, Shintani Y, Honda S, et al. Metastasis suppressor gene KiSS-1 encodes peptide ligand of a G-protein-coupled receptor. *Nature*. 2001;411:613–617.

34. Liu X, Lee K, Herbison AE. Kisspeptin excites gonadotropin-releasing hormone neurons through a phospholipase C/calcium-dependent pathway regulating multiple ion channels. *Endocrinology*. 2008;149:4605–4614.

35. Hrabovszky E, Ciofi P, Vida B, et al. The kisspeptin system of the human hypothalamus: sexual dimorphism and relationship with gonadotropin-releasing hormone and neurokinin B neurons. *Eur J Neurosci*. 2010;31:1984–1998.

36. Uenoyama Y, Inoue N, Pheng V, et al. Ultrastructural evidence of kisspeptin-gonadotrophin-releasing hormone (GnRH) interaction in the median eminence of female rats: implication of axo-axonal regulation of GnRH release. *J Neuroendocrinol*. 2011;23:863–870.

37. Messager S, Chatzidaki EE, Ma D, et al. Kisspeptin directly stimulates gonadotropin-releasing hormone release via G protein-coupled receptor 54. *Proc Natl Acad Sci USA*. 2005;102:1761–1766.

38. Lehman MN, Coolen LM, Goodman RL. Minireview: kisspeptin/neurokinin B/dynorphin (KNDy) cells of the arcuate nucleus: a central node in the control of gonadotropin-releasing hormone secretion. *Endocrinology*. 2010;151:3479–3489.

39. Skorupskaite K, George JT, Anderson RA. The kisspeptin-GnRH pathway in human reproductive health and disease. *Hum Reprod Update*. 2014;20:485–500.

40. Topaloglu AK, Semple RK. Neurokinin B signalling in the human reproductive axis. *Mol Cell Endocrinol*. 2011;346:57–64.

41. Marques P, Skorupskaite K, George JT, et al. Physiology of GNRH and gonadotropin secretion. [Updated 2018 Jun 19]. In: Feingold KR, Anawalt B, Boyce A, et al., eds. *Endotext [Internet]*. MDText.com, Inc.; 2000–. Available from: www.ncbi.nlm.nih.gov/books/NBK279070/.

42. Pinilla L, Aguilar E, Dieguez C, Millar RP, Tena-Sempere M. Kisspeptins and reproduction: physiological roles and regulatory mechanisms. *Physiol Rev*. 2012;92:1235–1316.

43. Ikegami K, Minabe S, Ieda N, et al. Evidence of involvement of neurone-glia/neurone-neurone communications via gap junctions in synchronised activity of KNDy neurons. *J Neuroendocrinol*. 2017:29.

44. Dhillo W, Chaudhuri O, Patterson M, et al. Kisspeptin-54 stimulates the hypothalamic-pituitary-gonadal axis in human males. *J Clin Endocrinol Metab*. 2005;90:6609–6615.

45. Gutierrez-Pascual E, Martinez-Fuentes AJ, Pinilla L, Tena-Sempere M, Malagon MM, Castano JP. Direct pituitary effects of kisspeptin: activation of gonadotrophs and somatotrophs and stimulation of luteinising hormone and growth hormone secretion. *J Neuroendocrinol*. 2007;19:521–530.

46. Navarro VM, Bosch MA, Leon S, et al. The integrated hypothalamic tachykinin-kisspeptin system as a central coordinator for reproduction. *Endocrinology*. 2015;156:627–637.

47. Han SK, Gottsch ML, Lee KJ, et al. Activation of gonadotropin-releasing hormone neurons by kisspeptin as a neuroendocrine switch for the onset of puberty. *J Neurosci*. 2005;25:11349–11356.

48. de Roux N, Genin E, Carel JC, Matsuda F, Chaussain JL, Milgrom E. Hypogonadotropic hypogonadism due to loss of function of the KiSS1-derived peptide receptor GPR54. *Proc Natl Acad Sci USA*. 2003;100:10972–10976.

49. Topaloglu AK, Reimann F, Guclu M, et al. TAC3 and TACR3 mutations in familial hypogonadotropic hypogonadism reveal a key role for Neurokinin B in the central control of reproduction. *Nat Genet*. 2009;41:354–358.

50. Teles MG, Bianco SD, Brito VN, et al. GPR54-activating mutation in a patient with central precocious puberty. *N Engl J Med*. 2008;358:709–715.

51. Silveira LG, Noel SD, Silveira-Neto AP, et al. Mutations of the KISS1 gene in disorders of puberty. *J Clin Endocrinol Metab*. 2010;95:2276–2280.

52. Clarke SA, Dhillo WS. Kisspeptin across the human lifespan: evidence from animal studies and beyond. *J Endocrinol*. 2016;229:R83–R98.

53. Comninos AN, Dhillo WS. Emerging roles of kisspeptin in sexual and emotional brain processing. *Neuroendocrinology*. 2018;106:195–202.

54. Dudek M, Ziarniak K, Sliwowska JH. Kisspeptin and metabolism: the brain and beyond. *Front Endocrinol (Lausanne)*. 2018;9:145.

55. Navarro VM, Gottsch ML, Wu M, et al. Regulation of NKB pathways and their roles in the control of Kiss1 neurons in the arcuate nucleus of the male mouse. *Endocrinology*. 2011;152:4265–4275.

56. Shibata M, Friedman RL, Ramaswamy S, Plant TM. Evidence that down regulation of hypothalamic KiSS-1 expression is involved in the negative feedback action of testosterone to regulate luteinising hormone secretion

56. in the adult male rhesus monkey (*Macaca mulatta*). *J Neuroendocrinol.* 2007;19:432–438.
57. Smith JT, Dungan HM, Stoll EA, et al. Differential regulation of KiSS-1 mRNA expression by sex steroids in the brain of the male mouse. *Endocrinology.* 2005;146:2976–2984.
58. Rochira V, Zirilli L, Genazzani AD, et al. Hypothalamic-pituitary-gonadal axis in two men with aromatase deficiency: evidence that circulating estrogens are required at the hypothalamic level for the integrity of gonadotropin negative feedback. *Eur J Endocrinol.* 2006;155:513–522.
59. Raven G, de Jong FH, Kaufman JM, de Ronde W. In men, peripheral estradiol levels directly reflect the action of estrogens at the hypothalamo-pituitary level to inhibit gonadotropin secretion. *J Clin Endocr.* 2006;91:3324–3328.
60. Goodman RL, Coolen LM, Anderson GM, et al. Evidence that dynorphin plays a major role in mediating progesterone negative feedback on gonadotropin-releasing hormone neurons in sheep. *Endocrinology.* 2004;145:2959–2967.
61. Boutari C, Pappas PD, Mintziori G, et al. The effect of underweight on female and male reproduction. *Metabolism.* 2020;107:154229.
62. Mintziori G, Nigdelis MP, Mathew H, Mousiolis A, Goulis DG, Mantzoros CS. The effect of excess body fat on female and male reproduction. *Metabolism.* 2020;107:154193.
63. Jahan S, Bibi R, Ahmed S, Kafeel S. Leptin levels in infertile males. *J Coll Physicians Surg Pak.* 2014;21:393–397.
64. Quennell JH, Mulligan AC, Tups A, et al. Leptin indirectly regulates gonadotropin-releasing hormone neuronal function. *Endocrinology.* 2009;150:2805–2812.
65. Smith JT, Acohido BV, Clifton DK, Steiner RA. KiSS-1 neurones are direct targets for leptin in the ob/ob mouse. *J Neuroendocrinol.* 2006;4:298–303.
66. Yeo SH, Colledge WH. The role of Kiss1 neurons as integrators of endocrine, metabolic, and environmental factors in the hypothalamic-pituitary-gonadal axis. *Front Endocrinol (Lausanne).* 2018;9:188.
67. Farooqi IS, O'Rahilly S. Leptin: a pivotal regulator of human energy homeostasis. *Am J Clin Nutr.* 2009;89:980S–984S.
68. DiVall SA, Radovick S, Wolfe A. Egr-1 binds the GnRH promoter to mediate the increase in gene expression by insulin. *Mol Cell Endocrinol.* 2007;270:64–72.
69. Zhen S, Zakaria M, Wolfe A, Radovick S. Regulation of gonadotropin-releasing hormone (GnRH) gene expression by insulin-like growth factor I in a cultured GnRHexpressing neuronal cell line. *Mol Endocrinol.* 1997;11:1145–1155.
70. Farkas I, Vastagh C, Sárvári M, Liposits Z. Ghrelin decreases firing activity of gonadotropin-releasing hormone (GnRH) neurons in an estrous cycle and endocannabinoid signaling dependent manner. *PLoS ONE.* 2013;8: e78178.
71. Oakley AE, Breen KM, Clarke IJ, Karsch FJ, Wagenmaker ER, Tilbrook AJ. Cortisol reduces gonadotropin-releasing hormone pulse frequency in follicular phase ewes: influence of ovarian steroids. *Endocrinology.* 2009;150:341–349.
72. Kinsey-Jones JS, Li XF, Knox AM, et al. Down-regulation of hypothalamic kisspeptin and its receptor, Kiss1r, mRNA expression is associated with stress-induced suppression of luteinising hormone secretion in the female rat. *J Neuroendocrinol.* 2009;21:20–29.
73. Ducret E, Anderson GM, Herbison AE. RFamide-related peptide-3, a mammalian gonadotropin-inhibitory hormone ortholog, regulates gonadotropin-releasing hormone neuron firing in the mouse. *Endocrinology.* 2009;150:2799–2804.
74. Liu X, Herbison AE. Kisspeptin regulation of neuronal activity throughout the central nervous system. *Endocrinol Metabol.* 2016;31:193–205.
75. Cheng CK, Leung PC. Molecular biology of gonadotropin releasing hormone (GnRH)-I, GnRH-II, and their receptors in humans. *Endocr Rev.* 2005;26:283–306.
76. Kakar SS. Molecular structure of the human gonadotropin releasing hormone receptor gene. *Eur J Endocrinol.* 1997;137:183–192.
77. Grosse R, Schmid A, Schoneberg T, et al. Gonadotropin-releasing hormone receptor initiates multiple signaling pathways by exclusively coupling to Gq/11 proteins. *J Biol Chem.* 2000;275:9193–9200.
78. Stojilkovic SS, Reinhart J, Catt KJ. Gonadotropin-releasing hormone receptors: structure and signal transduction pathways. *Endocr Rev.* 1994;15:462–499.
79. Perrett RM, McArdle CA. Molecular mechanisms of gonadotropin-releasing hormone signaling: integrating cyclic nucleotides into the network. *Front Endocrinol (Lausanne).* 2013;4:180.
80. Padmanabhan V, McFadden K, Mauger DT, Karsch FJ, Midgley AR Jr. Neuroendocrine control of follicle-stimulating hormone (FSH) secretion. I. Direct evidence for separate episodic and basal components of FSH secretion. *Endocrinology.* 1997;138:424–432.
81. Kaiser UB, Jakubowiak A, Steinberger A, Chin WW. Differential effects of gonadotropin-releasing hormone (GnRH) pulse frequency on gonadotropin subunit and GnRH receptor messenger ribonucleic acid levels in vitro. *Endocrinology.* 1997;138:1224–1231.
82. Tsutsumi M, Laws SC, Rodic V, Sealfon SC. Translational regulation of the gonadotropin-releasing hormone receptor in T3-1 cells. *Endocrinology.* 1995;136:1128–1136.
83. McArdle CA, Franklin J, Green L, Hislop JN. Signaling, cycling and desensitization of gonadotropin-releasing hormone receptors. *J Endocrinol.* 2002;173:1–11.
84. Harris D, Chuderland D, Bonfil D, Kraus S, Seger R, Naor Z. Extracellular signal-regulated kinase and c-Src, but not Jun N-terminal kinase, are involved in basal and gonadotropin releasing hormone-stimulated activity of the glycoprotein hormone-subunit promoter. *Endocrinology.* 2003;144:612–622.
85. Lanciotti L, Cofini M, Leonardi A, Penta L, Esposito S. Up-to-date review about minipuberty and overview on hypothalamic-pituitary-gonadal axis activation in fetal and neonatal life. *Front Endocrinol.* 2018;9:410.
86. O'Donnell L, Stanton P, de Kretser DM. Endocrinology of the male reproductive system and spermatogenesis. [Updated 2017 Jan 11]. In: Feingold KR, Anawalt B, Boyce A, et al., eds. *Endotext*

87. Pitteloud N, Dwyer AA, DeCruz S, et al. Inhibition of luteinizing hormone secretion by testosterone in men requires aromatization for its pituitary but not its hypothalamic effects: evidence from the tandem study of normal and gonadotropin-releasing hormone-deficient men. *J Clin Endocrinol Metab*. 2008;93:784–791.

88. Sheckter CB, Matsumoto AM, Bremner WJ. Testosterone administration inhibits gonadotropin secretion by an effect directly on the human pituitary. *J Clin Endocrinol Metab*. 1989;68:397–401.

89. Hayes FJ, DeCruz S, Seminara SB, Boepple PA, Crowley WF Jr. Differential regulation of gonadotropin secretion by testosterone in the human male: absence of a negative feedback effect of testosterone on follicle-stimulating hormone secretion. *J Clin Endocrinol Metab*. 2001;86:53–58.

90. Rochira V, Madeo B, Diazzi C, Zirilli L, Daniele S, Carani C. Estrogens and male reproduction. [Updated 2016 Nov 24]. In: Feingold KR et al., eds. *Endotext [Internet]*. MDText.com, Inc.; 2000–. Available from www.ncbi.nlm.nih.gov/books/NBK278933/.

91. de Kretser DM, Robertson DM. The isolation and physiology of inhibin and related proteins. *Biol Reprod*. 1989;40:33–47.

92. Iliadou PK, Tsametis C, Kaprara A, Papadimas I, Goulis DG. The Sertoli cell: novel clinical potentiality. *Hormones (Athens)*. 2015;14:504–514.

93. Namwanje M, Brown CW. Activins and inhibins: roles in development, physiology, and disease. *Cold Spring Harb Perspect Biol*. 2016;8:a021881.

94. Burger LL, Dalkin AC, Aylor KW, Haisenleder DJ, Marshall JC. GnRH pulse frequency modulation of gonadotropin subunit gene transcription in normal gonadotropes-assessment by primary transcript assay provides evidence for roles of GnRH and follistatin. *Endocrinology*. 2002;143:3243–3249.

95. Kaiser UB, Lee BL, Carroll RS, Unabia G, Chin WW, Childs GV. Follistatin gene expression in the pituitary: localization in gonadotropes and folliculostellate cells in diestrous rats. *Endocrinology*. 1992;130:3048–3056.

96. Tsutsui K, Saigoh E, Ukena K, et al. A novel avian hypothalamic peptide inhibiting gonadotropin release. *Biochem Biophys Res Commun*. 2000;275:661–667.

97. Tsutsui K, Ukena K. Hypothalamic LPXRF-amide peptides in vertebrates: identification, localization and hypophysiotropic activity. *Peptides*. 2006;27:1121–1129.

98. Ubuka T, Morgan K, Pawson AJ, et al. Identification of human GnIH homologs, RFRP-1 and RFRP-3, and the cognate receptor, GPR147 in the human hypothalamic pituitary axis. *PLoS ONE*. 2009;4:e8400.

99. Hu KL, Chang HM, Li R, Yu Y, Qiao J. Regulation of LH secretion by RFRP-3: from the hypothalamus to the pituitary. *Front Neuroendocrinol*. 2019;52:12–21.

100. Hinuma S, Shintani Y, Fukusumi S, et al. New neuropeptides containing carboxy-terminal RFamide and their receptor in mammals. *Nat Cell Biol*. 2000;2:703–708.

101. Tsutsui K, Ubuka T, Son YL, Bentley GE, Kriegsfeld LJ. Contribution of GnIH research to the progress of reproductive neuroendocrinology. *Front Endocrinol (Lausanne)*. 2015;6:179.

102. George JT, Hendrikse M, Veldhuis JD, Clarke IJ, Anderson RA, Millar RP. Effect of gonadotropin-inhibitory hormone on luteinizing hormone secretion in humans. *Clin. Endocrinol*. 2017;86:731–738.

103. Anderson RC, Newton CL, Anderson RA, Millar RP. Gonadotropins and their analogs: current and potential clinical applications. *Endocr Rev*. 2018;39:911–937.

104. Jiang X, Liu H, Chen X, et al. Structure of follicle-stimulating hormone in complex with the entire ectodomain of its receptor. *Proc Natl Acad Sci USA*. 2012;109:12491–12496.

105. Hsueh AJ, He J. Gonadotropins and their receptors: coevolution, genetic variants, receptor imaging, and functional antagonists. *Biol Reprod*. 2018;99:3–12.

106. Teerds KJ, Huhtaniemi IT. Morphological and functional maturation of Leydig cells: from rodent models to primates. *Hum Reprod Update*. 2015;21:310–328.

107. Zirkin BR, Papadopoulos V. Leydig cells: formation, function, and regulation. *Biol Reprod*. 2018;99:101–111.

108. Wang Y, Chen F, Ye L, Zirkin B, Chen H. Steroidogenesis in Leydig cells: effects of aging and environmental factors. *Reproduction*. 2017;154:R111–R122.

109. Casarini L, Santi D, Brigante G, Simoni M. Two hormones for one receptor: evolution, biochemistry, actions, and pathophysiology of LH and hCG. *Endocr Rev*. 2018;39:549–592.

110. Santi D, Crépieux P, Reiter E, et al. Follicle-stimulating hormone (FSH) action on spermatogenesis: a focus on physiological and therapeutic roles. *J Clin Med*. 2020;9:1014.

111. Ruwanpura SM, McLachlan RI, Meachem SJ. Hormonal regulation of male germ cell development. *J Endocrinol*. 2010;205:117–131.

112. Xu HY, Zhang HX, Xiao Z, Qiao J, Li R. Regulation of anti-Müllerian hormone (AMH) in males and the associations of serum AMH with the disorders of male fertility. *Asian J Androl*. 2019;21:109–114.

113. Meachem SJ, Nieschlag E, Simoni M. Inhibin B in male reproduction: pathophysiology and clinical relevance. *Eur J Endocrinol*. 2001;145:561–571.

114. Huhtaniemi I. A short evolutionary history of FSH-stimulated spermatogenesis. *Hormones (Athens)*. 2015;14:468–478.

115. Griffin J, Wilson JD, Snyder PJ, Matsumoto AM, Martin KA. Male reproductive physiology. In: Post TW, ed. *UpToDate*. UpToDate; 2013.

116. Nieschlag E, Behre HM, Nieschlag S. *Andrology: Male Reproductive Health and Dysfunction*. 3rd ed. Springer-Verlag; 2010.

117. Matsumoto A, Bremner W. Male hypogonadism. In: Melmed S, Polonsky K, Larsen P, Kroneneberg H, eds. *Williams Textbook of Endocrinology*. 12th ed. Saunders; 2011:709–755.

118. Kanakis GA, Goulis DG. Classification and epidemiology of hypogonadism. In: Simoni M, Huhtaniemi I, eds. *Endocrinology of the Testis and Male Reproduction*. Springer; 2017:1–23.

119. Miller WL, Auchus RJ. The molecular biology, biochemistry, and physiology of human steroidogenesis and its disorders. *Endocr Rev*. 2011;32:81–151.
120. Miller WL. StAR search: what we know about how the steroidogenic acute regulatory protein mediates mitochondrial cholesterol import. *Mol Endocrinol*. 2007;21:589–601.
121. Tuckey RC, Cameron KJ. Catalytic properties of cytochrome P-450scc purified from the human placenta: comparison to bovine cytochrome P-450scc. *Biochim Biophys Acta*. 1993;1163:185–194.
122. Kim CJ, Lin L, Huang N, et al. Severe combined adrenal and gonadal deficiency caused by novel mutations in the cholesterol side chain cleavage enzyme, P450scc. *J Clin Endocrinol Metabol*. 2008;93:696–702.
123. Chung BC, Picado-Leonard J, Haniu M, et al. Cytochrome P450c17 (steroid 17 alpha-hydroxylase/17,20 lyase): cloning of human adrenal and testis cDNAs indicates the same gene is expressed in both tissues. *Proc Nat Acad Sci USA*. 1987;84:407–411.
124. Lachance Y, Luu-The V, Labrie C, et al. Characterization of human 3 beta-hydroxysteroid dehydrogenase/delta 5-delta 4-isomerase gene and its expression in mammalian cells. *J Biol Chem*. 1990;265:20469–20475.
125. Flück CE, Miller, WL, Auchus RJ. The 17, 20-lyase activity of cytochrome p450c17 from human fetal testis favors the delta5 steroidogenic pathway. *J Clin Endocrinol Metabol*. 2003;88:3762–3766.
126. Labrie F, Luu-The V, Lin SX, et al. The key role of 17 beta-hydroxysteroid dehydrogenases in sex steroid biology. *Steroids*. 1997;62:148–158.
127. Manna PR, Stetson CL, Slominski AT, Pruitt K. Role of the steroidogenic acute regulatory protein in health and disease. *Endocrine*. 2016;51:7–21.
128. Winters SJ, Troen P. Testosterone and estradiol are co-secreted episodically by the human testis. *J Clin Inv*. 1986;78:870–873.
129. Plymate SR, Tenover JS, Bremner WJ. Circadian variation in testosterone, sex hormone-binding globulin, and calculated non-sex hormone-binding globulin bound testosterone in healthy young and elderly men. *J Androl*. 1989;10:366–371.
130. Sheckter CB, Matsumoto AM, Bremner WJ. Testosterone administration inhibits gonadotropin secretion by an effect directly on the human pituitary. *J Clin Endocrinol Metabol*. 1989;68:397–401.
131. Morishima A, Grumbach MM, Simpson ER, Fisher C, Qin K. Aromatase deficiency in male and female siblings caused by a novel mutation and the physiological role of estrogens. *J Clin Endocrinol Metabol*. 1995;80:3689–3698.
132. Sansone A, Kliesch S, Isidori AM, Schlatt S. AMH and INSL3 in testicular and extragonadal pathophysiology: what do we know? *Andrology*. 2019;7:131–138.
133. Bay K, Hartung S, Ivell R, et al. Insulin-like factor 3 serum levels in 135 normal men and 85 men with testicular disorders: relationship to the luteinizing hormone-testosterone axis. *J Clin Endocrinol Metabol*. 2005;90:3410–3438.
134. Ferlin A, Garolla A, Rigon F, Rasi Caldogno, L, Lenzi A, Foresta C. Changes in serum insulin-like factor 3 during normal male puberty. *J Clin Endocrinol Metabol*. 2006;91:3426–3431.
135. de Kretser DM, Buzzard JJ, Okuma Y, et al. The role of activin, follistatin and inhibin in testicular physiology. *Mol Cell Endocrinol*. 2004;225:57–64.
136. Boepple PA, Hayes FJ, Dwyer AA, et al. Relative roles of inhibin B and sex steroids in the negative feedback regulation of follicle-stimulating hormone in men across the full spectrum of seminiferous epithelium function. *J Clin Endocrinol Metabol*. 2008;93:1809–1814.
137. Anawalt BD, Bebb RA, Matsumoto AM, et al. Serum inhibin B levels reflect Sertoli cell function in normal men and men with testicular dysfunction. *J Clin Endocrinol Metabol*. 1996;81:3341–3335.
138. Jamin SP, Arango NA, Mishina Y, Hanks MC, Behringer RR. Genetic studies of the AMH/MIS signaling pathway for Müllerian duct regression. *Mol Cell Endocrinol*. 2003;211:15–19.
139. Sofikitis N, Giotitsas N, Tsounapi P, Baltogiannis D, Giannakis D, Pardalidis N. Hormonal regulation of spermatogenesis and spermiogenesis. *J Steroid Biochem Mol Biol*. 2008;109:323–330.
140. Hammond GL. Diverse roles for sex hormone-binding globulin in reproduction. *Biol Reprod*. 2011:85:431–441.
141. Manni A, Pardridge WM, Cefalu W, et al. Bioavailability of albumin-bound testosterone. *J Clin Endocrinol Metabol*. 1985;61:705–710.
142. Giton F, Fiet J, Guéchot J, et al. Serum bioavailable testosterone: assayed or calculated? *Clin Chem*. 2006;52:474–481.
143. Goldman, AL, Bhasin S, Wu FCW, Krishna, M, Matsumoto, AM, Jasuja R. A reappraisal of testosterone's binding in circulation: physiological and clinical implications. *Endocr Rev*. 2017;38:302–324.
144. Joseph DR. Structure, function, and regulation of androgen-binding protein/sex hormone-binding globulin. *Vitamins Hormones*. 1994;49:197–280.
145. Stone J, Folkerd E, Doody D, et al. Familial correlations in postmenopausal serum concentrations of sex steroid hormones and other mitogens: a twins and sisters study. *J Clin Endocrinol Metabol*. 2009:94:4793–4800.
146. Bhasin S, Cunningham GR, Hayes FJ, et al. Testosterone therapy in men with androgen deficiency syndromes: an Endocrine Society clinical practice guideline. *J Clin Endocrinol Metabol*. 2018;103:1–30.
147. de Ronde W, van der Schouw YT, Pols HAP, et al. Calculation of bioavailable and free testosterone in men: a comparison of 5 published algorithms. *Clin Chem*. 2006;52:1777–1784.
148. Schiffer L, Arlt W, Storbeck K-H. Intracrine androgen biosynthesis, metabolism and action revisited. *Mol Cell Endocrinol*. 2018:465:4–26.
149. Imperato-McGinley J, Zhu Y-S. Androgens and male physiology the syndrome of 5alpha-reductase-2 deficiency. *Mol Cell Endocrinol*. 2002;198:51–59.
150. Bertelloni S, Baldinotti F, Russo G, et al. 5α-reductase-2 deficiency: clinical findings, endocrine pitfalls, and genetic features in a large Italian cohort. *Sex Develop*. 2016;10:28–36.
151. Swerdloff RS, Dudley RE, Page ST, Wang C, Salameh WA.

Dihydrotestosterone: biochemistry, physiology, and clinical implications of elevated blood levels. *Endocr Rev.* 2017;38:220–254.

152. Wilson EM, French FS. Binding properties of androgen receptors. Evidence for identical receptors in rat testis, epididymis, and prostate. *J Biol Chem.* 1976;251:5620–5629.

153. Lombardi G, Zarrilli S, Colao A, et al. Estrogens and health in males. *Mol Cell Endocrinol.* 2001;178:51–55.

154. Bélanger A, Pelletier G, Labrie F, Barbier O, Chouinard S. Inactivation of androgens by UDP-glucuronosyltransferase enzymes in humans. *Trends Endocrinol Metab.* 2003;14:473–479.

155. Rey RA, Grinspon RP, Gottlieb S, et al. Male hypogonadism: an extended classification based on a developmental, endocrine physiology-based approach. *Andrology.* 2013;1:3–16.

156. Shukla GC, Plaga AR, Shankar E, Gupta S. Androgen receptor-related diseases: what do we know? *Andrology.* 2016;4:366–381.

157. Lee DK, Chang C. Molecular communication between androgen receptor and general transcription machinery. *J Steroid Biochem Mol Biol.* 2003;84:41–49.

158. Brinkmann AO, Faber PW, van Rooij HC, et al. The human androgen receptor: domain structure, genomic organization and regulation of expression. *J Steroid Biochem.* 1989;34:307–310.

159. Zitzmann M. Pharmacogenetics of testosterone replacement therapy. *Pharmacogenomics.* 2009;10:1341–1349.

160. Foradori CD, Weiser MJ, Handa RJ. Non-genomic actions of androgens. *Front Neuroendocrinol.* 2008;29:169–181.

161. Gorczynska E, Handelsman DJ. Androgens rapidly increase the cytosolic calcium concentration in Sertoli cells. *Endocrinology.* 1995;136:2052–2059.

162. Cheng J, Watkins SC, Walker WH. Testosterone activates mitogen-activated protein kinase via Src kinase and the epidermal growth factor receptor in Sertoli cells. *Endocrinology.* 2007;148:2066–2074.

163. Hammes A, Andreassen TK, Spoelgen R, et al. Role of endocytosis in cellular uptake of sex steroids. *Cell.* 2005;122:751–762.

164. Tapanainen J, Kellokumpu-Lehtinen P, Pelliniemi L, Huhtaniemi I. Age-related changes in endogenous steroids of human fetal testis during early and midpregnancy. *J Clin Endocrinol Metabol.* 1981;52:98–102.

165. Grumbach MM. A window of opportunity: the diagnosis of gonadotropin deficiency in the male infant. *J Clin Endocrinol Metabol.* 2005;90:3122–3127.

166. Patton GC, Viner R. Pubertal transitions in health. *Lancet.* 2007;369:1130–1139.

167. Gray A, Feldman HA, McKinlay JB, Longcope C. Age, disease, and changing sex hormone levels in middle-aged men: results of the Massachusetts Male Aging Study. *J Clin Endocrinol Metab.* 1991;73:1016–1025.

168. Andersson AM, Toppari J, Haavisto AM, et al. Longitudinal reproductive hormone profiles in infants: peak of inhibin B levels in infant boys exceeds levels in adult men. *J Clin Endocrinol Metabol.* 1998;83:675–681.

169. Grinspon RP, Rey RA. New perspectives in the diagnosis of pediatric male hypogonadism: the importance of AMH as a Sertoli cell marker. *Arq Brasil Endocrinol Metabol.* 2011;55:512–519.

Section 2 The Biology of Male Reproduction and Infertility

Chapter 6

Sperm Chromatin Packaging and the Toroid Linker Model

Hubert Szczygieł, Anna Ung, Hieu Nguyen, and W. Steven Ward

6.1 Introduction: Revised Toroid Loop Model for Sperm Chromatin Structure

Mammalian sperm chromatin is the most highly condensed DNA known. It is packaged by protamines, which are essentially poly-arginine polypeptides whose positive charges neutralize the negative charge of the DNA phosphodiester backbone [1]. This neutralization of the DNA's negative charges allows the DNA to condense into large toroids with up to 50 kb of DNA [2,3], a primary chromatin structure that is vastly different from the nucleosomes into which histones fold most eukaryotic DNA [4]. The folding of DNA into toroids by protamines is similar to an interaction between DNA and multivalent cations such as cobalt [5,6].

We have shown that sperm chromatin is also organized into loops of 25–50 kb in size that are attached at their bases to a proteinaceous nuclear matrix [7,8]. This loop domain organization was first seen in somatic cells [9,10] and somatic mitotic chromosomes [11]. Later publications demonstrated that topoisomerase II was located at the bases of these loops as part of the nuclear matrix [12,13], and subsequent work showed that the topoisomerase II enzymes cleaved the DNA during apoptosis in somatic cells [14]. We proposed a model for sperm DNA packaging in which each protamine toroid represented one loop of DNA [15–17]. We found evidence of a luminal nuclease that is present in sperm epididymal and vas deferens fluid that digests sperm DNA when activated with Mn2+ [18–20].

One aspect of this model that we have described is the possibility that topoisomerase II was located at the bases of the sperm DNA loop domains, just as they are in somatic cells, and that they could be activated to cleave sperm DNA [21]. We based this evidence on experiments in which the luminal nuclease digestion of sperm chromatin appeared to be reversed by treatment with ethylenediaminetetraacetic acid (EDTA), a hallmark of the reversible cleavage of topoisomerase II [14,22]. However, as we report here, we have obtained recent evidence to suggest that what we had previously interpreted as reversal of topoisomerase cleavage was, in fact, inhibition of the luminal nuclease digestion. Our confusion resulted from the fact that the sperm luminal nuclease remains active in sodium dodecyl sulfate (SDS) long enough to digest DNA. This unexpected result – that the luminal fluid of the epididymis and the vas deferens has a nuclease that is active in SDS for a short time – has important implications for sperm chromatin structure and for the prevention of sperm chromatin degradation by endogenous nucleases when analyzing sperm DNA damage.

6.2 Methods

Mature C57BL/6J male, 7–10 weeks old, were used to collect epididymis and vas deferens spermatozoa in 25 mM Tris, pH 7.4 and 0.25% Triton X-100 on ice. Six mice were used per experiment. The luminal fluid was diluted to obtain a final concentration of 1 to 2 × 108 sperm per mL. The suspensions were either treated with $MnCl_2$, SDS, or EDTA, at 37°C as described in figure legends and then plugged in agarose or plugged in agarose without treatment. To plug the sperm suspensions, 50 μL of the sperm suspension was mixed with 50 μL of low melting agarose at 54°C and cooled in plugging wells. The sperm plugs were then incubated in digestion buffer (10 mM Tris, 100 mM NaCl, 0.5% SDS, 50 mM dithiothreitol (DTT), and 50 μg/mL proteinase K) for one hour at 54°C. The agarose plugs were then loaded into a 1% pulsed-field gel electrophoresis (PFGE) gel and run with 0.5 × TBE buffer using a BIO-RAD CHEF Mapper XA System run at 14°C for 16 hours using the auto-alignment algorithm with a molecular weight range of 5–200K, included angle of 120°, initial switch time of 1 second, and a final switch time of 25 seconds. Finally, the gel was analyzed with LAS-3000.

6.3 Sperm Luminal Nuclease Is Active in SDS for a Short Time

We became suspicious that the luminal nuclease in the epididymal and vas deferens luminal fluid might be active in SDS while conducting further experiments on the luminal nuclease. To clearly test this, we isolated mouse luminal fluids from the cauda epididymis or from the vas deferens, and put them into low melting agar to form plugs for PFGE, using methods described previously [16]. These plugs contained both the sperm and the luminal fluid in which they were suspended. The plugs were then incubated in digestion buffer (D) that includes 0.5% SDS and 1 mM DTT. In these plugs, the DNA in both sperm from the epididymis and from the vas deferens remained intact so that it did not even enter the gel (Figure 6.1, lanes 1 and 6). However, when the plug was incubated in digestion buffer that had 10 mM MnCl$_2$, the DNA was degraded to less than 50 kb fragments in epi-sperm (Figure 6.1, lane 2) and the vas-sperm DNA was degraded even further (Figure 6.1, lane 7. In this case, most of the DNA was digested to such small fragments that it exited the gel). Under these conditions, the Mn2+ and the SDS both diffused into the plug at the same time. The luminal nuclease had to be active, at least partially, during this incubation. A similar result was obtained when Mn2+ was incubated with the plug before SDS (Figure 6.1, lanes 3 and 8), but in this case, we could not discern whether the luminal nuclease activity occurred before or after SDS digestion. Also, the digestion appeared to be less most likely because the Mn2+ started diffusing out of the gel as the SDS was diffusing in, reducing the luminal nuclease's activity. We next tested whether the sperm luminal nuclease could be inhibited by incubation in SDS for 30 minutes before the addition of Mn2+, and found that it could (Figure 6.1, lanes 4 and 9). These data suggested that the sperm luminal nuclease, that we have reported before [19,20], is inhibited by prolonged incubation in SDS, as are most nucleases, but that the luminal nuclease can remain active in SDS for a time. We tested the length of time the luminal nuclease could remain active in SDS by incubating the sperm plugs in SDS for 0.5–30 minutes in SDS before adding manganese. We found that the luminal nuclease remained very active for 2 minutes in SDS, but that 30 minutes incubation in SDS was sufficient to inhibit all the luminal nuclease digestion (Figure 6.2).

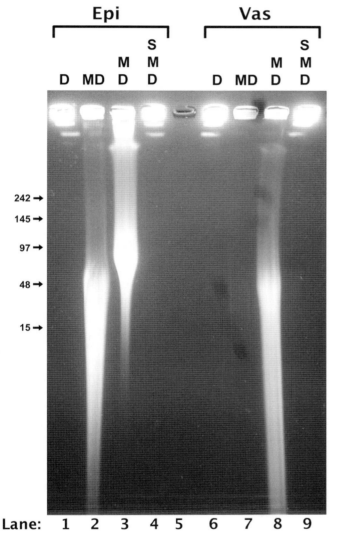

Figure 6.1 Epididymal and vas deferens luminal nuclease is active in SDS, but is inhibited by prolonged exposure to SDS. Epididymal (lanes 1–4) or vas deferens (lanes 6–9) luminal fluid suspensions containing sperm were treated in various ways and plugged in agarose for PFGE analysis. (Lanes 1 and 6) Control: sperm plugs were incubated immediately in digestion buffer (D, 0.5% SDS, 1 mM DTT, 10 mM, 1 mM EDTA Tris, pH 7.4). (Lanes 2 and 7) Evidence that the luminal nuclease is active in SDS: sperm plugs were incubated in digestion buffer containing 10 mM MnCl$_2$ (M). (Lanes 3 and 8) Sperm suspensions were incubated in MnCl$_2$ before being plugged and incubated in digestion buffer. The luminal nuclease activity is slightly decreased because the Mn2+ diffuses out of the plug when put into a tube containing the digestion buffer. (Lanes 4 and 9) Sperm suspensions were incubated in 0.5% SDS for 30 minutes before treatment with Mn2+, then plugged. Incubation of the luminal fluid in SDS effectively inhibits luminal nuclease activity.

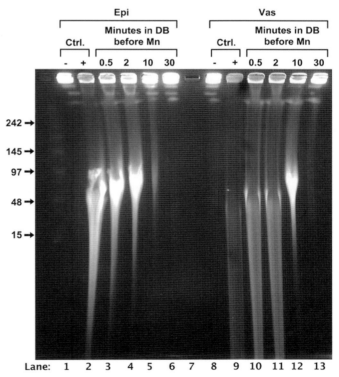

Figure 6.2 Time course of SDS in activation of luminal nuclease. Epididymal (lanes 1–6) or vas deferens (lanes 8–13) luminal fluid suspensions containing sperm were plugged in agarose. The plugs were then incubated in digestion buffer (0.5% SDS, 10 mM DTT) with 0.5% SDS for 0–30 minutes (lanes 3–6 and 10–13) and then 10 mM MnCl$_2$ was added for an additional 30 minutes at 37°C before being digested fully by incubation at 54°C for 1 hour. Lanes 1 and 8 were negative controls with no Mn2+, and lanes 2 and 9 were positive controls with no preincubation in SDS. The luminal nuclease was completely inhibited when incubated in SDS for 30 minutes.

6.4 Protection of DNA from Nucleases by Protamines

In previous publications, we interpreted the extensive DNA degradation of sperm chromatin in the vas deferens as an ability of the luminal nuclease to digest sperm chromatin in situ, with the protamines still attached. However, our new understanding of the action of the luminal nuclease suggested a different sequence of events. It was now clear that some DNA degradation was not only possible in the SDS digestion buffer, but that the SDS seemed to enhance the degradation of the DNA, perhaps by removing protamines to expose more DNA. We previously reported that the vas deferens luminal fluid contained a higher concentration of luminal nuclease activity than epididymal luminal fluid [20]. This is likely the reason that vas-sperm DNA is always more extensively degraded than epi-sperm DNA (compare lanes 2 and 3 to 9 and 10 in Figure 6.2). However, this more extensive degradation seemed contradictory to other data that showed that protamines protected sperm DNA from even high concentrations of DNase I [16,23]. The data presented above offer a new explanation that reconciles both sets of data: The more extensive degradation that occurred in vas deferens sperm was due to the higher concentration of luminal nuclease in the vas deferens luminal fluid and the fact that this luminal nuclease activity is active in SDS for up to 10 minutes. Thus, the SDS and DTT in the digestion buffer may have extracted some protamines, allowing the luminal nuclease that was still active to digest the vas-sperm DNA longer.

One aspect of the toroid-loop model for sperm chromatin structure is that the toroid linkers – the DNA between protamine toroids that is not predicted to be protamine-bound – is sensitive to nuclease digestion. Thus, the DNA in the toroid linkers that separates the protamine toroids can be biochemically isolated from the protamine-bound DNA by nuclease digestion. Our new experiments offered us a way to design nuclease digestion that is controlled and clearly inhibited before SDS and DTT completely disrupted the protective coating of DNA by the protamines. In our previous studies, we hypothesized that topoisomerase II reversibly cleaved the DNA and that EDTA would reverse this cleavage [14,22]. Thus, we did not add EDTA to stop the reaction, but rather assumed SDS would digest the luminal nuclease and topoisomerase that was causing the digestion. In our older model, we hypothesized that topoisomerase II works in concert with luminal nucleases to digest sperm chromatin in a manner similar to somatic cells during apoptosis [14,24–26].

However, our new data, described above, suggested a much simpler model. The new model does not require the action of topoisomerase II to interpret the data. We now propose that the luminal nuclease that is present in the luminal fluid of both epididymal and vas deferens fluid can only digest the DNA that is not bound to protamine in in situ sperm chromatin. The protamines protect the DNA from degradation even in the higher concentrations of luminal nuclease in the vas deferens.

We tested this model by altering our procedure for the experiment. We made agarose plugs that contained the sperm, then incubated these plugs in Mn2+ for 30 minutes, then in 50 mM EDTA for 30 minutes before incubating them in digestion buffer. In this experiment, the luminal nuclease digestion of both epididymal and vas deferens sperm DNA was limited to loop-sized fragments that we hypothesize correspond to protamine toroids (Figure 6.3, lanes 4 and 10, respectively). As predicted, EDTA did not inhibit the luminal nuclease permanently. When Mn2+ was added after EDTA was taken away, the luminal nuclease digestion could still proceed (Figure 6.3, lanes 3 and 9). When EDTA was *not* removed, it protected the DNA from luminal nuclease digestion in the presence of Mn2+ (Figure 6.3, lanes 5 and 11). Note that when the digestion of vas deferens sperm DNA is allowed to continue in the presence of SDS (Figure 6.3, lane 9) the DNA is digested to much smaller fragments than when the luminal nuclease digestion is halted by EDTA before SDS extraction (compare lanes 3 to 4 and 9 to 10 in Figure 6.3). We interpret these data to indicate that when the protamines have not been extracted, they confer luminal nuclease protection, and only the protamine linker regions – the DNA that connects two protamine toroids – are susceptible to nuclease attack.

6.5 Two Steps in Luminal Nuclease Digestion

Taken together, these experiments revealed two different steps in digestion by the luminal nuclease. First, the luminal nuclease can digest the sperm chromatin when it is fully condensed into loop-sized fragments (Figure 6.3, lanes 4 and 10). This in situ digestion occurs only at the toroid linker regions and histone bound DNA (Figure 6.4B). The protamine-bound DNA is protected from this luminal nuclease digestion. This in situ luminal nuclease digestion is the most important for investigating sperm chromatin structure. The second step in the luminal nuclease digestion, unprotected digestion, is when the luminal nuclease remains active (because of Mn2+) in the presence of the digestion buffer that contains SDS and DTT. The digestion buffer begins to remove the protamines, allowing the luminal nuclease to digest DNA that was previously protected by the protamines as long as the nuclease remains active (Figure 6.1, lanes 2, 3, 7 and 8; Figure 6.4C). We therefore now had a set of conditions that allowed us to separate in situ luminal nuclease digestion (in which the sperm chromatin structure is intact) from unprotected luminal nuclease digestion (in which sperm chromatin structure is being disrupted by protamine extraction). In situ luminal nuclease digestion occurs when sperm are incubated with Mn2+ for 30 minutes, then the luminal nuclease digestion is halted by a high concentration of EDTA, then incubated in SDS and DTT to remove the protamines for DNA analysis. The DNA is digested only to loop-sized fragments (Figure 6.3, lanes 4 and 10).

These data, together with our previously published data documenting that the vas deferens luminal fluid contains

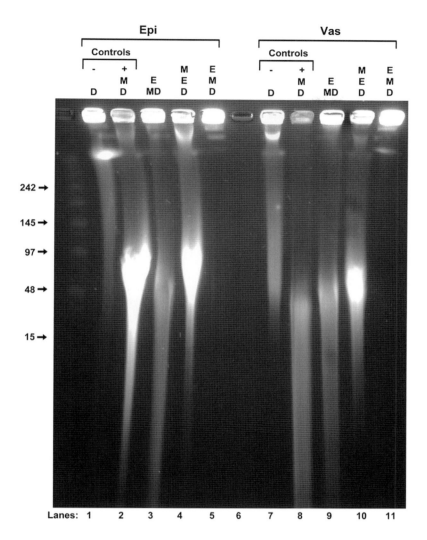

Figure 6.3 EDTA arrests luminal nuclease activity. Epididymal (lanes 1–5) or vas deferens (lanes 7–11) luminal fluid suspensions were treated in various ways as indicated on the top of the lanes, then plugged in agarose and analyzed by PFGE. (D, lanes 1 and 7) Negative controls, no treatment. (M, D, lanes 2 and 8) Positive controls, sperm suspensions were incubated with 10 mM MnCl$_2$ for 30 minutes at 37°C, then plugged in agarose and incubated in digestion buffer. The sperm DNA was maximally digested suggesting the luminal nuclease was still active as the digestion buffer removed the protamines. (E, MD, lanes 3 and 9) Sperm suspensions were incubated with 50 mM EDTA at 37°C before plugging agarose. The plugs were then incubated in digestion buffer with 10 mM MnCl$_2$. The EDTA could not fully prevent digestion because it diffused out of the plug as the SDS and Mn2+ was diffusing in. (M, E, D, lanes 4 and 10) Sperm suspension were incubated in 10 mM MnCl$_2$ for 30 minutes at 37°C, then 50 mM EDTA was added and allowed to incubate for 30 minutes at 37°C, and the suspensions were plugged and incubated in digestion buffer. The luminal nuclease digestion was limited to loop-sized fragments of 25–100 kb, suggesting it was restricted to sperm DNA that was not protected by protamines, and was inhibited before incubation in SDS. (E, M, D, lanes 5 and 11) EDTA inhibits the luminal nuclease. Sperm suspensions were incubated in 50 mM EDTA for 30 minutes at 37°C, then 10 mM MnCl$_2$ was added and incubated for another 30 minutes. EDTA prevented luminal nuclease digestion because it remained in the suspension preventing Mn2+ from activating the luminal nuclease.

much higher amounts of the luminal nuclease than the epididymal luminal fluid [20], also explain why in situ luminal nuclease digestion appears similar in epididymal and vas deferens sperm (Figure 6.3, lanes 4 and 10), but unprotected luminal nuclease digestion is much more extensive in vas deferens sperm (Figure 6.3, lanes 2 and 8, and Figures 6.1 and 6.2).

6.6 Implications for Sperm Chromatin Structure

The major implication for studying sperm chromatin structure conferred by these data is that it is now possible to use the endogenous sperm luminal nuclease activity that degrades only the toroid linker regions to examine protamine packaging (Figure 6.4). A similar question has been addressed by many different laboratories that focused on extracting histones from in situ sperm chromatin to identify the histone-bound DNA [27–29]. The goal in these studies was to determine whether the 1–10% of histones that remained in the sperm nucleus were bound to specific DNA sequences or not, and most studies have concluded that they are. However, all of these studies found large tracts of DNA that were bound to histones, and we have suggested that these large tracts represent entire loops that were not replaced by histones (Figure 6.4A). These previous studies were restricted to nucleases that could only digest linker regions of histone nucleosomes so that the nucleosomal DNA could be analyzed. While we have predicted that the protamine toroid linker DNA is bound to histones, there is no evidence to support this other than its nuclease sensitivity. It is possible that the protamine linker DNA is not associated with either protamines or histones, or that it is so short, compared to the larger tracts of histone-bound DNA, that the smaller, much more diverse toroid linker regions are not prominent in the analyses. If true, endogenous luminal nuclease digestion of all the toroid linkers, as we predict occurs in in situ luminal nuclease digestions, would provide a picture of the specificity matrix attachment regions and protamine toroid placement.

A. Toroid Loop Model for Sperm Chromatin Structure

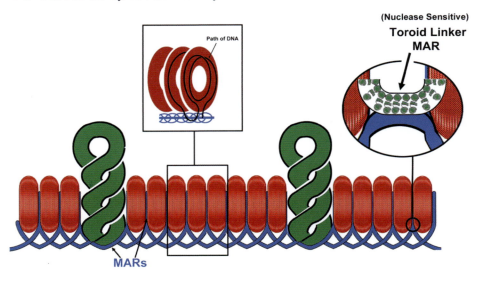

B. In Situ Luminal Nuclease Digestion

Histone bound DNA and Toroid Linkers digested.

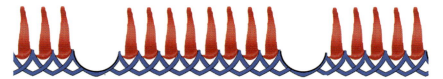

C. Unprotected Luminal Nuclease Digestion

Protamines are partially extracted allowing nuclease to digest more DNA.

Figure 6.4 Protamine loop domain model for sperm chromatin structure and luminal nuclease digestion. (A) Model: This model was first described fully in Ward, 2010, and the figure is based on a figure from that publication [17]. DNA is organized into loop domains, from 25 to 100 kb in size, that are anchored at their bases on the nuclear matrix (blue) at matrix attachment regions (MARs). Each loop domain is condensed by protamines into one toroid (red, left inset). The DNA that links the protamine toroids is called toroid linker DNA and is nuclease sensitive (right inset). Based on data published from other laboratories [27-29] we hypothesized that in some cases, the histones in entire loops are not replaced by protamines and remain in the sperm chromatin (green). (B) In Situ Luminal Nuclease Digestion: The luminal nuclease can only digest DNA that is not bound to protamines, which is the histone-bound DNA and the toroid linkers (which may also be histone-bound). The DNA in the protamine toroids is still protected. (C) Unprotected Luminal Nuclease Digestion: When the luminal nuclease is not inactivated by EDTA before SDS extracts the protamines, the DNA that was protected by the protamines is now exposed to the luminal nuclease action for as long as it remains active.

6.7 Implications for Sperm DNA Damage Assays

The relationship between the endogenous luminal nuclease that is present in the epididymal and vas deferens luminal fluid to human clinical assisted reproductive technology is not easy to assess, but we do believe our studies may issue a warning that should be considered. It is not clear whether semen contains a similar or the same luminal nuclease that is present in vas deferens luminal fluid, but it is possible that the ejaculate would include some of the activity. Most assays for sperm DNA damage that are used in clinical settings include some form of sperm isolation, such as swim-up separation or brief Percoll gradient centrifugation. This should separate the sperm chromatin from most of the luminal nuclease that is present in the extracellular ejaculate. However, it is possible that some would remain. Our data indicate that this luminal nuclease is active in 0.5% SDS for up to 30 minutes, so it is important, especially for COMET assays that use SDS to denature sperm chromatin, to ensure that any luminal nuclease that is retained would be neutralized before the DNA. Our data suggest that high concentrations of EDTA before SDS is introduced are key to clearly identifying DNA lesions that were present in the sperm when it was intact.

6.8 Conclusion

The luminal nuclease that is present in the epididymis and vas deferens remains active in SDS, complicating DNA damage analyses of sperm chromatin. However, high concentrations of EDTA can prevent digestion from occurring during protamine extraction, reducing artefactual DNA damage while analyzing sperm DNA.

References

1. Balhorn R. A model for the structure of chromatin in mammalian sperm. *J Cell Biol*. 1982;93:298–305.
2. Hud NV, Allen MJ, Downing KH, Lee J, Balhorn R. Identification of the elemental packing unit of DNA in mammalian sperm cells by atomic force microscopy. *Biochem Biophys Res Commun*. 1993;193:1347–1354.
3. Hud NV, Downing KH, Balhorn R. A constant radius of curvature model for the organization of DNA in toroidal condensates. *Proc Natl Acad Sci U S A*. 1995;92:3581–3585.
4. Smith MM. Histone structure and function. *Curr Opin Cell Biol*. 1991;3:429–437.
5. Hud NV, Downing KH. Cryoelectron microscopy of lambda phage DNA condensates in vitreous ice: the fine structure of DNA toroids. *Proc Natl Acad Sci U S A*. 2001;98:14925–14930.
6. Conwell CC, Vilfan ID, Hud NV. Controlling the size of nanoscale toroidal DNA condensates with static curvature and ionic strength. *Proc Natl Acad Sci U S A*. 2003;100:9296–9301.
7. Ward WS, Partin AW, Coffey DS. DNA loop domains in mammalian spermatozoa. *Chromosoma*. 1989;98:153–159.
8. Nadel B, de Lara J, Finkernagel SW, Ward WS. Cell-specific organization of the 5S ribosomal RNA gene cluster DNA loop domains in spermatozoa and somatic cells. *Biol Reprod*. 1995;53:1222–1228.
9. Pardoll DM, Vogelstein B, Coffey DS. A fixed site of DNA replication in eucaryotic cells. *Cell*. 1980;19:527–536.
10. Vogelstein B, Pardoll DM, Coffey DS. Supercoiled loops and eucaryotic DNA replication. *Cell*. 1980;22:79–85.
11. Paulson JR, Laemmli UK. The structure of histone-depleted metaphase chromosomes. *Cell*. 1977;12:817–828.
12. Earnshaw WC, Halligan B, Cooke CA, Heck MM, Liu LF. Topoisomerase II is a structural component of mitotic chromosome scaffolds. *J Cell Biol*. 1985;100:1706–1715.
13. Earnshaw WC, Heck MM. Localization of topoisomerase II in mitotic chromosomes. *J Cell Biol*. 1985;100:1716–1725.
14. Li TK, Chen AY, Yu C, Mao Y, Wang H, Liu LF. Activation of topoisomerase II-mediated excision of chromosomal DNA loops during oxidative stress. *Genes Dev*. 1999;13:1553–1560.
15. Ward WS. Chromosome organization in mammalian sperm nuclei. In: Barratt CL, de Jong JH, Mortimer D, Parinaud J, eds. *Genetics of Human Male Fertility*. Editions E.D.K.; 1997:147–163.
16. Sotolongo B, Lino E, Ward WS. Ability of hamster spermatozoa to digest their own DNA. *Biol Reprod*. 2003;69:2029–2035.
17. Ward WS. Function of sperm chromatin structural elements in fertilization and development. *Mol Hum Reprod*. 2010;16:30–36.
18. Shaman JA, Yamauchi Y, Ward WS. Sperm DNA fragmentation: awakening the sleeping genome. *Biochem Soc Trans*. 2007;35:626–628.
19. Boaz SM, Dominguez KM, Shaman JA, Ward WS. Mouse spermatozoa contain a nuclease that is activated by pretreatment with EGTA and subsequent calcium incubation. *J Cell Biochem*. 2008;103:1636–1645.
20. Gawecka JE, Boaz S, Kasperson K, Nguyen H, Evenson DP, Ward WS. Luminal fluid of epididymis and vas deferens contributes to sperm chromatin fragmentation. *Hum Reprod*. 2015;30:2725–2736.
21. Shaman JA, Prisztoka R, Ward WS. Topoisomerase IIB and an extracellular nuclease interact to digest sperm DNA in an apoptotic-like manner. *Biol Reprod*. 2006;75:741–748.
22. Liu LF, Rowe TC, Yang L, Tewey KM, Chen GL. Cleavage of DNA by mammalian DNA topoisomerase II. *J Biol Chem*. 1983;258:15365–15370.
23. Sotolongo B, Huang TF, Isenberger E, Ward WS. An endogenous nuclease in hamster, mouse and human spermatozoa cleaves DNA into loop-sized fragments. *J Androl*. 2005;26:272–280.
24. Lagarkova MA, Iarovaia OV, Razin SV. Large-scale fragmentation of mammalian DNA in the course of apoptosis proceeds via excision of chromosomal DNA loops and their oligomers. *J Biol Chem*. 1995;270:20239–20241.
25. Solovyan VT, Bezvenyuk ZA, Salminen A, Austin CA, Courtney MJ. The role of topoisomerase II in the excision of

DNA loop domains during apoptosis. *J Biol Chem.* 2002;277:21458–21467.

26. Widlak P, Garrard WT. Discovery, regulation, and action of the major apoptotic nucleases DFF40/CAD and endonuclease G. *J Cell Biochem.* 2005;94:1078–1087.

27. Brykczynska U, Hisano M, Erkek S, et al. Repressive and active histone methylation mark distinct promoters in human and mouse spermatozoa. *Nat Struct Mol Biol.* 2010;17:679–687.

28. Hammoud SS, Nix DA, Zhang H, Purwar J, Carrell DT, Cairns BR. Distinctive chromatin in human sperm packages genes for embryo development. *Nature.* 2009;460:473–478.

29. Arpanahi A, Brinkworth M, Iles D, et al. Endonuclease-sensitive regions of human spermatozoal chromatin are highly enriched in promoter and CTCF binding sequences. *Genome Res.* 2009;19:1338–1349.

Section 2 The Biology of Male Reproduction and Infertility

Chapter 7

Ejaculation and Sperm Transport
Physiology and Clinical Concerns

Christopher Koprowski, Garrick Greear, and Tung-Chin Hsieh

7.1 Introduction

Ejaculation was historically an essential step in human reproduction. Advancements in intracytoplasmic sperm injection (ICSI) and surgical sperm retrieval, as well as other assisted reproductive technologies (ART) have resulted in a shift in the focus of research in reproductive medicine. As such, interest has shifted away from ejaculatory disorders in part due to the tremendous success of assisted reproduction [1]. Certainly, an understanding of the physiology and pathophysiology of ejaculation and sperm transportation remains crucial in the practice of urology, recognizing that much remains to be uncovered in this area. Ejaculatory disorders in particular are poorly understood and frequently misdiagnosed [2]. While sperm retrieval procedures are highly effective in achieving the goal of reproduction, there is a key role of accurate diagnosis and management of these disorders to attempt to spare this associated morbidity and minimize complexity of ART required. Additionally, many of these pathophysiologic states induce distress in patients, despite having any concerns involving fertility.

7.1.1 Physiology

Ejaculation represents the climax of the sexual cycle and comprises emission (secretion of semen) and expulsion (propulsion of semen) phases [3]. On the contrary, orgasm refers to the central nervous system phenomenon coinciding with ejaculation. Orgasm is a cerebral and cortical occurrence and should not be confused with ejaculation [1]. The ejaculatory phases of emission and expulsion will be reviewed, along with some comments on neurophysiology.

7.1.2 Emission

Emission refers to the delivery of seminal fluid to the posterior urethra [4]. This is a coordinated process involving the bladder neck, the prostatic urethra, the seminal vesicles, the vas deferens, and the distal epididymis [1]. Sympathetic nervous system innervation first initiates closure of the bladder neck. The prostatic urethra then collects the mixture of secretions arising from the seminal vesicles, the prostate, the vas deferens, and Cowper's glands.

The thoracolumbar spine (levels T10–L2) principally mediates emission. Sympathetic fibers give rise to the lumbar sympathetic trunk ganglia. On the right side, these fibers travel through the interaortocaval space, whereas on the left, they pass lateral to the aorta. These disparate bundles of nerve fibers later coalesce into the superior hypogastric plexus, anterior to the sacrum. From here, they innervate the bladder neck, seminal vesicles, prostate, and vas deferens. Sympathetic innervation is key in emission; parasympathetic innervation is not thought to be contributory [1,5,6].

The composition of seminal fluid has been further characterized. The seminal vesicles contribute the most toward ejaculate volume (65–75%). This mixture is an alkaline solution rich with fructose, citrate, and prostaglandins, which help to facilitate sperm motility. The prostate contributes approximately 30–35% of the ejaculatory volume. Serine proteases, such as prostate-specific antigen (PSA), are abundant in this acidic mixture that helps to liquify coagulated semen. Vasal fluid, or fluid contributed by the vas deferens, represents a minority (5–10%) of total ejaculate volume and is principally composed of spermatozoa. Finally, the bulbourethral glands emit pre-ejaculate, with primary ingredients including galactose and mucous (1–2%) [1,7].

7.1.3 Expulsion

Expulsion is a neurologically mediated pathway via somatic fibers whose result is the propulsion of semen out of the meatus [1]. First, the external urethral sphincter relaxes. Contractions of the prostatic smooth muscle then work in tandem with the bulbocavernosus, ischiocavernosus, levator ani, and transverse perineal muscles in order to advance semen along the length of the urethra until it meets the meatus [8]. In order to effectively achieve this goal, synchronization is key for effective antegrade flow of semen.

Currently, expulsion is best understood as a process mediated by sacral somatic nerve fibers, with contributions from sympathetic and sensory inputs. Primary sensory inputs include the dorsolateral and ventrolateral penile branches of the perineal branch of the pudendal nerve [4]. The synchronization of the muscle contractions of the bulbospongiosus muscle followed by relaxation of the external sphincter and subsequent prostatic and seminal vesicle contractions is mediated through complex reflex arcs [9]. Aforementioned afferent perineal sensory nerve fibers synapse in the nucleus of

Onuf with pudendal motor neurons in addition to spinal interneurons (T10–L2) in order to first achieve emission, which then leads to direct muscle innervation of the bulbospongiosis muscle via the perineal nerve [1,10].

7.1.4 Cerebral Control and Neurotransmission

The neurobiology of ejaculation continues to be an area of active research. Cerebral control of ejaculation is complex. Multiple areas are thought to actively participate and include the posteromedial division of the bed nucleus of the striaterminals, the posterodorsal area of the amygdala, the posterodorsal pre-optic nucleus as well as the parvicellular aspect of the subparafascicular thalamus [11].

Important excitatory neural pathways involve the pre-optic medial area and its projections into the paraventricular hypothalamus, which later gives rise to axons in communication with autonomic fibers in the medullar ejaculation centers. Conversely, major inhibitory pathways involve neurons in the gigantocellular nuclei and ventral raphe in the ventral medulla, with notable activity in the thalamus and cerebral cortex during ejaculation [11,12].

Critical neurotransmitters are best divided into three groups: peripheral, medullar, and central mediators. Peripheral neurotransmitters are by far the more robust group and include norepinephrine (contraction of seminal vesicles via α-1 receptors in smooth muscle), acetylcholine (contraction of seminal vesicles via muscarinic receptors), nitric oxide (contraction of seminal vesicles), oxytocin (contraction of seminal apparatus), purines (contraction of vas deferens via adenosine triphosphate dependent pathways), and serotonin (expulsion reflex with 5HT2 receptors). Medullar control is primarily achieved by GABA (in CNS; GABA antagonists prevent ejaculation), oxytocin (inhibits ejaculation, poorly understood), and substance P (sensory transmission via NK1 receptors). Finally, central neurotransmitters include serotonin (delay ejaculation via 5-HT receptors), dopamine (pro-ejaculatory via D2 receptors), opioids (inhibits ejaculation), and oxytocin (stimulates ejaculation) [11]. The complex neurobiology of ejaculation is only beginning to be understood.

7.2 Pathophysiology

Ejaculatory dysfunction is a heterogenous group of disorders. Accurate diagnosis to better understand the pathophysiology is key to effective management.

7.2.1 Diagnosis of Ejaculatory Dysfunction

A thorough history and physical is crucial in the evaluation of ejaculatory dysfunction. When patients describe issues with ejaculation, one should consider circumstantial factors (sexual arousal) in addition to their medical, surgical, and social history. Congenital ejaculatory dysfunction should be differentiated from acquired. Laboratory workup may include FSH, LH, testosterone, TSH, prolactin, and HBA1c. Post-ejaculate urinalysis can be performed if retrograde ejaculation is suspected [1].

7.2.2 Premature Ejaculation

Multiple definitions exist for premature ejaculation (PE). The *Diagnostic and Statistical Manual of Mental Disorders, Fifth Edition* (DSM-V) defines it as "persistent and recurrent ejaculatory pattern of intravaginal ejaculatory latency time (IELT) of 1 minute or less after vaginal penetration or before the desire of the individual," with a duration of more than six months that causes clinically relevant stress [13]. The International Society for Sexual Medicine defines premature ejaculation as "ejaculation that occurs always or almost always within the first minute after vaginal penetration since the first sexual intercourse or a clinical significative reduction in IELF, usually within 3 minutes of penetration" [14]. The prevalence of PE is difficult to estimate, with 38 papers from 1998 to 2004 estimating from 3% (when defined as IELT <1 minute) to 83.7% (when defined as occasional occurrence of involuntary ejaculation) [15].

Premature ejaculation can be further divided into primary versus secondary PE. Primary PE is present since the first sexual intercourse and continues in at least 80–90% of future encounters without a significant change in IELT with age. More than 85% of men ejaculate within one minute and the remaining men ejaculate between the first and second minute [16]. Secondary PE begins later in life with a superior IELT relative to primary PE, generally up to three minutes [14]. Other authors further distinguish PE with variable (normal variant) and subjective subtypes (cultural or abnormal psychological constructs) [17].

Etiologies for PE differ based on whether it is primary or secondary. In primary PE, some authors have proposed a relationship with low serotonin levels, with no clear inheritance pattern [16]. Others have identified specific genetic polymorphisms such as 5-HTTLPR, where in 89 patients with this polymorphism, 83 ejaculated in less than one minute [18]. Other implicated polymorphisms include the C(1019)G polymorphism of the 5HT1A receptor as well as the Cys23Ser polymorphism of the 5HT1C receptor [19–21]. Risk factors for secondary PE include psychorelational factors, sexual dysfunction, endocrine (low testosterone, low prolactin, hyperthyroidism), and chronic prostatitis [21].

Diagnosis is done through a good patient history. Physical exam will generally be normal, with the exception of certain cases of secondary PE if they are suspected to be secondary to hypogonadism, frenulum breve, phimosis, venereal disease, or prostatitis [21]. The toll of PE on patients can be quite severe, as it has been linked to high levels of personal stress, difficulty maintaining relationships, low self-esteem and self-confidence, and anxiety related to sexual encounters [22].

7.3 Treatment

Multiple treatment strategies have been described. Behavioral techniques are the least invasive way to address PE. Sensory abstraction with thought redirection, precoital masturbation, and use of climax control condoms have all been widely employed techniques. Sexual therapy aimed at achieving better partner communication, reducing anxiety, and improving confidence has been found to be effective, though quantitative data are challenging to find in the literature [21,23]. Squeezing the glans to reduce sensation and using coital or masturbation suspension has also been described with reportedly high success (up to 95%) [24].

If the etiology is thought to be due to an underlying medical condition, it can be specifically targeted. For example, starting a regular exercise program, management of underlying endocrinopathies, achieving excellent glycemic control, abstaining from drug use, and managing suspected contributing bacterial infections (prostatitis) with antibiotics are all appropriate strategies [25]. While not robustly studied, one report did show that managing hyperthyroidism decreased prevalence of PE in a cohort of patients from 50% to 15% [25].

Local anesthesia is another commonly used treatment. Theoretically, by reducing sensation to cutaneous nerve fibers, IELT may be prolonged. One of the more recent formulations introduced on the market is a mixture of lidocaine (150 mg/mL) and prilocaine (50 mg/mL). This solution is sprayed onto the glans and is rapidly absorbed, within five minutes of initial application. Consistent efficacy was demonstrated in 88% of patients with a median increase in basal IELT of six times [26]. Topical anesthetics are well-tolerated, and rarely noted to have local side effects including hypoesthesia, loss of erection, genital erythema, or burning [21,26].

Oral medications generally include selective serotonin reuptake inhibitors (SSRIs) or off-label use of tricyclic antidepressants. Within the SSRI class, dapoxetine is an attractive option as it has a quick onset and offset, with peak serum levels achieved within 1–3 hours and a 95% clearance by 24 hours [27]. It has been used in both primary and secondary PE with a 2.5–3 times increase in mean IELT [28]. Important contraindications include severe hepatic disease, heart failure, ischemic cardiac disease, and carriers of pacemakers [28]. Dapoxetine is generally used as an "on-demand" agent, and side effects are minimal, generally limited to headache, dizziness, nausea, and, rarely, diarrhea. Daily use of SSRIs is sometimes used, especially in situations of couples with an active sexual life. Of course, the side effects are increased with daily versus as needed usage.

Common medications used on a daily basis include paroxetine (increase of IELT by up to 8.8 times), sertraline, fluoxetine, and citalopram [27]. Some have even used tramadol for its neuromodulatory properties on the serotonin/norepinephrine cascades with increases of basal IELT observed from 2.4 to 12.6 times baseline [28]. Tramadol, however, has addictive properties which are well known and can cause serotonin syndrome if combined with other agents in this class [28]. The most common tricyclic antidepressant used for PE is clomipramine, which can have cardiac side effects including palpitations and arrhythmias [21].

7.4 Retrograde Ejaculation and Failure of Emission

Propulsion of seminal fluid from the posterior urethra into the bladder, called retrograde ejaculation (RE), is classically understood to result from impairment of bladder neck closure during expulsion. Failure of emission (FE) is characterized by the lack of deposition of vasal and seminal vesicle fluid into the prostatic urethra. These two conditions are best considered as a spectrum of ejaculatory dysfunction, with FE as the most severe manifestation, but may be readily discerned by post-masturbatory urinalysis. RE and FE occur in a number of clinical settings, which can be characterized into several categories of dysfunction: neurogenic, pharmacologic, and congenital or acquired bladder neck incompetence [29].

Any neurologic insult or pathology that interrupts sympathetic outflow at the level of the spinal cord, sympathetic chain, hypogastric plexus, or postganglionic fibers may impair ejaculatory function. Spinal lesions or iatrogenic injury, as in retroperitoneal lymphadenectomy (RPLND), aortoiliac surgery, or abdominoperineal resection, are common etiologies of neurogenic ejaculatory dysfunction. Mild or unilateral injury may present with only decreased ejaculate secondary to partial denervation of the bladder neck, while complete disruption may manifest as FE. Refinement in surgical technique has greatly reduced the risk of ejaculatory dysfunction, at least with respect to RPLND. Modern series report preserved ejaculation in >95% of patients undergoing bilateral nerve-sparing primary dissection and >80% in those undergoing nerve-sparing post-chemotherapy dissection [30].

RE or FE may also be found in men with poorly controlled diabetes who have developed autonomic neuropathy. The prevalence of RE or FE in a young male diabetic population was found to be 6% [31], but has been reported in up to 32% of men with diabetes overall [32].

Identification of ejaculatory dysfunction in men with diabetes is generally straightforward, but an emphasis should be placed on the thorough evaluation of infertility. Men with diabetes are at increased risk of metabolic syndrome and hypogonadism, and thus the possibility of a multifactorial etiology of male infertility cannot be understated.

Many pharmacologic agents with sympatholytic properties may induce ejaculatory dysfunction, especially alpha-receptor antagonists, tricyclic antidepressants, or atypical antipsychotics. The most common offending medications are alpha-adrenergic antagonists, as used in the treatment of hypertension or lower urinary tract symptoms. For years, it was assumed that these medications caused retrograde ejaculation by impairment of bladder neck closure. In fact, alpha blockers appear to result in FE. A well-conducted randomized control trial comparing the effect of tamsulosin, alfuzosin, and placebo on semen parameters demonstrated decreased ejaculate in the tamsulosin group. Surprisingly, post-masturbatory urinalysis revealed no differences in sperm concentration recovered between the treatment and placebo groups, indicating that FE, rather than RE, is more descriptive of this pathology [33]. The mechanism appears to be related to the high concentrations of the alpha-1a adrenergic receptor and associated mRNA observed in the seminal vesicles and vasa deferentia, which is suspected to mediate their contraction to facilitate emission [34]. The degree to which men experience ejaculatory dysfunction with alpha-blocker therapy is proportional to the selectivity of the drug for the 1a-subtype, though it should be noted that this adverse effect of therapy occurs in a minority of treated patients overall (2.6–7.7%) [35]. Combination therapy of alpha-blocker with 5-alpha reductase inhibitor appears to increase the risk of ejaculatory dysfunction, though the mechanism remains unclear [36].

Mechanical incompetence of the bladder neck may be congenital, arising from exstrophy or its variants, posterior urethral malformations, or utricular cysts. More commonly, bladder neck incompetence is acquired, following surgical intervention for outlet obstruction related to prostatic enlargement. There is considerable ambiguity in the reporting of ejaculatory dysfunction after outlet reduction surgery and the assumption that postoperative ejaculatory dysfunction represents RE is commonly encountered. Indeed, we were unable to identify any study that provided proof of RE after outlet reduction (i.e., post-masturbatory urinalysis). With this caveat, we will continue to use the common terminology of RE to refer to ejaculatory dysfunction after outlet reduction for the sake of consistency.

Surgical approaches to outlet reduction are numerous and are associated with variable rates of RE. Historically, retrograde ejaculation after transurethral resection of the prostate (TURP) has been reported in up to 80% of patients [37]. Holmium laser enucleation of prostate (HoLEP) also commonly (70–88%) results in retrograde ejaculation [38]. Prospective comparison of TURP and HoLEP has confirmed equivalent rates: 78.3% in both groups at 24 months follow-up [39]. Photo-selective vaporization of prostate (PVP) appears to impart a lower risk of retrograde ejaculation than TURP or HoLEP: approximately 22–34.7% (PVP) vs. 60.5–65% (TURP) or 88% (HoLEP) in comparative randomized controlled trials [38]. In smaller glands (less than 30 cc), transurethral incision of prostate has been associated with much lower rates of retrograde ejaculation (approximately 0–35%, overall 28.2%) [40]. Finally, minimally invasive non-ablative techniques, including the prostatic urethral lift, convective water-vapor thermal therapy, and prostate artery embolization have all demonstrated near-complete preservation of antegrade ejaculation in prospective studies [41].

It should be noted that the classic paradigm that closure of the bladder neck is required for antegrade ejaculation has been challenged in recent years by modifications to ablative techniques that have resulted in higher rates of preserved ejaculatory function than have been previously reported. Proponents of these techniques describe a "high-pressure ejaculatory area" around the verumontanum that is principally responsible for antegrade expulsion of the ejaculate. Indeed, dynamic ultrasound during ejaculation in a small number of healthy volunteers demonstrated not only bladder neck closure, but also conformal changes in the verumontanum that may facilitate antegrade propulsion of seminal fluid [42]. In these ejaculation-preserving techniques, resection or vaporization of the median lobe is stopped 1 cm proximal to the verumontanum, and the lateral lobes carefully treated without damaging paracollicular tissue. The bladder neck is resected in the standard fashion. Prospective studies of these techniques were associated with only a 9–20% rate of retrograde ejaculation while preserving efficacy with respect to improvement in urinary symptoms [43,44]. Similarly, Aquablation is a novel technique with a low reported rate of retrograde ejaculation (approximately 10%) that employs ultrasound-based conformal planning and limits destruction of tissue around the verumontanum [45]. The association of these verumontanum-sparing techniques with preserved ejaculatory function implies a need to reconsider our understanding of the relative contributions of bladder neck closure and conformal changes of the verumontanum to the physiologic process of expulsion.

7.4.1 Treatment of Retrograde Ejaculation and Failure of Emission

Treatment for RE or FE begins with a careful assessment of the suspected etiology, and should be tailored to the degree to which the condition is causing distress or infertility. In cases of pharmacologically induced RE or FE, cessation of the offending agent may restore normal ejaculatory function after an appropriate washout period. Medical therapy and sperm recovery procedures with or without penile vibratory stimulation or electroejaculation may also be considered in various scenarios.

Various alpha agonists, anticholinergic, and antihistaminic drugs have been employed as potential treatments for neurogenic RE. The most commonly employed is imipramine, a tricyclic antidepressant, which may restore antegrade ejaculation in about 46% of cases [46]. Milodrine, an alpha agonist, appears to have similar efficacy (53%). Medical therapy for FE in patients without spinal cord injury (SCI) is generally less successful: imipramine (38%) or milodrine (18%). Parasympathomimetics have been studied in patients with FE and SCI, but carry the risk of severe side effects and must be administered in a monitored setting [46].

When the goal of treatment is the acquisition of sperm for use in assisted reproduction techniques, post-masturbatory urine collection and sperm washing may be performed. Urine is alkalinized prior to collection and can be accomplished by ingestion of sodium bicarbonate. The post-masturbatory urine specimen is obtained by voiding or catheterization, Overall pregnancy rate per cycle using sperm obtained in this method was 15% [47].

In men with SCI who possess an intact ejaculatory reflex arc, penile vibratory stimulation (PVS) may be considered first-line treatment. PVS has been reported successful in 86% of cases in the context of level of injury T10 or higher [48]. Electroejaculation (EEJ) is generally successful when PVS fails, but must be performed under general anesthesia and is thought to generate lower-quality semen for insemination than that produced by PVS [49]. However, similar pregnancy and live birth rates are observed using sperm collected by PVS or EEJ when compared to in vitro fertilization [50].

7.5 Conclusion

Ejaculation is a complex physiologic phenomenon. While ejaculation may have been historically necessary to achieve pregnancy, the advent of ART has circumvented this in most cases. Nonetheless, ejaculatory dysfunction remains a heterogenous group of conditions that can have significant quality of life implications for patients. The evaluation of this entity requires a careful history and physical in order to help determine an accurate diagnosis and appropriate treatment strategy. Thoughtful individualized workup and treatment can result in high levels of patient satisfaction. More research is needed to better understand this group of disorders and how best to manage them.

References

1. Revenig L, Leung A, Hsiao W. Ejaculatory physiology and pathophysiology: assessment and treatment in male infertility. *Transl Androl Urol.* 2014;3(1):41–49. doi:10.3978/j.issn.2223-4683.2014.02.02
2. Althof SE. Prevalence, characteristics and implications of premature ejaculation/rapid ejaculation. *J Urol.* 2006;175(3 Pt 1):842–848. doi:10.1016/S0022-5347(05)00341-1
3. Giuliano F. Neurophysiology of erection and ejaculation. *J Sex Med.* 2011;8 (Suppl 4):310–315. doi:10.1111/j.1743-6109.2011.02450.x
4. Abdel-Hamid IA, Ali OI. Delayed ejaculation: pathophysiology, diagnosis, and treatment. *World J Mens Health.* 2018;36(1):22–40. doi:10.5534/wjmh.17051
5. Giuliano F, Clement P. Neuroanatomy and physiology of ejaculation. *Annu Rev Sex Res.* 2005;16:190–216.
6. Lipshultz LI, Howards SS, Niederberger CS. *Infertility in the Male.* 4th ed. Cambridge University Press; 2009.
7. Hafez ESE. *Human Semen and Fertility Regulation in Men.* Mosby; 1976.
8. Vaucher L, Bolyakov A, Paduch DA. Evolving techniques to evaluate ejaculatory function. *Curr Opin Urol.* 2009;19(6):606–614. doi:10.1097/MOU.0b013e3283318ee2
9. Yang CC, Bradley WE. Innervation of the human anterior urethra by the dorsal nerve of the penis. *Muscle Nerve.* 1998;21(4):514–518. doi:10.1002/(sici)1097-4598(199804)21:4<514::aid-mus10>3.0.co;2-x
10. Wieder JA, Brackett NL, Lynne CM, Green JT, Aballa TC. Anesthetic block of the dorsal penile nerve inhibits vibratory-induced ejaculation in men with spinal cord injuries. *Urology.* 2000;55(6):915–917. doi:10.1016/s0090-4295(99)00608-1
11. Clement P, Giuliano F. Physiology and pharmacology of ejaculation. *Basic Clin Pharmacol Toxicol.* 2016;119(Suppl 3):18–25. doi:10.1111/bcpt.12546
12. Educational Committee of the ESSM. *The ESSM Manual of Sexual Medicine.* 2nd updated ed: Medix; 2015.
13. David Prologo J, Snyder LL, Cherullo E, Passalacqua M, Pirasteh A, Corn D. Percutaneous CT-guided cryoablation of the dorsal penile nerve for treatment of symptomatic premature ejaculation. *J Vasc Interv Radiol.* 2013;24(2):214–219. doi:10.1016/j.jvir.2012.09.015
14. Serefoglu EC, McMahon CG, Waldinger MD, et al. An evidence-based unified definition of lifelong and acquired premature ejaculation: report of the Second International Society for Sexual Medicine Ad Hoc Committee for the Definition of Premature Ejaculation. *J Sex Med.* 2014;11(6):1423–1441. doi:10.1111/jsm.12524
15. Patrick DL, Althof SE, Pryor JL, et al. Premature ejaculation: an observational study of men and their partners. *J Sex Med.* 2005;2(3):358–367. doi:10.1111/j.1743-6109.2005.20353.x
16. Lorentzen SS, Papoutsakis C, Myers EF, Thoresen L. Adopting nutrition care process terminology at the national level: the Norwegian experience in evaluating compatibility with international statistical classification of diseases and related health problems, 10th revision, and the existing Norwegian coding system. *J Acad Nutr Diet.* 2019;119(3):375–393. doi:10.1016/j.jand.2018.02.006
17. Parnham A, Serefoglu EC. Classification and definition of premature ejaculation. *Transl Androl Urol.* 2016;5(4):416–423. doi:10.21037/tau.2016.05.16
18. Bernard S. Premature ejaculation: a review of 1130 cases. *J Urol.* 1943:374–379.
19. Waldinger MD. The pathophysiology of lifelong premature ejaculation. *Transl Androl Urol.* 2016;5(4):424–433. doi:10.21037/tau.2016.06.04
20. Gao J, Zhang X, Su P, et al. Prevalence and factors associated with the complaint of premature ejaculation and the four premature ejaculation syndromes: a large observational study in China. *J Sex Med.* 2013;10(7):1874–1881. doi:10.1111/jsm.12180
21. Pereira-Lourenço M, Brito DVE, Pereira BJ. Premature ejaculation: from physiology to treatment. *J Family Reprod Health.* 2019;13(3):120–131.
22. Lindau ST, Schumm LP, Laumann EO, Levinson W, O'Muircheartaigh CA, Waite LJ. A study of sexuality and health among older adults in the United States. *N Engl J Med.* 2007;357(8):762–774. doi:10.1056/NEJMoa067423
23. Öztürk M, Koca O, Tüken M, Keleş MO, Ilktaç A, Karaman MI. Hormonal evaluation in premature ejaculation. *Urol Int.* 2012;88(4):454–458. doi:10.1159/000336137
24. Patrick DL, Giuliano F, Ho KF, Gagnon DD, McNulty P, Rothman M. The Premature Ejaculation Profile: validation of self-reported outcome measures for research and practice. *BJU Int.* 2009;103(3):358–364. doi:10.1111/j.1464-410X.2008.08041.x
25. Barnes T, Eardley I. Premature ejaculation: the scope of the problem. *J Sex Marital Ther.* 2007;33(2):151–170. doi:10.1080/00926230601098472
26. Frühauf S, Gerger H, Schmidt HM, Munder T, Barth J. Efficacy of psychological interventions for sexual dysfunction: a systematic review and meta-analysis. *Arch Sex Behav.*

27. Melnik T, Althof S, Atallah AN, Puga ME, Glina S, Riera R. Psychosocial interventions for premature ejaculation. *Cochrane Database Syst Rev.* 2011;(8): CD008195. doi:10.1002/14651858.CD008195.pub2

28. Althof SE, McMahon CG, Waldinger MD, et al. An update of the International Society of Sexual Medicine's guidelines for the diagnosis and treatment of premature ejaculation (PE). *Sex Med.* 2014;2(2):60–90. doi:10.1002/sm2.28

29. Hershlag A, Schiff SF, DeCherney AH. Retrograde ejaculation. *Hum Reprod.* 1991;6(2):255–258. doi:10.1093/oxfordjournals.humrep.a137317

30. Mano R, Di Natale R, Sheinfeld J. Current controversies on the role of retroperitoneal lymphadenectomy for testicular cancer. *Urol Oncol.* 2019;37 (3):209–218. doi:10.1016/j.urolonc.2018.09.009

31. Gaunay G, Nagler HM, Stember DS. Reproductive sequelae of diabetes in male patients. *Endocrinol Metab Clin North Am.* 2013;42(4):899–914. doi:10.1016/j.ecl.2013.07.003

32. Dunsmuir WD, Holmes SA. The aetiology and management of erectile, ejaculatory, and fertility problems in men with diabetes mellitus. *Diabet Med.* 1996;13(8):700–708. doi:10.1002/(SICI) 1096-9136(199608)13:8<700::AID-DIA174>3.0.CO;2-8

33. Hellstrom WJ, Sikka SC. Effects of acute treatment with tamsulosin versus alfuzosin on ejaculatory function in normal volunteers. *J Urol.* 2006;176(4 Pt 1):1529–1533. doi:10.1016/j.juro.2006.06.004

34. Hisasue S, Furuya R, Itoh N, Kobayashi K, Furuya S, Tsukamoto T. Ejaculatory disorder caused by alpha-1 adrenoceptor antagonists is not retrograde ejaculation but a loss of seminal emission. *Int J Urol.* 2006;13 (10):1311–1316. doi:10.1111/j.1442-2042.2006.01535.x

35. Gacci M, Ficarra V, Sebastianelli A, et al. Impact of medical treatments for male lower urinary tract symptoms due to benign prostatic hyperplasia on ejaculatory function: a systematic review and meta-analysis. *J Sex Med.* 2014;11(6):1554–1566. doi:10.1111/jsm.12525

36. DeLay KJ, Nutt M, McVary KT. Ejaculatory dysfunction in the treatment of lower urinary tract symptoms. *Transl Androl Urol.* 2016;5 (4):450–459. doi:10.21037/tau.2016.06.06

37. Rassweiler J, Teber D, Kuntz R, Hofmann R. Complications of transurethral resection of the prostate (TURP): incidence, management, and prevention. *Eur Urol.* 2006;50(5):969–979; discussion 980. doi:10.1016/j.eururo.2005.12.042

38. Cornu JN, Ahyai S, Bachmann A, et al. A systematic review and meta-analysis of functional outcomes and complications following transurethral procedures for lower urinary tract symptoms resulting from benign prostatic obstruction: an update. *Eur Urol.* 2015;67(6):1066–1096. doi:10.1016/j.eururo.2014.06.017

39. Briganti A, Naspro R, Gallina A, et al. Impact on sexual function of holmium laser enucleation versus transurethral resection of the prostate: results of a prospective, 2-center, randomized trial. *J Urol.* 2006;175 (5):1817–1821. doi:10.1016/S0022-5347 (05)00983-3

40. Marra G, Sturch P, Oderda M, Tabatabaei S, Muir G, Gontero P. Systematic review of lower urinary tract symptoms/benign prostatic hyperplasia surgical treatments on men's ejaculatory function: time for a bespoke approach? *Int J Urol.* 2016;23(1):22–35. doi:10.1111/iju.12866

41. Lebdai S, Chevrot A, Doizi S, et al. Do patients have to choose between ejaculation and miction? A systematic review about ejaculation preservation technics for benign prostatic obstruction surgical treatment. *World J Urol.* 2019;37 (2):299–308. doi:10.1007/s00345-018-2368-6

42. Gil-Vernet JM, Alvarez-Vijande R, Gil-Vernet A. Ejaculation in men: a dynamic endorectal ultrasonographical study. *Br J Urol.* 1994;73(4):442–448. doi:10.1111/j.1464-410x.1994.tb07612.x

43. Ronzoni G, De Vecchis M. Preservation of anterograde ejaculation after transurethral resection of both the prostate and bladder neck. *Br J Urol.* 1998;81(6):830–833. doi:10.1046/j.1464-410x.1998.00658.x

44. Alloussi SH, Lang C, Eichel R, Alloussi S. Ejaculation-preserving transurethral resection of prostate and bladder neck: short- and long-term results of a new innovative resection technique. *J Endourol.* 2014;28(1):84–89. doi:10.1089/end.2013.0093

45. Gilling P, Barber N, Bidair M, et al. WATER: a double-blind, randomized, controlled trial of Aquablation. *J Urol.* 2018;199(5):1252–1261. doi:10.1016/j.juro.2017.12.065

46. Kamischke A, Nieschlag E. Update on medical treatment of ejaculatory disorders. *Int J Androl.* 2002;25 (6):333–344. doi:10.1046/j.1365-2605.2002.00379.x

47. Jefferys A, Siassakos D, Wardle P. The management of retrograde ejaculation: a systematic review and update. *Fertil Steril.* 2012;97(2):306–312. doi:10.1016/j.fertnstert.2011.11.019

48. Brackett NL, Ibrahim E, Iremashvili V, Aballa TC, Lynne CM. Treatment for ejaculatory dysfunction in men with spinal cord injury: an 18-year single center experience. *J Urol.* 2010;183 (6):2304–2308. doi:10.1016/j.juro.2010.02.018

49. Brackett NL. Semen retrieval by penile vibratory stimulation in men with spinal cord injury. *Hum Reprod Update.* 1999;5(3):216–222. doi:10.1093/humupd/5.3.216

50. Kathiresan AS, Ibrahim E, Aballa TC, et al. Comparison of in vitro fertilization/intracytoplasmic sperm injection outcomes in male factor infertility patients with and without spinal cord injuries. *Fertil Steril.* 2011;96(3):562–566. doi:10.1016/j.fertnstert.2011.06.078

Section 2 The Biology of Male Reproduction and Infertility

Chapter 8: Genetic Aspects of Male Infertility

Albert Salas-Huetos and Kenneth I. Aston

8.1 Introduction

Male infertility can take many forms, from apparently normal sperm production with some uncharacterized molecular defect that renders sperm incapable to fertilize an oocyte or support normal embryonic development, to the complete absence of sperm production or severe disorders of sexual development. Infertility phenotypes can be categorized as pretesticular, testicular, and posttesticular. Pretesticular disorders include ejaculatory disorders, erectile dysfunction, and hypogonadotrophic hypogonadism. Testicular disorders refer to diminished testicular function and may be related to altered testicular environment (e.g., cryptorchidism or varicocele), injury, gonadotoxic medications, or genetic factors that result in the loss or diminished function of germ cells or supporting niche cells. Posttesticular disorders include obstruction, dysfunction, or absence of the vas deferens [1]. Further, infertility may be congenital or acquired. Congenital causes are of particular importance in the search for genetic causes of male infertility.

8.2 Advances in Tools for Genetic Analysis

Molecular genetics is a relatively young field. Heritability patterns were first recognized and documented by Gregor Mendel in the mid-1800s, and chromosomes were first described by Heinrich Waldeyer several decades later. Important incremental discoveries by the likes of Friederich Meischer, Phoebus Levene, and Erwin Chargaff to characterize the chemical nature of DNA and advances in X-ray imaging by Maurice Wilkins, Rosalind Franklin, and Raymond Gosling paved the way for James Watson and Francis Crick to describe the three-dimensional structure of DNA in 1953 [2]. Shortly thereafter, the 46-chromosome human karyotype was first described and a relationship between abnormal chromosome number and human disease was demonstrated, first with trisomy 21 and soon after with Klinefelter syndrome [3]. A fundamental understanding of the composition of DNA and the role of genetic material in human disease was a critical step in the progression of the field of medical genetics.

Equally important was the development of molecular assays including polymerase chain reaction and Sanger sequencing that finally enabled investigation of the DNA sequence at single-base resolution. Subsequent application of those and other tools led to the completion of the draft human genome reference sequence in 2001 following a herculean effort by hundreds of researchers over a period of 13 years and a cost of approximately $2.7 billion [4]. While many important discoveries of human genetic variation preceded the completed Human Genome Project, a full assembly of the human genome was a fundamental foundation in characterizing human genetic variation and identifying genetic signatures underlying disease states.

Significant advances in sequencing platforms dramatically reduced the time and costs associated with sequencing whole genomes and exomes, resulting in an explosion in the publicly available human genome sequence data. To date it is estimated that more than 1,000,000 human genomes have been sequenced, with a number of initiatives currently underway to sequences hundreds of thousands to millions more genomes in the coming decade. These efforts have been, and will continue to be, critical in defining normal genetic variation and attributing genetic variants to specific disease states.

8.3 History of Male Infertility Genetics

A genetic component of male infertility has long been recognized, beginning with the recognition that Klinefelter syndrome was caused by an extra X chromosome just four years after the normal human karyotype was described [3], and the same year that trisomy 21 was first characterized. Fewer than two decades later, karyotype analysis successfully identified a deletion of the distal portion of Yq11 in six men with azoospermia, a region later named the azoospermia factor (AZF) region [5]. Subsequently, in the late 1980s, mutations in the cystic fibrosis transmembrane conductance regulator (CFTR) were found to underly cystic fibrosis, and later it was determined that CFTR mutations caused obstructive azoospermia due to congenital bilateral absence of vas deferens [6].

Following these important findings, researchers in the field applied the best available tool, Sanger sequencing of genes known to be required for spermatogenesis, in an effort to identify novel genetic causes of male infertility. These studies typically involved sequencing of a single gene in cohorts of tens to several hundred infertile men – most often azoospermic or severely oligozoospermic men, along with normozoospermic controls, to identify any polymorphisms or rare variants that might confer increased risk for, or cause spermatogenic defects. These efforts were largely though not entirely unsuccessful in identifying clinically relevant variants [7,8].

Subsequently array-based techniques were applied to more broadly investigate the role of common single nucleotide polymorphisms and copy number variants (CNVs) in male infertility, again with very limited success [9–14]. These genome-wide approaches did reveal several important features of male infertility: first, that common polymorphisms do not contribute appreciably to the phenotype, and second, and more interestingly, several CNV studies reported increased CNV burden in infertile men, suggesting reduced genomic stability associated with infertility. However, a few important variants, primarily CNVs, were identified by this approach, initially in the context of globozoospermia [15,16] and more recently for nonobstructive azoospermia (NOA) [17,18].

Based on these findings, it quickly became clear that the application of approaches that allowed the identification of rare or novel variants on a genome-wide scale was necessary. As has occurred across the spectrum of complex diseases, the use of next-generation exome and whole-genome sequencing approaches for male infertility has quickly expanded over the past several years, albeit with some lag compared with many other complex diseases (Figure 8.1), yielding a significant number of novel discoveries during the same period. As illustrated in Figure 8.1, the use of exome sequencing in male infertility studies has exploded over the past few years, and whole-genome sequencing is expected to follow a similar trend as the technology becomes more accessible due to decreasing costs. Importantly, the cost to sequence an entire human genome today is approximately the same as the cost to sequence a human exome just five years ago.

8.4 Common Male Infertility Genetic Factors

This chapter will describe some of the most frequent known genetic causes of male infertility as well as a few noteworthy recent discoveries; however, the field is advancing so quickly that a review of all genetic causes of male infertility would be outdated shortly after publication. We would point the reader to an excellent recent systematic review of the subject [19]. Dr. Veltman, senior author for this review, is working to coordinate annual updates through the International Male Infertility Genomics Consortium due to recent rapid advances in the field.

8.4.1 Pretesticular Infertility

Pretesticular forms of male infertility generally involve defects in genes involved in sexual differentiation and development, and disrupted endocrine signaling due to hypothalamic, pituitary, or adrenal gland dysfunction. Numerous genetic variants have been implicated in both disorders of sexual development [20] and hypogonadotropic hypogonadism (HH) [21]. Importantly, a genetic cause can be identified in over 40% of male patients with disorders of sexual development [22] and half of patients with congenital HH [23].

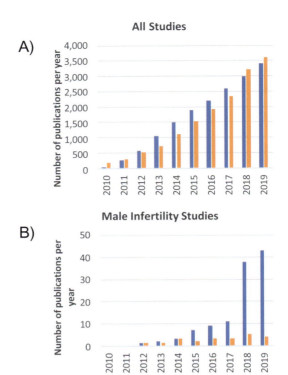

Figure 8.1 Growth in the number of PubMed citations for whole-genome and whole-exome sequencing over a 10-year period. (A) All studies: The number of PubMed citations each year that include the keyword "whole-genome sequencing" OR "exome sequencing." Note that the number of references for whole-genome sequencing has surpassed exome sequencing for the past two years. (B) Male infertility studies: The number of PubMed citations each year that include the keyword "whole-genome sequencing" OR "exome sequencing" AND "male infertility."

8.4.2 Obstructive Azoospermia

Obstructive azoospermia is caused by defects in the ejaculatory ducts that impede sperm transport and accounts for approximately 40% or azoospermic cases [24]. Obstructions can be due to several factors including infection, injury, vasectomy, or congenital anomalies. The most common known genetic variants associated with congenital bilateral absence of the vas deferens include biallelic mutations in *CFTR* that are identified in up to 80% of men displaying congenital bilateral absence of the vas deferens [25]. Several studies have also implicated mutations in the X-linked adhesion G-protein-coupled receptor G2 (*ADGRG2*) gene [26,27].

8.4.3 Quantitative Sperm Defects

Reduced sperm production (oligozoospermia) or the lack of sperm production (NOA) are relatively common in infertile men. NOA encompasses a broad range of spermatogenic defects, from the complete absence of germ cells in the testis, referred to as Sertoli cell-only syndrome, to meiotic arrest of spermatogenesis that can occur at any stage of meiosis. This diversity of phenotypes explains in part the challenge in identifying genetic factors underlying spermatogenic impairment, as oligozoospermia and the various subclasses of NOA are almost certainly the result of disruption of different genes [28].

The most common genetic causes of NOA and severe oligozoospermia are Klinefelter syndrome, identified in 5–15% of infertility cases [29] and deletions of the AZF region of the Y chromosome, present in 5–10% of that patient group [30]. In addition, chromosomal translocations and inversions are approximately ten times more common in oligozoospermic men than in normozoospermic men [31], suggesting underlying genomic instability associated with severe spermatogenic defects. This is supported by several CNV studies that found increased CNV burden in infertile men [13,17,32].

Progress in the discovery of bona fide novel genetic causes for quantitative spermatogenic defects has benefited significantly by the application of next-generation sequencing approaches. In the past several years, the number of likely causal variants for NOA has expanded rapidly, with a few noteworthy examples being variants in *FANCM* [33], *FANCA* [34], and *M1AP* [35], all identified through whole-exome sequencing. The list of genetic variants underlying NOA is sure to increase rapidly as more groups utilize next-generation sequencing approaches to interrogate the genomes of larger groups of infertile men as single-base resolution.

8.4.4 Qualitative Sperm Defects

Qualitative sperm defects include reduced sperm motility and morphological defects of the sperm head and tail. While a genetic cause for quantitative sperm defects remains unresolved in a significant proportion of cases, progress in characterizing the genetic basis for qualitative sperm defects, particularly morphological defects, has accelerated significantly in recent years due largely to the power of family-based studies and the utilization of genome-wide approaches. Morphological defects in sperm that have been investigated include globozoospermia, acephalia, primary ciliary dyskinesia, and multiple morphological abnormalities of the sperm flagella (MMAF). Investigation of the genetic basis for some of these abnormalities has proven extremely successful, likely due in large part to the discrete nature of the phenotypes. For example, an underlying genetic cause for globozoospermia, most commonly mutations in *DPY19L2* and *SPATA16*, can be identified in approximately 70% of cases [16,36,37]. Further, genetic defects are identified in *DNAH1*, several *CFAP* genes, or *FSIP2* in approximately 20% of men with MMAF (38–40).

8.5 Challenges in Male Infertility Genetic Studies

There are numerous challenges in efficiently identifying the underlying genetic causes of male infertility. Principal among the challenges is the complexity of spermatogenesis and the overwhelming number of genes involved in the process. Based on gene and protein expression metrics, spermatogenesis ranks among the most complex processes in the human body. Based on data collected by the Genotype-Tissue Expression (GTEx) project, the testis is the most transcriptionally diverse tissue among the 49 tissues evaluated, with more than 19,000 genes expressed (Figure 8.2). Moreover, the Human Protein Atlas reports that transcripts for 84% (n = 16,598) of all human proteins (n = 19,670) are expressed in the testis, and 2,274 of these genes show an elevated expression in testis compared to other tissue types (Figure 8.3; www.proteinatlas.org/). The transcriptional and translational complexity of the testis greatly expands the list of possible genes that might be implicated in spermatogenic defects. In addition, the involvement of several thousand genes, many working in concert with one another, means that some forms of male infertility are likely polygenic in nature.

In addition to the inherent complexity of spermatogenesis, "male infertility" encompasses an incredibly broad set of phenotypes and disease states. Moreover, currently available tools to phenotype and categorize male infertility are largely limited, with endocrine assays and semen analysis being the most widely utilized. These tools can effectively identify endocrine disruption as well as some spermatogenic defects such as impaired sperm production, reduced or absent sperm motility or viability, and morphological defects. However, the underlying causes for those defects are undoubtedly as diverse as the repertoire of genes regulating the process.

Finally, the lack of available tools for in vitro studies of spermatogenesis limits our ability to study the effects of specific gene variants in a robust manner. This limitation can be overcome in part with the use of in vitro and in vivo experiments using available culture systems and animal models. However, in spite of the importance of these systems, species-specific differences in spermatogenesis and reproductive processes somewhat limit the generalizability of model organism experiments in male infertility research.

8.6 Resources for Genetic Studies

In spite of the challenges associated with the discovery of genetic variants associated with male infertility, there are a number of resources and new and improving technologies that have become invaluable for the field. These include extensive reference datasets, improved sequencing platforms, a growing number of analytical tools, and powerful tools for evaluating the functional consequence of specific variants of interest in model systems.

8.6.1 Data Resources

Information on frequency of a specific variant within a population, the role of a specific gene in spermatogenesis, and the functional consequences of a variant are all necessary to enable the prioritization of genomic variants from an exome or whole-genome dataset. The human genome contains several million variants, making it imperative to narrow down variants of interest to a manageable number. This is often done

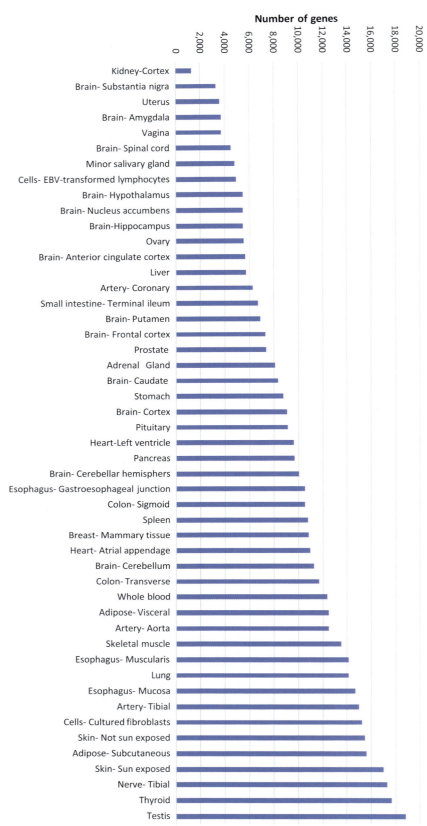

Figure 8.2 The number of genes expressed in each of 49 human tissues as assessed by the GTEx project. More genes are expressed in the testis than in any other tissue analyzed.

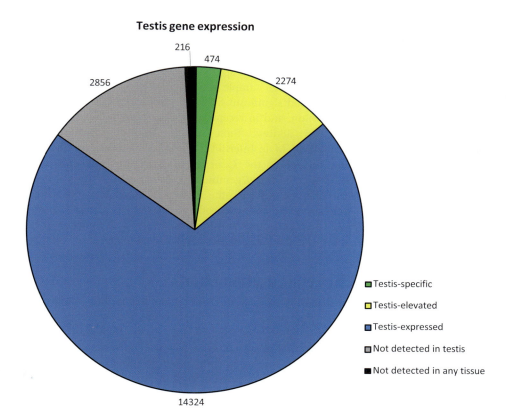

Figure 8.3 Protein Atlas data indicate that 84% of transcripts that code for proteins are expressed in the testis, with 474 being testis-specific and an additional 2,274 being enriched in the testis relative to other tissues.

with the help of reference datasets that enable the elimination of common variants, variants in genes that are not expressed in the tissue of interest, or genes whose ablation in model organisms is not associated with the disease or phenotype of interest.

The Genome Aggregation Database (gnomAD; https://gnomad.broadinstitute.org/) is a database that includes whole-genome sequence data for more than 87,000 unrelated individuals and exome data for more than 141,000 unrelated individuals. The depth of sequence data across such a large number of individuals makes this database an invaluable resource for determining relative variant frequency in a population. In the context of male infertility research, it is common to eliminate variants from consideration based on allele frequency of >1% in variant databases.

Other useful tools used for filtering variants include gene and protein expression atlases. For example, the Human Protein Atlas (www.proteinatlas.org/) contains data on relative expression of more than 15,000 proteins in 44 normal human tissues, including the testis, epididymis, and accessory glands. This can allow the further narrowing of variants based on enrichment or lack of expression of a specific protein in reproductive tissues. Additionally, a number of high-resolution single-cell RNA sequence (scRNA-seq) reference datasets in testis tissue have been generated over the past several years, both in mouse [41] and human [42], and useful browser interfaces based on these datasets are in development https://conradlab.shinyapps.io/HISTA/. As with protein expression data, gene expression data can be extremely valuable in determining whether a variant in a specific gene might underly the infertility phenotype of interest. Not only can this resource help to implicate a specific gene in infertility, it can also be useful in predicting the specific phenotype that would be expected. For example, disruption of a gene that is expressed during early meiosis would be expected to result in early maturation arrest. Proof-of-principal of this approach was recently demonstrated in by performing scRNA-seq in mouse models with known gene disruptions underlying gonadal defects [41].

With the ability to generate terabytes of genome sequence data at relatively low cost, clearly data analysis has in recent years become the bottleneck for variant discovery. Numerous tools exist to support data analysis efforts and to integrate many of the datasets mentioned above [43,44]; however, most of these tools lack the specificity to efficiently study the broad list of phenotypes underlying male infertility. However, recently, a male infertility-specific analysis framework was developed, and this tool continues to be refined by the developers [45].

8.6.2 Model Systems

In addition to powerful data resources, in vitro and in vivo models have become an indispensable tool for the discovery and validation of variants involved in male infertility. These models rely on reliable and specific gene editing tools, of which CRISPR/Cas methods have emerged as a clear favorite over the past few years because they are inexpensive and relatively simple to apply. In vitro systems are particularly valuable because they enable the testing large numbers of variants in an efficient and cost-effective manner. Unfortunately, while in vitro systems that support spermatogenesis in mice have been successfully developed, a similar system in human does not yet exist [46]. Efforts continue in this area, and ultimately successful development of this tool will enable the recapitulation of the exact mutation identified through genomic approaches to evaluate the functional effects and would potentially enable the in vitro correction of variants that disrupt spermatogenesis for therapeutic use [47,48].

Some in vivo systems that have proven useful in the study of male infertility include yeast for the study of meiotic genes and unicellular flagellated and ciliated organisms including *Tetrahymena*, *Trypanisoma*, and *Chlamydomonas* for the evaluation of functional consequences of variants involved in sperm flagellar assembly and function [49–51].

Moving up to more advanced organisms, *Drosophila melanogaster* has been successfully used in male infertility studies. Given the reproductive capacity of flies and the spermatogenesis similarities shared with human, this is an important model for high throughput functional screening to identify genes important in spermatogenesis by RNA interference. For example, Yu et al. screened 22 drosophila orthologues based on associations identified in a large genome-wide association study and found that 7 showed a reproductive phenotype in *Drosophila* [52].

In addition, Zebrafish (*Danio rerio*) has been used increasingly as a model to study the genetics of complex disease, including male infertility, owing to a number of advantages. These include relatively simple and inexpensive housing requirements, reproductive physiology that shares many similarities with mammals, greater genomic similarities to humans compared with lower model species, easy embryonic manipulation, and prolific reproductive capacity. An example of the utility of zebrafish models in male infertility research is a recent study in which CRISPR gene editing was used to systematically evaluate the role of 17 different *Fanconi anemia* genes in reproduction [53].

Of course the most widely utilized model used in the study of male infertility is the mouse. Early discovery studies utilized N-ethyl-N-nitrosourea (ENU), an alkylating agent that induces mutagenesis at random loci throughout the genome to induce disease phenotypes. Once a specific phenotype is identified, the mutation is mapped to the genome and confirmatory studies conducted to implicate the role of a gene in a specific disease. This forward-genetics strategy proved very useful in identifying numerous genes necessary for spermatogenesis and male fertility [54]. More recently, mouse models using gene editing techniques have been employed to test the impact of specific mutations on male fertility based on variants identified using genomic approaches in humans [55,56].

8.7 Collaborative Approaches

A common feature of essentially all successful efforts to characterize the underlying etiology of complex diseases is a collaborative approach. Multi-institutional collaboration is necessary to provide the resources and expertise needed to achieve sufficient power to study the genomic basis of complex diseases using big-data approaches because these studies typically require large sample sets, diverse clinical and analytical expertise, and significant financial resources. Male infertility is no exception, and in recent years a number of consortia have arisen to address these needs. Examples include the International Male Infertility Genomics Consortium (IMIGC; www.imigc.org/), the Genetics of Male Infertility Initiative (GEMINI; https://gemini.conradlab.org/), ReproUnion (https://reprounion.eu/), the Andrology Research Consortium (ARC), and the Male Reproductive Health Initiative (MRHI) [57]. These and other collaborative efforts will continue to be critical in making significant strides in male infertility research.

8.8 Gene Curation Efforts

The discovery of male infertility genes has rapidly accelerated in the past several years due to the many technological advances and collaborative efforts discussed above. However, the number of genes confidently linked to male infertility is still extremely limited in comparison to other genetic diseases that significantly limits the clinical utility of genomics in male reproductive medicine [58]. In addition, male infertility literature is littered with hundreds of reported genetic associations that are either never pursued for validation in larger studies or fail subsequent validation. This is not necessarily due to "bad science," rather it is a result of limited resources and practical limitations of earlier genetic tools such as Sanger sequencing. The diverse body of existing male infertility genetics literature and the wide range of evidence for the involvement of specific variants in the disease make organized gene curation efforts absolutely imperative. Fortunately, two recent efforts aim to systematically address this data issue.

Recently, the group of Veltman et al. published a systematic review and standardized clinical validity assessment of male infertility genes according the gene–disease scoring system of Smith et al. [59] to curate all available information on the genetics of human male infertility from 1958 through December 2018 [19]. A current effort led by IMIGC aims to apply this methodology on a regular basis to prepare an up-to-date paper to be published at the end of each year starting in 2020.

The Smith methodology is based on a gene–disease scoring system ranging from 1 to 17 to assess the strength of evidence for the relationship between a gene and a type of male infertility. If the score is 1–2 the level is considered "without evidence," 3–8 with "limited" level of evidence, 9–12 "moderate," 13–15 "strong," and 16–17 "definitive." The scoring system has two distinct components. The first considers sequencing and variant information, taking into account the number of unrelated patients described with an inheritance pattern, the number of variants described with a likely-pathogenic or pathogenic classification, and the number of independent publications reporting independent individuals with variants of uncertain significance, or likely-pathogenic, or pathogenic variants. The second evaluates functional evidence for the gene described. Criteria include whether the gene is expressed in the correct tissue/cell type (according the testis RNAseq information: https://conradlab.shinyapps.io/HISTA/ or Human ProteinAtlas: www.proteinatlas.org/), the physical interaction with genes previously related with the same disease (according STRING: https://string-db.org/), the determination of mutational mechanisms, or the existence of animal models confirming the pathology in humans, among others.

8.8.1 ClinGen Initiative

In parallel, the Clinical Genome Resource Initiative (ClinGen; https://clinicalgenome.org/) is currently assembling an expert panel to curate genes and variants associated with male infertility based on standardized methodologies. ClinGen is a National Institutes of Health–funded resource dedicated to building a central resource that defines the clinical relevance of genes and variants for use in precision medicine and research. This initiative is based in a recently published, rigorous classification system [60] that will be applied by a group of experts in male infertility.

Like the Smith methodology, this methodology is also based in gene–disease scoring, but in this case with a scoring range between 1 and 18. If the score is 1–6 the gene is considered to have "limited," 7–11 "moderate," and 12–18 "strong" evidence for involvement in a specific disease. The curation is dynamic, so a gene–disease score initially classified as strong can be reclassified as "definitive" if the relationship is replicated over time. Using this classification, and for the purposes of scoring, genetic evidence is divided into two categories: case-level data and case-control data. Again, two parts are clearly differentiated. The first part considers the genetic evidence (if the case-level, family- segregation, or case-control data support the gene–disease association), and the second part evaluates the functional/experimental evidence (gene-level experimental evidence that support the gene–disease association).

These two significant and complementary efforts are critical to bringing routine genomic screening to routine use in male infertility diagnostics [61].

8.9 Conclusions

This is an exciting era in genomic medicine. With the rapidly increasing accessibility of genomic tools and resources and the concomitant increasing application of these resources to male infertility, we have seen a significant increase in the rate of new discoveries in the field over the past several years. With increasingly large study cohorts and a greater emphasis on collaborative approaches, these trends are sure to continue in the coming years. The clinical utility of genomic discoveries in male reproductive medicine will be dependent on robust clinical and functional validation and careful gene and variant curation efforts. As progress continues in this space, and in vitro tools for gene editing and tissue culture continue to improve, clinicians and patients benefit not only from expanded diagnostic options, but potentially from the ability to fix specific genetic lesions and restore fertility in the coming years.

References

1. Krausz C. Male infertility: pathogenesis and clinical diagnosis. *Best Pract Res Clin Endocrinol Metab.* 2011;25:271–285.
2. Watson JD, Crick FH. Molecular structure of nucleic acids; a structure for deoxyribose nucleic acid. *Nature.* 1953;171:737–738.
3. Jacobs PA, Strong JA. A case of human intersexuality having a possible XXY sex-determining mechanism. *Nature.* 1959;183:302–303.
4. Lander ES, Linton LM, Birren B, et al. Initial sequencing and analysis of the human genome. *Nature.* 2001;409:860–921.
5. Tiepolo L, Zuffardi O. Localization of factors controlling spermatogenesis in the nonfluorescent portion of the human Y chromosome long arm. *Hum Genet.* 1976;34:119–124.
6. Chillon M, Casals T, Mercier B, et al. Mutations in the cystic fibrosis gene in patients with congenital absence of the vas deferens. *N Engl J Med.* 1995;332:1475–1480.
7. Aston KI. Genetic susceptibility to male infertility: news from genome-wide association studies. *Andrology.* 2014;2:315–321.
8. Tuttelmann F, Rajpert-De Meyts E, Nieschlag E, Simoni M. Gene polymorphisms and male infertility – a meta-analysis and literature review. *Reprod Biomed Online.* 2007;15:643–658.
9. Aston KI, Carrell DT. Genome-wide study of single-nucleotide polymorphisms associated with azoospermia and severe oligozoospermia. *J Androl.* 2009;30:711–725.
10. Aston KI, Conrad DF. A review of genome-wide approaches to study the genetic basis for spermatogenic defects. *Methods Mol Biol.* 2013;927:397–410.
11. Fruhmesser A, Vogt PH, Zimmer J, et al. (2013) Single nucleotide polymorphism array analysis in men with idiopathic azoospermia or oligoasthenozoospermia syndrome. *Fertil Steril.* 100:81–87.
12. Hu Z, Xia Y, Guo X, et al. A genome-wide association study in Chinese men identifies three risk loci for non-obstructive azoospermia. *Nature Genetics.* 2012;44:183–186.
13. Krausz C, Giachini C, Lo Giacco D, et al. High resolution X chromosome-specific array-CGH detects new CNVs in infertile males. *PLoS ONE.* 2012;7: e44887.
14. Stouffs K, Vandermaelen D, Massart A, et al. Array comparative genomic hybridization in male infertility. *Hum Reprod.* 2012;27:921–929.

15. Dam AH, Koscinski I, Kremer JA, et al. Homozygous mutation in SPATA16 is associated with male infertility in human globozoospermia. *Am J Hum Genet*. 2007;81:813–820.
16. Koscinski I, Elinati E, Fossard C, et al. DPY19L2 deletion as a major cause of globozoospermia. *Am J Hum Gen*. 2011;88:344–350.
17. Lopes AM, Aston KI, Thompson E, et al. Human spermatogenic failure purges deleterious mutation load from the autosomes and both sex chromosomes, including the gene DMRT1. *PLoS Genetics*. 2013;9: e1003349.
18. Yatsenko AN, Georgiadis AP, Ropke A, et al. X-linked TEX11 mutations, meiotic arrest, and azoospermia in infertile men. *N Engl J Med*. 2015;372:2097–2107.
19. Oud MS, Volozonoka L, Smits RM, Vissers L, Ramos L, Veltman JA. A systematic review and standardized clinical validity assessment of male infertility genes. *Hum Reprod*. 2019;34:932–941.
20. Delot EC, Papp JC, DSD-TRN Genetics Workgroup, Sandberg DE, Vilain E. Genetics of disorders of sex development: the DSD-TRN experience. *Endocrinol Metab Clin North Am*. 2017;46:519–537.
21. Bianco SD, Kaiser UB. The genetic and molecular basis of idiopathic hypogonadotropic hypogonadism. *Nat Rev Endocrinol*. 2009;5:569–576.
22. Eggers S, Sadedin S, van den Bergen JA, et al. Disorders of sex development: insights from targeted gene sequencing of a large international patient cohort. *Genome Biol*. 2016;17:243.
23. Boehm U, Bouloux PM, Dattani MT, et al. Expert consensus document: European Consensus Statement on congenital hypogonadotropic hypogonadism – pathogenesis, diagnosis and treatment. *Nat Rev Endocrinol*. 2015;11:547–564.
24. Jarow JP, Espeland MA, Lipshultz LI Evaluation of the azoospermic patient. *J Urol*. 1989;142:62–65.
25. Yu J, Chen Z, Ni Y, Li Z. CFTR mutations in men with congenital bilateral absence of the vas deferens (CBAVD): a systemic review and meta-analysis. *Hum Reprod*. 2012;27:25–35.
26. Patat O, Pagin A, Siegfried A, et al. Truncating mutations in the adhesion G protein-coupled receptor G2 gene ADGRG2 cause an X-linked congenital bilateral absence of vas deferens. *Am J Hum Genet*. 2016;99:437–442.
27. Yang B, Wang J, Zhang W, et al. Pathogenic role of ADGRG2 in CBAVD patients replicated in Chinese population. *Andrology*. 2017;5:954–957.
28. Kasak L, Laan M. Monogenic causes of non-obstructive azoospermia: challenges, established knowledge, limitations and perspectives. *Hum Genet*. 2021;140:135–154.
29. Vockel M, Riera-Escamilla A, Tuttelmann F, Krausz C. The X chromosome and male infertility. *Hum Genet*. 2021;140:203–215.
30. Punab M, Poolamets O, Paju P, et al. Causes of male infertility: a 9-year prospective monocentre study on 1737 patients with reduced total sperm counts. *Hum Reprod*. 2017;32:18–31.
31. Krausz C, Riera-Escamilla A. Genetics of male infertility. *Nat Rev Urol*. 2018;15:369–384.
32. Tuttelmann F, Simoni M, Kliesch S, et al. Copy number variants in patients with severe oligozoospermia and Sertoli-cell-only syndrome. *PLoS ONE*. 2011;6:e19426.
33. Kasak L, Punab M, Nagirnaja L, et al. Bi-allelic recessive loss-of-function variants in FANCM cause non-obstructive azoospermia. *Am J Hum Genet*. 2018;103:200–212.
34. Krausz C, Riera-Escamilla A, Chianese C, et al. From exome analysis in idiopathic azoospermia to the identification of a high-risk subgroup for occult Fanconi anemia. *Genet Med*. 2019;21:189–194.
35. Wyrwoll MJ, Temel SG, Nagirnaja L, et al. Bi-allelic mutations in M1AP are a frequent cause of meiotic arrest and severely impaired spermatogenesis leading to male infertility. *Am J Hum Genet*. 2020;107:342–351.
36. Dam AH, Feenstra I, Westphal JR. Ramos L, van Golde RJ, Kremer JA. Globozoospermia revisited. *Hum Reprod Update*. 2007;13:63–75.
37. Harbuz R, Zouari R, Pierre V, et al. A recurrent deletion of DPY19L2 causes infertility in man by blocking sperm head elongation and acrosome formation. *Am J Hum Genet*. 2011;88:351–361.
38. Amiri-Yekta A, Coutton C, Kherraf ZE, et al. Whole-exome sequencing of familial cases of multiple morphological abnormalities of the sperm flagella (MMAF) reveals new DNAH1 mutations. *Hum Reprod*. 2016;31:2872–2880.
39. Sha YW, Wang X, Xu X, et al. Novel mutations in CFAP44 and CFAP43 cause multiple morphological abnormalities of the sperm flagella (MMAF). *Reprod Sci*. 2017:1933719117749756.
40. Wang WL, Tu CF, Tan YQ. Insight on multiple morphological abnormalities of sperm flagella in male infertility: what is new? *Asian J Androl*. 2020;22:236–245.
41. Jung M, Wells D, Rusch J, et al. Unified single-cell analysis of testis gene regulation and pathology in five mouse strains. *Elife*. 2019;8.
42. Guo J, Grow EJ, Mlcochova H, et al. The adult human testis transcriptional cell atlas. *Cell Res*. 2018;28:1141–1157.
43. Grabowski P, Rappsilber J. A primer on data analytics in functional genomics: how to move from data to insight? *Trends Biochem Sci*. 2019;44:21–32.
44. Langmead B, Nellore A. Cloud computing for genomic data analysis and collaboration. *Nat Rev Genet*. 2018;19:208–219.
45. Wilfert AB, Chao KR, Kaushal M, et al. Genome-wide significance testing of variation from single case exomes. *Nat Genet*. 2016;48:1455–1461.
46. Komeya M, Sato T, Ogawa T. In vitro spermatogenesis: a century-long research journey, still half way around. *Reprod Med Biol*. 2018;17:407–420.
47. Ibtisham F, Wu J, Xiao M, et al. Progress and future prospect of in vitro spermatogenesis. *Oncotarget*. 2017;8:66709–66727.
48. Sato T, Katagiri K, Gohbara A, et al. In vitro production of functional sperm in cultured neonatal mouse testes. *Nature*. 2011;471:504–507.
49. Coutton C, Vargas AS, Amiri-Yekta A, et al. Mutations in CFAP43 and CFAP44 cause male infertility and flagellum defects in Trypanosoma and human. *Nat Commun*. 2018;9:686.
50. Duquesnoy P, Escudier E, Vincensini L, et al. Loss-of-function mutations in the

human ortholog of *Chlamydomonas reinhardtii* ODA7 disrupt dynein arm assembly and cause primary ciliary dyskinesia. *Am J Hum Genet*. 2009;85:890–896.

51. Kherraf ZE, Amiri-Yekta A, Dacheux D, et al. A homozygous ancestral SVA-insertion-mediated deletion in WDR66 induces multiple morphological abnormalities of the sperm flagellum and male infertility. *Am J Hum Genet*. 2018;103:400–412.

52. Yu J, Wu H, Wen Y, et al. Identification of seven genes essential for male fertility through a genome-wide association study of non-obstructive azoospermia and RNA interference-mediated large-scale functional screening in Drosophila. *Hum Mol Genet*. 2015;24:1493–1503.

53. Ramanagoudr-Bhojappa R, Carrington B, Ramaswami M, et al. Multiplexed CRISPR/Cas9-mediated knockout of 19 Fanconi anemia pathway genes in zebrafish revealed their roles in growth, sexual development and fertility. *PLoS Genet*. 2018;14:e1007821.

54. Jamsai D, O'Bryan MK. Mouse models in male fertility research. *Asian J Androl*. 2011;13:139–151.

55. Geister KA, Timms AE, Beier DR. Optimizing genomic methods for mapping and identification of candidate variants in ENU mutagenesis screens using inbred mice. *G3 (Bethesda)*. 2018;8:401–409.

56. Kennedy CL, O'Bryan MK. N-ethyl-N-nitrosourea (ENU) mutagenesis and male fertility research. *Hum Reprod Update*. 2006;12:293–301.

57. De Jonge C, Barratt CLR. The present crisis in male reproductive health: an urgent need for a political, social, and research roadmap. *Andrology*. 2019;7:762–768.

58. Tuttelmann F, Ruckert C, Ropke A. Disorders of spermatogenesis: perspectives for novel genetic diagnostics after 20 years of unchanged routine. *Med Genet*. 2018;30:12–20.

59. Smith ED, Radtke K, Rossi M, et al. Classification of genes: standardized clinical validity assessment of gene-disease associations aids diagnostic exome analysis and reclassifications. *Hum Mutat*. 2017;38:600–608.

60. Strande NT, Riggs ER, Buchanan AH, et al. Evaluating the clinical validity of gene-disease associations: an evidence-based framework developed by the clinical genome resource. *Am J Hum Genet*. 2017;100:895–906.

61. Laan M. Systematic review of the monogenetic causes of male infertility: the first step towards diagnostic gene panels in the andrology clinic. *Hum Reprod*. 2019;34:783–785.

Section 2 The Biology of Male Reproduction and Infertility

Chapter 9: The Mechanistic and Predictive Utility of Sperm Epigenetics

Timothy G. Jenkins

9.1 Introduction

In the past, the male contribution to fertility and offspring health has been largely overlooked.

However, in recent years, sperm epigenetic signatures and their ties to fertility outcomes have received a great deal of attention in the literature. Many findings in the past few decades have contributed to this interest. Among the most compelling reasons for studying the male's contribution to fertility and offspring health are the data regarding the steady decline in fertility in men. In fact, recent studies have shown that sperm counts and other notable metrics for male fertility have been falling for many decades [1]. In one recent systematic review, it was found that sperm counts have fallen by nearly half over the past 40 years [2]. It is not surprising then that as many as 15% of couples experience infertility and approximately 50% of these cases have some male factor contribution [3]. Compounding the issues of rapidly declining fertility in men, because of social and economic pressures, couples are waiting longer to attempt conception and thus advancing paternal age is an increasingly common issue. Of particular interest to individuals studying sperm epigenetics are epidemiological studies that have linked these patterns of advancing paternal age to various neuropsychiatric abnormalities in the offspring [4]. Taken as a whole the data quite clearly demonstrate that the male contribution to fertility extends beyond the delivery of the paternal genome to the egg.

This recent emphasis on male infertility has brought to light a long known but not thoroughly addressed issue in the field. Simply put, we don't have an ideal method to assess, in a clinically meaningful way, male infertility. While clinicians and andrology labs can and do perform basic semen analyses often, the results from these analyses are poorly correlated with reproductive outcomes for a couple. The glaring exception to this rule is a diagnosis of azoospermia. Outside of this diagnosis however, the vast majority of findings and diagnoses provided based on semen analysis data are not useful in predicting the most meaningful endpoint of attempted conception (with or without assisted reproductive technologies), namely a viable pregnancy. If any sperm are present, even if those sperm are of low quality (by our conventional motility/morphology-based approaches), there is a chance that the individual will be able to father a child. Further, in cases where basic semen analysis metrics look completely normal, it is not uncommon to find men who still are unable to yield a viable pregnancy. It is essential that we identify new and better targets for diagnosis for male infertility that are able to guide the clinical path of a couple or the individual patient. As of today, findings on a semen analysis are rarely meaningful in clinical management. However, there are multiple intriguing new lines of research focused on the development of improved male fertility diagnostics. Among the most promising candidates for this purpose are epigenetic alterations to sperm as these are modifiable throughout life, can exist even in "normal" sperm (based on standard clinical assessments), and have the potential to be passed on to the offspring.

This chapter will provide important background information on the sperm epigenetic marks, how they are unique, and what opportunities and challenges they present in their study. Unique marks in the sperm such as DNA methylation, nuclear proteins and associated modifications, and various RNA species will all be described. Further, the chapter will discuss what we have learned from a great deal of work assessing these marks and, just as important, what we have yet to learn.

9.2 The Unique Sperm Epigenetic Landscape

9.2.1 DNA Methylation

DNA methylation occurs in all cell types in mammals and is a key gene regulator of human gene activity. This modification is the addition of a methyl group to the 5 carbon of cytosine residues in the DNA specifically in the context of cytosine phosphate guanine dinucleotides (CpGs). The importance of this CpG context is seen in the fact methylation (or lack thereof) at a C in the CG dinucleotide pair typically occurs on both strands of the DNA. This is possible because the antiparallel complementary base paring of the CG sequence on one strand is also a CG sequence on the complementary strand (both being read 5' to 3'). This mark can thus be maintained throughout DNA replication. DNA methylation is thought to play many roles in terms of gene regulation but is most often described as having an inhibitory affect when present at gene promoters where it is able to block transcriptional machinery. Importantly, this mark is sensitive to many different epigenetic modifiers and can be altered throughout the lifetime of an individual and impact cellular and organismal phenotypes.

The sperm methylome is among the most unique of any cell type. It can be easily distinguished from all somatic cell types and behaves significantly different than does somatic tissue when exposed to various epigenetic modifiers (aging, toxin exposures, etc.). This is particularly important in the study of DNA methylation marks in sperm. While DNA methylation in all cell types is highly polarized with most CpGs either being highly methylated (>80%) or unmethylated (<20%), the polarization is even more exaggerated in sperm where intermediate methylation levels are quite rare. As one example of the unique nature of sperm DNA methylation signatures, through the aging process the modifications that occur to DNA methylation are entirely distinct in sperm and in somatic cells. In fact, while aging causes a global reduction in DNA methylation levels in somatic tissue on average and a bias toward increased methylation locally with age, the exact opposite appears to be true in sperm. In the male gamete there is a marked increase in average methylation globally and a bias toward methylation loss locally with age [5,6]. These unique marks have made the study of DNA methylation in sperm both extremely informative and challenging.

Sperm DNA methylation has been demonstrated in many studies to be associated with various forms of infertility. This has been shown in both animal models and in humans. Targeted studies using the DNA methyltransferase blocking compound 5-azacytidine and 5-deoxycytodine have established that a shotgun approach to generating sperm DNA methylation perturbations in mice results at a minimum in reduced fertility, increased incidence of embryo mortality, reduced fertilization rates, and increased preimplantation loss [7]. The impacts on offspring and fertilization are compelling evidence that sperm DNA methylation patterns play a vital role in not only the production of sperm, but in their competence to generate a viable pregnancy. Additional studies in humans have found that patients with specific semen analysis metrics (reduced motility, morphology, or count) also appear to have distinct abnormalities in their sperm DNA methylation signatures [8]. Still other studies have found that reduced fecundity is associated with specific DNA methylation alterations in sperm at two related genes, HSP1L and HSP1B [9]. Further studies have also found DNA methylation alterations, specifically at imprinted loci, are associated with male infertility phenotypes [10].

It is clear that sperm DNA methylation signatures are both highly unique and extremely important for normal sperm function including fertilization and embryo development. Despite the clear link, to date there is very little data that enables us to understand the mechanism that drives the link between DNA methylation signatures and particular fertility phenotypes. More work needs to be done to elucidate why certain regions of the DNA methylome are altered with certain phenotypes and if these associations are clinically meaningful.

9.2.2 Nuclear Proteins

Likely the most striking epigenetic feature in mammalian sperm is the incorporation of protamine proteins into the chromatin. These proteins are only found in sperm and are essential for the incredibly tight compaction that occurs in the sperm nucleus. This condensation event creates a nuclear structure that is as much as 20 times more compact than histone bound chromatin [7]. The protamination process (the replacement of histone proteins with protamines), occurs in a stepwise fashion during spermatogenesis in humans where histones are first replaced by transition proteins and transition proteins are replaced by protamine 1 (P1) and protamine 2 (P2). Both P1 and P2 are incorporated in equal amounts into the mature sperm (in a ratio of 1:1) and any alteration to this ratio appears to be detrimental to chromatin compaction and subsequent fertility [11]. While extremely unique and essential for normal sperm function, it is important to note that removal of histones is not without consequence as histones are important regulators of gene activity. Histone tail modifications are capable of affecting gene transcription in multiple ways. These modifications come in many forms including methylation, phosphorylation, ubiquitination, and acetylation, all of which are able to affect gene activity depending on their location.

While the replacement of histones with protamines is essential to normal sperm function, it is well known that this process is not complete. In fact, between 5 and 15% of the genome remains nucleosome/histone bound [12]. This small amount of retention leaves open the possibility that sperm may be capable of handing down important histones with their associated tail modifications to the offspring. This is supported by the fact that the distribution of retained histones is not random in nature but that these loci of histone retention are enriched at sites important in development [13]. Interestingly, the distribution of these histones is that their respective marks closely reflect those seen in the embryonic stem cells. Specifically, sperm contain bivalent histone modifications at developmental promoters, which is highly suggestive that the sperm nuclear proteins actually do contribute epigenetic marks to early embryogenesis.

Based on the above information, it is not surprising to note that alterations to histones or protamines in sperm result in significant alterations and various forms of infertility. A common assessment of nuclear proteins in sperm is a protamine ratio analysis. Effectively, both P1 and P2 are quantified and the ratio of P1 to P2 compared. In patients with impaired fertility, abnormal P1:P2 ratios are common. Specifically, it has been shown that in severe forms of male infertility, there is a significant amount of variability in protamine content between sperm cells. This alteration in protamine content results in decreased viability and decreased DNA integrity. These are understandable outcomes as the alterations seen therein likely lead to a less compacted DNA that is thus more susceptible to damage from a variety of sources. It has been suggested that a portion of these alterations is driven by abnormal protamine expression and even novel polymorphisms in protamine genes [14]. The protamines are not the only nuclear proteins that can be altered to yield abnormal sperm. Abnormal histone retention patterns are also related to various infertility forms. Specifically, it has been shown that abnormal histone retention patterns at developmental and imprinted genes are more frequently seen in the sperm of infertile men.

It is clear that nuclear protein content is tightly regulated in sperm and needed for both the safe delivery of the paternal genome to the oocyte and proper embryogenesis. Thus, even small modifications to this important epigenetic mark can result in significant abnormalities in the sperm and the embryo.

9.2.3 RNAs

The most widely distributed and variable aspect of the sperm epigenome are the various RNA species. While not as easy to study as some of the other marks presented in the chapter, microRNAs and other unique RNA species offer the profound possibility of targeted and well-controlled studies of mechanisms, something that is not possible with current technologies with DNA methylation and histone retention/modification. For this reason, these small molecules provide some of the most exciting opportunities for diagnostics and interventions in male infertility. While not a tremendous amount of data is currently available, the volume of studies is ever increasing and is painting an interesting and highly complex story.

One of the keys to understanding the role of RNAs in male infertility is their origin. Many studies have assessed the role of various RNA species in various reproductive tissues including mature sperm, testes, seminal plasma, and in the epididymis [15]. The distribution of RNAs in these various tissues is quite distinct and the findings from each tissue are important to sperm function and male fertility in general for different reasons. Among many interesting developing stories in the search for ties to fertility and offspring health is that of epididymal RNAs and RNAs found in exosomes of the epididymis (termed epididymosomes). Epididymosomes have become a recent area of interest as a result of studies that have begun to suggest that there is a link between various noncoding RNA (ncRNA) species found within the epididymosome and the potential role these play in embryo health/competency and in epigenetic inheritance patterns whose mechanisms have long been elusive [16]. This work is at the cutting edge of male fertility studies as well as studies of transgenerational inheritance and thus requires special attention moving forward. A thorough review of the current state of knowledge and the directions being taken forward for epididymal and epididymosomal RNAs is found in a recent review by James et al. [16].

Various RNA species in the mature sperm represent potentially the most logical and straightforward place to assess for links to different forms of male infertility. While a great deal has been learned, much like other epigenetic areas of interest, there is still much work that needs to be done and the data are still incomplete. It is clear that certain small noncoding RNAs are consistently present in the mature sperm and that this can be altered in certain types of infertility. Among the most common microRNA found in sperm is the family of mir-34 and most notably mir 34-c. Multiple studies have identified this miRNA in sperm and have suggested that it has the most prominent small RNA [15]. However, the data surrounding the utility of this transcript have been called into question with some reporting it as being essential to embryogenesis (specifically the first cleavage) and others suggesting that it is not needed [15]. Interestingly, a recent report suggested that it is not the presence of any single RNA that matters for the downstream functionality of the sperm (competence to fertilize and coordinate embryogenesis) [17]. Instead, it has been proposed that fertility is reliant on a large group of RNA elements in the sperm and not a disproportionate contribution from a single RNA. These studies have shown that if the entire group of RNA elements is not present in the sperm, then fertility decline is likely. This would also help to explain the lack of findings for a single particular RNA or a small handful of RNA species that alone drive fertility.

Previously held beliefs that RNA species in the mature sperm were largely the remanent of what was present during spermatogenesis and maturation in the epididymis have been largely overcome. The current body of literature establishes that this outdated view was limited in scope and that RNAs in sperm appear to drive or contribute to many important processes in the sperm and the embryo. A further description of how powerful this relationship may be can be found in the discussion of clinical utility in Section 9.3.

9.3 Clinical Utility

A key endpoint to any study of molecular or genetic biomarkers of complex disease is implementation, utility, and efficacy in the clinic. The study of male infertility and ties to embryogenesis and offspring health is no different. The study of this complex disease is particularly important as it is on the rise both in terms of severity and incidence and as such needs improved tools for diagnosis, treatment, and prevention. However, the current body of literature on sperm epigenetic patterns has yet to yield extremely clear and concise mechanistic insights into disease etiology. This is not surprising as it is extremely difficult to study the mechanisms of infertility when the cell being studied is quiescent and the outcome of the complex disease in question is the formation of a unique and genetically independent tissue to which two cells from different individuals contribute. Despite the challenges, a great deal of work has repeatedly established that a relationship between sperm epigenetic signatures and fertility outcomes does exist, though the nature of the relationship still requires elucidation.

The distinction between a mechanistic understanding and predictive capacity is important in this discussion as many are reluctant to implement clinical tests if they do not first understand the mechanism that drives the predictive capacity of a diagnostic. However, these mechanisms are difficult to define in sperm as mentioned above and while concrete mechanisms involving epigenetic marks driving infertility have been elusive, the predictive capacity of sperm epigenetic signatures is becoming more and more clear. By no means is this effort complete, nor are there firmly established tools available today that are able to predict with a high degree of accuracy the likelihood of success that any given couple may have in IVF based on epigenetic signatures alone. However, consistent and measurable progress is being made toward predative models that may significantly improve male factor infertility diagnosis.

Two major lines of questioning are beginning to bring us closer to the above realization, namely a tool that is able to aid in clinical decision-making for patients with male factor infertility. One is a focus on RNA and the other on DNA methylation. Each has distinct advantages and drawbacks. Among the most promising studies using RNA is that assessing the utility of RNA elements in predicting fertility outcomes [17]. In a recent study, Jodar et al. found that the likelihood of achieving a pregnancy with timed intercourse or intrauterine insemination when missing any of the required RNA elements in the sperm decreased significantly (from 73% to 27%). However, this could be overcome with the use of in vitro fertilization. Thus, if such a signal was repeatable and implementable in clinic this type of information could guide patients' decision-making with moving directly to IVF and, regardless of the results, could save patients time and money. In a similar study using sperm DNA methylation, Aston et al. utilized machine-learning techniques to identify specific patterns that were seen in IVF patients compared to sperm donors [18]. The results of the study also suggested that embryo quality may be able to be predicted with sperm DNA methylation signatures in the absence of female factors. Further data in couples with no known fertility issues also found distinct epigenetic signatures at specific genomic loci that were associated with time to pregnancy [9]. Taken together it is clear that there is a great degree of potential for this work in generating viable diagnostic tests.

9.4 Conclusion: What We Know, What We Don't, and Where We Go from Here

It is clear from the above examples that progress is being made toward the realization of creating new and improved diagnostics for male factor infertility. However, there are still tremendous gaps in knowledge regarding the nature of the relationship between sperm epigenetic marks and infertility phenotypes. Indeed, we do not know if the alterations we have been able to detect are in some way causative or if these are simply correlations (Figure 9.1). Despite the incomplete nature of the story to date, it is likely that we will have opportunities to predict outcomes in the near future. The question then becomes: Are we willing to accept a predictive test for which we don't fully understand the mechanism that drives the process?

One interesting recent example exists with sperm epigenetics and aging, though implementation has largely been in research and not in the clinic. In 2014 we identified specific sites in the sperm epigenome that become altered throughout the aging process [6]. However, we have not been able to define the exact mechanism that causes this modification – we have only been able to prove that it occurs consistently. Without understanding the mechanism fully, using machine learning we were able to apply what we learned in 2014 to construct an age prediction model for sperm specifically that is highly reliable and can predict an individual's age with ~94% accuracy with only sperm DNA methylation signatures [19]. This

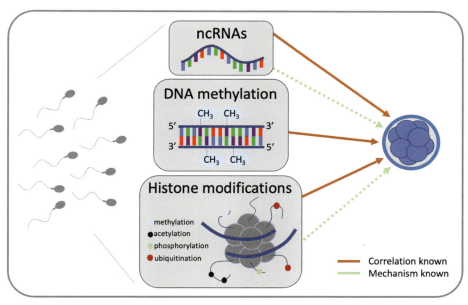

Figure 9.1 Descriptive chart illustrating what is known about the impacts of various epigenetic modifications in sperm and their association with fertility outcomes (including embryogenesis). In effect, while we have defined a number of associations between the epigenetic marks in sperm and fertility, clear mechanisms involving the sperm epigenome that cause poor fertility outcomes have not been elucidated.

calculation has been highly useful in research studies and similar calculators exist and are used in research studies for somatic cells as well. Despite the widespread use, we still do not know what drives these signatures or if they can be modified in any way.

As studies continue to move forward, there will be a time when decisions need to be made among clinicians as to whether or not certain diagnostics are worth implementing in clinical workflow. For the improvement of male factor infertility diagnostics, we must decide how much accuracy in prediction is required to be useful and if predictive power in the absence of mechanistic understanding is enough. The bar for male factor infertility diagnostics is currently quite low, but that does not mean that subpar new diagnostics are ok simply because they offer a slight or even perceived improvement. Instead, it is imperative that significant effort is made in putting together all aspects of male fertility assessment and capturing as large a number of sample sizes as possible to identify the ideal and most efficacious diagnostic testing pipelines. This will require a great degree of collaborative efforts from many different experts to truly improve the current state of male fertility diagnosis and treatment. The potential for increased predictive power is clear, but a great degree of work still needs to be performed particularly when it is unlikely that the mechanistic underpinnings of sperm epigenetics and links to fertility will be fully understood in the near future.

Disclosures:
Timothy G. Jenkins is a shareholder in Inherent Biosciences (an epigenetics company) and Advanced Conceptions (a microfluidics company specializing in sperm isolation).

References

1. Sengupta P, Borges E, Dutta S, Krajewska-Kulak E. Decline in sperm count in European men during the past 50 years. *Hum Exp Toxicol*. 2018;37(3):247–255.
2. Levine H, Jørgensen N, Martino-Andrade A, et al. Temporal trends in sperm count: a systematic review and meta-regression analysis. *Hum Reprod Update*. 2017;23(6):646–659.
3. Ravitsky V, Kimmins S. The forgotten men: rising rates of male infertility urgently require new approaches for its prevention, diagnosis and treatment. *Biol Reprod*. 2019;101(5):872–874.
4. Jenkins TG, Aston KI, Carrell DT. Sperm epigenetics and aging. *Transl Androl Urol*. 2018. 7(Suppl 3):S328–S335.
5. Johnson AA, Akman K, Calimport SRG, et al. The role of DNA methylation in aging, rejuvenation, and age-related disease. *Rejuvenation Res*. 2012;15(5):483–494.
6. Jenkins TG, Aston KI, Pflueger C, Cairns BR, Carrell DT. Age-associated sperm DNA methylation alterations: possible implications in offspring disease susceptibility. *PLoS Genet*. 2014;10(7):e1004458.
7. Jenkins TG, Carrell DT. The sperm epigenome and potential implications for the developing embryo. *Reproduction*. 2012;143(6):727–734.
8. Jenkins TG, Aston KI, Hotaling JM, Shamsi MB, Simon L, Carrell DT. Teratozoospermia and asthenozoospermia are associated with specific epigenetic signatures. *Andrology*. 2016;4(5):843–849.
9. Jenkins TG, Aston KI, Meyer TD, et al. Decreased fecundity and sperm DNA methylation patterns. *Fertil Steril*. 2016;105(1):51–7-e1–3.
10. Nanassy L, Carrell DT. Analysis of the methylation pattern of six gene promoters in sperm of men with abnormal protamination. *Asian J Androl*. 2011;13(2):342–346.
11. Aoki VW, Emery BR, Liu L, Carrell DT. Protamine levels vary between individual sperm cells of infertile human males and correlate with viability and DNA integrity. *J Androl*. 2006;27(6):890–898.
12. Wykes SM, Krawetz SA. The structural organization of sperm chromatin. *J Biol Chem*. 2003;278(32):29471–29477.
13. Hammoud SS, Nix DA, Zhang H, Purwar J, Carrell DT, Cairns BR. Distinctive chromatin in human sperm packages genes for embryo development. *Nature*. 2009;460(7254):473–478.
14. Aoki VW, Liu L, Carrell DT. A novel mechanism of protamine expression deregulation highlighted by abnormal protamine transcript retention in infertile human males with sperm protamine deficiency. *Mol Hum Reprod*. 2006;12(1):41–50.
15. Salas-Huetos A, James ER, Aston KI, Carrell DT, Jenkins TG, Yeste M. The role of miRNAs in male human reproduction: a systematic review. *Andrology*. 2020;8(1):7–26.
16. James ER, Carrell DT, Aston KI, Jenkins TG, Yeste M, Salas-Huetos A. The role of the epididymis and the contribution of epididymosomes to mammalian reproduction. *Int J Mol Sci*. 2020;21(15):5377.
17. Jodar M, Sendler E, Moskovtsev SI, et al. Absence of sperm RNA elements correlates with idiopathic male infertility. *Sci Transl Med*. 2015;7(295):295re6.
18. Aston KI, Uren PJ, Jenkins TG, et al. Aberrant sperm DNA methylation predicts male fertility status and embryo quality. *Fertil Steril*. 2015;104(6):1388–1397 e1–5.
19. Jenkins TG, Aston KI, Cairns B, Smith A, Carrell DT. Paternal germ line aging: DNA methylation age prediction from human sperm. *BMC Genomics*. 2018;19(1):763.

Section 2 The Biology of Male Reproduction and Infertility

Chapter 10: Aging and Environmental Interactions with the Sperm Epigenome

Albert Salas-Huetos and Douglas T. Carrell

10.1 Introduction

In the early 1940s, Conrad Waddington introduced the term epigenetics to describe the branch of biology that studies the causal interactions between genes and their products that bring the phenotype into being [1,2]. Over the following years, the definition of epigenetics has been redefined and today is generally accepted as the study of heritable factors, other than DNA base pair coding, that regulate gene expression [3]. The main difference is the introduction of the term heritable, because in that sense, epigenetic alterations not only can affect the health of the primary individuals but also can affect the future progeny via transgenerational effects.

In this chapter, we briefly review the main epigenetic factors that exist in spermatozoa (e.g., histone and chromatin modifications, DNA methylation, and noncoding RNAs [ncRNAs]) and underline the associations and effects of aging, adiposity, and some lifestyle and environmental factors on the sperm epigenome.

10.2 Sperm Epigenome

From sperm homunculus (seventeenth century) conception to the actual knowledge of the sperm cell, a lot of reproductive theories have been refuted [4]. Only two decades before, for instance, there was the misconception that the sperm only had one function, to deliver the paternal DNA to the oocyte. However, nowadays we know that the male gamete is a very differentiated cell with specialized functions that carry hundreds of RNA molecules, proteins, and methylation signatures. The scientific society acknowledges that sperm cells have a unique epigenome that allows the essential functions of this cell and early embryogenesis [5]. The main epigenetic factors that exist in spermatozoa are histone and chromatin modifications, DNA methylation, and ncRNAs (Figure 10.1).

10.2.1 Histone and Chromatin Modifications

Histones are highly conserved proteins in mammals that can become post-translationally modified at amino acid residues located on their N- and C-terminal tails. There are four core histones: histone 2A (H2A), histone 2B (H2B), histone 3 (H3), and histone 4 (H4), and one linker histone, histone 1 (H1) [6]. The DNA in somatic cells is usually compacted with repeating structural (and functional) units of chromatin, formatting the nucleosome. However, the DNA in spermatozoa is organized in a different way, mainly wrapped around protamines (protamine 1; PRM1 and protamine 2; PRM2) instead of histones. Protamines are arginine-rich, nuclear proteins essential for sperm head ultra-condensation and DNA stabilization. However, spermatic DNA is not 100% compacted with protamines, in fact, during mammalian spermatogenesis, sperm cells undergo dramatic chromatin structural rearrangements and approximately 85–90% of histones are replaced by protamines [7]. Importantly, this distribution of protamine–histone compaction is nonrandom in human sperm [8]. Some studies demonstrate that gene sequences and repetitive elements that have the potential to be involved in the early embryo are mainly less compacted (histone-compacted) [9,10].

10.2.2 DNA Methylation

DNA methylation is a heritable epigenetic mark involving the covalent transfer of a methyl group (CH_3) to the cytosine ring of DNA. This process is regulated by the DNA methyltransferases (DNMTs) family: DNMT1, DNMT2, DNMT3A, DNMT3B, and DNMT3L [11]. Methylation is a critical modification that provides regulation of tissue-specific gene expression patterns. In mammalian development, DNA methylation is typically removed during zygote formation and then reestablished during implantation. In human sperm, the methylome is highly homogeneous and relatively hypermethylated in comparison to the hypomethylated patterns seen in oocytes [12]. A recent meta-analytic study demonstrated a strong association between male infertility and alterations in sperm methylation at *H19*, *MEST*, and *SNRPN*.

10.2.3 Noncoding RNAs

An ncRNA is a functional RNA molecule that is transcribed from DNA but not translated into proteins and includes microRNAs (miRNAs), piwiRNAs (piRNAs), long noncoding RNAs (lncRNAs), and tRNA fragments (tRFs).

10.2.3.1 miRNAs

The miRNAs are small transcripts of 21–26 nucleotides that form imperfect complementary stem-loop structures in the 3' untranslated region of their target messenger RNA (mRNA) [13]. The canonical biogenesis pathway is the dominant

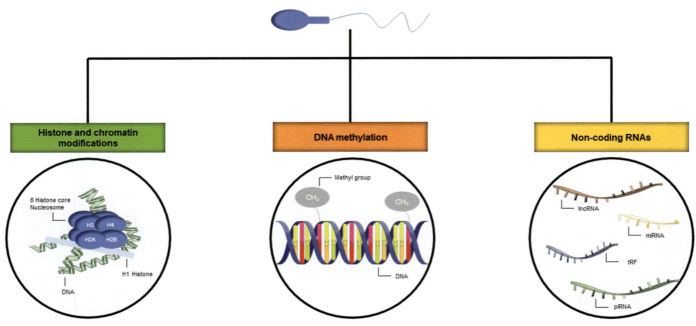

Figure 10.1 Representation of the main epigenetic factors that exist in spermatozoa: histone and chromatin modifications, DNA methylation, and ncRNAs (long noncoding RNAs, lncRNAs; microRNAs, miRNAs; transfer RNA-derived RNA fragments, tRFs; and piwi-RNAs, piRNAs).

pathway by which miRNAs are processed and begins with the generation of the pri-miRNA transcript. The complex Drosha-DGCR8 cleaves the pri-miRNA to produce the 60–70-nt miRNA precursor (pre-miRNA). The pre-miRNA is then exported to the cytoplasm via Exportin 5 and processed to produce the mature miRNA duplex. The miRNA function is performed by miRNA-induced silencing complex (miRISC) that contains the Argonaute (AGO) family proteins [14]. Until now, 1,982 miRNAs have been identified in humans (miRBase v.22.1; www.mirbase.org) [15] and more than 220 are consistently present in human sperm [16].

10.2.3.2 piRNAs

The piRNAs are approximately 30 nucleotides in length expressed during spermatogenesis, mostly in spermatids. piRNAs are associated with MIWI (murine [mouse] ortholog), a spermatogenesis-specific PIWI (P-element induced WImpy testis in Drosophila) subfamily member of the AGO family [17]. The main difference between miRNAs and piRNAs is their biogenesis (although this is not yet fully understood in humans) and associated proteins. It is likely that piRNAs are derived from either the repeated DNA sequence elements or complex DNA sequence elements [18]. Nowadays, up to 8 million piRNAs have been identified in humans (piRBase v.2.0; www.regulatoryrna.org/database/piRNA/index.html) [19] and approximately 1,000 are present in human sperm [20].

10.2.3.3 lncRNAs

The lncRNAs are defined as nonprotein-coding transcripts longer than 200 nucleotides that can interact with DNA, other RNAs, and proteins, including epigenetic modifiers [21]. Some lncRNAs are related to genomic imprinting and are associated with chromatin-modifying complexes that can regulate gene transcription in spermatogenesis of mammals [22]. The biogenesis of lncRNAs is cell type and stage type specific and are transcribed by RNA Polymerase II/III at several loci of the genome. Depending on the origin different lncRNAs nomenclatures exist: enhancer associated, promoter associated, exonic/sense, long intergenic, or antisense lncRNAs [23]. Until now, 127,802 lncRNAs have been identified in humans (LNCpedia v.5.2; https://lncipedia.org/) [24], and specifically in human sperm, more than 57,000 lncRNAs [25].

10.2.3.4 tRFs

The tRFs are approximately 14–30 nucleotides in length generated from precursor tRNA (pre-tRNA), which contain extra bases at their 5′- and 3′-ends called leader and trailer sequences, and usually cleaved by RNase Z [26]. Finally, a nontemplated single "CCA" sequence is added to the 3′-ends of the trailer-free tRNAs by the enzyme tRNA nucleotidyl transferase and mature tRFs are exported to the cytoplasm with the help of a nuclear export receptor [27]. Currently, 28,824 tRFs have been identified in humans (MINTbase v.2.0; https://cm.jefferson.edu/MINTbase) [28] and about 1,900 tRFs were contained in mature human sperm [29]. tRFs are scarce in testicular sperm, but are gained as sperm mature in the epididymis due to the action of epididymosomes [30].

The main epigenetic elements contained in sperm (ncRNAs) and the different modifications and signatures (histone/chromatin modifications and DNA methylation) demonstrate extreme plasticity throughout spermatogenesis as a consequence of cellular reprogramming and have also been shown to be modifiable by age, adiposity, lifestyle, and environmental factors as will be discussed in this chapter.

10.3 Age

Nowadays most people can expect to live into their 60s and beyond [31]. When we combine the highest life expectancy with falling fertility rates and decline in sperm quality [32], the populations around the world are suffering a rapid aging [33].

In terms of the relation between aging and sperm epigenome, a study conducted in 2014 in 17 fertile sperm donors who provided samples in the 1990s and then again in 2008, identified 139 differentially hypomethylated regions and 8 hypermethylated regions associated with age. The authors also revealed that sperm DNA methylation changes were located at genes previously associated with schizophrenia and bipolar disorder, establishing the first non-causative relationship between paternal aging and the incidence of neuropsychiatric and other disorders in offspring [34]. The same group also analyzed 16 patients with older (>40 years of age) paternal grandfathers and 16 patients with younger (<25 years of age) grandfathers to investigate if the age-associated sperm DNA methylation patterns persist transgenerationally. The authors found an extremely small trend toward a lower sperm DNA methylation change present between the young grandfather paternal age and old grandfather paternal age groups that resemble the aging pattern in older sperm. However, the authors concluded that these changes could be almost biologically inert [35].

To our knowledge, only one study has been published investigating the association between aging and miRNAs expression. The authors found a single miRNA (hsa-miR-34b-3p) that was positively associated with age, in a cohort of 40 semen samples from different fertile (n = 10) and infertile individuals (n = 30) [36]. This relationship between aging and miRNA expression (higher expression in older individuals) is in line with the results in DNA methylation studies.

10.4 Adiposity

It is well-known that unhealthy adiposity is related with several diseases like cancers and cardiovascular diseases, among others [37]. Moreover, a recent systematic review and meta-analysis undoubtedly indicated that overweight, obesity, and underweight categories were associated with lower sperm quality [38], suggesting that maintaining a healthy body weight is critical for male fertility. However, the associations/effects of adiposity on the sperm epigenome are still a matter of debate [39].

The latest results in humans come from a cohort of 69 healthy volunteers comparing some sperm DNA methylation signatures (*MEG3-IG, MEG3, PEG1/MEST, IGF2, H19, GRB10, NNAT, NDN, SNRPN, SGCE/PEG10, PEG3*, and *PLAGL1*) of obese/overweight volunteers (n = 23) versus normal weight men (n = 46). This study suggested that male overweight/obesity status is traceable in the sperm epigenome, because after adjusting for age and fertility patient status, semen from overweight/obese men had significantly lower methylation percentages at the *MEG3, NDN, SNRPN*, and *SGCE/PEG10*, and a slight increase at the *MEG3-IG* and *H19* regions [40]. Moreover, an experimental mouse study comparing the miRNA expression profile of mice fed either a high-fat diet (n = 10), inducing paternal obesity with a 21% increase in adiposity, or a control diet (n = 10) for a period of 10 weeks reveals that expression of 11 miRNAs were affected in the testis of the F0-generation mice initiating metabolic disturbances in the next two generations and altering the transcriptional profile of testis and sperm [41]. Future studies investigating sperm epigenetic aberrations due to paternal adiposity status are warranted.

10.5 Lifestyle and Environmental Factors

Several studies and meta-regression analyses reported a significant decline in sperm counts (~50–60% decline) between 1973 and 2011 in certain geographic regions of the world (e.g., Australia, New Zealand, Europe, and North America) [32,42]. Therefore, more research on causes of this decline is urgently needed. There are multiple possible causes of this decline; the most plausible seems to be related to environmental and lifestyle factors such as diet and smoking.

10.5.1 Diet

Several observational studies, systematic reviews, and meta-analysis suggested that specific foods (e.g., fish, shellfish and seafood, poultry, cereals, vegetables and fruits, and low-fat dairy) [43,44], some nutrients and dietary supplements (e.g., omega-3, CoQ10, selenium, zinc, and carnitines) [43,45], and some dietary patterns (e.g., the Mediterranean diet) [43,46] may improve male sperm quality parameters.

However, only a few studies have been published assessing the impact of diet on the sperm epigenetic signatures. The effect of some nutrients, like folic acid and vitamin D, special diets (e.g., high-fat or low-protein diets), and foods (e.g., nuts) were analyzed in nine different studies in mammals, including humans [47–55].

In terms of nutrient intake, only one study tested the effect of vitamin D on the mice sperm epigenome [47]. The authors revealed that depletion of vitamin D for five weeks prior to mating mice resulted in 15,827 differentially sperm methylated loci (69% loss of methylation), mainly localized in regions enriched for developmental and metabolic genes and pathways. On the other hand, four different studies tested the effect of folic acid supplementation in sperm epigenome. Firstly, Lambrot and collaborators described that low paternal dietary folate not only alters the mouse sperm epigenome but also is associated with negative pregnancy outcomes. Compared with folate sufficient males, mice receiving a folate-deficient diet displayed alteration of 57 genomic regions [48]. However, in humans, low-dose folic acid supplementation has very little or no effect on human sperm DNA methylation in either short-term (90 days) or long-term exposures [49]. In fact, some studies in humans revealed that the administration of a high daily dose of folic acid (up to 10 times the daily recommended dose) for six months can alter the sperm methylome but that could be influenced by the presence of the *MTHFR* C677T polymorphism [50,51].

Other authors suggested that special diets and dietary patterns can modulate the sperm epigenome. For example, Watkins and collaborators developed a mouse paternal low-protein diet model for eight weeks, and, compared with control mice, this diet leads to sperm global DNA hypomethylation associated with reduced testicular expression of DNA methylation and folate-cycle regulators. The authors also discovered that all offspring derived from paternal low-protein diet sperm and/or seminal plasma became heavier with increased adiposity, glucose intolerance, perturbed hepatic gene expression symptomatic of nonalcoholic fatty liver disease, and altered gut bacterial profiles [52]. This is not the only study suggesting there are some sperm epigenome regions/markers that could respond to diet with the potential to alter the offspring. In fact, Claycombe-Larson et al. [53] in mice, and Nätt et al. [54] in humans recently described that human sperm shows rapid responses involving several sperm miRNAs expression and/or concentration to different diets.

To the best of our knowledge, the only foods that have been tested in humans are in the context of the FERTINUTS randomized clinical trial (RCT) study with nuts [55]. The FERTINUTS study was a 14-week RCT parallel trial with a total of 119 healthy men. The healthy, nonsmoking men were allocated to one of two intervention groups: One group was fed the usual Western-style diet enriched with 60 g of a mixture of raw nuts/d (almonds, hazelnuts, and walnuts), and the other was fed the usual Western-style diet avoiding nuts. Interestingly, the researchers found an improvement of the main sperm quality parameters in the nuts group (e.g., sperm count, vitality, motility, and morphology), and also observed a significant reduction in the hsa-miR-34b-3p expression level in the group supplemented with nuts compared with the control group. Taken together, these results suggest that the sperm epigenome (mainly methylation and miRNAs) can be modulated by some diet supplementation or changes in the diet.

10.5.2 Smoking
Cigarettes are smoked by nearly 800 million men and smoking is considered a worldwide health problem because it has been demonstrated that it causes many diseases (cardiovascular and respiratory diseases, cancers, etc.). Moreover, some meta-analysis recently described that cigarette smoking also has an overall negative effect on semen parameters [56].

Presently only a few studies assessing the impact of cigarette smoking on the sperm epigenetic signature have been published. Regarding the miRNAs, one small case-control study (6 smokers and 7 nonsmokers human participants) described 28 miRNAs differentially expressed in smokers compared with nonsmokers. The researchers also described that the validated targets of the differentially expressed miRNAs were involved in cellular proliferation, differentiation, and cell death pathways [57]. Regarding the DNA methylation, in the last few years, two different groups have published some interesting works. On one hand, the Hammadeh group described significantly lower global sperm DNA methylation in nonsmokers (n = 54) compared with smoker individuals (n = 55) [58] and, in a smaller population (14 smokers and 14 proven nonsmokers) the same authors described 11 CpGs differentially methylated [59]. On the other hand, the Aston and collaborators group analyzed sperm DNA methylation patterns in 78 men who smoke and 78 nonsmokers and identified 141 significantly differentially methylated CpGs [60]. None of the groups described if the differentially methylated CpGs were associated with a specific biologic pathway. Finally, Aston and collaborators performed an experiment with cigarette smoking exposed versus nonexposed (n = 10–12) mice, in order to further explore the previous results. In that experiment the authors described that smoking induces DNA methylation changes in F0 sperm, and impacted DNA methylation and gene expression changes in F1 brains. Interestingly, the authors also used $Nrf2^{-/-}$ mice (the nuclear factor [erythroid-derived 2]-like 2 [*NRF2*] pathway is the primary cellular defense against the cytotoxic effects of oxidative stress) and described that the effects observed in cigarette smoking–exposed offspring are similar to those in $Nrf2^{-/-}$ offspring [61].

Taken together, these results suggest that smoking exposure could have negative reproductive epigenetic health consequences, not only for the exposed individuals, but also for the descendants of those who are exposed.

10.6 Conclusions
This chapter contributes in several ways to our understanding of the main epigenetic factors that exist in spermatozoa and the associations and effects of aging, adiposity, and some lifestyle and environmental factors on the sperm epigenome and provides a basis for new well-designed animal and human studies. Further work needs to be done to establish whether the changes of sperm epigenome triggered by aging, adiposity, diet, and smoking can have not only implications for reproductive health but also for future offspring.

Acknowledgments:
The authors would like to thank Servier Medical Art for its image bank used to assist the creation of Figure 10.1.

References

1. Waddington CH. The epigenotype. 1942. *Int J Epidemiol.* 2012;41(1):10–13.
2. Waddington CH. Towards a theoretical biology. *Nature.* 1968;218:525–527.
3. Santana V, Salas-Huetos A, James ER, Carrell DT. The effect of endocrine disruptors and environmental and lifestyle factors on the sperm epigenome. In: Aitken RJ, Mortimer D, Kovacs G, eds. *Male and Sperm Factors That Maximize IVF Success.* Cambridge University Press; 2020:41–58.
4. Jones RE, Lopez KH. *Human Reproductive Biology.* 4th ed. Academic Press; 2004.
5. Schagdarsurengin U, Paradowska A, Steger K. Analysing the sperm epigenome: roles in early embryogenesis and assisted reproduction. *Nat Rev Urol.* 2012;9(11):609–619.
6. Bowman GD, Poirier MG. Post-translational modifications of histones that influence nucleosome dynamics. *Chem Rev.* 2015;115(6):2274–2295.
7. Oliva R. Protamines and male infertility. *Hum Reprod Update.* 2006;12(4):417–435.
8. Oliva R, Castillo J, Estanyol J, Ballescà J. Human sperm chromatin epigenetic potential: genomics, proteomics, and male infertility. *Asian J Androl.* 2015;17(4):601–609.
9. Hammoud SS, Nix DA, Zhang H, Purwar J, Carrell DT, Cairns BR. Distinctive chromatin in human sperm packages genes for embryo development. *Nature.* 2009;460(7254):473–478.
10. Brykczynska U, Hisano M, Erkek S, et al. Repressive and active histone methylation mark distinct promoters in human and mouse spermatozoa. *Nat Struct Mol Biol.* 2010;17(6):679–687.
11. Jin B, Li Y, Robertson KD. DNA methylation: superior or subordinate in the epigenetic hierarchy? *Genes Cancer.* 2011;2(6):607–617.
12. Camprubí C, Cigliano RA, Salas-Huetos A, Garrido N, Blanco J. What the human sperm methylome tells us. *Epigenomics.* 2017;9(10):1299–1315.
13. Ha M, Kim VN. Regulation of microRNA biogenesis. *Nat Rev Mol Cell Biol [Internet].* 2014 [cited 2014 Jul 17];15(8):509–524. Available from: www.ncbi.nlm.nih.gov/pubmed/25027649
14. O'Brien J, Hayder H, Zayed Y, Peng C. Overview of microRNA biogenesis, mechanisms of actions, and circulation. *Front Endocrinol (Lausanne).* 2018;9:1–12.
15. Kozomara A, Griffiths-Jones S. miRBase: integrating microRNA annotation and deep-sequencing data. *Nucleic Acids Res.* 2011;39:D152–D157.
16. Salas-Huetos A, Blanco J, Vidal F, Mercader JM, Garrido N, Anton E. New insights into the expression profile and function of micro-ribonucleic acid in human spermatozoa. *Fertil Steril.* 2014;102(1):213–222.
17. Grivna ST, Beyret E, Wang Z, Lin H. A novel class of small RNAs in mouse spermatogenic cells. *Genes Dev.* 2006;20(13):1709–1714.
18. He Z, Kokkinaki M, Pant D, Gallicano GI, Dym M. Small RNA molecules in the regulation of spermatogenesis. *Reproduction.* 2009;137(6):901–911.
19. Wang J, Zhang P, Lu Y, et al. PiRBase: a comprehensive database of piRNA sequences. *Nucleic Acids Res.* 2019;47(D1):D175–D180.
20. Krawetz SA, Kruger A, Lalancette C, et al. A survey of small RNAs in human sperm. *Hum Reprod.* 2011;26(12):3401–3412.
21. Pedroso Ayub AL, D'Angelo Papaiz D, da Silva Soares R, Galvonas JM. The function of lncRNAs as epigenetic regulators. In: L Tutar, S Aras, E Tutar, eds. *Non-Coding RNAs.* IntechOpen; 2020:1–20.
22. Zhang X, Gao F, Fu J, Zhang P, Wang Y, Zeng X. Systematic identification and characterization of long non-coding RNAs in mouse mature sperm. *PLoS ONE.* 2017;12(3):e0173402.
23. Dahariya S, Paddibhatla I, Kumar S, Raghuwanshi S, Pallepati A, Gutti RK. Long non-coding RNA: classification, biogenesis and functions in blood cells. *Mol Immunol.* 2019;112:82–92.
24. Volders PJ, Anckaert J, Verheggen K, et al. Lncipedia 5: towards a reference set of human long non-coding RNAs. *Nucleic Acids Res.* 2019;47(D1):D135–D139.
25. Zhang X, Zhang P, Song D, et al. Expression profiles and characteristics of human lncRNA in normal and asthenozoospermia sperm. *Biol Reprod.* 2019;100(4):982–993.
26. Zhu L, Ge J, Li T, Shen Y, Guo J. tRNA-derived fragments and tRNA halves: the new players in cancers. *Cancer Lett [Internet].* 2019;452:31–37. Available from: doi.org/10.1016/j.canlet.2019.03.012
27. Kumar P, Kuscu C, Dutta A. Biogenesis and function of transfer RNA related fragments (tRFs). *Trends Biochem Sci.* 2016;41(8):679–689.
28. Pliatsika V, Loher P, Magee R, et al. MINTbase v2.0: a comprehensive database for tRNA-derived fragments that includes nuclear and mitochondrial fragments from all the Cancer Genome Atlas projects. *Nucleic Acids Res.* 2018;46(D1):D152–D159.
29. Hua M, Liu W, Chen Y, et al. Identification of small non-coding RNAs as sperm quality biomarkers for in vitro fertilization. *Cell Discov.* 2019;5(1):20.
30. Trigg NA, Eamens AL, Nixon B. The contribution of epididymosomes to the sperm small RNA profile. *Reproduction.* 2019;157:R209–R223.
31. Beard JR, Officer A, De Carvalho IA, et al. The world report on ageing and health: a policy framework for healthy ageing. *Lancet.* 2016;387(10033):2145–2154.
32. Levine H, Jørgensen N, Martino-Andrade A, et al. Temporal trends in sperm count: a systematic review and meta-regression analysis. *Hum Reprod Update.* 2017;23(6):646–659.
33. Vollset SE, Goren E, Yuan C, et al. Fertility, mortality, migration, and population scenarios for 195 countries and territories from 2017 to 2100: a forecasting analysis for the Global Burden of Disease Study. *Lancet.* 2020;396(10258):1285–1306.
34. Jenkins TG, Aston KI, Pflueger C, Cairns BR, Carrell DT. Age-associated sperm DNA methylation alterations: possible implications in offspring disease susceptibility. *PLoS Genet.* 2014;10(7):e1004458.
35. Jenkins TG, James ER, Aston KI, et al. Age-associated sperm DNA methylation patterns do not directly persist trans-generationally. *Epigenetics Chromatin.* 2019;12:74.
36. Salas-Huetos A, Blanco J, Vidal F, et al. Spermatozoa from patients with

seminal alterations exhibit a differential micro-ribonucleic acid profile. *Fertil Steril.* 2015;104(3):591–601.

37. Bhaskaran K, Douglas I, Forbes H, Dos-Santos-Silva I, Leon DA, Smeeth L. Body-mass index and risk of 22 specific cancers: a population-based cohort study of 5·24 million UK adults. *Lancet.* 2014;384(9945):755–765.

38. Salas-Huetos A, Maghsoumi-Norouzabad L, James ER, et al. Male adiposity, sperm parameters and reproductive hormones: an updated systematic review and collaborative meta-analysis. *Obes Rev.* 2021;22(1): e13082.

39. Craig JR, Jenkins TG, Carrell DT, Hotaling JM. Obesity, male infertility, and the sperm epigenome. *Fertil Steril.* 2017;107(4):848–859.

40. Soubry A, Guo L, Huang Z, et al. Obesity-related DNA methylation at imprinted genes in human sperm: results from the TIEGER study. *Clin Epigenetics.* 2016;8(1):1–11.

41. Fullston T, Ohlsson Teague EMC, Palmer NO, et al. Paternal obesity initiates metabolic disturbances in two generations of mice with incomplete penetrance to the F2 generation and alters the transcriptional profile of testis and sperm microRNA content. *FASEB J.* 2013;27(10):4226–4243.

42. Merzenich H, Zeeb H, Blettner M. Decreasing sperm quality: a global problem? *BMC Public Health.* 2010;10 (24):1–5.

43. Salas-Huetos A, Bulló M, Salas-Salvadó J. Dietary patterns, foods and nutrients in male fertility parameters and fecundability: a systematic review of observational studies. *Hum Reprod Update.* 2017;23(4):371–389.

44. Gaskins AJ, Chavarro JE. Diet and fertility: a review. *Am J Obstet Gynecol.* 2017;218(4):379–389.

45. Salas-Huetos A, Rosique-Esteban N, Becerra-Tomás N, Vizmanos B, Bulló M, Salas-Salvadó J. The effect of nutrients and dietary supplements on sperm quality parameters: a systematic review and meta-analysis of randomized clinical trials. *Adv Nutr An Int Rev J.* 2018;9(6):833–848.

46. Salas-Huetos A, Babio N, Carrell DT, Bulló M, Salas-Salvadó J. Adherence to the Mediterranean diet is positively associated with sperm motility: a cross-sectional analysis. *Sci Rep.* 2019;9 (1):3389.

47. Xue J, Gharaibeh RZ, Pietryk EW, et al. Impact of vitamin D depletion during development on mouse sperm DNA methylation. *Epigenetics.* 2018;13 (9):959–974.

48. Lambrot R, Xu C, Saint-Phar S, et al. Low paternal dietary folate alters the mouse sperm epigenome and is associated with negative pregnancy outcomes. *Nat Commun.* 2013;4:2889.

49. Chan D, McGraw S, Klein K, et al. Stability of the human sperm DNA methylome to folic acid fortification and short-term supplementation. *Hum Reprod.* 2017;32(2):272–283.

50. Aarabi M, Christensen KE, Chan D, et al. Testicular MTHFR deficiency may explain sperm DNA hypomethylation associated with high dose folic acid supplementation. *Hum Mol Genet.* 2018;27(7):1123–1135.

51. Aarabi M, San Gabrie MC, Chan D, et al. High-dose folic acid supplementation alters the human sperm methylome and is influenced by the MTHFR C677T polymorphism. *Hum Mol Genet.* 2015;24 (22):6301–6313.

52. Watkins AJ, Dias I, Tsuro H, et al. Paternal diet programs offspring health through sperm- and seminal plasma-specific pathways in mice. *Proc Natl Acad Sci U S A.* 2018;115 (40):10064–10069.

53. Claycombe-Larson KG, Bundy AN, Roemmich JN. Paternal high-fat diet and exercise regulate sperm miRNA and histone methylation to modify placental inflammation, nutrient transporter mRNA expression and fetal weight in a sex-dependent manner. *J Nutr Biochem.* 2020;81:108373.

54. Nätt D, Kugelberg U, Casas E, et al. Human sperm displays rapid responses to diet. *PLoS Biol.* 2019;17(12): e3000559.

55. Salas-Huetos A, Moraleda R, Giardina S, et al. Effect of nut consumption on semen quality and functionality in healthy men consuming a Western-style diet: a randomized controlled trial. *Am J Clin Nutr.* 2018;108(5):953–962.

56. Sharma R, Harlev A, Agarwal A, Esteves SC. Cigarette smoking and semen quality: a new meta-analysis examining the effect of the 2010 World Health Organization laboratory methods for the examination of human semen. *Eur Urol.* 2016;70(4):635–645.

57. Marczylo EL, Amoako AA, Konje JC, Gant TW, Marczylo TH. Smoking induces differential miRNA expression in human spermatozoa: a potential transgenerational epigenetic concern? *Epigenetics.* 2012;7(5):432–439.

58. Hamad MF, Dayyih WAA, Laqqan M, AlKhaled Y, Montenarh M, Hammadeh ME. The status of global DNA methylation in the spermatozoa of smokers and non-smokers. *Reprod Biomed Online.* 2018;37(5):581–589.

59. Alkhaled Y, Laqqan M, Tierling S, Lo Porto C, Amor H, Hammadeh ME. Impact of cigarette-smoking on sperm DNA methylation and its effect on sperm parameters. *Andrologia.* 2018;50 (4):e12950.

60. Jenkins TG, James ER, Alonso DF, et al. Cigarette smoking significantly alters sperm DNA methylation patterns. *Andrology.* 2017;5(6):1089–1099.

61. Murphy PJ, Guo J, Jenkins TG, et al. NRF2 loss recapitulates heritable impacts of paternal cigarette smoke exposure. *PLoS Genet.* 2020;16(6): e1008756.

Section 2 The Biology of Male Reproduction and Infertility

Chapter 11: The Effects of Aging on Male Fertility and the Health of Offspring

Alex M. Kasman, Francesco Del Giudice, and Michael L. Eisenberg

11.1 Introduction

As the population ages and the age at which couples proceed with conception continues to rise, it is important that we understand the potential impact this may have on reproduction [1]. Paternal age has increased over the last several decades, and there is concern that this may have negative reproductive effects including alterations in semen parameters and detrimental health outcomes in offspring via a variety of mechanisms including epigenetic changes that may occur during spermatogenesis. While advanced maternal age has been well established to negatively impact fertility as well as peripartum and neonatal outcomes, the effect of advanced paternal age has been less well characterized. Increasing evidence has suggested that age-related occurrences may negatively impact a father's semen quality while increasing age has been suggested to be a negative predictor of offspring health, particularly neurodevelopmental disorders. Questions have also arisen as to whether delaying fatherhood may lead to a longer time to pregnancy and, if needed, impact assisted reproductive technique outcomes. This chapter seeks to explore the impact that an aging father has on his own fertility, semen parameters, pregnancy outcomes, assisted reproductive technique outcomes, and offspring's health.

11.2 Effect of Age on Male Fertility

The maternal age effect on reproductive outcomes is well documented and as such prenatal counseling has adapted to reflect advancing maternal age as a risk factor for adverse pregnancy outcomes [2]. As maternal age increases, there are lower rates of natural conception and successful artificial reproductive technology (ART) outcomes. With temporal increases in paternal age, there has been an increasing focus on whether paternal age may have a similar negative effect on fertility and related outcomes. In the following sections the impact that an age has on a father's fertility through epigenetic, genetic, and functional disorders associated with age will be explored.

11.2.1 Age and Epigenetic/Genetic Alterations in Sperm

There have been increased data that examine the potential negative impact changes in the sperm epigenome and DNA fragmentation in parallel with increasing paternal age may have on fertility, embryogenesis, and offspring health.

As sperm may retain histones at important developmental genes and DNA methylation patterns can persist after delivery, this may be a potential mechanism that can impact offspring health. In a study of 17 fertile sperm donors who provided 2 semen samples separated by 9–19 years, the authors examined global changes in methylation status [3]. As donor age increased, the researchers found that 139 regions were significantly hypomethylated while 8 regions were hypermethylated, which impacted up to 117 genes within the sperm genome. It was noted that several genes affected had been previously shown to be associated with bipolar disorder and schizophrenia within these regions. Similarly, within 37 semen samples from a known fertile population there were significantly increased global methylation changes in 5-methylcytosine and 5-hydroxymethylcytosine levels as paternal age increased [4]. These studies suggest that as age increases in fathers, there can be global changes in sperm epigenetics, which could impact fertility and potentially offspring health.

Sperm DNA damage increases as males age and this finding has been confirmed a number of times within the literature [5]. However, it remains unclear how this finding may translate to a male's fertility status and, even more unclear, their offspring's health. Sperm DNA fragmentation has been predominantly established within the infertility literature as a possible predictive measure of ART outcome success, however its application outside this field has yet to be well established. A systematic review and meta-analysis of 28 total studies found that infertile men, compared to either fertile controls or healthy donors, had significantly higher levels of sperm DNA fragmentation with an area under the curve of 0.844 ($p< 0.001$) for predicting an infertility diagnosis, representing a potential mechanism for male infertility [6]. While increasing DNA fragmentation may translate to reduced chance of conception, it may also negatively impact the pregnancy. A recent meta-analysis of 14 trials with 530 men undergoing sperm DNA fragmentation showed that higher levels of fragmentation were associated with increased chance of recurrent pregnancy loss suggesting that increased sperm DNA fragmentation impacts not only fertility but also embryonic development [7]. Prospective studies examining age, DNA damage, and pregnancy success have yet to be done to establish a causative link.

Elevated reactive oxygen species (ROS) are known to cause DNA damage that can then lead to adverse outcomes during embryonic development (e.g., impaired implantation, spontaneous abortion) as well as during development of offspring if the damage were to be inherited. ROS are present in increased levels in the seminal ejaculates of older men and may increase the risk of DNA damage [8]. While DNA damage has been demonstrated to have the negative reproductive effects mentioned above, it has yet to be demonstrated that accumulated ROS is a contributing mechanism to impaired fertility in older men.

With regard to paternal age and offspring health, selfish spermatogonial selection has been proposed as a potential mechanism for adverse health outcomes in children of aged fathers [9]. Several paternal age affect (PAE) disorders such as Costello syndrome, Apert syndrome, and achondroplasia are caused by mutations within the male germline, specifically within components of the tyrosine kinase receptor/RAS/MAPK signaling pathway. The mutations that cause these PAE disorders occur during mitosis of the spermatogonal stem cells and appear to give these spermatozoa a selective advantage, allowing these clones to selectively overpopulate seminiferous tubules. This advantage is termed selfish spermatogonial selection and, while it can occur in all men, it is more common in older men suggesting a possible cause for adverse health outcomes in offspring of older men.

As such, as a father ages there may be epigenetic and genetic changes that can lead to changes in expression of genes during embryonic development that may therefore impact fertility and, possibly, the outcome of offspring health. However, much of these data remain to be demonstrated in prospective trials and it requires further investigation to determine a definitive link between the aging father, alternations in the sperm epigenome and/or genome, fertility, and offspring health.

11.2.2 Functional Disorders of Urology

The delivery of sperm into the female reproductive tract requires adequate erectile function and ejaculatory function while any disruption during this process may lead to functional male infertility. Erectile dysfunction (ED) has been shown to increase in prevalence as men age with 18.4% of US men over the age of 18 suffering from ED. As ED is associated with microvascular disease, it increases further in prevalence with development of age-related conditions such as hypertension or cardiovascular disease [10]. Therefore, as men age they are at increasing risk of inability to adequately penetrate for delivery of semen. Furthermore, ED may predispose a man to longer abstinence time that can lead to increased rates of sperm DNA fragmentation [11].

Ejaculatory dysfunction (EjD), other than premature ejaculation, comprises a range of disorders that include several conditions that may lead to functional infertility such as delayed ejaculation, anejaculation, and retrograde ejaculation. Natural fertilization requires normal antegrade ejaculatory function that may not always occur in older men. For antegrade ejaculation to occur there must be emission (closure of the bladder neck and ejection of prostatic secretions into the urethra) and expulsion (ejection of semen through the urethra via coordination of pelvic and penile musculature). Any disease process or medication that may disrupt either emission or expulsion may cause infertility through inadequate delivery of semen. The mean age of EjD is 52 years and the prevalence increases with age suggesting that as men age these conditions may contribute to infertility albeit likely a small subset [12]. While most reports suggest these conditions remain relatively uncommon within the population (~1–4% of men suffering from either delayed ejaculation, anejaculation, or retrograde ejaculation), it is unclear how much these contribute to clinical infertility. However, data suggest ejaculatory disorders are likely vastly underreported with estimates as high as 24% of men [13].

Finally, a number of common urologic conditions that men may experience as they age could contribute to infertility. Benign prostatic hypertrophy (BPH) and lower urinary tract symptoms (LUTS) increase with age and have been highly associated with EjD with 41% of those with mild LUTS reporting some degree of sexual dysfunction, rising to 76% in those with severe LUTS [14]. As such, men with LUTS may be at risk of impaired fertility through EjD as discussed previously. Similarly, alpha blockers utilized in the treatment of BPH and LUTS disrupt the emission phase of ejaculation leading to retrograde ejaculation through relaxation of the bladder neck. However, there is variance in the degree of EjD between alpha blockers for example – sildosin and tamsulosin have a significantly higher degree of EjD while doxazosin and terazosin have minimal to no EjD in the placebo-controlled trials. As with medications to treat BPH, surgical treatment such as transurethral resection of the prostate and various laser ablative techniques (e.g., GreenLight) may disrupt the bladder neck leading to retrograde ejaculation (up to 70%) and/or cauterization of the ejaculatory ducts leading to stricture or obstruction. Alternative surgeries for BPH may offer less of a risk of functional infertility such as UroLift, transurethral microwave thermoablation and needle ablation, and transurethral incision of prostate; however, further studies are necessary to confirm. In the treatment of prostatic and bladder malignancy, the incidence of which increases with age, the complete removal of the prostate during prostatectomy and cystoprostatectomy disrupts the reproductive tract and requires sperm banking prior or surgical sperm retrieval after for men interested in fertility. In addition, alternative treatments such as radiation or hormonal therapy may either cause EjD or suppression of spermatogenesis. More broadly, as the risk of malignancy increases with age for most cancer types, fertility-related effects associated with treatment (e.g., chemotherapy or radiotherapy) should be discussed with men interested in future fertility. Finally, exogenous testosterone reduces the secretion of gonadotropins (luteinizing hormone and follicle-stimulating hormone) from the pituitary causing a reduction in intratesticular testosterone and spermatogenesis [15]. As serum testosterone levels decline with age, exogenous supplementation for symptomatic hypogonadism may lead to infertility. While most cases are reversible within six months of cessation, continued or permanent suppression has been associated with years of use or increased age at testosterone therapy initiation [16]. Many of the potential causes of infertility can be avoided with careful counseling prior to initiation of treatment or through the use of ART if treatment is deemed necessary or has already been delivered.

11.3 Paternal Age Effect on Fertility

11.3.1 Changes in Semen Parameters

Semen analysis is utilized as the main diagnostic tool for male fertility status. The normal ranges of semen parameters continue to evolve based on population studies and the World Health Organization laboratory manual for the examination and processing of human semen, from which "normal" ranges are defined, is currently on its fifth edition. While changes within the semen analysis may not always reflect clinical fertility status and certain controversy exists regarding the importance of various parameters, there remains no better test for fertility for men [17]. However, studies attempting to link aging in men to alterations in various semen parameters have often been conflicting. Many of these studies are limited in sample size, sample source, mean age of the study participants, and lack of abstinence timing.

Consistent across most all studies is an age-related decline in seminal volume. Two large systematic reviews have identified decreases in volume by up to 22% and an effect size of −0.103 with the greatest effect as men entered their fifth decade of life [5,18]. When Kidd et al. examined motility and percent normal sperm they found a decrease of 3–37% and 4–18%, respectively [18]. Johnson et al., adding to these findings, found a similarly significant decline with age in total count, motility, and morphology [5]. They were unable to find a significant effect on concentration, which they attributed to the age-related decline in seminal volume. Several more recent studies have been published since these systematic reviews and meta-analysis were conducted and while some have echoed these findings, others have found no significant age effect on semen parameters. A study of 71,623 men in China found no effect of age on semen parameters; however, this is likely because the population were predominantly infertile men, while Priskorn et al. found no significant effect of paternal age on any semen parameter in a retrospective review of 10,965 men undergoing fertility evaluation at the Copenhagen Sperm Analysis Laboratory [19,20]. On the contrary, Verón et al. echoed similar findings to prior studies and reviews when they examined semen parameters of 11,706 men undergoing routine semen analysis [21]. There was a negative correlation of age with semen volume, sperm count, and motility as age increased with no effect in sperm concentration. The authors also noted, for the first time, that there was also a negative impact of male age on sperm vitality and peroxidase-positive cells.

Overall, there is a trend in the literature suggesting that as a man ages there is a decline in at least seminal volume, motility, and sperm count with no effect on sperm concentration. Until future prospective studies are done with adequate power, adequate selection of study groups, and controlling for confounders such as abstinence time men may need to be counseled on potential detrimental effect of age on semen quality.

11.3.2 Effect on Natural Conception

The human female ovary contains a fixed number of nongrowing follicles (NGFs), defined as the ovarian reserve, established before birth that decline with increasing age culminating in the menopause at 50–51 years [2]. With approximately 450 ovulatory monthly cycles in the normal human reproductive lifespan, this progressive decline in NGF numbers is attributed to follicular death by apoptosis. The *reproductive female potential* is therefore the ability of a woman to conceive in the absence of pathophysiologic changes in her reproductive system. As the maternal age increases, this reproductive potential may frequently be met leading to a growing number of patients to present for fertility evaluation and treatment. Additionally, the reproductive female potential has clear impacts on offspring perinatal and long-term health. However, the reproductive potential of the aging male is less well characterized.

On the male side, this colloquially named concept of a fertility "biologic clock" has been less well described in terms of age limits and therefore less is known about the *male reproductive potential*. In 1935, Seymour et al. described a case report of the oldest known man with documented paternity in medical literature achieving an unassisted conception at the age of 94 years old [22]. The semen analysis of this subject was defined as: "within average limits, with entirely normal conformation and great motility." Quantitative studies since the 1980s have revealed that semen parameters tend to decline with age and therefore spermatogenesis may be considered as susceptible to aging similar to the female reproductive potential (Figure 11.1) [18,23,24]. Nevertheless, the production of sufficient fertile spermatozoa by the testis of aging men is increasingly relevant as couples wait longer to have children, and the average age of paternity increases [25]. The impact of paternal age on pregnancy rate has been less studied, compared to maternal age. This contrast may be due to the different biological background that gametes (i.e., men vs women) are exposed to and as direct consequence a lack of consensus on the definition of advanced paternal age.

The most commonly implemented limit to define advanced paternal age is men >40 years at time of conception [25]. If we assume this cutoff, it becomes immediately clear how important male age may be in the success of natural conception. In an analysis of over 168 million US births, Khandwala et al. found

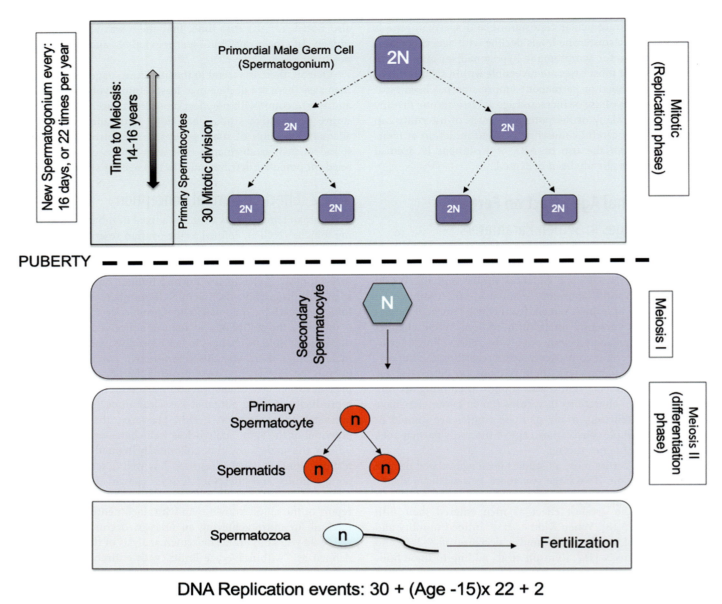

Figure 11.1 Male meiosis and development of spermatozoa. Figure adapted from Conti and Eisenberg (2016) [24].

that the mean paternal age increased from 27.4 to 30.9 years over a 40-year period with similar trends reported in European countries such as Germany and the United Kingdom [26,27]. Moreover, in the most recent years, 8.9% of all births were sired to men at least 40 years of age. As happened for maternal studies, the association of older paternal age with adverse perinatal outcomes has been more investigated over the years both in terms of genetics and development factors affecting the early and long-term consequences on the offspring [28]. However, less is known about the relevance of this aging epidemiological trend in terms of increased pregnancy rates. The most commonly studied association regards the delay in the achievement of pregnancies when comparing younger versus older men in combination with the effect of maternal age. The Avon Longitudinal Study of Pregnancy and Childhood (ALSPAC Study Team) examined the effect of paternal age on the likelihood of delayed conception using data derived from a geographically defined UK population during pregnancy [29]. The likelihood of conception within 6 or 12 months was lower in older men. In their multivariable logistic regression analysis, after adjusting for maternal age, BMI, smoking habit, level of education, paternal alcohol consumption and other relevant variables, the odds ratio for conception in ≤ 12 months was 0.51 (0.31, 0.86) in men aged ≥ 40 years. Similarly, Hassan et al. demonstrated that increasing men's age was associated with a longer time to pregnancy and declining conception rates [30]. In this report, the odds were even higher (men >45 years were 4.6-fold and 12.5-fold more likely to have experienced >1 or >2 years' time to pregnancy). To date, the largest multi-institutional European population-based sample focused on this topic was a retrospective cohort analysis that included 6,188 European women (from Denmark, Italy, Spain, and Germany) aged 25–44 years randomly selected from census registers in 1991–1993 [31]. This study identified a mutual association for specific paternal and maternal age groups that were independent risk factors for delayed pregnancy success. Only the combination of men aged >40 years with the female partner within the 35–39 range compared to younger men (<40 years) was found indeed to be independently associated with both delayed pregnancy (OR of 2.21; 95% CI: 1.13–4.33) and overall risk of conception failure within 12 months or delivery of a stillbirth (OR of 3.02; 1.56–5.85). In contrast, greater paternal age in combination with younger female partner (<35 years) was not associated with fecundability outcome.

In conclusion, the current evidence suggests the existence of a link between advanced paternal age and delayed time to pregnancy as well as overall decline in the couple's reproductive success. However, the magnitude of the effect of paternal age still remains a question of debate with limitations associated with the relatively low to moderate level of evidence available in the medical literature on this specific topic.

11.3.3 Effect on ART Conception

As infertility continues to rise in Western countries, couples are turning to ART for help with conception. To date, ART might be considered as the most successful treatment for infertility but does require a physical and financial cost [32]. Part of this high rate of success, however, is explained by the patient selection process, peri-treatment counseling, and the increasing social and personal consciousness of available therapeutic choices. As it is for natural conception, the effectiveness of ART also depends on age with evidence demonstrating that conception rates start declining when the woman is over 30 years of age while the impact of male age is less well understood [33].

The effect of male age on ART outcomes is better characterized than within the unassisted conception literature. The investigation of this topic in the ART setting has focused primarily on two different type of study designs: 1) population-based retrospective cohort studies studying the gametes of the infertile couple and 2) oocyte donation cycles implemented to minimize the confounding of maternal factors or impaired semen parameters that may necessitate ART. In the first analyses, the role of increased paternal age was independently associated with ART failure, most of the time in parallel with the effect of maternal age both for the intrauterine insemination and the in vitro fertilization (IVF) techniques [34]. Once again, the threshold age value for predicting adverse pregnancy and live birth rates was >40 years old for fathers.

However, some investigators reported that the paternal age effect was not significant if the mother was more than 35 years old. In data from 4,057 IVF or intracytoplasmic sperm injection (ICSI) cycles, the probability of pregnancy was reduced by 10% for women who were 35 years old with a male donor over 40 years versus women aged 35 years with a donor under 30 years old [35]. Additionally, a retrospective Chinese study on 9,991 IVF cycles observed that the effect of paternal age was associated with implantation and pregnancy rate only in cases where the female partners were 30–34 years of age [36]. Importantly, no associations with male age were found if the female partner was under 30. Furthermore, the study revealed that paternal age was not associated with other ART outcomes such as fertilization rate, embryo quality at the cleavage stage, and miscarriage rate. Why does paternal age seem to independently influence the pregnancy rate of IVF in such a specific female age group? A possible explanation for this phenomenon could be the combination of genetic aberrations that affect both the oocyte and the spermatozoa at certain ages in human biology. Of note, none of the aforementioned experiences adjust for semen quality as well as other possible confounding factors such as underlying comorbidities or reason for seeking IVF. Finally, another experience by Kaarouch et al. selected 83 couples undergoing IVF treatment on the basis of documented male factor infertility and identified the male age of 40 years as a threshold for male donors during ART [37]. In this study the two groups of younger versus older males undergoing IVF were not significantly different in semen quality, but showed differences in genetic and epigenetic markers such as DNA sperm fragmentation, chromatin decondensation, and global DNA methylation changes specifically within paternal imprinted genes such as *H19-DMR* and *PEG 1/MEST-DMR* [38,39].

As previously mentioned, in order to interpret the effect of paternal age on IVF outcome independently of maternal factors or abnormal semen parameters, several studies were designed using the "oocyte donation model." De la Rochebrochard et al. and Robertshaw et al. demonstrated lower ART success rates when paternal age was higher than 40 years old with a decreased probability of a live birth rate for each 5-year increase in paternal age respectively [40,41]. In contrast, other studies did not reach the same conclusions using the donor oocyte model. For example, a study of 4,887 oocyte donation cycles carried out with ICSI fertilization technique by Beguería et al showed that there were no differences in any reproductive outcomes analyzed (biochemical pregnancy, clinical pregnancy, miscarriage, and live birth) in all male age groups from <25 to >60 years [42]. A possible explanation for this apparent discrepancy given by the authors may be related to embryo culture duration [43]. However, the reasons for these disparate findings remain unknown.

Given the heterogeneity in the literature, it is difficult to determine the association between paternal age and ART outcomes. However, stratifying for the techniques adopted (ICSI vs. IVF) or selecting donor oocyte studies, the evidence suggests a more limited impact of advanced paternal age compared to maternal age with regard to the success rate of ART [44]. While a significant statistical correlation between increasing paternal age and ART outcomes cannot be obtained, the trend among reduced semen quality and older age was prevalent in the majority of the studies. However, while the importance of the routine semen analysis evaluation is of greatest relevance in the case of natural conception attempt, these measures do not necessarily correlate with functional sperm fertilization potential. Therefore, in future the efforts will need to determine the association between paternal age, semen quality, and different reproductive outcomes themselves such as fertilization, implantation, pregnancy, spontaneous miscarriage, and livebirth.

11.4 Paternal Age Effect on Offspring Health

As the age of motherhood worldwide continues to rise, the complications relating to advanced maternal age in pregnancy and later in childhood have long been a focus while the full scope of the impact of increased paternal age on offspring health recently gained traction within the last decade. Much research has been done with particular attention focused upon neuropsychiatric disorders and perinatal outcomes including birth defects and chromosomal disorders. While a number of conditions have increased risk among fathers with advanced paternal age (e.g., schizophrenia, autism spectrum disorders, and overall birth defects), it is important to note that the absolute risk of many of these conditions remains low [28,45].

11.4.1 Perinatal, Neonatal, and Obstetric Outcomes

Several measures of obstetric and neonatal outcomes have been examined in association with advanced paternal age. Few studies have undertaken an examination of perinatal outcomes and those that have have typically been underpowered or were limited by the upper limit of the age of the fathers. From their systematic review and meta-analysis, Oldereid et al. were unable to find a significant association with advanced paternal age and low birth weight or being small for gestational age [28]. However, there was a small but significant increase in odds of preterm birth (OR 1.02, 95% CI 1.00–1.05) and stillbirth (OR 1.19, 95% CI 1.10–1.30). More recently, Khandwala et al. found in an analysis of over 40,000,000 births within the United States that increased paternal age (i.e., fathers >45) had higher odds of infants born prematurely (OR 1.14, 95% CI 1.13–1.15), lower APGAR score (<8, OR 1.14, 95% CI 1.08–1.20), and had a 14% greater risk of a birth weight less than 2,500 g [1]. A similar study noted increased chance of stillbirth in those infants fathered by older men with particular risk occurring after the paternal age of 39 though the maternal effect was notably larger [46].

11.4.2 Birth Defects

Overall, the risk of any birth defect in the offspring of an older father appears to be low with an odds ratio of 1.05 (95% CI 1.02–1.07) [28]. These odds appear to be most pronounced in fathers more than 45 years old though they are significant after the age of 35 years. Much of the literature examining the overall risk has also included chromosomal abnormalities into its assessment, which may skew results toward a finding of increased risk. Individually, particular attention has been paid to congenital heart defects, orofacial abnormalities (e.g., cleft lip/palate), gastroschisis, and spina bifida although the odds of these in offspring fathered from older men do not appear to be statistically significant. The exception to this is orofacial abnormalities from fathers more than 45 years old (OR 1.14, 95% CI 1.02–1.29).

11.4.3 Chromosomal and Genetic Abnormalities

In addition to the PAE disorders mentioned previously (Costello syndrome, Apert syndrome, achondroplasia) that can be caused by distinct mutations within the tyrosine kinase receptor/RAS/MAPK signaling pathway, trisomies have also been investigated in association with advanced paternal age. While assessment of trisomy 13 and 18 has been done within other studies, these remain small and inconclusive. In contrast, studies on trisomy 21 demonstrate increased odds in the offspring of older fathers (OR 1.13, 95% CI 1.05–1.23) with the risk beginning at 40 years of age [28].

11.4.4 Neurodevelopmental Disorders

Numerous studies have examined the risk of neurodevelopmental disorders in offspring of older fathers such as autism spectrum disorders (ASD), schizophrenia, and attention deficit hyperactivity disorder (ADHD). Single nucleotide variants associated with age have been implicated in the development of a number of these conditions via whole-exome sequencing data [47]. While intellectual disability has been examined from a maternal age viewpoint, there have been few studies examining the risk of intellectual disability in those children born to older fathers. Both schizophrenia and ASD have been extensively studied and demonstrate an increased odds with increasing paternal age. Overall, the odds of development of an ASD are 1.26 (95% CI 1.20–1.30) with the highest odds in those fathers over the age of 45; however, the odds appear to begin as early as age 35 (OR 1.07, 95% CI 1.02–1.12) [28]. This is interesting as previous reports have seen the opposite from mothers with mothers younger than 20 having an increased risk of having a child with schizophrenia while the risk with older maternal age appears to be unclear [45]. A similar trend among older fathers is noted for schizophrenia and related schizoaffective disorders with overall odds of 1.31 (95% CI 1.23–1.38) with the odds increasing at a paternal age of 35 (OR 1.06, 95% CI 1.01–1.12). These findings are similarly true for psychosis and psychotic-like symptoms. Interestingly, with regard to ADHD there appear to be conflicting reports with younger fathers having a higher risk of affected offspring. With regard to bipolar disorder, there have been several US- and European-based population studies with either no or minimal association with paternal age [45].

11.4.5 Childhood Cancer and Mortality

With cancer as the leading cause of death in children under 14 years old, the association between older parental age and development of childhood cancer is an interesting area of research. Two separate population-based studies, one in the USA and one in Denmark, have examined the overall risk of childhood cancer in offspring born to older fathers [48,49]. No overall risk was found in the Danish cohort, while in the US cohort children born to older fathers had a slightly increased odds of development of cancer (OR 1.03, 95% 1.02–1.05). The Danish cohort findings are in line with a recent systematic review and meta-analysis [28]. Similar to overall cancer risk, it is unclear whether older fathers have children with an increased risk of acute lymphoblastic leukemia (ALL) or lymphoma, as conflicting studies exist. Overall, if there are increased odds it is likely small [45]. Wang et al. did find increased odds in their Danish cohort of non-Hodgkin lymphoma with OR 1.10 (95% CI 1.02–1.19) while they did not find an association with ALL [28,49].

When examining the association between paternal age and mortality of offspring, studies have been heterogenous with varying follow-up times from less than 5 years of age up to 40 years. Therefore, it is difficult to draw firm conclusions [28].

11.5 Conclusion

The effect of aging on male fertility has become increasingly relevant both for clinicians and patients due to the increasing paternal age especially in the Western countries. Current available evidence suggests a decline in male fertility with age. It is not clear if this decline may lead to inferior ART outcomes. As such, men seeking preconception care may benefit from counseling on the possible risks of later conception including impaired perinatal outcomes and childhood outcomes.

Acknowledging the existence of a male "biological clock" could increase awareness and potentially motivate younger men to seek earlier workup for semen analysis and fertility evaluation. Moreover, given the literature suggesting the role of impaired fertility status as a biomarker for future later health, optimizing patient consciousness on the association between health and reproduction may be an opportunity to both improve conception and prevent later morbidity and mortality [50–52]. Thus, the clinician's role in men's health is evolving, as is the interdisciplinary management of the infertile couple.

References

1. Khandwala YS, Baker VL, Shaw GM, Stevenson DK, Lu Y, Eisenberg ML. Association of paternal age with perinatal outcomes between 2007 and 2016 in the United States: population based cohort study. *BMJ*. 2018;363:1–8. doi:10.1136/bmj.k4372
2. Sauer MV. Reproduction at an advanced maternal age and maternal health. *Fertil Steril*. 2015;103 (5):1136–1143. doi:10.1016/j.fertnstert.2015.03.004
3. Jenkins TG, Aston KI, Pflueger C, Cairns BR, Carrell DT. Age-associated sperm DNA methylation alterations: possible implications in offspring disease susceptibility. *PLoS Genet*. 2014;10(7):1–13. doi:10.1371/journal.pgen.1004458
4. Jenkins TG, Aston KI, Cairns BR, Carrell DT. Paternal aging and associated intraindividual alterations of global sperm 5-methylcytosine and 5-hydroxymethylcytosine levels. *Fertil Steril*. 2013;100(4):945–951.e2. doi:10.1016/j.fertnstert.2013.05.039
5. Johnson SL, Dunleavy J, Gemmell NJ, Nakagawa S. Consistent age-dependent declines in human semen quality: a systematic review and meta-analysis. *Ageing Res Rev*. 2015;19:22–33. doi:10.1016/j.arr.2014.10.007
6. Santi D, Spaggiari G, Simoni M. Sperm DNA fragmentation index as a promising predictive tool for male infertility diagnosis and treatment management – meta-analyses. *Reprod Biomed Online*. 2018;37(3):315–326. doi:10.1016/j.rbmo.2018.06.023
7. Tan J, Taskin O, Albert A, Bedaiwy MA. Association between sperm DNA fragmentation and idiopathic recurrent pregnancy loss: a systematic review and meta-analysis. *Reprod Biomed Online*. 2019;38(6):951–960. doi:10.1016/j.rbmo.2018.12.029
8. Cocuzza M, Athayde KS, Agarwal A, et al. Age-related increase of reactive oxygen species in neat semen in healthy fertile men. *Urology*. 2008;71 (3):490–494. doi:10.1016/j.urology.2007.11.041
9. Maher GJ, Goriely A, Wilkie AOM. Cellular evidence for selfish spermatogonial selection in aged human testes. *Andrology*. 2013;2:304–314. doi:10.1111/j.2047-2927.2013.00175.x
10. Selvin E, Burnett AL, Platz EA. Prevalence and risk factors for erectile dysfunction in the US. *Am J Med*. 2007;120:151–157. doi:10.1016/j.amjmed.2006.06.010
11. Agarwal A, Gupta S, Plessis S Du, et al. Abstinence time and its impact on basic and advanced semen parameters. *Urology*. 2016;94:102–110. doi:10.1016/j.urology.2016.03.059
12. Paduch D, Polzer P, Morgentaler A, et al. Clinical and demographic correlates of ejaculatory dysfunctions other than premature ejaculation: a prospective, observational study. *J Sex Med*. 2015;12:2276–2286. doi:10.1111/jsm.13027
13. Kasman AM, Bhambhvani HP, Eisenberg ML. Ejaculatory dysfunction in patients presenting to a men's health clinic: a retrospective cohort study. *Sex Med*. 2020;8(3):454–460. doi:10.1016/j.esxm.2020.05.002
14. Avellino G, Theva D, Oates RD. Common urologic diseases in older men and their treatment: how they impact fertility. *Fertil Steril*. 2017;107 (2):305–311. doi:10.1016/j.fertnstert.2016.12.008
15. Mahabadi V, Amory JK, Swerdloff RS, et al. Combined transdermal testosterone gel and the gonadotropins in men. *J Clin Endocrinol Metab*. 2009;94(7):2313–2320. doi:10.1210/jc.2008-2604
16. Kohn TP, Louis MR, Pickett SM, et al. Age and duration of testosterone therapy predict time to return of sperm count after human chorionic gonadotropin therapy. *Fertil Steril*.

2017;107(2):351–357.e1. doi:10.1016/j.fertnstert.2016.10.004

17. Wang C, Swerdloff RS. Limitations of semen analysis as a test of male fertility and anticipated needs from newer tests. *Fertil Steril.* 2014;102(6):1502–1507. doi:10.1016/j.fertnstert.2014.10.021

18. Kidd SA, Eskenazi B, Wyrobek AJ. Effects of male age on semen quality and fertility: a review of the literature. *Fertil Steril.* 2001;75(2):237–248. doi:10.1016/s0015-0282(00)01679-4

19. Li WN, Jia MM, Peng YQ, Ding R, Fan LQ, Liu G. Semen quality pattern and age threshold: a retrospective cross-sectional study of 71,623 infertile men in China, between 2011 and 2017. *Reprod Biol Endocrinol.* 2019;17 (107):1–8. doi:10.1186/s12958-019-0551-2

20. Priskorn L, Jensen TK, Lindahl-Jacobsen R, Skakkebæk NE, Bostofte E, Eisenberg ML. Parental age at delivery and a man's semen quality. *Hum Reprod.* 2014;29(5):1097–1102. doi:10.1093/humrep/deu039

21. Verón GL, Tissera AD, Bello R, Beltramone F, Estofan G, Molina RI, Vazquez-Levin MH. Impact of age, clinical conditions, and lifestyle on routine semen parameters and sperm kinematics. *Fertil Steril.* 2018;110 (1):68–75e3. doi:10.1016/j.fertnstert.2018.03.016.

22. Seymour F, Duffy C, Koerner A. A case of authenticated fertility in a man, aged 94. *JAMA.* 1935;105(18):1423–1424.

23. Johnson S, Dunleavy J, Gemmell N, Nakagawa S. Consistent age-dependent declines in human semen quality: a systematic review and meta-analysis. *Ageing Res Rev.* 2015;19:22–33. doi:10.1016/j.arr.2014.10.007

24. Conti SL, Eisenberg ML. Paternal aging and increased risk of congenital disease, psychiatric disorders, and cancer. *Asian J Androl.* 2016;18(3):420–424. doi:10.4103/1008-682X.175097

25. Hamilton B, Hoyert D, Martin J, Strombino D, Guyer B. Annual summary of vital statistics: 2010–2011. *Pediatrics.* 2013;131(3):548–558. doi:10.1542/peds.2012-3769

26. Khandwala Y, Zhang C, Lu Y, Eisenberg M. The age of fathers in the USA is rising: an analysis of 168,867,480 births from 1972 to 2015. *Hum Reprod.* 2017;32(10):2110–2116. doi:10.1093/humrep/dex267

27. Mazur DJ, Lipshultz LI. Infertility in the aging male. *Curr Urol Rep.* 2018;19 (7):54. doi:10.1007/s11934-018-0802-3

28. Oldereid NB, Wennerholm U, Pinborg A, et al. The effect of paternal factors on perinatal and paediatric outcomes: a systematic review and meta-analysis. *Hum Reprod Update.* 2018;24 (3):320–389. doi:10.1093/humupd/dmy005

29. Ford W, North K, Taylor H, Farrow A, Hull M, Golding J. Increasing paternal age is associated with delayed conception in a large population of fertile couples: evidence for declining fecundity in older men. The ALSPAC Study Team (Avon Longitudinal Study of Pregnancy and Childhood). *Hum Reprod.* 2000;15(8):1703–1708. doi:10.1093/humrep/15.8.1703

30. Hassan M, Killick S. Effect of male age on fertility: evidence for the decline in male fertility with increasing age. *Fertil Steril.* 2003;79(Suppl. 3):1520–1527. doi:10.1016/s0015-0282(03)00366-2

31. de la Rochebrochard E, Thonneau P. Paternal age >or=40 years: an important risk factor for infertility. *Am J Obs Gynecol.* 2003;189(4):901–905. doi:10.1067/s0002-9378(03)00753-1

32. Dain L, Auslander R, Dirnfeld M. The effect of paternal age on assisted reproduction outcome. *Fertil Steril.* 2011;95(1):1–8. doi:10.1016/j.fertnstert.2010.08.029

33. Whitcomb B, Levens E, Turzanski-Fortner R, et al. Contribution of male age to outcomes in assisted reproductive technologies. *Fertil Steril.* 2011;95(1):147–151. doi:10.1016/j.fertnstert.2010.06.039

34. Mathieu C, Ecochard R, Bied V, Lornage J, Czyba J. Cumulative conception rate following intrauterine artificial insemination with husband's spermatozoa: influence of husband's age. *Hum Reprod.* 1995;10 (5):1090–1097. doi:10.1093/oxfordjournals.humrep.a136100

35. McPherson N, Zander-Fox D, Vincent A, Lane M. Combined advanced parental age has an additive negative effect on live birth rates – data from 4057 first IVF/ICSI cycles. *J Assist Reprod Genet.* 2018;35(2):279–287. doi:10.1007/s10815-017-1054-8

36. Wu Y, Kang X, Zheng H, Liu H, Liu J. Effect of paternal age on reproductive outcomes of in vitro fertilization. *PLoS ONE.* 2015;10(9):1–9. doi:10.1371/journal.pone.0135734

37. Kaarouch I, Bouamoud N, Madkour A, et al. Paternal age: negative impact on sperm genome decays and IVF outcomes after 40 years. *Mol Reprod Dev.* 2018;85(3):271–280. doi:10.1002/mrd.22963

38. Hajj N, Zechner U, Schneider E, et al. Methylation status of imprinted genes and repetitive elements in sperm DNA from infertile males. *Sex Dev.* 2011;5:60–69. doi:10.1159/000323806

39. Montjean D, Ravel C, Benkhalifa M, et al. Methylation changes in mature sperm deoxyribonucleic acid from oligozoospermic men: assessment of genetic variants and assisted reproductive technology outcome. *Fertil Steril.* 2013;100(5):1241–1247.

40. de la Rochebrochard E, de Mouzon J, Thepot F, Thonneau P, French National IVF Registry (FIVNAT) Association. Fathers over 40 and increased failure to conceive: the lessons of in vitro fertilization in France. *Fertil Steril.* 2006;85(5):1420–1424. doi:10.1016/j.fertnstert.2005.11.040

41. Robertshaw I, Khoury J, Abdallah ME, Warikoo P, Hofmann GE. The effect of paternal age on outcome in assisted reproductive technology using the ovum donation model. *Reprod Sci.* 2014;21(5):590–593. doi:10.1177/1933719113506497

42. Begeria R, Garcia D, Obradors A, Poisot F, Vassena R, Vernaeve V. Paternal age and assisted reproductive outcomes in ICSI donor oocytes: is there an effect of older fathers? *Hum Reprod.* 2014;29(10):2114–2122. doi:10.1093/humrep/deu189

43. Frattarelli JL, Miller KA, Miller BT, et al. Male age negatively impacts embryo development and reproductive outcome in donor oocyte assisted reproductive technology cycles. *Fertil Steril.* 2008;90(1):97–103. doi:10.1016/j.fertnstert.2007.06.009

44. Sagi-dain L, Sagi S, Dirnfeld M. Effect of paternal age on reproductive outcomes in oocyte donation model: a systematic review. *Fertil Steril.* 2015;104 (4):857–865.e1. doi:10.1016/j.fertnstert.2015.06.036

45. Bergh C, Pinborg A, Wennerholm U. Parental age and child outcomes. *Fertil Steril.* 2019;111(6):1036–1046. doi:10.1016/j.fertnstert.2019.04.026

46. Mayo JA, Lu Y, Stevenson DK, Shaw GM, Eisenberg ML. Parental age and stillbirth: a population-based cohort of nearly 10 million California deliveries from 1991 to 2011. *Ann Epidemiol.* 2019;31:32–37.e2. doi:10.1016/j.annepidem.2018.12.001

47. Taylor JL, Debost JPG, Morton SU, et al. Paternal-age-related de novo mutations and risk for five disorders. *Nat Commun.* 2019;10(3043):1–9. doi:10.1038/s41467-019-11039-6

48. Contreras ZA, Hansen J, Ritz B, Olsen J, Yu F, Heck JE. Parental age and childhood cancer risk: a Danish population-based registry study. *Cancer Epidemiol.* 2017;49:202–215. doi:10.1016/j.canep.2017.06.010

49. Wang R, Metayer C, Morimoto L, et al. Parental age and risk of pediatric cancer in the offspring: a population-based record-linkage study in California. *Am J Epidemiol.* 2017;186(7):843–856. doi:10.1093/aje/kwx160

50. Kasman AM, Giudice D, Eisenberg ML. New insights to guide patient care: the bidirectional relationship between male infertility and male health. *Fertil Steril.* 2020;113(3):469–477. doi:10.1016/j.fertnstert.2020.01.002

51. Del Giudice F, Kasman A, De Berardinis E, Busseto G, Belladelli F, Eisenberg ML. Association between male infertility and male specific malignancies: systematic review and metanalysis of the population-based retrospective cohort studies. *Fertil Steril.* 2020;114(5):984–996. doi:10.1016/j.fertnstert.2020.04.042

52. Del Giudice F, Kasman A, Ferro M, et al. Clinical correlation among male infertility and overall male health: a systematic review of the literature. *Investig Clin Urol.* 2020;61(4):355–371. doi:10.4111/icu.2020.61.4.355

Section 3 Clinical Evaluation and Treatment of Male Infertility

Chapter 12 Office Evaluation of the Infertile Male

Kevin J. Campbell, John F. Sullivan, and Larry I. Lipshultz

12.1 Introduction

The evaluation of the infertile male is often a multistep process for clinicians and patients alike. Infertility is a disease process that affects approximately 15% of couples who attempt to conceive. Male factor infertility may be attributable to approximately 50% of infertile relationships: 30% of couples due to a significant male factor alone and 20% with combined male and female factors [1]. Infertility may be considered to exist after 12 months of attempted conception without contraception. This consideration is in the setting that pregnancy rates by intercourse in couples are approximately 20–25% per month and 90% at one year [2]. Thus, the male who presents for an infertility workup should be evaluated with the primary goal of identifying reversible conditions that may improve the male's fertility, as well as finding irreversible conditions which may relegate candidates to assisted reproductive techniques (ART) or identify nontreatable genetic causes. Those patients with irreversible conditions not amenable to ART may be appropriately counseled.

12.2 History and Physical Examination

12.2.1 History

Obtaining a thorough history is a critical part of the office evaluation. The fertility workup requires the concurrent assessment of each partner with an appreciation by the specialist of the sensitive and anxiety-provoking nature of the process. Both partners should be present.

A myriad of conditions contribute to male reproductive dysfunction and a structured and methodical format to the history is key to uncover all potential causes including genetic, congenital, medical, surgical, environmental, and psychosocial etiologies. The use of structured questionnaires completed at home or in the office prior to consultation can assist in this regard.

One full cycle of spermatogenesis lasts, on average, 74 days [3] so careful attention is required to historical results over the preceding 2–3 months; if a clear temporal etiology is identified, a repeat evaluation should be undertaken in a further 3 months.

It is best to begin questioning with discussion of the duration of the couple's infertility, previous attempted treatments, and prior pregnancies. A thorough reproductive and sexual history should follow, as well as identifying contributory past medical and surgical history, social and family history, as well as review of systems.

One should discuss the couple's sexual behavior, as commonly there are misconceptions regarding the optimum timing and frequency of intercourse. Often it is not appreciated that semen parameters peak after 2–3 days of abstinence, but waiting longer than this actually may result in poorer sperm quality [4]. The authors recommend that intercourse should be performed every other day beginning 5 days before expected ovulation until 5 days after. At this juncture questioning regarding lubricants commonly used during intercourse should be broached, as some may cause impaired sperm motility and viability.

The interview should elicit information on relevant past medical and surgical histories, even those from childhood. Report of genitourinary anomalies or reconstructive surgery may prove important. In utero or childhood exposure to chemotherapy, radiation, or hormones may result in defects in spermatogenesis [5]. Cryptorchidism and a delay in its treatment can be associated with testicular failure, and surgery for testicular torsion or pediatric hernia repair can similarly affect future paternity.

Questions probing other common diseases of adulthood, including diabetes mellitus, sleep apnea, sexually transmitted infections, neurologic disorders, and trauma should be identified. All these illnesses may have implications for fertility, affecting emission, ejaculation, or potentially resulting in obstruction of the male reproductive tract [5].

In patients with a history of malignancy, questions should include use of chemotherapeutic agents, including treatment duration, dose, and concurrent sperm banking. Likewise, patients treated with radiation should be queried about dose, duration, and any efforts toward gonadal shielding, as recovery of spermatogenesis can be unpredictable [6]. In men with a history of testicular cancer any retroperitoneal surgery should be detailed.

Time should be spent discussing family history and the presence of genetic syndromes known to be related to reproductive dysfunction such as cystic fibrosis.

Pharmacologic and environmental exposures should be addressed. Environmental toxins may include synthetic estrogens associated with pesticide use, organic solvents in paints or inks, ionizing radiation in nuclear power plants, and heavy metals in manufacturing [5]. Time regularly spent in saunas, hot tubs, and prolonged laptop usage should be elucidated as these putative perturbations in scrotal temperature may be associated with deranged spermatogenesis.

Prescription and recreational drugs can also impair sperm production and function. Tobacco and nicotine may impair sperm motility and morphology and increase DNA fragmentation rates. Alcohol and marijuana excess similarly have gonadotoxic effects, whereas narcotics are known to affect gonadotropin secretion, which results in lower serum and intratesticular testosterone [5].

Antihypertensives and their association with erectile dysfunction, antipsychotics and decreased libido, opioids and decreased testosterone production, anti-inflammatory agents, and PDE 5 inhibitors are all potentially harmful. Exposure to exogenous anabolic steroids suppresses serum gonadotropins and intratesticular testosterone levels that will impair spermatogenesis. Cessation can result in a reversal of spermatogenic arrest; however, complete recovery can take up to two years [5].

Additional questioning of the female partner should include age, history of pelvic surgery or infections, and known uterine or tubal abnormalities. In addition, exposure to gonadotoxins, and a history of endometriosis or ovulatory irregularity should be queried. Importantly infertility issues or success with other partners should be noted.

12.2.2 Physical Examination

The physical exam is a key part of the initial office evaluation, beginning with a general evaluation of the patient's appearance. The patient's body habitus may reveal the patient's androgen status. A lack of virilization may result in sparse distribution of body hair, eunuchoid proportions, or gynecomastia, though many men with 47, XXY karyotype do not display a gynecoid appearance. Obesity and excessive adipose tissue may contribute to elevated estradiol levels as a result of the peripheral conversion from testosterone by an abundance of the enzyme aromatase.

The genital exam then progresses to visual inspection of the groin and genitals. Previous surgical scars may indicate prior testicular surgery, hernia repair, or trauma. The phallus is inspected noting the presence of phimosis, abnormal curvature, and location of the meatus. Hypospadias or significant curvature may result in improper delivery of semen in the vaginal vault.

The testicles are evaluated for size, consistency, and location. Measurements are recommended with an orchidometer or calipers for accuracy. In a normal adult male, the testicle measures at least 4.6 cm in length, 2 cm in width, and 20 cm3 in volume. Decreased testicular size or soft, boggy consistency may indicate impaired spermatogenesis as the normal sperm-producing seminiferous tubules make up 85% of testicular volume [7]. High-riding testes or their location in close proximity to the thighs may produce an insufficient temperature difference (normally <2°F) between the body and scrotal contents. The presence of a varicocele may also lead to temperature changes and impaired spermatogenesis and can be found

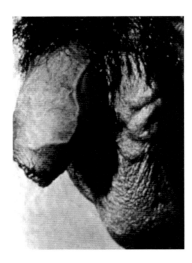

Figure 12.1 Demonstration of a grade 3 left-sided varicocele, visible without need for Valsalva by patient

in up to one-third to one-half of infertile males [8]. Varicoceles are graded as small (grade 1) if palpable when standing only with the Valsalva maneuver, moderate (grade 2) if palpable while standing without performing the Valsalva maneuver but not visible, or large (grade 3) if the veins are visible through the scrotal skin (Figure 12.1). Subclinical varicoceles are those only found with an ancillary technique and not clearly identified but suggested on physical evaluation.

The spermatic cord also should be carefully palpated for the presence of or absence of the vas deferens bilaterally. Unilateral absence of the vas deferens could point to Wolffian duct developmental abnormalities and ipsilateral renal agenesis. Bilateral absence of the vas deferens is highly suggestive of cystic fibrosis gene mutations and the need for specific genetic testing.

Palpation of the epididymis may reveal fullness indicative of obstruction while tenderness could reflect an infectious process and/or an inflammatory reaction. Spermatoceles and epididymal cysts may also be palpated but do not generally cause obstruction.

A digital rectal exam should be performed to evaluate for prostatic enlargement, size, seminal vesicle induration, or midline cysts; however, the majority of abnormalities found on transrectal ultrasound are not found on physical examination.

12.3 Initial Laboratory Assessment

12.3.1 Semen Analysis

The semen analysis is the cornerstone laboratory evaluation of the male undergoing an infertility workup. At minimum, 2–3 semen analyses should be obtained, maintaining a similar duration of abstinence for consistency. The ideal abstinence period is 2–3 days. Shorter periods may affect concentration, whereas longer periods may affect motility. Specimens are optimally obtained in a wide-mouthed container that should be clean, but not necessarily sterile, and devoid of spermicidal chemicals. Collection may be from masturbation, coitus interruptus, or following the use of special collection condoms.

Table 12.1 Bulk semen analysis

Semen characteristic	Lower reference limit
Semen volume (mL)	1.5
Sperm concentration (million/mL)	15
Total number (million/mL)	39
Total motility (%)	40
Progressive motility (%)	32
Normal forms (%)	4
Vitality (%)	58

Modified from WHO reference values 2010 [8].

Semen samples should be transported to the laboratory at room or body temperature within one hour from the time of ejaculation.

The semen is evaluated for several key parameters. Reference ranges are set out by the World Health Organization (WHO) with the most recent iteration from 2010 (Table 12.1) (9). A 95% confidence limit defines the limits of normalcy.

Ejaculate volume is mostly derived from the seminal vesicles. Markedly reduced volume is suspicious for incomplete collection, ejaculatory duct obstruction (complete or partial), seminal vesicle agenesis, androgen deficiency, or retrograde ejaculation. Fructose is a product of the seminal vesicles and its presence in the ejaculate generally rules out complete obstruction. For semen volumes below 1 mL, a postejaculate urine sample should be obtained to rule out retrograde ejaculation. Seminal vesicle agenesis, often confirmed with transrectal ultrasound (TRUS), is often accompanied by ipsilateral vasal agenesis [10].

Seminal viscosity is evaluated to determine if liquefaction has occurred or if there is presence of hyperviscous semen. Semen is a coagulum that liquefies 5–25 minutes after ejaculation due to prostatic proteolytic enzymes. A postcoital test to evaluate the adequacy of sperm in the cervical mucus may be obtained if hyperviscous or nonliquifying semen is reported.

Sperm concentration is a measure of density, reported as millions of sperm per milliliter of semen. An accompanying parameter is the total sperm count, which refers to the total number of sperm in the entire ejaculate. A normal germinal epithelium produces 100–300 million sperm per day [11]. Approximately 3 months are required for the production and maturation of sperm within the seminiferous tubules and another 3–10 days are needed for transport through the male reproductive tract. In general, a sperm density of between 60 and 80 million/mL is reported as average. A variety of methods are used to determine the sperm count, though most employ the use of a grid. If there are no sperm identified in the sample, the sample should be centrifuged and the resultant pellet examined for the presence of spermatozoa. No sperm in the centrifuged pellet confirms true azoospermia.

Azoospermia is the complete absence of sperm in the ejaculate and occurs in 8% of men who present to the infertility clinic. If diagnosed, azoospermia must be determined to be either obstructive or nonobstructive (NOA). Obstructive azoospermia typically is associated with normal testicular size and no detectable endocrinopathy. Nonobstructed patients typically have small or soft testicles, elevated follicle-stimulating hormone (FSH) levels, and abnormal biopsy findings, including maturation arrest, severe hypospermatogenesis, or germ cell aplasia.

Sperm motility refers to the percentage of sperm demonstrating any motion whereas forward progression is a qualitative assessment of the relative speed with which spermatozoa move in a forward direction. Motility is scored using a five-point scale, with a rating of 0 indicating no motility, 1 as sluggish or nonprogressive movement, 2 as slow, meandering, forward progression, 3 as a reasonably straight line with moderate speed, and 4 with high speed in a straight line [5]. If the motility is less than 5–10%, a viability stain should be used to determine if the immotile sperm are alive or represent necrospermia. Alive but nonmotile sperm would suggest the presence of an ultrastructural abnormality, such as primary ciliary dyskinesia that may be confirmed with electron microscopy.

Round cells without tails may indicate immature germ cells or white blood cells. Excessive numbers of round cells should be noted and may be differentiated with subsequent assays. Significant amounts of sperm agglutination are suggestive of antisperm antibodies.

Following WHO 2010 guidelines evaluation of sperm morphology classifies sperm as being normal (oval), amorphous (including large and small sperm), tapered, duplicated, and immature [9]. Strict morphology is usually the morphological test of choice [12].

12.3.2 Endocrine Evaluation

Endocrine causes of male infertility are present in less than 3% of cases [13]. Most endocrinopathies are found in men with sperm concentrations of less than 10 million sperm/mL. The initial hormone assessment should include a serum FSH and testosterone, drawn in the morning given its well-described diurnal variation.

A more comprehensive endocrine evaluation that includes luteinizing hormone (LH), prolactin, estradiol, free testosterone, and sex hormone binding globulin should be obtained when abnormalities are present on the initial evaluation. Additional markers such as Inhibin B and anti-Müllerian hormone are still largely investigational in the United States, and incremental improvement in accuracy is typically small.

With assessment of testosterone, FSH, and LH, differentiation between hypergonadotropic hypogonadism (primary testicular failure), hypogonadotropic hypogonadism (secondary testicular failure), androgen resistance, and hyperprolactinemia is possible (Table 12.2).

Table 12.2 Interpretation of various hormone profiles

Condition	FSH	LH	Testosterone
Normal spermatogenesis	=	=	=
Delayed spermatogenesis	= / ↑	=	= / ↓
Hypergonadotropic hypogonadism	↑	↑	↓
Hypogonadotropic hypogonadism	↓	↓	↓
Pituitary tumor	= / ↓	= / ↓	↓

12.4 Imaging in the Male Infertility Office Evaluation

Clinically significant varicoceles are typically diagnosed by physical examination alone; however, the ancillary use of color Doppler ultrasound may be required in patients in whom the physical examination is challenging due to obesity, tight or small scrotums, following previous surgery, or with altered anatomy. Reversal of blood flow with a Valsalva maneuver and the presence of spermatic veins greater than 3 mm are accepted ultrasound criteria for the diagnosis of varicocele [14]. However, we believe this threshold is changing with the advent of standing scrotal ultrasounds (Figure 12.2).

Ultrasonography may also identify additional pathologic conditions affecting fertility, including testicular tumors, spermatoceles, seminal vesicle atresia, ejaculatory cysts, and renal disorders associated with congenital bilateral absence of the vas deferens (CBAVD). In men with CBAVD, TRUS may reveal absence of the ampullae of the vas deferens or seminal vesicle abnormalities.

TRUS is also frequently used in patients with low-volume azoospermia, severe unexplained oligoasthenospermia, palpable abnormalities on digital rectal examination, and when ejaculatory duct obstruction (EDO) is suspected.

EDO can be the result of infection or inflammation leading to stenosis, compression from median cysts, or atonic or enlarged seminal vesicles such as those in patients with diabetes and adult polycystic kidney disease, respectively. Visualization of seminal vesicles greater than 1.5 cm in anteroposterior diameter is considered suggestive of EDO, and seminal vesicle aspiration to confirm sperm may be performed concurrently to confirm the diagnosis [15].

Other imaging modalities, including MRI, are used selectively. MRI may prove valuable in patients with renal, seminal vesicle, vasal, urethral, or other pelvic abnormalities not fully visualized with ultrasound. However, an MRI is more commonly used in the workup of profound hypogonadism and hyperprolactinemia to rule out pituitary adenoma.

The utility of vasography is diminishing and has been almost completely superseded by modalities such as TRUS and MRI, while venography is still important when performing percutaneous ablation.

12.5 Interpretation of the Initial Evaluation

Much of the fertility evaluation can be organized into an algorithmic approach. The semen analysis is evaluated on individual parameters inclusive in the test. No single reference range parameter is an absolute discriminator of fertility, except a sperm density of zero. Thirty percent of infertile men have "normal" semen parameters [1]. There are, however, multiple functional assay tests that may be employed when indicated.

If no functional sperm defects are identified, contributing female factors should be ruled out and intrauterine insemination (IUI) or IVF may be considered. Men with normal semen parameters should be counseled regarding coital timing and lifestyle changes such as discouragement of certain lubricants, hot tubs, and saunas.

12.6 Defects in Isolated Semen Parameters

12.6.1 Volume

Volume disorders may be due to abnormalities of the ejaculatory process. A volume decrease may be due to a number of factors, such as retrograde ejaculation from medical or surgical bladder outlet therapies, neurologic disorders such as spinal cord injury and diabetes, or sympathetic nerve injury from retroperitoneal or colonic surgeries.

It is key to differentiate ejaculatory failure (aspermia) from azoospermia and anorgasmia. Low-volume ejaculates are most commonly due to incomplete collection. Patients at risk for retrograde ejaculation and those with volumes less than 1.0 mL should undergo postejaculate urinalysis [10]. Any sperm found on the urinalysis is also useful in ruling out complete ejaculatory duct obstruction. If there is complete absence of sperm in the urinalysis in the setting of normal-sized testes and normal FSH/testosterone, EDO should be suspected. A typical EDO semen analysis is acidic, low volume, and fructose-negative. TRUS can be performed to rule out EDO through evaluation of semen volume and characterized in an obstructed state with >1.5cm anteroposterior diameter [16]. If dilated vesicles are found, they should be aspirated for sperm. Partial EDO may present as low volume, oligoasthenospermia with normal testes size, and normal hormonal evaluation. Patients with partial EDO typically have enough sperm for ART in their antegrade samples, though transurethral dilation of stenotic ejaculatory ducts may be beneficial.

12.6.2 Oligospermia

WHO defines significant oligospermia as <15 million/mL sperm. Eight percent of men presenting with infertility will have isolated oligospermia. Men with fewer than 10 million sperm/mL should undergo testing with at a minimum serum FSH and testosterone, as most will have clinically significant endocrinopathies [17]. Severe oligospermia as defined as fewer than

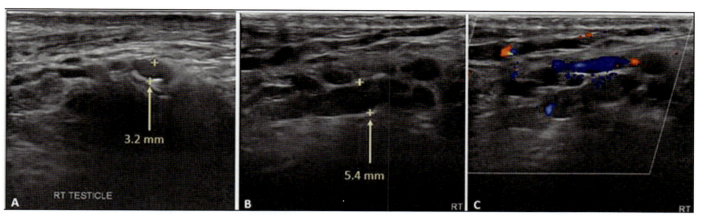

Figure 12.2 Testicular ultrasound demonstrating increase in varicocele diameter from supine (A) to standing (B) position. Reversal of flow (C) is demonstrated in the standing position.

5 million/mL should be screened for genetic abnormalities with a karyotype and Y-chromosome microdeletion analysis.

12.6.3 Azoospermia

Azoospermia accounts for approximately 10% of cases of male infertility and is suspected to affect 2% of men in the general population [18]. Nonobstructive versus obstructive azoospermia must be delineated. NOA is a deficiency of spermatogenesis whereas OA represents adequate production with ductal obstruction. The physical exam noting testis size and presence of vasa can assist with differentiation. Complete endocrine evaluation as well as high-definition karyotype and Y-chromosome microdeletion analysis should be performed.

NOA generally presents with atrophic testes and an elevated FSH indicative of failure of spermatogenesis [17]. Normal testes size and normal FSH suggests the possibility of OA that may be caused by CBAVD, EDO, and vasal or epididymal obstruction. The finding of CBAVD requires additional testing for cystic fibrosis transmembrane conductance regulator (CFTR) gene mutations as well as the 5T allele. If genetic abnormalities are found during the infertility workup, referral for genetic counseling should be offered before proceeding with ART.

12.6.4 Motility

Asthenospermia refers to a low percentage of sperm demonstrating any movement and is often found in conjunction with poor forward progression and oligospermia. Causes may include prolonged abstinence, partial EDO, genital tract infections, pyospermia, antisperm antibodies (ASAs), ultrastructural sperm defects, or varicoceles. The presence of agglutination suggests the presence of ASAs that may be specifically assayed or in association with leukocytospermia denoting excessive white blood cells in the ejaculate. If no treatable cause of severe asthenospermia is present (<10% movement), patients are usually directed to ART. Nonmotile sperm are typically nonviable, but if in high numbers, should be confirmed with vital staining. Necrospermia denotes that all sperm are nonviable. Absent or low (5–10%) motility and normal viability levels may suggest ultrastructural defects that should be examined with electron microscopy [1]. The most common of these ultrastructural defect disorders is primary ciliary dyskinesia.

12.6.5 Morphology

Teratospermia denotes defects in sperm morphology and is commonly idiopathic. The predictive value of strict morphology in successful reproductive techniques has been inconsistent [19]. Isolated abnormalities should not immediately prompt IVF, since natural conception and IUI remain possible for these couples. Thirty-seven percent of men presenting for infertility will have defects in two or more semen parameters [1]. Oligoasthenoteratospermia (OAT) denotes semen analysis abnormalities in sperm density, motility, and morphology. Varicoceles are the most common cause of OAT on semen analysis. Additionally, OAT may be caused by fever, gonadotoxic exposures, certain medications, prior cryptorchidism, and partial EDO.

Leukocytospermia is defined by the WHO as greater than 1 million/mL white blood cells in the semen. Men with findings of leukocytospermia should have a semen culture performed. Empiric antibiotic therapy is irrational and generally does not provide significant benefit [20]. In patients with negative semen cultures, nonsteroidal anti-inflammatory medications, and frequent ejaculations are appropriate next steps with refractory cases considered for sperm processing followed by IUI.

12.7 Additional Semen Tests

12.7.1 Reactive Oxygen Species

Reactive oxygen species (ROS) include superoxide anion, the hydroxyl radical, and the hypochlorite radical, which are important mediators of normal sperm physiology; however,

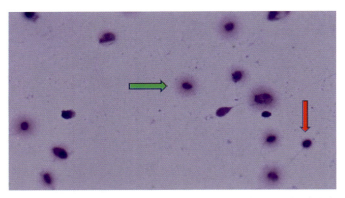

Figure 12.3 Brightfield microscopy slide at x20 power (Zeiss AXIO Lab A1). Image displays sperm after acid denaturing of nuclear proteins. When absence of DNA fragmentation exists a large halo is evident (green arrow). Conversely, if significant DNA fragmentation is present, sperm without any halo can be seen (red arrow).

they retain the potential to damage aerobic cellular systems. Normal physiologic levels are involved in cell signaling, tight junction regulation, production of hormones, capacitation, sperm motility, zona pellucida binding, and the acrosome reaction. When seminal antioxidants, such as superoxide dismutase and catalase, are depleted, excess ROS levels can adversely affect spermatogenesis and have been seen to be elevated in up to 40% of infertile patients [21].

The presence of high ROS concentrations can have widespread effects on most seminal parameters, including elevations in levels of DNA fragmentation, and improvements in ROS levels following varicocelectomy have been demonstrated [5].

Therapy, however, has been primarily directed at increasing levels of antioxidants in the semen using nutraceuticals. Unfortunately, most studies have been uncontrolled or have indirect end points of success. Further research is required to determine the optimal composition and preparation of antioxidants to protect sperm from oxidative stress.

12.7.2 DNA Fragmentation

The stability and integrity of sperm DNA is important for fertilization and resultant healthy embryo development and is normally maintained by disulfide cross-links between protamines, allowing for condensation and protection of nuclear chromatin.

DNA fragmentation refers to denatured and damaged DNA, which is not able to be repaired and can result from a multitude of factors, including abnormal protamination, mutations altering DNA compaction, the presence of a varicocele, and other toxic environmental exposures [10].

Elevated DNA fragmentation rates have been shown to be more common in infertile men compared with fertile donors [10] and can lead to impairment of natural conception, IUI, and IVF with intracytoplasmic sperm injection (ICSI).

Both direct and indirect assays have been developed to quantify sperm DNA fragmentation rates. Single-cell gel electrophoresis (COMET) and terminal deoxynucleotidyl transferase-mediated deoxyuridine triphosphate nick-end labeling (TUNEL) are direct assays that analyze the number of breaks in the DNA.

In contrast, indirect assays, such as the sperm chromatin structure assay (SCSA), measure the susceptibility of sperm nuclear DNA to acid-induced DNA denaturation in situ [19]. The sperm chromatin dispersion (SCD) assay has results comparable to the SCSA but is easier and cheaper to perform. This SCD assay relies on the fact that sperm containing high amounts of fragmented DNA do not produce a halo of DNA loops as unfragmented sperm do when pretreated with acid (to remove nuclear proteins) (Figure 12.3). Limited studies suggest that sperm retrieved from the testicle have better DNA quality in men with abnormal levels of DNA fragmentation in ejaculated sperm. These data suggest that men with high levels of DNA damage in ejaculated sperm should be considered for microsurgical testicular sperm extraction (micro-TESE) for ICSI [19].

Nutraceuticals have also been associated with improvements in sperm DNA fragmentation, although this has not always translated into improvements in pregnancy rates. In patients with a palpable varicocele and an abnormal semen analysis, varicocele repair has been shown to result in a significant decrease in sperm DNA fragmentation rates. This effect has translated, in some cases, to higher spontaneous and ART-associated pregnancy rates. In general, therapeutic considerations for the infertile man with elevated DNA fragmentation include avoidance of gonadotoxins, antioxidant supplementation, treatment of semen infection, and varicocele repair [19].

12.7.3 Fluorescent in Situ Hybridization

Fluorescent in situ hybridization (FISH) is used to directly assess sperm aneuploidy, which can result in increased risks of embryo loss and fetal anomalies. The most frequent sperm chromosomal anomaly in infertile men is diploidy [22]. Current indications for FISH testing include couples with recurrent pregnancy loss and unexplained, persistent IVF failure. Rates of sperm aneuploidy are highest in men with NOA, ultrastructural sperm defects, chromosomal translocations, and karyotypic abnormalities [22]. FISH testing in these men may help assess the relative risks of ICSI and to understand whether to proceed with ICSI or consider preimplantation genetic diagnosis testing.

12.8 The Genetic Evaluation

Identifiable genetic abnormalities contribute 15–20% of the more severe forms of male infertility. Genetic testing is indicated when the sperm density is less than 5 million/mL, NOA is present, or there are clinical suggestions of a genetic abnormality. The most commonly used tests are reviewed.

12.8.1 Congenital Bilateral Absence of the Vas Deferens and Cystic Fibrosis Gene Mutations

Congenital bilateral absence of the vas deferens (CBAVD) is diagnosed on physical examination and is usually due to a mutation in the CFTR gene located on chromosome 7 [23]. Almost all men with clinically detected cystic fibrosis demonstrate CBAVD. Eighty percent of azoospermic men with CBAVD and one-third of men with unexplained obstruction will have CFTR mutations [23]. In patients found to have an abnormality on CFTR testing, the partner should be screened. Failure to detect a CFTR mutation in either partner does not exclude the presence of a mutation that is not always identifiable by most current methods; therefore, the progeny of the couple remains at some risk. There are over 2,000 described mutations to date, with currently available CFTR screening panels typically including 25–40 of the most common mutations [23]. The most frequent mutation is p.F508del, with a worldwide frequency of 66% [24]. Another common mutation, IVS9–5T allele, leads to the formation of only 10% of the normal protein and causes malformation of the vas deferens. In addition to a spectrum of phenotypes due to CFTR mutations, there is also a wide variance in frequency among race. Approximately 1 in 25 people of European descent, and one in 30 of Caucasian Americans, carry a CF mutation, compared to 1 in 46 Hispanics, 1 in 65 Africans, and 1 in 90 Asians. Ireland has the world's highest prevalence of CF disease, at 1 in 1,353 [24].

12.8.2 Karyotype-Associated Abnormalities

The prevalence of chromosomal abnormalities is known to be higher in infertile men and is inversely related to sperm concentration. In men with azoospermia, the prevalence is 10–15%, whereas in men with severe oligospermia, defined as fewer than 5 million sperm/mL, the rate approaches 5%. This is in stark contrast to men with normal sperm concentrations who demonstrate a less than 1% prevalence [25].

In azoospermic men, sex chromosome abnormalities predominate, whereas in oligospermic men, autosomal anomalies (i.e., Robertsonian and reciprocal translocations) are more frequent [26]. In light of these findings, men with azoospermia, severe oligospermia, or clinical evidence of a chromosomal syndrome should undergo karyotype testing before ART.

Klinefelter syndrome (KS) represents the most common karyotypic abnormality in infertile men (47, XXY), and is present in 11% of men with azoospermia and 1 in 500 live births [25]. Ninety-five percent of affected men present in adulthood with infertility, but only 25% demonstrate the characteristic gynecomastia, tall stature, and small firm testes. KS results from a meiotic nondisjunction event in most cases; however, up to 3% of men with KS are mosaic 46,XX/47,XXY. Micro-TESE, coupled with ICSI, is a successful strategy for some patients with azoospermia and KS. Sperm retrieval rates approach 72% per micro-TESE, and 69% of men have adequate sperm for ICSI [23]. It is imperative to remember that couples in which the man has a karyotypic abnormality are at a higher risk of miscarriage and the transmission of chromosomal and congenital defects.

12.8.3 Y-chromosome Microdeletions

Two percent of normal men exhibit deletions of clinically relevant regions of the Y chromosome; in contrast, these microdeletions are found in 7% of men with impaired spermatogenesis. The incidence of these microdeletions increases to 16% in men with severe oligospermia or azoospermia [23]. These microdeletions are not detectable with standard karyotype testing. Instead, identifying these deletions require polymerase chain reaction techniques to analyze sequence tagged sites along the Y chromosome.

Within the long arm of the Y chromosome (Yq11) are three important regions that influence spermatogenesis and are known as the azoospermia factor (AZF) regions. These regions include AZFa, (proximal), AZFb (central), and AZFc (distal) (Figure 12.4) [23]. There may be other, yet undiscovered, regions that contain genes necessary for spermatogenesis. Of the three regions, AZFc deletions are the most common, being seen in 13% of men with NOA and 6% of severely oligospermic men.

A deletion in the azoospermia (DAZ) gene, which encodes a transcription factor present in men with normal fertility, resides in the AZFc region. The location of these deletions affects the likelihood of the presence of spermatogenesis and is prognostic in regard to the success of micro-TESE. Men with AZFc microdeletions have quantitatively impaired spermatogenesis with variable expressions of either severe oligospermia or azoospermia. The level of spermatogenesis is typically stable among individuals, and micro-TESE with ICSI remains a therapeutic option. In contrast, deletions of the AZFa or AZFb regions portend a very poor prognosis for sperm retrieval. Men with Y-chromosome microdeletions will pass the abnormality to their sons who consequently may also be infertile.

12.9 Future Horizons

The future is optimistic in the evaluation and treatment of male infertility. Mouse spermatogonial stem cells have been shown to be capable of spermatogenesis after long-term cryopreservation (~12 years). Subsequent testicular transplantation has been reported without apparent genetic or epigenetic errors in the produced sperm [27]. Spermatogonial stem cell treatment also has implications for oncofertility as prepubertal boys set to undergo gonadotoxic chemotherapeutics may benefit from spermatogonial stem cell banking as they do not yet produce mature sperm cells.

Epigenetic abnormalities have been shown to have a clear relationship to male infertility. Abnormal protamine protein ratios of P1 and P2 have been suggested as a cause of poor semen parameters due to alterations in density and localization

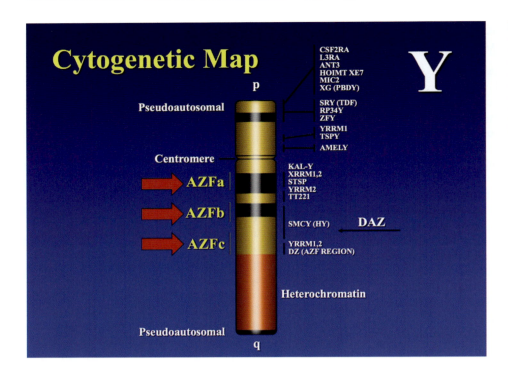

Figure 12.4 Y chromosome, with its "short arm – p" and a "long arm – y." Most deletions causing azoospermia or oligozoospermia occur in regions of the long arm known as the azoospermia factor (AZF), divided into AZFa, AZFb, and AZFc regions. These regions, and likely others on the Y chromosome yet undiscovered, contain genes necessary for normal sperm production, with deletion resulting in defects in spermatogenesis.

of histone marks and associated tail modifications [29]. Additionally, men with idiopathic male infertility have been reported to possess differential methylation signatures at various sperm promoter regions.

Recently, exosomes that affect spermatozoa motility and capacitation have been isolated and characterized in seminal plasma of men with severe asthenozoospermia [29]. The analysis and use of these compact genetic transmitters will be useful in the future.

References

1. Sigman M, Lipshultz LI, Howards S. Office evaluation of the subfertile male. In: Lipshultz L, Howards S, Niederberger C, eds. *Infertility in the Male*. 4th ed. Cambridge University Press; 2009:153–176.
2. Spira A. Epidemiology of human reproduction. *Hum Reprod*. 1986;1(2):111–115.
3. Misell LM, Holochwost D, Boban D, et al. A stable isotope-mass spectrometric method for measuring human spermatogenesis kinetics in vivo. *J Urol*. 2006;175(1):242–246; discussion 6.
4. Levitas E, Lunenfeld E, Weiss N, et al. Relationship between the duration of sexual abstinence and semen quality: analysis of 9,489 semen samples. *Fertil Steril*. 2005;83(6):1680–1686.
5. Burrows PJ, Schrepferman CG, Lipshultz LI. Comprehensive office evaluation in the new millennium. *Urol Clin North Am*. 2002;29(4):873–894.
6. De Palma A, Vicari E, Palermo I, D'Agata R, Calogero AE. Effects of cancer and anti-neoplastic treatment on the human testicular function. *J Endocrinol Invest*. 2000;23(10):690–696.
7. Chipkevitch E, Nishimura RT, Tu DG, Galea-Rojas M. Clinical measurement of testicular volume in adolescents: comparison of the reliability of 5 methods. *J Urol*. 1996;156(6):2050–2053.
8. Fretz PC, Sandlow JI. Varicocele: current concepts in pathophysiology, diagnosis, and treatment. *Urol Clin North Am*. 2002;29(4):921–937.
9. Cooper TG, Noonan E, von Eckardstein S, et al. World Health Organization reference values for human semen characteristics. *Hum Reprod Update*. 2010;16(3):231–245.
10. Practice Committee of the American Society for Reproductive Medicine. Diagnostic evaluation of the infertile male: a committee opinion. *Fertil Steril*. 2015;103(3):e18–25.
11. Kim ED, Lipshultz LI. Advances in the evaluation and treatment of the infertile man. *World J Urol*. 1997;15(6):378–393.
12. van der Merwe FH, Kruger TF, Oehninger SC, Lombard CJ. The use of semen parameters to identify the subfertile male in the general population. *Gynecol Obstet Invest*. 2005;59(2):86–91.
13. Sigman M, Jarow JP. Endocrine evaluation of infertile men. *Urology*. 1997;50(5):659–664.
14. Chiou RK, Anderson JC, Wobig RK, et al. Color Doppler ultrasound criteria to diagnose varicoceles: correlation of a new scoring system with physical examination. *Urology*. 1997;50(6):953–956.
15. Jurewicz M, Gilbert BR. Imaging and angiography in male factor infertility. *Fertil Steril*. 2016;105(6):1432–1442.
16. Belker AM, Steinbock GS. Transrectal prostate ultrasonography as a diagnostic and therapeutic aid for ejaculatory duct obstruction. *J Urol*. 1990;144(2 Pt 1):356–358.

17. Jarow JP. Endocrine causes of male infertility. *Urol Clin North Am.* 2003;30(1):83–90.
18. Ghieh F, Mitchell V, Mandon-Pepin B, Vialard F. Genetic defects in human azoospermia. *Basic Clin Androl.* 2019;29:4.
19. Smith RP, Coward RM, Lipshultz LI. The office visit. *Urol Clin North Am.* 2014;41(1):19–37.
20. Yanushpolsky EH, Politch JA, Hill JA, Anderson DJ. Antibiotic therapy and leukocytospermia: a prospective, randomized, controlled study. *Fertil Steril.* 1995;63(1):142–147.
21. Aitken RJ, Buckingham D, West K, Wu FC, Zikopoulos K, Richardson DW. Differential contribution of leucocytes and spermatozoa to the generation of reactive oxygen species in the ejaculates of oligozoospermic patients and fertile donors. *J Reprod Fertil.* 1992;94(2):451–462.
22. Egozcue S, Blanco J, Vendrell JM, et al. Human male infertility: chromosome anomalies, meiotic disorders, abnormal spermatozoa and recurrent abortion. *Hum Reprod Update.* 2000;6(1):93–105.
23. Oates RD, Lamb DJ. Genetic aspects of infertility. In: Lipshultz L, Howards S, Niederberger C, eds. *Infertility in the Male.* 4th ed. Cambridge University Press; 2009:171–189.
24. de Souza DAS, Faucz FR, Pereira-Ferrari L, Sotomaior VS, Raskin S. Congenital bilateral absence of the vas deferens as an atypical form of cystic fibrosis: reproductive implications and genetic counseling. *Andrology.* 2018;6(1):127–135.
25. Ravel C, Berthaut I, Bresson JL, Siffroi JP, Genetics Commission of the French Federation of CECOS. Prevalence of chromosomal abnormalities in phenotypically normal and fertile adult males: large-scale survey of over 10,000 sperm donor karyotypes. *Hum Reprod.* 2006;21(6):1484–1489.
26. Van Assche E, Bonduelle M, Tournaye H, et al. Cytogenetics of infertile men. *Hum Reprod.* 1996;11(Suppl. 4):1–24; discussion 5–6.
27. Wu X, Goodyear SM, Abramowitz LK, et al. Fertile offspring derived from mouse spermatogonial stem cells cryopreserved for more than 14 years. *Hum Reprod.* 2012;27(5):1249–1259.
28. James E, Jenkins TG. Epigenetics, infertility, and cancer: future directions. *Fertil Steril.* 2018;109(1):27–32.
29. Murdica V, Giacomini E, Alteri A, et al. Seminal plasma of men with severe asthenozoospermia contain exosomes that affect spermatozoa motility and capacitation. *Fertil Steril.* 2019;111(5):897–908 e2.

Section 3 **Clinical Evaluation and Treatment of Male Infertility**

Chapter 13

Medical Management of Male Infertility

Jason R. Kovac

13.1 Introduction

The inability to conceive after approximately 12 months of unprotected sexual intercourse has been traditionally characterized as an inflection point in the diagnosis of infertility. While 10–15% of couples trying to conceive take this much time (or longer), many individuals are seeking the assistance of reproductive professionals earlier in the course of their fertility journey [1]. In many situations, the false societal stigma of fertility being a "woman's" condition leads the female partner to initially seek the services of a gynecologist and/or reproductive endocrinologist. At this point, it is hoped that the male partner would either present themselves, or with the assistance of the involved physicians/stakeholders, for assessment. Since male factors can be identified as the primary cause of infertility in 20–30% of cases, and a contributory cause in 50–60% of couples [2], a simple semen analysis can result in rapid diagnosis and treatment of male partner issues. While delays in therapy are common, continued failure of conception results in emotional discomfort and distress for couples. As awareness grows, many family physicians, gynecologists, and reproductive endocrinologists are now moving to prompt investigations and referral to a urologist/andrologist/male infertility specialist in order to facilitate improved outcomes.

The primary test to investigate male fertility that is most known to everyone, specialists and patients alike, is the semen analysis. The spectrum of results ranges from a complete lack of sperm production (azoospermia), poor sperm production (oligospermia), abnormal morphology (teratospermia), and onto normal production [3]. Male factor issues can present in any of these classifications with variations in samples, days of abstinence, and lifestyle factors all contributing. The causes can be just as diverse consisting of concurrent medical conditions [4], anatomic abnormalities [5], advanced paternal age [6,7], physical obstruction post vasectomy [8], and genetic aberrations [2,9]. Most frustrating for patients, however, is that the most common etiology remains unknown and classified as idiopathic [10]. Even in cases of acceptable semen analyses, normal hormones, and idiopathic etiologies, many lifestyle changes and medical therapies have the potential to evoke efficacious improvements in male fertility potential.

Over the years, many options for medical management have been investigated, evaluated, and used in improving male fertility [11,12]. There are typically two interconnected methodologies that, when used in concert, yield the most gains: improvements in lifestyle factors and medical management via hormonal manipulation through pharmaceuticals.

A complex interplay of hormones under the control of gonadotropin-releasing hormone (GnRH) regulates spermatogenesis [13]. The pulsatile secretion of GnRH from the hypothalamus stimulates the release of follicle stimulating hormone (FSH) and luteinizing hormone (LH) from the anterior pituitary. Testicular Sertoli cells regulate spermatogenesis and Leydig cells control testicular androgen secretion. Indeed, these aforementioned hormones serve as the primary drivers for spermatogenesis and, thus, act as the primary players in pharmaceutical and medical management strategies in the treatment of male fertility [14].

Unfortunately, male partners are typically hesitant to seek care and occasionally have difficulty understanding that there are options for treatment. This may be due to their incorrect perceptions of infertility resulting in the male being less "of a man" and a "failure" or simply due to a lack of understanding about what happens at the office of a male infertility specialist [15]. Furthermore, many men seem fixated on testicular surgery as the only way to improve sperm production and are hesitant to have any physicians interacting with their scrotal/testicular region. It is hoped that this chapter will illustrate that both lifestyle and pharmaceutical treatment options exist and are effective in improving both semen parameters and increasing the chances of natural pregnancy/conception.

13.2 Lifestyle Factors

Modifiable lifestyle factors are a part of the management of the infertile male. While variable and difficult to control, improvements to factors like diet, exercise, and smoking have been shown to assist with male fertility and improve spermatogenesis [16].

Smoking has also been found to have a negative effect on conception in general with numerous studies finding that cigarette smokers exhibit sub-fertility. For example, a 19% reduction in sperm concentration was observed in men smoking >20 cigarettes per day [17]. In another study, semen analyses in men who were smokers had decreased sperm density (15.3%), counts (17.5%), and total motile sperm (16.6%) versus values compared to nonsmokers [18].

While the specific pathology in how smoking affects spermatogenesis is unknown, evidence suggests that nicotine may be involved [16]. In support of this concept, oral nicotine alone, without smoking, yielded significant decreases in sperm motility and counts in rats [19]. Furthermore, elevated levels of nicotine metabolites in seminal plasma corresponded to worsening sperm morphologies [20].

With regards to conception using assisted reproduction specifically, smoking has been shown to result in decreased success of in vitro fertilization [16]. As such, both male and female partners should be counseled to quit smoking to assist in their chances of conception whether it is via natural or assisted means.

Diet is critical in the medical management of male infertility. A Mediterranean diet resulted in improved semen quality [21] and diets low in fruit, vegetables, legumes, and grains were more likely to have abnormal sperm concentrations, counts, and motility [21]. Indeed, the traditional Western diet of processed meats, refined grains, pizza, and sweets was compared to a "prudent diet" (i.e., fish, chicken, vegetables, legumes, whole grains) with progressively motile sperm being higher in the latter [22]. Higher consumption of sugar-sweetened beverage intake resulted in lower sperm motilities [23] with habitual and binge drinking in excess of 25 units per week resulting in decreased sperm quality [24,25].

A sedentary lifestyle and low physical activity has been associated with poor semen quality and lower sperm counts [26,27] while conversely, high levels of vigorous activity have been found to be significantly associated with improved total sperm counts and concentration [28]. Bicycling (>1.5–5 hours per week), given the sustained mechanical pressures of the bicycle seat on the perineum and increased gonadal temperatures [29], has been associated with reduced sperm concentrations and motility [30,31].

Tight, restrictive clothing and underwear (i.e., briefs, boxer briefs, boxers, and no underwear) have not been negatively associated with semen analysis values patterns [32]. Studies on cellular phone use in humans and animals have found associated poor prognostic factors including worsening of sperm morphology [33] counts, motility, and viability [34,35]. Further work confirmed that mobile phone exposure [36] and computer laptop use with wireless wi-fi internet connections [37] negatively impacted sperm quality.

As such, manipulation and cessation of the above-mentioned lifestyle factors should remain an initial first step in any discussion on how to improve semen parameters.

13.3 Gonadotropin Therapy

Gonadotropins include the hypothalamic releasing-hormone, GnRH, as well as the downstream, anterior pituitary hormones LH and FSH [38]. Impaired or absent GnRH secretion rarely contributes to male infertility (<1%); however, impaired secretion of LH, FSH, and GnRH [38] routinely does.

As such, treatment of male fertility in this context can be achieved through two different, but inclusive pathways. Since GnRH stimulates the release of gonadotropins (i.e., LH, FSH) [39,40], it is possible to treat male patients with GnRH analogues to then indirectly increase LH/FSH secretion. More commonly, medications can be used to either directly stimulate LH and FSH release by bypassing GnRH altogether, or pharmacologically mimicking the downstream LH and FSH products.

Indeed, it has been shown that GnRH analogues alone induce both androgenization and spermatogenesis [41]. The agents may be administered subcutaneously [38], intranasally [42], or through an intravenous prolonged continuous pulsatile application [38,43] – the latter modality being particularly inconvenient. Overall, a summary of the research suggests no improvements over the cheaper, downstream gonadotropin (LH and FSH) therapies discussed exist.

Specifically, one such modality is therapy with FSH. Unfortunately, the data detailing the effectiveness of long-term FSH therapy in male patients is underwhelming. In men set to undergo intracytoplasmic sperm injection (ICSI), 75 IU of FSH per day for ≥ 50 days were administered with fertilization and pregnancy rates not reaching statistical significance [44]. Several years later, a randomized, single-blind study evaluated the effects of recombinant human FSH (hFSH) on seminal parameters of infertile men with idiopathic oligospermia (<10 million/mL) and normal serum FSH levels [45]. Men were administered 50 or 100 IU of r-hFSH intramuscularly (q2 days × 3 months) [45]. Plasma FSH levels were evaluated with no increase in sperm concentration in the untreated group and the 50IU r-hFSH group [45]; however, the 100 IU r-hFSH group showed significant increases in sperm concentration (73% doubling) [45]. No other improvements in seminal parameters were noted; however, an increased number of spermatogonia and spermatocytes in the r-hFSH treated groups were found suggesting stimulation of spermatogenesis by FSH. Correspondingly, FSH plasma levels increased with 100 IU of r-hFSH but not 50 IU [45] – mimicking the results seen in the testicular data.

A 2005 follow-up study, performed on a prospective, controlled, randomized population evaluated the effects of FSH on seminal parameters and spontaneous pregnancy rates in infertile men with idiopathic oligozoospermia [46]. The treatment group received r-hFSH 100 IU IM on alternate days for three months. Semen analysis identified improvements after three months of therapy with the responder group exhibiting significantly higher spontaneous pregnancy rates [46]. This demonstrated that in a properly selected group of patients (i.e., patients with normal plasma FSH and absence of maturation arrest), administration of FSH had benefits on sperm counts and pregnancy rates. Higher dose r-hFSH therapy (300 IU) was evaluated in men with infertility over a four-month period and, while sperm concentration tripled during therapy, it declined following treatment. This highlighted that the improvements noted with FSH occurred only during therapy and were not durable [47]. A meta-analysis examining sperm concentrations and pregnancy rates, both unassisted and via artificial reproductive techniques, improved in men given FSH [48]. It has also been noted that in men post testosterone therapy who have suffered testosterone induced-inhibition of spermatogenesis, the use of FSH at 75 or 150 IU every other day is effective at helping to restore semen analysis [49]. The recent 2021 American Urological Association (AUA) male infertility guidelines [50,51] suggest that treatment with FSH, while not FDA-approved, is an option. Men with normal FSH and testosterone levels appear to have the best improvements in spermatogenesis and, while the changes appear transient, and the treatment expensive, the option exists for difficult-to-treat male infertility.

Another option for gonadotropin therapy is human chorionic gonadotropin, or hCG (brand names Novarel or Pregnyl). This medication is most commonly injected subcutaneously and acts as an LH analogue that functions to stimulate testosterone production by direct action on testicular Leydig cells. Administration of hCG can maintain intratesticular testosterone in the face of gonadotropin suppression [52] and increase testosterone in normal men [49]. hCG therapy can not only maintain spermatogenesis in the face of concurrent testosterone or anabolic steroid use [53], it may also improve the return of sperm to the ejaculate in men with a history of suppression [54]. As such, hCG can be used as monotherapy in hypogonadal men with symptomology and should be used in conjunction with testosterone therapy in all men of fertile age who are considering future paternity. Unfortunately hCG, like FSH, has several drawbacks including cost, a subcutaneous route of administration, and relatively short half-life (33 hours) necessitating several injections per week [49,52]. Indeed, the 2021 AUA male infertility guidelines support a conditional recommendation for the use of hCG in the medical management of male infertility [50,51].

13.4 Selective Estrogen Modulators

Selective estrogen modulators (SERMs) have the ability to indirectly stimulate the secretion of the pituitary hormones FSH and LH. As such, these medications have the potential to improve spermatogenesis via the actions of these hormones on the testicular tissue. SERMs are a class of medications that act on the estrogen receptor. Although not FDA-approved for use in men, the main anti-estrogen SERMs used to enhance fertility are tamoxifen and clomiphene citrate (Clomid). While exerting variable effects on tissues, one mode of action is on the hypothalamus and pituitary where they result in an increased GnRH secretion and, subsequently, an enhanced release of FSH and LH from the anterior pituitary.

Multiple studies have identified benefits using tamoxifen (brand name Nolvadex) with regards to improvements in sperm parameters. Tamoxifen was approved in the 1970s for the management of breast cancer given its tissue-specific actions as an estrogen receptor blocker in breast tissue. Other documented agonist effects in bone along with its estrogen antagonist effects in the hypothalamus and pituitary gland highlighted its primary roles [55].

In 1997, Adamopoulos and colleagues [56] published a prospective randomized study of 80 men with idiopathic oligozoospermia. The authors established four treatment groups including a control group and a group where men only received tamoxifen. Total sperm concentrations increased from onset to six months in the tamoxifen ($19.2 \times 10^6 \pm 13$ vs. $42.4 \times 10^6 \pm 21.7$) group when compared to placebo ($19.2 \times 10^6 \pm 14$ vs. $24.2 \times 10^6 \pm 15.5$) [56]. Another study utilizing tamoxifen 10 mg twice daily identified improvements in sperm density and number of live spermatozoa after three months of therapy [57]. Other studies have found benefits in sperm concentration in infertile men using tamoxifen [58–61] with the added benefit of a lack of intrinsic estrogenic effect – making monitoring of the estrogen levels less necessary.

Another SERM anti-estrogen-like compound that has been utilized since the 1970s in the management of male infertility is clomiphene citrate (or Clomid). Clomid, at a dose of 12.5, 25, or 50 mg per day, works primarily as an estrogen antagonist at the level of the pituitary gland and stimulates LH and FSH release [55]. Given this mode of action, Clomid is less effective at raising testosterone levels in men who are already in gonadal failure with elevated LH levels [55]. As such, men with lower LH and FSH are more likely to benefit from Clomid therapy. It is a very well-tolerated medication with side effects including gastrointestinal distress, dizziness, hair loss, gynecomastia, and weight gain as well as vision changes including blurry vision, photophobia, and diplopia – changes reversible with stoppage of the medication [62].

Several comparative studies have been performed to determine the role on clomiphene in male infertility. In 1983, Wang et al. [63] examined 46 men (ages 28–45 years) randomly assigned to six months of therapy. More pregnancies occurred in the clomiphene citrate group with men also demonstrating increased sperm concentrations and elevated FSH, LH, and testosterone levels compared to placebo. No added benefits were identified by using 50 mg clomiphene dose over the 25 mg dose [63]. In 2010, a prospective, randomized, double-blinded, placebo-controlled trial of 60 men (ages 20–40 years) was conducted examining the relationship between placebo (n = 30) and the combination (n = 30) of clomiphene citrate (25mg/d) plus vitamin E (400 mg/day) [64]. Following a six-month treatment period, sperm concentrations and number of pregnancies were significantly higher in the combination therapy group compared to the placebo group [64].

Not all studies on clomiphene citrate have been favorable. Indeed, Roth and colleagues in 2013 [65] reviewed the available evidence for the use of clomiphene citrate in management of male infertility. Primarily, the authors discuss the study performed by the World Health Organization (WHO) in 1992 [66] that found no improvements in pregnancy rates or semen parameters compared to placebo after six months of treatment [65,66]. Another meta-analysis by Chua and colleagues [67] using randomized clinical trials comparing clomiphene citrate and tamoxifen to placebo/no treatment [67] was conducted in 2013. Eleven trials were included in their meta-analysis (n = 903 men; ages 20–49) with all included men exhibiting some form of compromised semen analysis. The pooled effects estimated benefits on pregnancy outcomes and modest, significant increases in sperm concentration and motility [67].

Interestingly, the 2021 AUA guidelines on the treatment on the infertile male [50,51] suggest that the benefits of SERMs on idiopathic male infertility are small and are outweighed by the distinct advantages offered by other forms of medically assisted reproduction (i.e. in vitro fertilization or IVF). In reality, SERMs represent a very cost-effective (Clomid costs $30 for two months – Jan 2021 [www.goodrx.com] vs. $25,000 for IVF), safe, well-tolerated, and effective medication that has a strong potential to stimulate improved spermatogenesis. Coupled with that fact that there are no significant long-term detriments to spermatogenesis, and it is easily accessible to a large proportion of the population, it is tempting to speculate that SERMs should be, in fact, *first-line* medical therapy for all males with infertility.

13.5 Aromatase Inhibitors

The aromatase enzyme regulates the conversion of testosterone and androstenedione to estradiol and estrone respectively. Pharmacological inhibitors of this enzyme, aromatase inhibitors (AIs), limit estrogen production and thus elevate testosterone. The resultant decrease of estradiol then serves to remove the inhibitory effects of aromatase at the site of the hypothalamic-pituitary axis resulting in an increased release of both LH and FSH and subsequent theoretical improvements in spermatogenesis [55]. This testosterone to estrogen blockage occurs inside adipocytes as well as within the testicles [55].

There are two types of AIs that are divided into steroidal (testolactone), and nonsteroidal (letrozole and anastrazole). The nonsteroidal AIs are more effective in increasing the testosterone to estrogen (T/E) ratio and are less likely to interfere with the adrenal axis. Side effects include hot flashes, night sweats, muscle and joint pain as well as potential negative effects on bone density resulting in increased osteoporosis risk and joint disorders after greater than five years of use.

Early work showed the effectiveness of AIs as a way to increase testosterone and decrease estradiol in men with hypogonadism [68]. Based on the physiological principles detailed above, AIs have increased in popularity as an off-label option in the medical management of male infertility. Along this vein, the effects of testolactone and anastrozole on the hormonal and semen profiles of 140 men with abnormal baseline T/E ratios were examined [69]. The men who had lower baseline T/E ratios had them improved with AIs while also showing increased sperm concentrations from approximately 5.5 to 11–16 million sperm/mL [69]. Another 2001 study examined infertile men and found that testolactone resulted in improved semen parameters [70]. Similarly, Saylam et al. [71] treated 27 infertile males with a T/E ratio <10 and found testosterone increased and 20% of oligospermic men conceived naturally. More recently, a study by Gregoriou et al. [72] compared the effects of 2.5 mg Letrozole with 1 mg Anastrozole daily in 29 male patients with low (<10) T/E ratios. Significant improvements in T/E ratios in both groups as well as increased sperm counts were identified [72]. Indeed, while the majority of the aforementioned studies show benefits with treatment using aromatase inhibition, randomized controlled trials as well as pregnancy outcomes would further solidify their role in the treatment of male fertility.

13.6 Prolactin Modulators

Evaluation of prolactin levels is critical in the management of the infertile male since elevations cause male infertility in approximately 11% of oligospermic males [73]. Prolactin is a polypeptide hormone that is secreted by the lactotroph cells of the pituitary gland. Regulation is accomplished by the hypothalamic dopaminergic neurons that provide dopamine to the anterior pituitary and tonically suppress prolactin release [74]. Excess secretion of prolactin, or hyperprolactinemia, can cause hypogonadal symptoms (low libido, fatigue, sexual dysfunction, etc.), galactorrhea and abnormal hormone levels with resultant decreases in LH and FSH release and spermatogenesis [75]. Possible causes include pituitary tumors, altered thyroid levels, renal failure, growth hormone anomalies as well as medications that can decrease dopamine inhibition of prolactin secretion including opioids, antidepressants, and antihypertensives [50,51]. Typical antipsychotic medications are primary culprits causing sustained hyperprolactinemia due to their high affinity for the D2 dopamine receptor [74].

With regards to the diagnosis and medical management of male fertility, if a prolactin is checked and found to be only mildly elevated (<1.5 times normal) then a repeat level should be drawn to rule out a falsely elevated level caused by anxiety, stress, or environmental factors [75]. For persistently elevated levels, an MRI of the pituitary should be obtained to rule out an adenoma/tumor [76] followed by serum testing to rule out alternative causes. Treatment is variable and dependent upon the etiology; however, dopamine agonists are first-line and include Dostinex (cabergoline) [77]. Cabergoline (at a dose of 0.5–2 mg weekly) is typically recommended over other dopamine agonists due to its higher efficacy in normalizing prolactin levels, improved frequency of pituitary tumor shrinkage, and lower side-effect profile [75]. Bromocriptine remains an alternative modality but approximately 25% of patients are resistant to the medication and, once, switched to cabergoline, 80% will achieve prolactin normalization [75]. Findings on MRI should warrant referral to a neurosurgeon or neurology for future evaluation and potential surgery.

13.7 Conclusions

Numerous factors affect a male's fertility potential. When considering management, lifestyle improvements as well as medical management options should be discussed and employed. Male members of an infertile couple should always be referred to a specialist for management. This review details the majority of the medications involved in medical management of male infertility including gonadotropins, SERMs, AIs, and regulation of prolactin.

References

1. Bhasin S, de Kretser DM, Baker HW. Clinical review 64: pathophysiology and natural history of male infertility. *J Clin Endocrinol Metab.* 1994;79:1525–1529.
2. Kovac JR, Pastuszak AW, Lamb DJ. The use of genomics, proteomics, and metabolomics in identifying biomarkers of male infertility. *Fertil Steril.* 2013;99:998–1007.
3. Madhukar D, Rajender S. Hormonal treatment of male infertility: promises and pitfalls. *J Androl.* 2009;30:95–112.
4. Kovac JR, Flood D, Mullen JB, Fischer MA. Diagnosis and treatment of azoospermia resulting from testicular sarcoidosis. *J Androl.* 2012;33:162–166.
5. Kovac JR, Golev D, Khan V, Fischer MA. Case of the month # 168: seminal vesicle cysts with ipsilateral renal dysgenesis. *Can Assoc Radiol J.* 2011;62:223–225.
6. Kovac JR, Smith RP, Lipshultz LI. Relationship between advanced paternal age and male fertility highlights an impending paradigm shift in reproductive biology. *Fertil Steril.* 2013;100:58–59.
7. Kovac JR, Addai J, Smith RP, Coward RM, Lamb DJ, Lipshultz LI. The effects of advanced paternal age on fertility. *Asian J Androl.* 2013;15:723–728.
8. Hakky TS, Coward RM, Smith RP, Kovac JR, Lipshultz LI. Vasovasostomy: a step-by-step surgical technique video. *Fertil Steril.* 2014;101:e14.
9. Lehmann KJ, Kovac JR, Xu J, Fischer MA. Isodicentric Yq mosaicism presenting as infertility and maturation arrest without altered SRY and AZF regions. *J Assist Reprod Genet.* 2012;29:939–942.
10. Kovac JR, Lipshultz LI. Interaction between oviductal epithelial cells and spermatozoa underlies a systems biology approach to treating infertility. *Fertil Steril.* 2013;99:1207–1208.
11. Patel DP, Chandrapal JC, Hotaling JM. Hormone-based treatments in subfertile males. *Curr Urol Rep.* 2016;17:56.
12. Hwang K, Walters RC, Lipshultz LI. Contemporary concepts in the evaluation and management of male infertility. *Nat Rev Urol.* 2011;8:86–94.
13. McLachlan RI. The endocrine control of spermatogenesis. *Baillieres Best Pract Res Clin Endocrinol Metabol.* 2000;14:345–362.
14. Plant TM, Marshall GR. The functional significance of FSH in spermatogenesis and the control of its secretion in male primates. *Endocr Rev.* 2001;22:764–786.
15. Mehta A, Nangia AK, Dupree JM, Smith JF. Limitations and barriers in access to care for male factor infertility. *Fertil Steril.* 2016;105:1128–1137.
16. Kovac JR, Khanna A, Lipshultz LI. The effects of cigarette smoking on male fertility. *Postgrad Med.* 2015;127:338–341.
17. Ramlau-Hansen CH, Thulstrup AM, Aggerholm AS, Jensen MS, Toft G, Bonde JP. Is smoking a risk factor for decreased semen quality? A cross-sectional analysis. *Hum Reprod.* 2007;22:188–196.
18. Kunzle R, Mueller MD, Hanggi W, Birkhauser MH, Drescher H, Bersinger NA. Semen quality of male smokers and nonsmokers in infertile couples. *Fertil Steril.* 2003;79:287–291.
19. Oyeyipo IP, Raji Y, Emikpe BO, Bolarinwa AF. Effects of nicotine on sperm characteristics and fertility profile in adult male rats: a possible role of cessation. *J Reprod Infertil.* 2011;12:201–207.
20. Wong WY, Thomas CM, Merkus HM, Zielhuis GA, Doesburg WH, Steegers-Theunissen RP. Cigarette smoking and the risk of male factor subfertility: minor association between cotinine in seminal plasma and semen morphology. *Fertil Steril.* 2000;74:930–935.
21. Karayiannis D, Kontogianni MD, Mendorou C, Douka L, Mastrominas M, Yiannakouris N. Association between adherence to the Mediterranean diet and semen quality parameters in male partners of couples attempting fertility. *Hum Reprod.* 2017;32:215–222.
22. Gaskins AJ, Colaci DS, Mendiola J, Swan SH, Chavarro JE. Dietary patterns and semen quality in young men. *Hum Reprod.* 2012;27:2899–2907.
23. Chiu YH, Afeiche MC, Gaskins AJ, et al. Sugar-sweetened beverage intake in relation to semen quality and reproductive hormone levels in young men. *Hum Reprod.* 2014;29:1575–1584.
24. Jensen TK, Gottschau M, Madsen JO, et al. Habitual alcohol consumption associated with reduced semen quality and changes in reproductive hormones; a cross-sectional study among 1221 young Danish men. *BMJ Open.* 2014;4:e005462.
25. Jensen TK, Swan S, Jorgensen N, et al. Alcohol and male reproductive health: a cross-sectional study of 8344 healthy men from Europe and the USA. *Hum Reprod.* 2014;29:1801–1809.
26. Magnusdottir EV, Thorsteinsson T, Thorsteinsdottir S, Heimisdottir M, Olafsdottir K. Persistent organochlorines, sedentary occupation, obesity and human male subfertility. *Hum Reprod.* 2005;20:208–215.
27. Stoy J, Hjollund NH, Mortensen JT, Burr H, Bonde JP. Semen quality and sedentary work position. *Int J Androl.* 2004;27:5–11.
28. Gaskins AJ, Mendiola J, Afeiche M, Jorgensen N, Swan SH, Chavarro JE. Physical activity and television watching in relation to semen quality in young men. *Br J Sports Med.* 2015;49:265–270.
29. Jozkow P, Rossato M. The impact of intense exercise on semen quality. *Am J Mens Health.* 2016;11:654–662.
30. Gaskins AJ, Afeiche MC, Hauser R, et al. Paternal physical and sedentary activities in relation to semen quality and reproductive outcomes among couples from a fertility center. *Hum Reprod.* 2014;29:2575–2582.
31. Wise LA, Cramer DW, Hornstein MD, Ashby RK, Missmer SA. Physical activity and semen quality among men attending an infertility clinic. *Fertil Steril.* 2011;95:1025–1030.
32. Sapra KJ, Eisenberg ML, Kim S, Chen Z, Buck Louis GM. Choice of underwear and male fecundity in a preconception cohort of couples. *Andrology.* 2016;4:500–508.
33. Wdowiak A, Wdowiak L, Wiktor H. Evaluation of the effect of using mobile phones on male fertility. *Ann Agric Environ Med.* 2007;14:169–172.
34. Agarwal A, Deepinder F, Sharma RK, Ranga G, Li J. Effect of cell phone usage on semen analysis in men attending infertility clinic: an observational study. *Fertil Steril.* 2008;89:124–128.
35. Liu K, Li Y, Zhang G, et al. Association between mobile phone use and semen quality: a systemic review and

36. Adams JA, Galloway TS, Mondal D, Esteves SC, Mathews F. Effect of mobile telephones on sperm quality: a systematic review and meta-analysis. *Environ Int.* 2014;70:106–112.

37. Avendano C, Mata A, Sanchez Sarmiento CA, Doncel GF. Use of laptop computers connected to internet through wi-fi decreases human sperm motility and increases sperm DNA fragmentation. *Fertil Steril.* 2012;97:39–45 e2.

38. Liu PY, Handelsman DJ. The present and future state of hormonal treatment for male infertility. *Hum Reprod Update.* 2003;9:9–23.

39. Naor Z, Shacham S, Harris D, Seger R, Reiss N. Signal transduction of the gonadotropin releasing hormone (GnRH) receptor: cross-talk of calcium, protein kinase C (PKC), and arachidonic acid. *Cell Mol Neurobiol.* 1995;15:527–544.

40. Kiesel LA, Rody A, Greb RR, Szilagyi A. Clinical use of GnRH analogues. *Clin Endocrinol.* 2002;56:677–687.

41. Mortimer CH, McNeilly AS, Fisher RA, Murray MA, Besser GM. Gonadotrophin-releasing hormone therapy in hypogonadal males with hypothalamic or pituitary dysfunction. *Br Med J.* 1974;4:617–621.

42. Klingmuller D, Schweikert HU. Maintenance of spermatogenesis by intranasal administration of gonadotropin-releasing hormone in patients with hypothalamic hypogonadism. *J Clin Endocrinol Metabol.* 1985;61:868–872.

43. Blumenfeld Z, Makler A, Frisch L, Brandes JM. Induction of spermatogenesis and fertility in hypogonadotropic azoospermic men by intravenous pulsatile gonadotropin-releasing hormone (GnRH). *Gynecol Endocrinol.* 1988;2:151–164.

44. Ashkenazi J, Bar-Hava I, Farhi J, et al. The role of purified follicle stimulating hormone therapy in the male partner before intracytoplasmic sperm injection. *Fertil Steril.* 1999;72:670–673.

45. Foresta C, Bettella A, Merico M, Garolla A, Ferlin A, Rossato M. Use of recombinant human follicle-stimulating hormone in the treatment of male factor infertility. *Fertil Steril.* 2002;77:238–244.

46. Foresta C, Bettella A, Garolla A, Ambrosini G, Ferlin A. Treatment of male idiopathic infertility with recombinant human follicle-stimulating hormone: a prospective, controlled, randomized clinical study. *Fertil Steril.* 2005;84:654–661.

47. Paradisi R, Natali F, Fabbri R, Battaglia C, Seracchioli R, Venturoli S. Evidence for a stimulatory role of high doses of recombinant human follicle-stimulating hormone in the treatment of male-factor infertility. *Andrologia.* 2014;46:1067–1072.

48. Santi D, Granata AR, Simoni M. FSH treatment of male idiopathic infertility improves pregnancy rate: a meta-analysis. *Endocr Connect.* 2015;4: R46–R58.

49. Tatem AJ, Beilan J, Kovac JR, Lipshultz LI. Management of anabolic steroid-induced infertility: novel strategies for fertility maintenance and recovery. *World J Mens Health.* 2020;38:141–150.

50. Schlegel PN, Sigman M, Collura B, et al. Diagnosis and treatment of infertility in men: AUA/ASRM guideline part II. *Fertil Steril.* 2021;115:62–69.

51. Schlegel PN, Sigman M, Collura B, et al. Diagnosis and treatment of infertility in men: AUA/ASRM guideline part I. *Fertil Steril.* 2021;115:54–61.

52. Coviello AD, Matsumoto AM, Bremner WJ, et al. Low-dose human chorionic gonadotropin maintains intratesticular testosterone in normal men with testosterone-induced gonadotropin suppression. *J Clin Endocrinol Metab.* 2005;90:2595–2602.

53. Hsieh TC, Pastuszak AW, Hwang K, Lipshultz LI. Concomitant intramuscular human chorionic gonadotropin preserves spermatogenesis in men undergoing testosterone replacement therapy. *J Urol.* 2013;189:647–650.

54. Wenker EP, Dupree JM, Langille GM, et al. The use of HCG-based combination therapy for recovery of spermatogenesis after testosterone use. *J Sex Med.* 2015;12:1334–1337.

55. Rambhatla A, Mills JN, Rajfer J. The role of estrogen modulators in male hypogonadism and infertility. *Rev Urol.* 2016;18:66–72.

56. Adamopoulos DA, Nicopoulou S, Kapolla N, Karamertzanis M, Andreou E. The combination of testosterone undecanoate with tamoxifen citrate enhances the effects of each agent given independently on seminal parameters in men with idiopathic oligozoospermia. *Fertil Steril.* 1997;67:756–762.

57. Kotoulas IG, Cardamakis E, Michopoulos J, Mitropoulos D, Dounis A. Tamoxifen treatment in male infertility. I. Effect on spermatozoa. *Fertil Steril.* 1994;61:911–914.

58. AinMelk Y, Belisle S, Carmel M, Jean-Pierre T. Tamoxifen citrate therapy in male infertility. *Fertil Steril.* 1987;48:113–117.

59. Vermeulen A, Comhaire F. Hormonal effects of an antiestrogen, tamoxifen, in normal and oligospermic men. *Fertil Steril.* 1978;29:320–327.

60. Kadioglu TC, Koksal IT, Tunc M, Nane I, Tellaloglu S. Treatment of idiopathic and postvaricocelectomy oligozoospermia with oral tamoxifen citrate. *BJU Int.* 1999;83:646–648.

61. Buvat J, Ardaens K, Lemaire A, Gauthier A, Gasnault JP, Buvat-Herbaut M. Increased sperm count in 25 cases of idiopathic normogonadotropic oligospermia following treatment with tamoxifen. *Fertil Steril.* 1983;39:700–703.

62. Patel DP, Brant WO, Myers JB, et al. The safety and efficacy of clomiphene citrate in hypoandrogenic and subfertile men. *Int J Impot Res.* 2015;27:221–224.

63. Wang C, Chan CW, Wong KK, Yeung KK. Comparison of the effectiveness of placebo, clomiphene citrate, mesterolone, pentoxifylline, and testosterone rebound therapy for the treatment of idiopathic oligospermia. *Fertil Steril.* 1983;40:358–365.

64. Ghanem H, Shaeer O, El-Segini A. Combination clomiphene citrate and antioxidant therapy for idiopathic male infertility: a randomized controlled trial. *Fertil Steril.* 2010;93:2232–2235.

65. Roth LW, Ryan AR, Meacham RB. Clomiphene citrate in the management of male infertility. *Semin Reprod Med.* 2013;31:245–250.

66. World Health Organization. A double-blind trial of clomiphene citrate for the treatment of idiopathic male infertility. World Health Organization. *Int J Androl.* 1992;15:299–307.

67. Chua ME, Escusa KG, Luna S, Tapia LC, Dofitas B, Morales M. Revisiting oestrogen antagonists (clomiphene or tamoxifen) as medical empiric therapy for idiopathic male infertility: a meta-analysis. *Andrology*. 2013;1:749–757.
68. Burnett-Bowie SA, McKay EA, Lee H, Leder BZ. Effects of aromatase inhibition on bone mineral density and bone turnover in older men with low testosterone levels. *J Clin Endocrinol Metabol*. 2009;94:4785–4792.
69. Raman JD, Schlegel PN. Aromatase inhibitors for male infertility. *J Urol*. 2002;167:624–629.
70. Pavlovich CP, King P, Goldstein M, Schlegel PN. Evidence of a treatable endocrinopathy in infertile men. *J Urol*. 2001;165:837–841.
71. Saylam B, Efesoy O, Cayan S. The effect of aromatase inhibitor letrozole on body mass index, serum hormones, and sperm parameters in infertile men. *Fertil Steril*. 2011;95:809–811.
72. Gregoriou O, Bakas P, Grigoriadis C, Creatsa M, Hassiakos D, Creatsas G. Changes in hormonal profile and seminal parameters with use of aromatase inhibitors in management of infertile men with low testosterone to estradiol ratios. *Fertil Steril*. 2012;98:48–51.
73. Singh P, Singh M, Cugati G, Singh AK. Hyperprolactinemia: an often missed cause of male infertility. *J Hum Reprod Sci*. 2011;4:102–103.
74. Fitzgerald P, Dinan TG. Prolactin and dopamine: what is the connection? A review article. *J Psychopharmacol*. 2008;22:12–19.
75. Melmed S, Casanueva FF, Hoffman AR, et al. Diagnosis and treatment of hyperprolactinemia: an Endocrine Society clinical practice guideline. *J Clin Endocrinol Metabol*. 2011;96:273–288.
76. Bayrak A, Saadat P, Mor E, Chong L, Paulson RJ, Sokol RZ. Pituitary imaging is indicated for the evaluation of hyperprolactinemia. *Fertil Steril*. 2005;84:181–185.
77. Vilar L, Vilar CF, Lyra R, Freitas MDC. Pitfalls in the diagnostic evaluation of hyperprolactinemia. *Neuroendocrinology*. 2019;109:7–19.

Section 3 Clinical Evaluation and Treatment of Male Infertility

Chapter 14 Surgical Management of Male Infertility

Jesse B. Persily, Sameer Thakker, and Bobby B. Najari

14.1 Introduction

14.1.1 Male Factor Infertility

Infertility is defined as the inability to conceive despite 12 months of unprotected intercourse [1]. A male factor may contribute in up to 50% of these cases, resulting in a burden of male factor infertility of around 7% of the population [2]. Fortunately, as our understanding of the many causes of male infertility improves, so does our ability to manage and optimize fertility. These improvements include, but are not limited to, advancements in microsurgical reconstruction for obstruction, the refinement of varicocelectomy for improved spermatogenesis, and the adoption of techniques for sperm retrieval in combination with in vitro fertilization with intracytoplasmic sperm injection (IVF/ICSI) for nonobstructive azoospermia (NOA). IVF/ICSI has specifically expanded the potential of surgical intervention in the setting of previously hopeless cases, including nonreconstructable defects and NOA. However, given the financial and physical toll of IVF/ICSI, it has become increasingly important for providers to consider the full spectrum of surgical interventions for male-factor infertility, and to counsel male patients accordingly based on their desires, their anatomy and physiology, and the fertility status of their partner.

When considering the surgical interventions for male-factor infertility, one can broadly think of the options as 1) correction of physical defects in the setting of obstructive azoospermia, 2) restoration and optimization of testicular function and spermatogenesis through varicocele repair, and 3) sperm retrieval. It should be stated at the outset that for men who have multiple options for surgical management of their infertility, determination of the correct order of intervention is often a discussion that takes into account a partner's fertility status and the couple's goals for conception (timeline, number of desired offspring).

14.2 Improving Sperm Delivery through Correction of Male Reproductive Tract Obstruction

14.2.1 Correction of Vasal or Epididymal Obstruction

14.2.1.1 Background and Preoperative Considerations

There are a number of scenarios in which obstruction of the vas deferens or epididymis can be corrected with a surgical anastomosis, either through a vasovasostomy (VV) or a vasoepididymostomy (VE). Vasectomy is by far the most common cause of vasal obstruction in North America. National survey and insurance claims data estimate that 6–13% of couples utilize vasectomy as their primary form of contraception, with roughly 500,000 vasectomies performed annually [3,4]. However, up to 20% of vasectomized men may desire another child, and anywhere from 2% to 6% of vasectomized men pursue vasectomy reversal [5,6]. Surgically correctable vasa and epididymal obstruction may also be the result of genital infection, or of iatrogenic injury to the epididymis or vas deferens. Of course, sperm retrieval (discussed later) can be used in the setting of epididymal or vasal obstruction when there is insufficient viable tissue for reconstruction or if the reconstruction is unlikely to result in pregnancy due to female factors. The lack of viable anatomy for reconstruction may be secondary to extensive inguinal or scrotal surgical history or congenital bilateral absence of the vas deferens.

Pure obstructive azoospermia should be suspected in men with normal testis volume, normal hormones, and azoospermia. Detailed history taking is key to planning a successful reconstructive intervention. Though it has been taught that vasectomy reversal patency and success rates steeply decline around 10–15 years postvasectomy, there is evidence that similar patency outcomes may be achievable in cases even greater than 15 years after vasectomy, though pregnancy rates postreversal do still seem to decline meaningfully over time [7]. It is imperative to consider the partner's fertility status, because female factors, including female age, may significantly influence success rates [5]. Vasectomy reversal allows for natural conception after a single surgical procedure, which makes sense in the setting of a desire for multiple children with a partner without fertility issues. Reconstruction may make less sense in the setting of a man who struggled to conceive prior to vasectomy or whose partner's fertility status may make future IVF/ICSI cycles the most likely route to conception.

Though a summary of varicocele management will be presented in Section 14.3.1, it should be noted that a varicocele may be identified as a part of a thorough prereconstruction workup. There is weak evidence that in select patients, correction of varicocele at the time of vasectomy reversal may optimize pregnancy outcomes, but this option must be considered with caution. When a varicocelectomy is performed properly, the spermatic and, potentially the gubernacular, veins are ligated, leaving only the vasal veins for venous drainage. The vasal veins are often compromised by a vasectomy, and if not, by the reversal procedure. The integrity of the vasal artery is also likely to be affected by the reversal, so preservation of the testicular artery is of paramount importance in these cases. If time permits, a reasonable approach is to reconstruct first, assess semen quality, and then perform the varicocelectomy at a later date. This decision will also depend on prereconstruction hormonal panel and semen analysis, as evidence of testicular dysfunction may indicate more pressing need for varicocele repair.

Though the decision about when to perform a VE instead of a VV is typically made intraoperative with an assessment of the vasal fluid, there are a number of preoperative predictors of whether or not there will be a need for VE. These characteristics included older age, obstructive interval, and whether or not a previous vasectomy reversal had been attempted [8]. Though there are no hard and fast rules, these characteristics may influence both the type of reconstruction performed, and also the decision to proceed with simultaneous sperm retrieval at the time of reconstruction.

14.2.1.2 Procedure Notes

Both VV and VE are performed using an operative microscope, and surgeons typically begin the procedure with either a median raphe incision or bilateral small linear incisions. The dissection is taken down to the vas. The vas is then freed of surrounding connections, and transected proximal and distal to the defect. At this point, a microscopic analysis of the testicular-side vasal fluid is performed.

A more comprehensive assessment of vasal fluid characteristics can be found elsewhere, and even so, optimal fluid characteristics that drive the decision toward VV or VE have not been defined [9]. Recent data suggest excellent patency rates (>90%) when VV is performed for men with parts of sperm or whole sperm in the vasal fluid on microscopy [10]. This is in contrast to a more traditional approach, which also took the physical characteristics of the fluid into account. In general, if no sperm granuloma is present and multiple attempts yield no sperm, VE is performed. Complicating this decision is the more challenging nature of the VE procedure, widely considered the most technically challenging operations in male infertility surgery. If the surgeon does not have sufficient VE experience, VV can still be performed, but with bilateral absence of sperm in the vasal fluid, sperm is unlikely to return to the ejaculate [11].

If the choice is made to proceed with VV, there a number of key surgical considerations that help optimize outcomes. Though these may seem obvious, their importance should not be underestimated. These principles include achieving accurate mucosal approximation, which can be made challenging by physical changes in the vasal tissue after vasectomy. It is also imperative that the surgeon construct a leakproof anastomosis, not only for proper delivery of sufficient sperm, but also because sperm are high antigenic and can trigger a detrimental immune response if they end up outside the vasal lumen [12]. Finally, the delicate nature of the vasal tissue makes it imperative that the anastomosis is performed as atraumatically as possible, in order to prevent secondary fibrosis and resulting stricture. Practically, beyond following the above principles, the VV anastomosis is typically approached as a one-layer anastomosis or a multilayer anastomosis. While the authors favor a multilayer approach, a recent meta-analysis found no statistically significant difference in patency rates between the two procedures, and so choice of procedure is at the surgeon's discretion [13].

VE is considered the more challenging procedure, typically only performed by experienced microsurgeons. Of the numerous available techniques, end-to-side anastomoses, meaning the end of the vas to the side of the epididymis, are most common, as they are least traumatic to the epididymis and do not compromise the epididymal blood supply [14]. Epididymal obstruction can result in clear proximal tubule dilation, facilitating choice of anastomosis site. The procedure is made challenging by the need to approximate the vasal muscular layers and adventitia to the epididymal tunic [15]. Many groups favor the two-stitch longitudinal intussusception approach to facilitate the anastomosis, which involves, as the name implies, a longitudinal incision and the use of two double-sided sutures in the vas [16]. Once the vas is placed over the longitudinal opening in the epididymal tunica, the sutures can be pulled through and the vas secured.

14.2.1.3 Outcomes and Complications

Patency and pregnancy outcomes vary with age of the patient, duration of obstruction, and skill and experience of the surgeon performing the procedure. In skilled hands, and when sperm is found in the vasal fluid prior to the operation, patency after VV can approach 99%, though success rates may range from 70% to 99%, with natural pregnancy rates ranging from 35% to 70% [17,18]. Despite the technical challenge, patency after the intussusception VE technique exceeding 80% has been seen in some reports [19]. In general, major predictors of successful fertility appear to be shorter duration of obstruction, presence of sperm in the vasal fluid or a sperm granuloma preoperatively, partner age, and surgeon experience [5].

Aside from postoperative hematoma, a possible risk after these procedures is disruption of the testicular blood supply, particularly in the setting of previous scrotal or inguinal surgery that may have compromised the testicular artery, given that vasal surgery is likely to disrupt the vasal artery. A more prevalent risk is reobstruction. With experience, groups have managed to bring post-VV reobstruction rates down to as low as 5% [20]. VE reobstruction rates are around 25% with end-to-end or end-to-side approaches but may be as low as 10% with the modified intussusception approach, though further follow-up and larger series are necessary [21].

14.2.2 Correction of Ejaculatory Duct Obstruction

14.2.2.1 Background and Preoperative Considerations

Ejaculatory duct obstruction represents a potentially reversible cause of male infertility that is amenable to simple surgical intervention via transurethral resection of the ejaculatory ducts (TURED). Roughly 1–5% of infertile men have either partial or complete ejaculatory duct obstruction [22]. The presentation of this condition is highly variable. Men may be entirely asymptomatic or may present with ejaculatory abnormalities such as hemospermia or pain with ejaculation. Ejaculatory duct obstruction should be entertained in men with a combination of low-volume, low-fructose, acidic ejaculate (secondary to obstruction of the seminal vesicle alkaline semen contribution) and oligo- or azoospermia. Obstruction may be due to congenital atresia or stenosis of the ejaculatory duct or the result of stricture secondary to trauma, infection, or even repeat transrectal prostate biopsies [23]. Imaging with transrectal ultrasound that suggests dilated seminal vesicle or ejaculatory ducts is often used for preliminary assessment, and, in the setting of a picture that fits with ejaculatory duct obstruction, can be used as the main preoperative imaging modality [24]. The poor sensitivity and specificity of TRUS for the diagnosis has led some to suggest more invasive preoperative diagnostic techniques, most notably transrectal ultrasound guided seminal vesicle aspiration looking for sperm [25]. This set-up allows the surgeon to cryopreserve sperm if found, and to instill indigo carmine dye in order to identify resectable lesions without the need for formal preoperative vasography, which risks stricture and worsening of the obstruction [26].

14.2.2.2 Procedure Notes

The original technique, described by Farley and Barnes, is still performed today with minor modification [27]. It can typically be done in the outpatient setting. The enlarged seminal vesicles are visualized on transrectal ultrasound on the day of the procedure, and from this position, indigo carmine can be instilled into the seminal vesicles. A 24-F resectoscope is introduced into the urethra, and expulsion of the indigo carmine dye can aid in the identification of the ejaculatory ducts at the level of the verumontanum. Bilateral resection is performed, taking care to avoid damage to the bladder neck [28].

14.2.2.3 Outcomes and Complications

Case series and small studies have demonstrated significant improvement in semen parameters, semen volume, and the appearance of sperm in the ejaculate in up to 50–66% of men with preoperative azoospermia or significant oligospermia. While postprocedure pregnancy outcome data are still lacking, modern case series suggest pregnancy rates between 13% and 25% [24,29]. Unfortunately, this procedure is not without risk, and the complication rate of TURED may be as high as 33% [29]. Significant complications include reflux of urine into the seminal vesicles and vas deferens, which can result in caustic injury to the seminal vesicle contents and also to chronic epididymitis if urine reaches the epididymis. Retrograde ejaculation can also occur.

14.3 Optimization of Testicular Function

14.3.1 Varicocele Repair

14.3.1.1 Background and Preoperative Considerations

Varicocelectomy is the most common procedure performed for the treatment of male infertility. A varicocele is defined as an abnormal dilation of the testicular pampiniform plexus of veins, found in up to 15% of the male population but in roughly 35% of men with primary infertility and up to 81% of men with secondary infertility [30]. Varicoceles have been associated with both semen analysis abnormalities and alterations in serum reproductive hormone levels, and surgical correction of the varicocele can halt testicular damage and improve spermatogenesis and Leydig cell function [31,32].

Though most varicoceles are asymptomatic, men may present with dull, aching scrotal or inguinal pain. Varicoceles are diagnosed on physical exam and are graded by the Dubin and Amelar grading system from I to III [33]. Grade I varicoceles are only palpable during the Valsalva maneuver. Grade II varicoceles are palpable without Valsalva, and grade III are visible through the scrotal skin. Scrotal ultrasound with color flow Doppler is not a standard part of the varicocele workup, though it may aid diagnosis in patients whose body habitus makes physical exam challenging [34]. Varicoceles diagnosed only by ultrasound are considered subclinical, and while correction of subclinical varicoceles improves semen analysis parameters, it does not appear to improve fertility [35].

Varicocele correction is indicated if a man presents with: 1) document infertility, 2) a palpable varicocele, 3) at least one abnormal semen parameter (except isolated teratospermia) and/or hormonal abnormalities on initial infertility workup, and 4) his partner has documented normal fertility or correctable infertility [34]. In addition, a man with a palpable varicocele, an abnormal semen analysis or hormone profile, a desire for future fertility, or varicocele-related pain may also benefit from varicocele repair. Independent of infertility, given the impact of varicoceles on testosterone production, some advocate for varicocele repair in the setting of low testosterone alone, as well as in adolescent males with varicoceles and testicular size discrepancy [36].

Not all diagnosed varicoceles must be corrected, as not all men with varicoceles will have trouble conceiving. A varicocele discovered incidentally, in the context of a chief complaint of pain, or a subclinical varicocele diagnosed only with ultrasound are less likely to require or warrant intervention. However, there are some limited data that suggest that uncorrected varicocele may cause progressive decline in semen parameters or fertility over time [37]. Thus, lacking a chief complaint of infertility is not an absolute contraindication for varicocele repair at any time.

14.3.1.2 Procedure Notes

There are a number of approaches to the management of varicoceles. Table 14.1 summarizes their pros, cons, and

Table 14.1 Approaches to varicocelectomy [46]

Technique	General consideration	Recurrence (%)	Hydrocele (%)	Spontaneous pregnancy (%)
Retroperitoneal (Palomo)	Pros: Ease of spermatic vein ligation and spermatic artery preservation Cons: High recurrence rate compared to other methods; without microscope, difficult to preserve lymphatics	15 (7–35)	8.2 (6.4–10)	37.7 (25–55)
Laparoscopic	Pros: Magnification of the endoscope aids spermatic artery and lymphatic preservation Cons: Relatively high recurrence rate, potential for bowel or large vessel injury	4.3 (2.2–7.14)	2.84 (2–9.4)	30.1 (14.3–42)
Microscopic inguinal or subinguinal	Pros: Considered the gold standard technique. Sub-inguinal does not require opening of the inguinal canal, while the spermatic artery is less likely to have complicated branching structure in the inguinal approach Cons: Cost of the operative microscope	1.0 (0–3.6)	0.4 (0.2–1.6)	42.0 (33–56)
Conventional inguinal	Pros: Few veins to ligate given high level of cord Cons: Without a surgical microscope, lymphatics are difficult to preserve, and the resulting hydrocele rate can be quite high	2.63 (0–37)	7.3 (7.3)	36 (34–39)
Radiographic	Similar advantages and disadvantages to retroperitoneal and laparoscopic approach. High recurrence rate must be considered.	12.7 (2–24)	N/A	33.2 (20.6–40)

outcomes. Though there are a number of ways to categorize and think about these approaches, the simplest is to first contrast nonsurgical ablation with surgical approaches. Nonsurgical ablation of the spermatic vein, performed by an interventional radiologist, is the least invasive approach, and its isolated focus on the proximal testicular vein make injury to the testicular artery or lymphatic drainage unlikely. However, current case series suggest that 6.5–11% of patients fail an initial ablative attempt and must be converted to surgical varicocelectomy [38]. In addition, recurrence rates remain high, given the inability to ligate collateral veins.

Surgical approaches can be categorized by the requisite tools and the anatomic level at which the spermatic cord structures are isolated. Laparoscopic and open retroperitoneal approaches are similar, in that the cord structures can be dissected and ligated as they enter the internal inguinal ring. At this level, the testicular artery theoretically need not be spared, because distal collateral arterial supply is sufficient, but when possible it ought to be identified and spared with the aid of a laparoscopic Doppler probe [39]. However, similar to radiographic ablation, recurrence from distal collaterals is not preventable with retroperitoneal approaches. Additionally, when the vasculature bundle is ligated so proximally, lymphatics are more difficult to identify and spare, potentially resulting in hydrocele.

Additional surgical approaches include the open inguinal, microsurgical inguinal, and microsurgical subinguinal varicocelectomy. The latter has become the procedure of choice for experts trained in microsurgery, and it is the preferred technique of the authors of this chapter. The subinguinal approach spares the morbidity of opening the external ring, and the use of the operative microscope allows for superior identification and preservation of not only the testicular artery, but also the lymphatics, minimizing postoperative hydrocele formation. A Doppler probe aids in the identification of the testicular artery throughout the procedure. In addition to the dissection and ligation of the veins within the spermatic cord itself, the inguinal and subinguinal microsurgical approaches allow access to external spermatic veins and/or gubernacular veins if ligation of these distal vessels is required.

14.3.1.3 Outcomes and Complications

A number of recent meta-analyses have compared efficacy in terms of postoperative spontaneous pregnancy rates and postoperative recurrence and hydrocele formation rates. These have also been summarized in Table 14.1. Microsurgical approaches appear to have lower rates of hydrocele recurrence, and they may have a slight, albeit statistically insignificant, edge when it comes to resulting pregnancy rates. In addition, the surgical approaches (retroperitoneal, inguinal ligation, and subinguinal ligation) all show significant improvements in sperm count and motility after varicocelectomy [40].

Finally, a recent meta-analysis evaluated whether varicocele repair improves outcomes for couples utilizing ART when sperm retrieval was necessary [41]. Though the analysis was not robust enough to compare the different methods of sperm retrieval, the group found improved live birth and pregnancy rates with IVF/ICSI, and specifically found that varicocele

Table 14.2 Sperm retrieval techniques

	Pros	Cons
MESA	Ample motile sperm for cryopreservation. Decreased rates of hematoma and obstruction.	Microsurgical skill required. Operating time and cost. Not an option for men with NOA
PESA	Simple, fast, cheap. Can be done in the office. Minimal patient discomfort and recovery. No microsurgical skill.	Unlikely sufficient sperm for cryopreservation. Blind approach risks epididymal damage and higher complication rate. Not an option for men with NOA.
TESA	No microsurgical skill required. Simple, fast, cheap. Can be done under local anesthesia. Can be used for OA or NOA.	Risk of hematoma and testicular atrophy. May retrieve inadequate sperm for cryopreservation. Testicular sperm is less mature than epididymal sperm.
TESE	Fast and repeatable. Does not require microsurgical skill.	Longer recovery compared to other techniques. Risk of testicular atrophy. Increased cost and operative time compared to TESA.
Micro-TESE	Optimal technique for NOA. Allows for identification of larger tubules, which are more likely to yield sperm. Less damage to testicular tissue than other testicular sperm retrieval approaches. Minimal complications, including minimal damage to testicular arterial supply.	Requires microsurgical skill. Increased cost and operative time.

repair improved sperm retrieval rates, even in men who remained persistently azoospermic after varicocele repair. These findings suggest a significant role for varicocelectomy in men who may require sperm retrieval for IVF/ICSI. These findings should be factored into one's counseling of couples.

14.4 Sperm Retrieval in the Setting of Uncorrectable Obstructive Azoospermia and Nonobstructive Azoospermia

14.4.1 Sperm Retrieval

14.4.1.1 Background and Preoperative Considerations

With the advent of IVF/ICSI, sperm retrieval, either from the epididymis or the testis, has greatly expanded the fertility potential of many couples who may have previously been considered infertile. This is particularly true in men with reproductive tract abnormalities not amenable to reconstruction, for example, men with congenital bilateral absence of the vas deferens. In addition, men with NOA who either lack a correctable varicocele or who continue to be infertile despite varicocelectomy may also conceive with the help of sperm retrieval. Of course, men with correctable reproductive tract obstruction may opt for sperm retrieval in the setting of reconstructive failure or in the context of female factor infertility that will necessitate the use of IVF/ICSI.

The two epididymal sperm retrieval techniques, percutaneous epididymal sperm aspiration (PESA) and microsurgical epididymal sperm aspiration (MESA), are indicated in men with OA who have viable epididymal tissue. Epididymal sperm are more mature and may result in better IVF outcomes, even with ICSI [42]. Men with NOA, in contrast, have diminished spermatogenesis that necessitates testicular sperm retrieval, either through testicular sperm aspiration (TESA), testicular sperm extraction (TESE), or micro-TESE. These techniques will be outlined and compared below.

14.4.1.2 Procedural Notes and Outcomes

The major advantages and disadvantages of each of the sperm retrieval methods are highlighted in Table 14.2. A full technical explanation of each sperm retrieval method has been outlined elsewhere [43]. Briefly, PESA and TESA are blind procedures in which multiple passes of a fine-gauge needle allow the surgeon to attempt to retrieve adequate sperm. In contrast, MESA and TESE allow for better tubule visualization, are more focused, and often yield larger quantities of sperm. Of note, the authors rarely utilize TESA, as the multiple passes through the testicular tissue are more likely to result in postoperative hematoma and even testicular atrophy.

Micro-TESE offers the best option for men with NOA, as it allows the surgeon to seek out individual dilated tubules that are most likely to yield sufficient sperm for IVF/ICSI [44]. In a systematic review and meta-analysis, micro-TESE yielded higher sperm retrieval rates than conventional TESE, and conventional TESE yielded higher sperm retrieval rates than TESA [45].

14.5 Final Thoughts

The techniques surveyed in this chapter are not all encompassing, but instead serve to highlight some of the most powerful tools urologists have to surgically manage male infertility. The progress made thus far has allowed many infertile couples to conceive, and as more patients and providers continue to utilize these options, robust studies assessing the efficacy of the techniques, particularly sperm retrieval, in different subpopulations of infertile men will allow the urologic community to make more tailored recommendations.

References

1. Krausz C. Male infertility: pathogenesis and clinical diagnosis. *Best Pract Res Clin Endocrinol Metab*. 2011;25:271–285.
2. Brugh VM, 3rd, Lipshultz LI. Male factor infertility: evaluation and management. *Med Clin North Am*. 2004;88:367–385.
3. Ostrowski KA, Holt SK, Haynes B, et al. Evaluation of vasectomy trends in the United States. *Urology*. 2018;118:76–79.
4. Eisenberg ML, Lipshultz LI. Estimating the number of vasectomies performed annually in the United States: data from the National Survey of Family Growth. *J Urol*. 2010;184:2068–2072.
5. Belker AM, Thomas AJ, Jr., Fuchs EF, et al. Results of 1,469 microsurgical vasectomy reversals by the Vasovasostomy Study Group. *J Urol*. 1991;145:505–511.
6. Potts JM, Pasqualotto FF, Nelson D, et al. Patient characteristics associated with vasectomy reversal. *J Urol*. 1999;161:1835–1839.
7. Boorjian S, Lipkin M, Goldstein M. The impact of obstructive interval and sperm granuloma on outcome of vasectomy reversal. *J Urol*. 2004;171:304–306.
8. Fuchs ME, Anderson RE, Ostrowski KA, et al. Pre-operative risk factors associated with need for vasoepididymostomy at the time of vasectomy reversal. *Andrology*. 2016;4:160–162.
9. Silber SJ. Microscopic vasectomy reversal. *Fertil Steril*. 1977;28:1191–1202.
10. Kirby EW, Hockenberry M, Lipshultz LI. Vasectomy reversal: decision making and technical innovations. *Transl Androl Urol*. 2017;6:753–760.
11. Sheynkin YR, Chen ME, Goldstein M. Intravasal azoospermia: a surgical dilemma. *BJU Int*. 2000;85:1089–1092.
12. Hagan KF, Coffey DS. The adverse effects of sperm during vasovasostomy. *J Urol*. 1977;118:269–273.
13. Herrel LA, Goodman M, Goldstein M, et al. Outcomes of microsurgical vasovasostomy for vasectomy reversal: a meta-analysis and systematic review. *Urology*. 2015;85:819–825.
14. Thomas AJ, Jr. Vasoepididymostomy. *Urol Clin North Am*. 1987;14:527–538.
15. Schiff J, Chan P, Li PS, et al. Outcome and late failures compared in 4 techniques of microsurgical vasoepididymostomy in 153 consecutive men. *J Urol*. 2005;174:651–615; quiz 801.
16. Chan PT. The evolution and refinement of vasoepididymostomy techniques. *Asian J Androl*. 2013;15:49–55.
17. Goldstein M, Li PS, Matthews GJ. Microsurgical vasovasostomy: the microdot technique of precision suture placement. *J Urol*. 1998;159:188–190.
18. Namekawa T, Imamoto T, Kato M, et al. Vasovasostomy and vasoepididymostomy: review of the procedures, outcomes, and predictors of patency and pregnancy over the last decade. *Reprod Med Biol*. 2018;17:343–355.
19. Marmar JL. Modified vasoepididymostomy with simultaneous double needle placement, tubulotomy and tubular invagination. *J Urol*. 2000;163:483–486.
20. Sheynkin YR, Li PS, Magid ML, et al. Comparison of absorbable and nonabsorbable sutures for microsurgical vasovasostomy in rats. *Urology*. 1999;53:1235–1238.
21. Matthews GJ, Schlegel PN, Goldstein M. Patency following microsurgical vasoepididymostomy and vasovasostomy: temporal considerations. *J Urol*. 1995;154:2070–2073.
22. Jarow JP, Espeland MA, Lipshultz LI. Evaluation of the azoospermic patient. *J Urol*. 1989;142:62–65.
23. Netto NR, Jr., Esteves SC, Neves PA. Transurethral resection of partially obstructed ejaculatory ducts: seminal parameters and pregnancy outcomes according to the etiology of obstruction. *J Urol*. 1998;159:2048–2053.
24. Yurdakul T, Gokce G, Kilic O, et al. Transurethral resection of ejaculatory ducts in the treatment of complete ejaculatory duct obstruction. *Int Urol Nephrol*. 2008;40:369–372.
25. Engin G, Celtik M, Sanli O, et al. Comparison of transrectal ultrasonography and transrectal ultrasonography-guided seminal vesicle aspiration in the diagnosis of the ejaculatory duct obstruction. *Fertil Steril*. 2009;92:964–970.
26. Jarow JP. Seminal vesicle aspiration in the management of patients with ejaculatory duct obstruction. *J Urol*. 1994;152:899–901.
27. Farley S, Barnes R. Stenosis of ejaculatory ducts treated by endoscopic resection. *J Urol*. 1973;109:664–666.
28. Avellino GJ, Lipshultz LI, Sigman M, et al. Transurethral resection of the ejaculatory ducts: etiology of obstruction and surgical treatment options. *Fertil Steril*. 2019;111:427–443.
29. El-Assmy A, El-Tholoth H, Abouelkheir RT, et al. Transurethral resection of ejaculatory duct in infertile men: outcome and predictors of success. *Int Urol Nephrol*. 2012;44:1623–1630.
30. Gorelick JI, Goldstein M. Loss of fertility in men with varicocele. *Fertil Steril*. 1993;59:613–616.
31. Damsgaard J, Joensen UN, Carlsen E, et al. Varicocele is associated with impaired semen quality and reproductive hormone levels: a study of 7035 healthy young men from six European countries. *Eur Urol*. 2016;70:1019–1029.
32. Su LM, Goldstein M, Schlegel PN. The effect of varicocelectomy on serum testosterone levels in infertile men with varicoceles. *J Urol*. 1995;154:1752–1755.
33. Dubin L, Amelar RD. Varicocelectomy as therapy in male infertility: a study of 504 cases. *J Urol*. 1975;113:640–641.

34. Stahl P, Schlegel PN. Standardization and documentation of varicocele evaluation. *Curr Opin Urol.* 2011;21:500–505.
35. Kohn TP, Ohlander SJ, Jacob JS, et al. The effect of subclinical varicocele on pregnancy rates and semen parameters: a systematic review and meta-analysis. *Curr Urol Rep.* 2018;19:53.
36. Schlegel PN, Goldstein M. Alternate indications for varicocele repair: non-obstructive azoospermia, pain, androgen deficiency and progressive testicular dysfunction. *Fertil Steril.* 2011;96:1288–1293.
37. Chehval MJ, Purcell MH. Deterioration of semen parameters over time in men with untreated varicocele: evidence of progressive testicular damage. *Fertil Steril.* 1992;57:174–177.
38. Światłowski Ł, Pyra K, Kuczyńska M, et al. Selecting patients for embolization of varicoceles based on ultrasonography. *J Ultrason.* 2018;18:90–95.
39. Tu D, Glassberg KI. Laparoscopic varicocelectomy. *BJU Int.* 2010;106:1094–1104.
40. Schauer I, Madersbacher S, Jost R, et al. The impact of varicocelectomy on sperm parameters: a meta-analysis. *J Urol.* 2012;187:1540–1547.
41. Kirby EW, Wiener LE, Rajanahally S, et al. Undergoing varicocele repair before assisted reproduction improves pregnancy rate and live birth rate in azoospermic and oligospermic men with a varicocele: a systematic review and meta-analysis. *Fertil Steril.* 2016;106:1338–1343.
42. van Wely M, Barbey N, Meissner A, et al. Live birth rates after MESA or TESE in men with obstructive azoospermia: is there a difference? *Hum Reprod.* 2015;30:761–766.
43. Esteves SC, Miyaoka R, Orosz JE, et al. An update on sperm retrieval techniques for azoospermic males. *Clinics (Sao Paulo).* 2013;68(Suppl. 1):99–110.
44. Ashraf MC, Singh S, Raj D, et al. Micro-dissection testicular sperm extraction as an alternative for sperm acquisition in the most difficult cases of azoospermia: technique and preliminary results in India. *J Hum Reprod Sci.* 2013;6:111–123.
45. Bernie AM, Mata DA, Ramasamy R, et al. Comparison of microdissection testicular sperm extraction, conventional testicular sperm extraction, and testicular sperm aspiration for nonobstructive azoospermia: a systematic review and meta-analysis. *Fertil Steril.* 2015;104:1099–1103.e3.
46. Cayan S, Shavakhabov S, Kadioğlu A. Treatment of palpable varicocele in infertile men: a meta-analysis to define the best technique. *J Androl.* 2009;30:33–40.

Chapter 15
Varicocele Repair in the Era of IVF/ICSI

Jessica N. Schardein, Alexander W. Pastuszak, and James M. Hotaling

15.1 Introduction

Among couples struggling with infertility, a male factor plays a role in approximately 50% of cases [1]. While there are many causes of male factor infertility, varicoceles have been identified as the most common and correctable cause [2]. Men presenting to infertility clinics have varicoceles at 2–3 times the frequency of the general male population as well as compared to fertile men [2]. Up to 35% of men with primary infertility and as many as 81% of men with secondary infertility are diagnosed with a clinical varicocele [2].

Varicoceles are defined as a pathologic dilation of the pampiniform venous plexus of the spermatic cord [3]. The pathology may be associated with dysfunctional valves, increased venous pressure, and/or left renal vein compression between the superior mesenteric artery and the abdominal aorta [3]. Subclinical varicoceles are detected only by ultrasound, while clinical varicoceles can be detected on physical exam and range from Grade I to Grade III depending on severity. Grade I varicoceles are palpated with Valsalva, grade II varicoceles are palpated without Valsalva, and grade III varicoceles are readily visible without manipulations.

When a varicocele is identified, approximately 25% of men will have abnormal semen parameters [4]. Abnormal semen parameters may be due to poor testicular drainage that impairs sperm production and leads to testicular dysfunction [5]. Hyperthermia-induced damage is one theory based on an early study by Goldstein and Eid that observed higher intratesticular temperatures in men with varicoceles [6]. Other theories are based on studies that found men with varicoceles have more reflux of adrenal metabolites in penile blood, testicular hypoxia, and antisperm antibodies [7–9]. These different biochemical processes have been associated with testicular atrophy, higher levels of reactive oxygen species, and decreased testosterone production, which can result in impaired fertility [8,10,11].

Surgical correction of a varicocele via varicocelectomy has been shown to improve the chances of achieving a natural pregnancy (NP) in men with abnormal semen parameters in several randomized controlled trials and meta-analyses [10,12–14]. In addition, men with abnormal semen parameters who do not pursue surgical repair may have progressive deterioration of semen quality, including a decrease in sperm density, total sperm count, or total motile sperm count (TMSC) of >45% or deterioration of sperm motility or morphology of >20% [15]. The increase in TMSC following varicocelectomy is statistically significant [16]. While in some cases there may be little to no improvements seen in typical semen parameters on repeat semen analyses following varicocelectomy, several studies have demonstrated improvements in sperm DNA fragmentation and a decrease in reactive oxygen species, which may explain the increase in pregnancy rates and live birth rates observed in this cohort [17–22].

When an NP does not occur, infertile couples may pursue assisted reproductive technology (ART), including intrauterine insemination (IUI), in vitro fertilization (IVF), and intracytoplasmic sperm injection (ICSI), to achieve a pregnancy. A male partner with a varicocele may elect to pursue varicocelectomy prior to ART in an attempt to improve the possibility of pregnancy and live birth.

15.2 Varicocelectomy and ART

The benefits of varicocelectomy prior to ART have not been clearly defined due to the lack of high-level evidence. While there are several controlled trials, there are no randomized controlled trials so the results must be interpreted carefully due to potential bias. However, investigations to date support a positive effect of varicocele repair on pregnancy rates regardless of approach. Table 15.1 summarizes all the available controlled trials in the literature that address this topic.

The current literature indicates that varicocelectomy may allow for success with less invasive modalities of ART or result in higher overall pregnancy rates and live birth rates [5]. Specifically, Samplaski et al. found that for baseline TMSC <5 million, the mean TMSC increased from 2.32±1.50 million to 15.97±32.92 million (p = 0.0000002) allowing 58.8% of men to be upgraded from IVF candidacy to NP or IUI candidacy [16]. In another study, by Cayan et al., 540 infertile men with clinical varicoceles underwent microsurgical varicocelectomy and were followed for more than two years postoperatively [23]. Of preoperative IVF/ICSI candidates, 31% became NP or IUI candidates after varicocelectomy [23]. Of IUI candidates, 42% gained the potential for NP [23]. A more recent study in 2020 by Turgut evaluated pregnancy rates in men with severe oligospermia and found that TMSC increased in the

Table 15.1 Outcomes following ART

Pregnancy and live birth outcomes following IUI

	Treated varicocele			Untreated varicocele		
Study	Couples	PR	LBR	Couples	PR	LBR
Marmar et al. (1992) [27]	52	7.7%	NR	14	14.3%	NR
Daitch et al. (2001) [28]	34	35.3%	35.3%	24	16.7%	4.2%
Boman et al. (2008) [29]	12	50%	NR	10	10%	NR

Pregnancy and live birth outcomes for oligospermic men following IVF/ICSI

	Treated varicocele			Untreated varicocele		
Study	Couples	PR	LBR	Couples	PR	LBR
Ashkenazi et al. (1989) [31]	12	20%	NR	12	0%	NR
Esteves et al. (2010) [32]	80	60%*	46.2%*	162	45%*	31.4%*
Pasqualotto et al. (2012) [34]	169	30.9%	NR	79	31.1%	NR
Gokce et al. (2013) [33]	168	62.5%*	47.6%*	139	47.1%*	29%*

Pregnancy and live birth outcomes for nonobstructive azoospermia men following IVF/ICSI

	Treated varicocele				Untreated varicocele			
Study	Couples	SRR	PR	LBR	Couples	SRR	PR	LBR
Inci et al. (2009) [42]	66	53%*	31.4%	NR	30	30%*	22.2%	NR
Haydardedeoglu et al. (2010) [43]	31	60.8%*	74.2%*	64.5%*	65	38.5%*	52.3%*	41.5%*

Notes: PR: pregnancy rate; LBR: live birth rate; SRR: sperm retrieval rate; NR: not reported; *: statistically significant values.

varicocelectomy group from 4.5±2.8 million to 16.5±4.3 million [24]. Among the 52 men who underwent varicocelectomy, the pregnancy rate was 38.5% with 13.4% due to NP, 13.4% due to IUI, and 11.5% due to ICSI [24]. This is in comparison to the 36 men who did not undergo varicocelectomy and had a statistically significant lower pregnancy rate of 11.1% and required ART [24].

15.3 IUI after Varicocelectomy

Most infertile couples pursue IUI as the first ART in an attempt to achieve a pregnancy. Case series without control groups estimate that IUI pregnancy rates per couple following varicocelectomy range between 10% and 27% [25,26]. The few studies looking at pregnancy rates with IUI after varicocelectomy with control groups demonstrate a wide range of results.

In 1992, a retrospective study by Marmar et al. investigating the effectiveness of IUI after varicocelectomy found a higher rate of IUI success in men with untreated varicocele than in men after varicocelectomy [27]. This was based on data that showed 52 men with surgically corrected varicoceles underwent 145 cycles of IUI resulting in 4 pregnancies (2.8%) in comparison to 14 men with untreated varicocele who underwent 30 cycles of IUI resulting in 2 pregnancies (6.7%). This corresponds to a pregnancy rate of 7.7% and 14.3% for men with and without varicocelectomy, respectively.

The low overall pregnancy rates may be related to the lack of ovarian stimulation in women undergoing IUI. Other limitations of this early study include its retrospective nature and small sample size. Overall, this study does not suggest that varicocelectomy significantly impacts pregnancy rates of those undergoing IUI.

Another retrospective study in 2001 by Daitch et al. specifically evaluated men with clinical varicoceles and abnormal semen parameters and found that while varicocelectomy did not significantly improve typical semen parameters, it was associated with higher pregnancy rates and live birth rates after IUI [28]. Among the 34 men who underwent IUI after varicocelectomy, 101 IUI cycles resulted in 12 pregnancies (11.8%), which all resulted in live births (11.8%), corresponding to a pregnancy rate of 35.3% and a live birth rate of 35.3%. Among the 24 men who underwent IUI without varicocelectomy, 63 IUI cycles resulted in 4 pregnancies (6.3%) and 1 live birth (1.6%), corresponding to a pregnancy rate of 16.7% and a live birth rate of 4.2%.

Boman et al. retrospectively reviewed men with clinical varicoceles and asthenospermia in 2008 and found that there were significant improvements in TMSC in men following varicocelectomy from 29.6 million to 39.0 million (p<0.05) [29]. The pregnancy rate for the 12 couples attempting IUI after varicocelectomy was higher than in the 10 couples who did not undergo varicocelectomy, although the difference was not statistically significant (50% vs. 10%, p>0.05). The number of IUI cycles performed to achieve a pregnancy were not reported. Overall, the study was underpowered due to the small sample size, but suggests the possibility that varicocelectomy prior to IUI may improve pregnancy rates.

A systematic review and meta-analysis by Kirby et al. in 2016 observed that pregnancy rates were not significantly improved with varicocelectomy (OR: 1.989; 95% CI: 0.565–8.834), but live birth rates were significantly higher for patients undergoing IUI after varicocelectomy (OR: 8.360; 95% CI: 1.170–363.002) [30].

Based on the existing literature, pregnancy rate with IUI after varicocelectomy ranges between 7.7% and 50%, making it challenging to establish the true rate. The studies do not consistently report semen parameters, female age, duration of follow-up, number of cycles attempted in total or per couple, ovulation induction protocol, or time from varicocelectomy to pregnancy, all of which are important to characterize IUI success following varicocelectomy. Future studies are necessary to draw adequate conclusions regarding how varicocele affects IUI outcomes.

15.4 IVF/ICSI after Varicocelectomy

IVF with or without ICSI may be required in oligospermic men when IUI is not feasible to achieve a pregnancy. It is important to consider men with azoospermia separately given the more severe abnormality in semen parameters, which may not be comparable to men with oligospermia. The presence of a varicocele and the possibility of a different pathophysiology in these groups is also an important factor that supports examining these groups separately. Figure 15.1 summarizes the pregnancy rates and live birth rates for men with oligospermia with and without varicocelectomy for couples who pursue both IUI and IVF/ICSI. Figure 15.2 summarizes the sperm retrieval rates, pregnancy rates, and live birth rates for men with azoospermia with and without varicocelectomy for couples who pursue IVF/ISCI.

15.4.1 In Men with Oligospermia

The initial study that demonstrated that correcting a varicocele prior to IVF may improve pregnancy rates in men with oligospermia was performed by Ashkenazi et al. in 1989 [31]. In this study, 12 men with clinical varicoceles, oligospermia, and infertility followed for more than two years were unable to achieve a pregnancy with IVF before varicocelectomy, but 20% of these men achieved a pregnancy with their partner using IVF after varicocelectomy.

In 2010, Esteves et al. compared IVF/ICSI outcomes in men with and without varicocelectomy who had similar baseline characteristics with regard to female age, mean infertility duration, proportion with bilateral varicoceles, and proportion with Grade I, II, and III varicoceles [32]. They found that men who underwent varicocelectomy achieved clinical pregnancy with the use of IVF/ICSI in 60.0% of cases, with a live birth rate of 46.2%, and men with untreated varicoceles achieved a clinical pregnancy rate of 45.0% and a live birth rate of 31.4%. These differences were statistically significant for both pregnancy rates and live birth rates after varicocelectomy (OR: 1.82; 95% CI: 1.06–3.15 and OR: 1.87; 95% CI: 1.08–3.25, respectively). The mean time between surgical correction of the varicocele and IVF/ICSI cycles was 6.2 months.

The largest study, by Gokce et al. in 2013, supported findings from prior studies that varicocelectomy prior to IVF/ICSI improves pregnancy rates in oligospermic men [33]. In this study, patients with and without varicocelectomy were comparable in female age, male age, proportion of couples with concurrent female infertility diagnoses, and proportion with Grade I, II, or III varicoceles. A pregnancy was

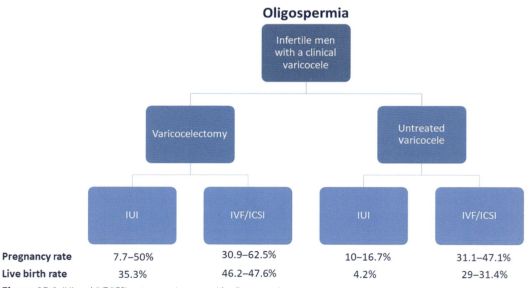

Figure 15.1 IUI and IVF/ICSI outcomes in men with oligospermia

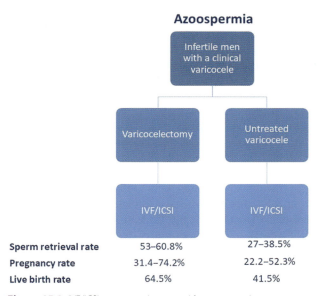

Figure 15.2 IVF/ICSI outcomes in men with azoospermia

achieved in 62.5% of the 168 couples with men who underwent varicocelectomy compared to 47.1% of the 138 couples with men who did not undergo varicocelectomy (p = 0.01). Live birth rates were 47.6% and 29.0%, respectively (p<0.001). The mean time between surgical correction of the varicocele and IVF/ICSI cycles was 7.2 months.

In contrast to these studies, a large retrospective study by Pasqualotto et al. in 2012 demonstrated no difference in IVF/ICSI success with or without varicocelectomy for a grade III varicocele [34]. Among the 169 men who underwent varicocele repair, 30.9% achieved a pregnancy compared to 31.1% of the 79 men who did not undergo varicocele repair (p = 0.97). Although pregnancy rates were not significantly different between the two groups, the time to pregnancy for couples who had undergone varicocelectomy was 6.0±0.5 years, whereas the time to pregnancy for couples with uncorrected varicoceles was 2.7±0.4 years (p<0.001). This longer duration of infertility implies that the varicocelectomy group may have had other factors contributing to greater difficulty in achieving a pregnancy, resulting in the null results of the study. The authors acknowledged prior studies that indicated varicocelectomy may be of benefit in some circumstances despite their results and recommended varicocelectomy be considered prior to ART due to this possibility.

The 2016 meta-analysis by Kirby et al. included all the prior studies to evaluate the effect of varicocelectomy on pregnancy rates and live birth rates with ART [30]. The authors estimated the pregnancy rates for oligospermic men undergoing IVF/ICSI after varicocelectomy to be 49.1% and 42.1% for men undergoing IVF/ICSI without varicocelectomy. The analysis revealed that pregnancy rates were not significantly improved following varicocelectomy (OR: 1.70; 95% CI: 0.95–3.02), but live birth rates were (OR: 1.70; 95% CI: 1.02–2.72). Overall, these results suggest that varicocelectomy prior to IVF/ICSI may be beneficial to improve the rate of live births in couples with infertility.

15.4.2 In Men with Nonobstructive Azoospermia

In men with nonobstructive azoospermia (NOA), varicocelectomy can improve semen parameters [35–38]. Varicocelectomy can be combined with testicular sperm extraction (TESE) or microdissection-TESE (m-TESE) for IVF/ICSI [35–38]. In men with a grade III varicocele and NOA, successful sperm retrieval in men who undergo m-TESE after varicocelectomy is 57.8% compared to 27% for men who have not undergone varicocelectomy (p<0.05) [39]. Following varicocelectomy, up to 44% of men have sufficient sperm in their ejaculate to proceed with IVF without need for TESE, making varicocelectomy a cost-effective strategy that reduces the number of invasive procedures [40,41].

Two controlled studies have been performed that support varicocelectomy in men with NOA if TESE with IVF/ICSI is indicated [42,43]. The study by Inci et al. in 2009 examined 66 men who underwent varicocelectomy prior to TESE with IVF/ICSI and 30 men who underwent TESE with IVF/ICSI without varicocelectomy and found that successful sperm retrieval occurred in 53% and 30% of men, respectively (p = 0.04) [42]. Pregnancy rates were 31.4% in the varicocelectomy group compared to 22.2% in the untreated varicocele group (p>0.05) [42]. Similarly, in 2010 Haydardedeoglu et al. found that among 31 men with varicocelectomy and 65 men without varicocelectomy, sperm retrieval rates were significantly higher for men who underwent varicocelectomy (60.8% vs. 38.5%, p = 0.01) [43]. The pregnancy rates and live birth rates were also significantly higher (74.2% and 64.5% vs. 52.3% and 41.5%, p<0.01) [43]. Together, these studies suggest that varicocelectomy prior to TESE can improve rates of sperm retrieval, pregnancy, and live birth.

The meta-analysis performed by Kirby et al. in 2016 confirmed the results of these controlled studies [30]. Overall, men with grade III varicoceles who underwent varicocelectomy had significantly higher rates of sperm retrieval (OR: 2.51; p<0.01) and pregnancy (OR: 2.34; 95% CI: 1.02–5.34), and near significant rates of live birth (OR:2.21; 95% CI: 0.99–4.90) when compared to men who did not undergo varicocelectomy.

Another 2016 meta-analysis by Esteves et al. incorporated the same studies and confirmed that sperm retrieval rates significantly increased in men with varicocelectomy compared to those without varicocelectomy (OR: 2.65; 95% CI: 1.69–4.14; p<0.001) [41]. There was a higher likelihood of sperm retrieval rates in men with hypospermatogenesis (HS) and maturation arrest (MA) histopathology compared to Sertoli cell-only (SCO) histopathology. In terms of the odds of finding sperm in postoperative ejaculate, there was a significant increase in odds for patients with HS compared to MA (OR: 2.35; 95% CI: 1.04–5.29; p = 0.04) and SCO (OR: 12.0; 95% CI: 4.34–33.17; p< = 0.001). Based on their analysis, although pregnancy rates and live birth rates with the use of testicular sperm retrieved by m-TESE favored the varicocelectomy group, neither had statistically significant odds ratios

(OR: 2.07; 95% CI: 0.92–4.65; p = 0.08 and OR: 2.19; 95% CI: 0.99–4.83; p = 0.05, respectively).

15.5 ART Considerations

The 2021 European Association of Urology guidelines on male sexual and reproductive health strongly recommend varicocelectomy for infertile men with a clinical varicocele, abnormal semen parameters, or otherwise unexplained infertility in a couple in which the female partner has a good ovarian reserve to improve the fertility rate and weakly recommend varicocelectomy for men with raised sperm DNA fragmentation with otherwise unexplained infertility or who have suffered from failed ART, including recurrent pregnancy loss or failure of embryogenesis and implantation [44]. The 2021 American Urological Association/American Society for Reproductive Medicine guidelines state that varicocelectomy should be considered in men attempting to conceive who have palpable varicocele(s), infertility, and abnormal semen parameters, except those with azoospermia [45]. Furthermore, the guidelines state that for men with clinical varicocele and NOA, couples should be informed of the absence of definitive evidence supporting varicocele repair prior to ART [45]. Current guidelines recommend against repair of subclinical varicoceles for infertility as varicocelectomy does not lead to clinically significant changes in semen parameters or improvements in pregnancy rates when compared to men without varicocelectomy [46]. Furthermore, there is currently no specific data evaluating varicocelectomy in patients with subclinical varicoceles pursuing ART [46]. The guidelines acknowledge the need to defer treatment with ART when undergoing varicocelectomy for clinical varicoceles, which is an important consideration for couples [44,45].

Varicocelectomy combined with IUI, IVF/ISCI, and/or TESE or m-TESE with IVF/ICSI can be a lengthy process. After varicocelectomy, sperm counts peak between three and six months postoperatively and have little to no additional improvement beyond six months, which is around the time NP or ART is pursued [47]. This confers additional time a couple must wait before trying to build their family, which may not be reasonable for couples with advanced maternal age. In addition, for men with NOA who undergo varicocelectomy, a gradual decline in spermatogenesis and return to azoospermia has been observed in up to 55.5% of men within one year after varicocelectomy so it is important for these couples to know a long-term benefit is uncertain if they wait too long or want additional children [48]. Of course, the couple's preference, age, desire for multiple children, baseline semen characteristics, tolerability of ART, and financial situation must all be used to individualize treatment.

Some couples may pursue varicocelectomy with the hope of pursuing less invasive ART modalities or avoiding the need for ART altogether afterwards. As previously discussed, varicocelectomy may allow for success with less invasive modalities of ART with between 26.8% and 58.8% of IVF candidates being upgraded to IUI or NP candidates and 42% of IUI candidates being upgraded to NP candidates [16,23,24]. These upgrades can significantly impact the cost associated with fertility treatment for both institutions and couples. The utilization of the least possible invasive modality offers several advantages to couples, including decreased out-of-pocket costs associated with ART.

Decision analysis models have been used by two authors in an attempt to determine the cost-effectiveness of varicocelectomy prior to ART. Based on their decision analysis model, Meng et al. determined that varicocelectomy is more cost-effective when the postoperative pregnancy rate is >14% in men with a preoperative TMSC <10 million sperm in the IVF/ICSI group and >45% in men with TMSC >10 million in the IUI group [49]. Lee et al. used a different decision analysis model with cost data from the USA in 2005 to evaluate the cost-effectiveness of varicocelectomy and found that despite the potential benefits of varicocele repair in NOA patients, varicocelectomy was not as cost-effective as straightforward micro-TESE with ICSI when direct and indirect costs per live delivery were calculated [50]. Varicocelectomy was found to be more cost-effective than TESE when the rate of NP after varicocelectomy is >40% or the rate of successful delivery after IVF/ICSI is <10% [50]. Costs at specific institutions, success rates of varicocelectomy and IVF/ISCI as well as insurance coverage would allow for more individualized results.

More recently, Dubin et al. evaluated men who underwent varicocelectomy for TMSC <2 million and performed a cost-effectiveness analysis of IUI and IVF/ICSI after varicocelectomy [40]. The authors found that 59% of the men who had severe oligospermia and underwent varicocelectomy had a TMSC >2 million at three months and could pursue less invasive ART. Varicocelectomy was determined to be a cost-effective procedure since the cost per pregnancy was approximately one-third the price in those who became eligible for IUI compared to those who required ICSI/IVF after varicocelectomy ($35,924 vs. $93,203). There were also substantial cost savings for the healthcare system when men pursued varicocelectomy in combination with IUI rather than simply advancing to IVF/ICSI without varicocelectomy ($35,924 vs. $45,795). While the number of children desired by the couples, the cost of birth defects, ART-related complications, and the differences in costs across countries and institutions all affect the objectivity of the results, varicocelectomy has the potential to be more cost-effective for both institutions and couples even in combination with ART.

15.6 Conclusion

Varicocelectomy prior to ART has the potential to improve semen parameters, pregnancy rates and live birth rates. Although not currently recommended by guidelines, varicocelectomy may even provide benefit to men with NOA, especially if healthy sperm can be recovered in the ejaculate. Further studies that evaluate preoperative factors that predict successful improvement in spermatogenesis following varicocelectomy are critical to determine which couples would benefit most from varicocelectomy prior to ART.

References

1. Irvine DS. Epidemiology and aetiology of male infertility. *Hum Reprod*. 1998;13(Suppl. 1):33–44.
2. Redmon JB, Carey P Pryor JL. Varicocele: the most common cause of male factor infertility? *Hum Reprod Update*. 2002;8(1):53–58.
3. Kohn TP, Kohn JR, Pastuszak AW. Varicocelectomy before assisted reproductive technology: are outcomes improved? *Fertil Steril*. 2017;108(3):385–391.
4. World Health Organization. The influence of varicocele on parameters of fertility in a large group of men presenting to infertility clinics. World Health Organization. *Fertil Steril*. 1992;57(6):1289–1293.
5. Pathak P, Chandrashekar A, Hakky TS, et al. Varicocele management in the era of in vitro fertilization/intracytoplasmic sperm injection. *Asian J Androl*. 2016;18(3):343–348.
6. Goldstein M, Eid JF. Elevation of intratesticular and scrotal skin surface temperature in men with varicocele. *J Urol*. 1989;142(3):743–745.
7. Ozbek E, Yurekli M, Soylu A, et al. The role of adrenomedullin in varicocele and impotence. *BJU Int*. 2000;86(6):694–698.
8. Hendin BN, Kolettis PN, Sharma RK, et al. Varicocele is associated with elevated spermatozoal reactive oxygen species production and diminished seminal plasma antioxidant capacity. *J Urol*. 1999;161(6):1831–1834.
9. Gilbert, BR, Witkin SS, Goldstein M. Correlation of sperm-bound immunoglobulins with impaired semen analysis in infertile men with varicoceles. *Fertil Steril*. 1989;52(3):469–473.
10. Abdel-Meguid TA, Farsi HM, Al-Sayyad A, et al. Effects of varicocele on serum testosterone and changes of testosterone after varicocelectomy: a prospective controlled study. *Urology*. 2014;84(5):1081–1087.
11. Mieusset R, Bujan L. Testicular heating and its possible contributions to male infertility: a review. *Int J Androl*. 1995;18(4):169–184.
12. Freire Gde C. Surgery or embolization for varicoceles in subfertile men. *Sao Paulo Med J*. 2013;131(1):67.
13. Kroese AC, de Lange NM, Collins J, et al. Surgery or embolization for varicoceles in subfertile men. *Cochrane Database Syst Rev*. 2012;10:CD000479.
14. Breznik R, Vlaisavljevic V, Borko E. Treatment of varicocele and male fertility. *Arch Androl*. 1993;30(3):157–160.
15. Chen SS, Chen LK. Risk factors for progressive deterioration of semen quality in patients with varicocele. *Urology*. 2012;79(1):128–132.
16. Samplaski MK, Lo KC, Grober ED, et al. Varicocelectomy to "upgrade" semen quality to allow couples to use less invasive forms of assisted reproductive technology. *Fertil Steril*. 2017;108(4):609–612.
17. Baazeem A, Belzile E, Ciampi A, et al. Varicocele and male factor infertility treatment: a new meta-analysis and review of the role of varicocele repair. *Eur Urol*. 2011;60(4):796–808.
18. Zini A, Azhar R, Baazeem A, et al. Effect of microsurgical varicocelectomy on human sperm chromatin and DNA integrity: a prospective trial. *Int J Androl*. 2011;34(1):14–19.
19. Smit M, Romijn JC, Wildhagen MF, et al. Decreased sperm DNA fragmentation after surgical varicocelectomy is associated with increased pregnancy rate. *J Urol*. 2013;189(1 Suppl):S146–S150.
20. Li F, Yamaguchi K, Okada K, et al. Significant improvement of sperm DNA quality after microsurgical repair of varicocele. *Syst Biol Reprod Med*. 2012;58(5):274–277.
21. Wang YJ, Zhang RQ, Lin YJ, et al. Relationship between varicocele and sperm DNA damage and the effect of varicocele repair: a meta-analysis. *Reprod Biomed Online*. 2012;25(3):307–314.
22. Chen SS, Huang WJ, Chang LS, et al. Attenuation of oxidative stress after varicocelectomy in subfertile patients with varicocele. *J Urol*. 2008;179(2):639–642.
23. Cayan S, Erdemir F, Ozbey I, et al. Can varicocelectomy significantly change the way couples use assisted reproductive technologies? *J Urol*. 2002;167(4):1749–1752.
24. Turgut H. The effect of varicocelectomy on the pregnancy rate in patients with severe oligospermia. *Niger J Clin Pract*. 2020;23(12):1744–1747.
25. Kamal KM, Jarvi K, Zini A. Microsurgical varicocelectomy in the era of assisted reproductive technology: influence of initial semen quality on pregnancy rates. *Fertil Steril*. 2001;75(5):1013–1016.
26. Grober ED, Chan PT, Zini A, et al. Microsurgical treatment of persistent or recurrent varicocele. *Fertil Steril*. 2004;82(3):718–722.
27. Marmar JL, Corson SL, Batzer FR, et al. Insemination data on men with varicoceles. *Fertil Steril*. 1992;57(5):1084–1090.
28. Daitch JA, Bedaiwy MA, Pasqualotto EB, et al. Varicocelectomy improves intrauterine insemination success rates in men with varicocele. *J Urol*. 2001;165(5):1510–1513.
29. Boman JM, Libman J, Zini A. Microsurgical varicocelectomy for isolated asthenospermia. *J Urol*. 2008;180(5):2129–2132.
30. Kirby EW, Wiener LE, Rajanahally S, et al. Undergoing varicocele repair before assisted reproduction improves pregnancy rate and live birth rate in azoospermic and oligospermic men with a varicocele: a systematic review and meta-analysis. *Fertil Steril*. 2016;106(6):1338–1343.
31. Ashkenazi J, Dicker D, Feldberg D, et al. The impact of spermatic vein ligation on the male factor in in vitro fertilization-embryo transfer and its relation to testosterone levels before and after operation. *Fertil Steril*. 1989;51(3):471–474.
32. Esteves SC, Oliveira FV, Bertolla RP. Clinical outcome of intracytoplasmic sperm injection in infertile men with treated and untreated clinical varicocele. *J Urol*. 2010;184(4):1442–1446.
33. Gokce A, Demirtas A, Ozturk A, et al. Association of left varicocoele with height, body mass index and sperm counts in infertile men. *Andrology*. 2013;1(1):116–119.
34. Pasqualotto FF, Braga DP, Figueira RC, et al. Varicocelectomy does not impact pregnancy outcomes following intracytoplasmic sperm injection procedures. *J Androl*. 2012;33(2):239–243.
35. Kim ED, Leibman BB, Grinblat DM, et al. Varicocele repair improves semen

35. parameters in azoospermic men with spermatogenic failure. *J Urol.* 1999;162 (3 Pt 1):737–740.
36. Matthews GJ, Matthews ED, Goldstein M. Induction of spermatogenesis and achievement of pregnancy after microsurgical varicocelectomy in men with azoospermia and severe oligoasthenospermia. *Fertil Steril.* 1998;70(1):71–75.
37. Schoysman R, Vanderzwalmen P, Nijs M, et al. Pregnancy after fertilisation with human testicular spermatozoa. *Lancet.* 1993;342(8881):1237.
38. Schlegel PN. Testicular sperm extraction: microdissection improves sperm yield with minimal tissue excision. *Hum Reprod.* 1999;14 (1):131–135.
39. Zampieri N, Bosaro L, Costantini C, et al. Relationship between testicular sperm extraction and varicocelectomy in patients with varicocele and nonobstructive azoospermia. *Urology.* 2013;82(1):74–77.
40. Dubin JM, Greer AB, Kohn TP, et al. Men with severe oligospermia appear to benefit from varicocele repair: a cost-effectiveness analysis of assisted reproductive technology. *Urology.* 2018;111:99–103.
41. Esteves SC, Miyaoka R, Roque M, et al. Outcome of varicocele repair in men with nonobstructive azoospermia: systematic review and meta-analysis. *Asian J Androl.* 2016;18 (2):246–253.
42. Inci K, Hascicek M, Kara O, et al. Sperm retrieval and intracytoplasmic sperm injection in men with nonobstructive azoospermia, and treated and untreated varicocele. *J Urol.* 2009. 182(4):1500–1505.
43. Haydardedeoglu B, Turunc T, Kilicdag EB, et al. The effect of prior varicocelectomy in patients with nonobstructive azoospermia on intracytoplasmic sperm injection outcomes: a retrospective pilot study. *Urology.* 2010;75(1):83–86.
44. Salonia A, Bettocchi C, Boeri L, et al. European Association of Urology Guidelines on Sexual and Reproductive Health – 2021 update: male sexual dysfunction. *Eur Urol.* 2021;80 (3):333–357.
45. Schlegel PN, Sigman M, Collura B, et al. Diagnosis and treatment of infertility in men: AUA/ASRM guideline part II. *Fertil Steril.* 2021;115(1):62–69.
46. Kohn TP, Ohlander SJ, Jacob JS, et al. The effect of subclinical varicocele on pregnancy rates and semen parameters: a systematic review and meta-analysis. *Curr Urol Rep.* 2018;19(7):53.
47. Al Bakri A, Lo K, Grober E, et al. Time for improvement in semen parameters after varicocelectomy. *J Urol.* 2012;187 (1):227–231.
48. Abdel-Meguid TA. Predictors of sperm recovery and azoospermia relapse in men with nonobstructive azoospermia after varicocele repair. *J Urol.* 2012;187 (1):222–226.
49. Meng MV, Greene KL, Turek PJ. Surgery or assisted reproduction? A decision analysis of treatment costs in male infertility. *J Urol.* 2005;174 (5):1926–1931; discussion 1931.
50. Lee R, Li PS, Goldstein M, et al. A decision analysis of treatments for nonobstructive azoospermia associated with varicocele. *Fertil Steril.* 2009;92 (1):188–196.

Section 3 Clinical Evaluation and Treatment of Male Infertility

Chapter 16

Implementing Genetic Testing of Male Infertility in the Clinic

Ahmad Majzoub, Chak Lam Cho, and Sandro C. Esteves

16.1 Introduction

Infertility is a global condition with pronounced implications on human health and longevity and the economic aspects of a given society. A systematic analysis of 277 health surveys from 190 countries reported a prevalence of primary and secondary infertility among couples of 1.9% and 10.5%, respectively [1]. Various male-related factors have been identified and may attribute to about 50% of infertility causes among couples [2]. Male factor infertility is prevalent in about 5–7% of the general male population and is believed to be rising due to the reported global decline in semen parameters [3]. Male infertility is didactically classified into pretesticular, testicular, and posttesticular etiologies and arises from genetic causes in 15–30% of cases [4]. Pretesticular causes are mainly endocrinological in nature and may result from mutations to genes regulating gonadotropin-releasing hormone (GnRH) secretion (e.g., Kallman syndrome). A number of chromosomal aberrations can also result in testicular failure (e.g., Klinefelter syndrome, XX male, chromosomal translocations, and Y chromosome microdeletion) while posttesticular male infertility can result from congenital absence of the vas deferens. Infertility may be the only presentation for patients with chromosomal abnormalities; however, these defects may influence the health and well-being of their carriers who are at risk for developing several malignant and nonmalignant medical diseases [5,6]. Despite infertility, sperm retrieval procedures coupled with assisted reproductive technology (ART) has allowed individuals with genetic defects to father children, but with the high risk of passing genetic disorders on to their offspring [7].

Moreover, the type of genetic abnormality detected can give insight into identifying the prognosis of sperm retrieval [4]. These points call for genetic testing for some men experiencing infertility for better sperm retrieval outcomes, genetic counseling for future health risks, and the effects on offspring. This chapter aims to unravel the various genetic etiologies of male infertility and provide an in-depth review of the utility of genetic testing methods in the clinic.

16.2 Indications of Genetic Testing

Genetic counseling and evaluation are usually recommended for infertile men with severe oligozoospermia (<5 million/mL) or azoospermia (8–13). For the latter, a proper patient evaluation conducted by a reproductive specialist usually provides an understanding of whether the azoospermia is obstructive or nonobstructive. Karyotype analysis and a Y-chromosome microdeletion assay are recommended in patients with suspicion of nonobstructive azoospermia (NOA) based on high serum follicle-stimulating hormone (FSH) levels and small testicular volume. In patients with unilateral or bilateral absence of the vas deferens, a cystic fibrosis transmembrane conductance regulator (CFTR) mutation analysis is advocated. The recent European Association of Urology (EAU) guidelines have proposed a new cut-off sperm count for recommending Y-chromosome microdeletion testing [10]. Based on the results of a meta-analysis revealing that 99% of deletions tend to occur in men with <1 million sperm/mL [14], the EAU guidelines have endorsed that Y-chromosome microdeletion testing should be offered for patients with a sperm count <5 million/mL and is necessarily tested in those with <1 million sperm/mL [10]. Other conditions for which genetic testing has been advocated, regardless of the semen analysis result, include patients with a history of recurrent spontaneous pregnancy loss, malformations, or mental retardation (Figure 16.1) [8–10]. However, genetic testing is not recommended for men with obstructive azoospermia (normal FSH and testicular volume), who had a previously documented sperm concentration >5 million/mL or prior toxic exposure to radiation or chemotherapy.

16.3 Genetic Tests for Nonobstructive Azoospermia/Severe Oligozoospermia

16.3.1 Karyotype Testing

A karyotype, which has proven useful in clinical settings since the 1950s, is a cytogenetic method that analyzes the characteristics and number of a patient's chromosomes [15]. Through this cytogenic evaluation, cultured peripheral blood lymphocytes are treated and arrested in mitosis. After exposure to a protease, the stained bands of the chromosomes are visualized and examined for abnormalities. This method provides low resolution and can only identify DNA abnormalities that are 4 million base pairs or larger [16].

16.3.1.1 Klinefelter Syndrome

Among infertile men with NOA and karyotypic abnormalities, 14% are attributed to Klinefelter syndrome (KS) alone [17].

127

Overall, KS is diagnosed in 1 in 600 men in the general population [18]. Furthermore, 80–90% of Klinefelter patients possess a 47,XXY karyotype, while the remainder 10–20% of men exhibit a mosaic karyotype, typically 46,XY/47,XXY [18]. In the case of mosaicism, extended karyotyping would be performed in order to determine true genomic mosaicism [19]. The supernumerary X chromosome in KS patients can equally arise from maternal or paternal origins (Figures 16.2 and 16.3). In the majority of cases, KS usually remains undetected until adulthood when patients present with infertility [13]. Previous reports show that viable ejaculated sperm can be found in up to 8.4% of KS patients, and natural pregnancy has been achieved [20]. However, NOA secondary to primary testicular failure is instead a typical presentation for KS patients who would require surgical sperm retrieval and intracytoplasmic sperm injection (ICSI) to achieve fatherhood. The reported sperm retrieval rate in patients with KS has been in the range of 30–50% [21–23]. Men with mosaic KS have a better chance of sperm retrieval and pregnancy than nonmosaic individuals. There have been some concerns regarding higher aneuploidy rates in the spermatozoa retrieved from KS patients; however, various reports demonstrated comparable fertilization, implantation, and pregnancy rates between KS and normal karyotype NOA patients with no aneuploid children reported [24–26]. While no single clinical variable can accurately predict sperm retrieval success in KS patients, it is generally believed that advancing age is associated with a higher likelihood of sperm aneuploidy and lower spermatogenesis potential in KS patients. Therefore, early diagnosis of KS is of paramount importance in fertility preservation, allowing early patient counseling. Sperm retrieval and banking at a younger age may represent a viable option for KS patients [27,28]. Early recognition of the condition is also crucial because KS patients face an increased risk of breast cancer, metabolic syndrome, osteoporosis, type 2 diabetes, and extragonadal germ cell tumors [6,18].

16.3.1.2 XX Male

Karyotype testing can also detect a less common chromosomal abnormality, 46,XX male syndrome, or testicular sex development disorder. This condition is prevalent in 1:20,000 males and is characterized by a mismatch between the patient's genotype and phenotype [29]. In roughly 80% of cases, 46,XX is usually caused by translocation of the sex-determining region (SRY) of the Y chromosome, which is the gene that induces and maintains dominant male phenotypes, into a sex chromosome or an autosome [30,31]. The remainder of cases in which fluorescent in-situ hybridization studies fail to locate an SRY region, presumed hidden mosaicism for the SRY gene or possible mutation of inhibitors of the male pattern have been postulated [30]. Phenotypically, 46,XX individuals possess male gonads but have smaller testes, shorter body habitus, and may have gynecomastia or cryptorchidism [13,32]. In general, men with 46,XX are universally infertile due to the absence of specific regions on the Y chromosome required for spermatogenesis, such as the azoospermia factor (AZF) regions [33]. Therefore, ART is not an option for these individuals, and they require donor sperm to father children.

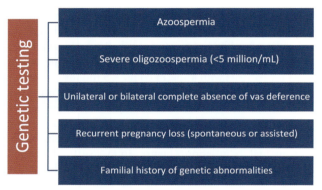

Figure 16.1 Indications for genetic testing

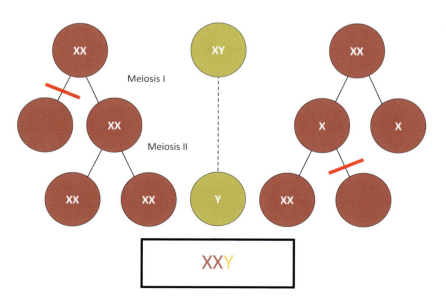

Figure 16.2 Klinefelter syndrome resulting from an extra maternal X chromosome. Nondisjunction can occur during the first or second meiotic divisions.

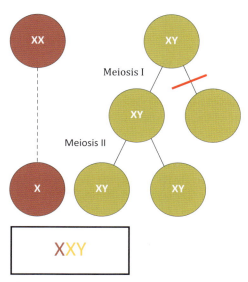

Figure 16.3 Klinefelter syndrome resulting from paternal X chromosome. Nondisjunction occurring only during the first meiotic division.

16.3.1.3 Chromosomal Translocations (Robertsonian/Reciprocal) and Inversions

Chromosomal translocations and inversions can also be detected with karyotype testing. According to previous cytogenetic evaluations, abnormal karyotypes and translocations are present in 13% of men with severely compromised semen parameters [34]. Robertsonian translocations usually occur due to centric fusion of the long arms of two nonhomologous acrocentric chromosomes (mostly chromosomes 13, 14, 15, 21, and 22). Male patients with these translocations are usually phenotypically normal but, due to abnormal chromosome pairing during meiosis, are prone to have embryos with acrocentric chromosome trisomies, uniparental disomies, or monosomies [35]. Reciprocal translocations, on the other hand, result from the exchange of genetic material between two chromosomes. Patients with these translocations have a normal number of chromosomes; however, their phenotypic presentation depends mainly on the particular translocation breakpoints that might disrupt the expression of specific genes [36]. Failure of chromosome pairing during meiosis places such patients at higher risk of unbalanced translocations or sperm aneuploidy, depending on the chromosome and breakpoint involved [37]. Therefore, men with Robertsonian translocations and other balanced translocations are more likely to result in a genetically abnormal embryo and are at increased risk of recurrent pregnancy loss [38]. Patients with chromosomal translocations require ICSI together with preimplantation genetic testing to achieve a successful pregnancy.

16.3.2 Y-Chromosome Microdeletion

Due to its low resolution and inability to detect details in specific genome regions, standard karyotyping should be supplemented by other cytogenetic methods for a comprehensive genetic evaluation of infertile men. Polymerase chain reaction (PCR) amplification with the use of DNA from the peripheral blood (blood assay) is used to examine the genetic content of the Y chromosome [39]. The Y chromosome contains many repetitive sequences, and due to its solitary nature is prone to genetic deletions during homologous recombination [40]. Approximately 95% of the Y chromosome possesses essential genes for male sex differentiation and sperm production [14]. Y chromosome microdeletions are particularly common along its long arm (Yq) in three distinct regions called AZF regions. The three AZF regions, AZFa, AZFb, and AZFc, are deleted in 5% of oligozoospermic men and 10% of azoospermic men [41]. The AZFa region contains genes necessary for spermatogenesis, including the USP9Y (ubiquitin specific peptidase 9 Y-linked) and DBY (DEAD box protein 3, Y-chromosomal) that when deleted result in loss of germ cells (Sertoli cell only) [42]. Deletions of the RBMY1 (Y chromosome RNA recognition motif 1) and PRY (protein-coding) genes of the AZFb region result in maturation arrest at the primary spermatocyte stage [4]. AZFc microdeletions are the most frequently observed AZF abnormality in infertile individuals (1:4,000 males) and are more heterogenous than AZFa or AZFb deletions [41]. The most commonly reported deletions reside in the DAZ (deleted in azoospermia) genes, followed by CDY (chromodomain protein, Y linked) and TSPY (testis-specific Y-encoded protein 1) (Figure 16.4) [43]. Isolated deletions in these AZFc regions would result in hypospermatogenesis, a less severe form of spermatogenic dysfunction [41]. In fact, a minority of men with AZFc microdeletion may still produce viable sperm in their ejaculate. Furthermore, the AZF regions are not distinctly separate from each other, but rather do overlap. Hence partial or a combination of deletions can be present. The type of Y-chromosome microdeletion provides important prognostic information for the success rate of surgical sperm retrieval [44,45]. While sperm retrieval has been rarely reported from patients with AZFa, AZFb, or AZFa/b deletions [46], it is generally believed that such deletions would invariably result in failed sperm retrieval [47]. On the other hand, a sperm retrieval rate of <10% has been reported from patients with partial AZFb with/without AZFc deletions [48]. Isolated AZFc deletions have the best prognostic outcome with a reported successful sperm retrieval rate in >50% of patients [23,47]. Genetic counseling is mandatory whereas preimplantation genetic testing may be recommended in these patients as their male offspring would undoubtedly have microdeletion of the AZFc region and possibly other regions.

16.3.3 Hypogonadotropic Hypogonadism

Hypogonadotropic hypogonadism is caused by acquired or idiopathic conditions and is characterized by a central deficiency of gonadotropins resulting in decreased androgen production and spermatogenesis failure [49]. Acquired causes are

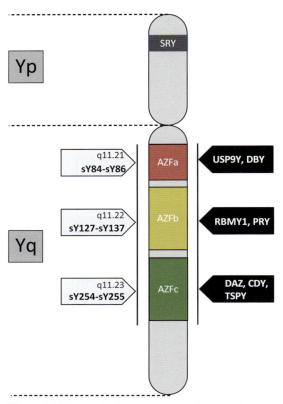

Figure 16.4 Human Y chromosome map depicting the short (Yp) and long (Yq) arms, AZF subregions, and gene content. The AZFa region maps from approximately 12.9 to 13.7 Mb of the chromosome and contains two single copy genes, USP9Y and DDY. AZFb spans from approximately 18 to 24.7 Mb of the chromosome and AZFc from approximately 23 to 26.7 Mb. Both regions contain multiple genes, the main ones identified in the right side (pentagons). The location of the basic set of sequence-tagged sites primers to be investigated in azoospermic men with spermatogenic failure, according to the European Association of Andrology and the European Molecular Genetics Quality Network 2013 guidelines, are identified in the left side (pentagons).

usually the result of a disease affecting the sella turcica (prolactinomas, craniopharyngiomas, other space-occupying lesions) [50]. In such cases, treatment of the underlying condition is usually warranted, and genetic testing is not indicated. However, this is not the case in congenital hypogonadotropic hypogonadism that either results from defects in the gonadotropin production cascade or failure of migration of gonadotropin-releasing hormone neurons from the olfactory placode to the hypothalamus [51]. The latter is observed in patients with Kallman's syndrome, an X-linked congenital disease characterized by delayed puberty, hypogonadism, infertility, and anosmia [52]. More than 20 genes for congenital hypogonadotropic hypogonadism (CHH) have been identified, the most common of which are reported in Table 16.1.

Patients with CHH generally respond well to gonadotropin replacement therapy, and the majority of them would regain sperm production and may proceed to natural conception [53]. However, genetic testing in such cases is recommended to explore the risks of disease inheritance to their offspring [13]. Preimplantation genetic testing may also be required for patients undergoing ICSI.

16.3.4 Polymorphisms in the Androgen Receptor

The androgen receptor (AR) gene is located on the long arm of the X chromosome (Xq11–12) [54]. It has two polymorphic trinucleotide microsatellites- a glutamine codon (CAG) with 8–60 repetitions and a glycine codon with 4–31 repetitions [55]. The average number of repetitions varies by ethnicity, and its polymorphisms have been associated with a number of disorders. Androgen insensitivity syndrome is one clinical condition caused by longer CAG repeats resulting in an altered function of the AR [56]. This condition results in the lack of responsiveness of tissues to the effect of androgens preventing the development of male secondary sexual characteristics during puberty. Nonetheless, the impaired function of the AR could vary and may only present with impairment of spermatogenesis [55]. However, the low frequency of AR mutations in men with severe semen abnormalities together with the presence of >400 mutations, and the need to conduct AR protein functional analysis to accurately diagnose the effect magnitude limit the routine testing of AR mutations during the evolution of infertile men.

16.4 Genetic Tests for Obstructive Azoospermia

16.4.1 Cystic Fibrosis Gene Mutation

Cystic fibrosis is one of the most common autosomal recessive diseases [57] and is caused by a mutation in the CFTR gene [58]. This gene encodes a transmembrane chloride channel and the function of which is regulation of exocrine epithelial cell secretion. Numerous mutations and polymorphisms of the CFTR gene have been described with variable sequelae depending on the involved transcription error [59]. Severe mutations may result in the complete absence of the CFTR protein, while milder mutations may impair CFTR protein function or reduce its synthesis. The phenotypic presentations of CFTR mutations range from an isolated complete bilateral absence of the vas deference (CBAVD) to clinically evident cystic fibrosis. Proper clinical examination can sufficiently identify patients with CBAVD. Additionally, these patients have an underdeveloped or absent epididymal tail, hypoplastic seminal vesicles, and an ejaculate of low volume and pH. The F508 deletion is the most prevalent CFTR mutation seen in 24% of men with cystic fibrosis [60]. The second most common mutation seen in 17% of men with cystic fibrosis involves polymorphisms of the 5T allele [20]. The CFTR screening panel usually includes 30–50 mutations commonly prevalent in cystic fibrosis patients. Given over 1,700 mutations have been found in the CFTR gene, the routine screening fails to detect genetic defects in a considerable number of CBAVD patients [59]. In fact, even with complete CFTR gene screening, genetic defects may be undetectable in about 25% of

Table 16.1 Common genes associated with CHH

Gene	Encoded protein	Function
ANOS1 (KAL1)	Anosmin 1	Neural cell adhesion and axonal migration
CHD7 (KAL5)	Chromodomain helicase DNA binding protein 7	Chromatin remodeling, perception of odors
FGF8 (KAL6)	Fibroblast growth factor 8	Cell division, regulation of cell growth and maturation, and development before birth
FGFR1 (KAL2)	Fibroblast growth factor receptor 1	Cell division, regulation of cell growth and maturation, formation of blood vessels, wound healing, and embryonic development
PROK2 (KAL4)	Prokineticin 2	Regulate cell function in various organs (small intestine, brain, and endocrine system)
PROKR2 (KAL3)	Prokineticin receptor 2	Regulate cell function in various organs (small intestine, brain, and endocrine system)
KISS1	Kisspeptins	Activates GnRH neurons
TAC3	Tachykinin-3	Neurotransmitter in the central and peripheral nervous system
TAC3R	Neurokinin B	Receptors for tachykinins
GnRH1	Peptide precursors for gonadoliberin-1 and GnRH-associated peptide 1	Stimulates the release of luteinizing and follicle-stimulating hormones

CBAVD patients [59,61]. However, both partners must be screened for CFTR gene mutations prior to assisted reproduction. Patients with CBAVD are ideal candidates for surgical sperm retrieval, with retrieval rates close to 100% [20,62, 63]. If both partners are confirmed carriers of this mutation, it is essential to conduct preimplantation genetic testing to avoid the transmission of cystic fibrosis to the offspring. A child of two parents carrying this mutation has a 25% chance of having cystic fibrosis.

Congenital unilateral absence of the vas deferens (CUAVD) is another rare condition prevalent in about 1% of the general population [64]. It is also associated with a CFTR gene mutation and with unilateral renal agenesis. It is unknown how CFTR mutations result in CUAVD or whether they contribute to renal agenesis. One study reported CFTR mutations in 25% of men with CUAVD and reported unilateral renal agenesis in another 25% who did not have any CFTR mutation [65]. Some have advocated that unilateral renal and vasal agenesis may instead result from an intrinsic Wolffian developmental defect [66]. Therefore, it is highly recommended that patients with CUAVD, and their partners, get genetic testing to screen for CFTR gene mutations and undergo a renal ultrasound to detect renal agenesis.

16.5 Future Directives in Genetic Testing
16.5.1 Epigenetics

One area that promises future advancement in understanding male infertility is epigenetics. Epigenetics refers to a series of modifications that alter gene expression, including DNA methylation of cytosine bases and/or chemical variations to histones [45]. Research has shown that records of an individual's spermatogenesis and information about embryonic development are contained within sperm epigenetics [67]. It can also give more insight into the mechanism of environmental impact on reproductive health. This signatures could be critical to understanding why environmental factors could be changing the epigenome, including age, diet, geography, and access to medications, to name a few [68]. Some research suggests that environmental factors may not only influence the risk of infertility but also pose risks to future children as well [69]. DNA methylation increases as people age and older men have an increased risk of having children with particular neuropsychiatric disorders [70,71]. DNA methylation is also found to be higher in infertile men than fertile men [72–74]. Also, in couples who experience recurring pregnancy loss, the male's sperm have greater histone retention and altered DNA methylation [75,76]. Additionally, since epigenetics could reflect the state of spermatogenesis, the test could potentially identify the etiology of impaired spermatogenesis and assess sperm quality in achieving normal embryogenesis.

16.5.2 Next-Generation DNA Sequencing

Next-generation DNA sequencing (NGS) is considered a breakthrough in DNA sequencing technology. It allows rapid parallel sequencing of DNA strands and has been used on targeted DNA regions (disease targeted sequencing), the entire exome (whole-exome sequencing, WES), or the entire genome (whole-genome sequencing, WGS). Specific DNA target regions of significant importance for the evaluation of infertile men have been identified. NGS was able to detect 100% of single nucleotide variations (SNV), copy number variations (CNV), autosomal/sex chromosomal abnormalities, and 94% of Y chromosome microdeletions [77]. With WES and WGS, extensive genetic variations testing may provide a broader investigation for a particular disease. However, the process could be quite overwhelming as millions of variations could be identified during WES with uncertain implications.

16.5.3 Microarray-Based Technologies

The microarray technology can detect SNA and CNV with high resolution (down to about 60 base pairs), offering a more robust analysis of genetic variations in comparison to standard genetic testing [78]. This advantage is most useful in the evaluation of small deletions of the Y chromosome. In fact, array comparative genomic hybridization (aCGH) could detect Y-chromosome microdeletions in patients who were not found to have any deletions with the standard PCR [78]. Furthermore, new deletions in regions other than the AZF region were identified in infertile men using aCGH [79]. Despite that, the number of sites that can be assessed with microarray technology is usually limited, hindering its ability to diagnose the problem. Furthermore, SNVs may vary according to ethnicity, and hence what is identified as an abnormality in one population could be a normal variant in another. CNVs may not necessarily correlate with gene expression and hence may not be meaningful in some circumstances [80].

16.6 Conclusion

Genetic testing is a critical investigation indicated in the evaluation of infertile men with severe derangement in semen parameters. It is also indicated in the evaluation of recurrent pregnancy loss. Karyotype testing and assessment of Y-chromosome microdeletions are the cornerstone genetic tests widely utilized in evaluating infertile men. Genetic testing allows the identification of conditions that may have negative implications for both patients and their offspring's health. The result of genetic evaluation provides relevant prognostic information regarding couples' chances of conception and facilitates genetic counseling.

References

1. Mascarenhas MN, Flaxman SR, Boerma T, Vanderpoel S, Stevens GA. National, regional, and global trends in infertility prevalence since 1990: a systematic analysis of 277 health surveys. *PLoS Med.* 2012;9:e1001356.
2. Brugh VM, Lipshultz LI. Male factor infertility: evaluation and management. *Med Clin North Am.* 2004;88:367–385.
3. Plaseska-Karanfilska D, Noveski P, Plaseski T, Maleva I, Madjunkova S, Moneva Z. Genetic causes of male infertility. *Balkan J Med Genet.* 2012;15:31–34.
4. Ferlin A, Raicu F, Gatta V, Zuccarello D, Palka G, Foresta C. Male infertility: role of genetic background. *Reprod Biomed Online.* 2007;14:734–745.
5. Turriff A, Macnamara E, Levy HP, Biesecker B. The impact of living with Klinefelter syndrome: a qualitative exploration of adolescents and adults. *J Genet Couns.* 2017;26:728–737.
6. Spaziani M, Radicioni AF. Metabolic and cardiovascular risk factors in Klinefelter syndrome. *Am J Med Genet C Semin Med Genet.* 2020;184:334–343.
7. O'Flynn O'Brien KL, Varghese AC, Agarwal A. The genetic causes of male factor infertility: a review. *Fertil Steril.* 2010;93:1–12.
8. Practice Committee of the American Society for Reproductive Medicine. Diagnostic evaluation of the infertile male: a committee opinion. *Fertil Steril.* 2015;103:e18–25.
9. Practice Committee of the American Society for Reproductive Medicine. Management of nonobstructive azoospermia: a committee opinion. *Fertil Steril.* 2018;110:1239–1245.
10. Salonia A, Bettocchi C, Carvalho J, et al. Guidelines on sexual and reproductive health - 2021 update: Male sexual dysfunction. *Eur Urol.* 2021;80(3):333–357.
11. Jarow J, Sigman M, Kolettis PN, et al. The optimal evaluation of the infertile male: AUA best practice statement. In: AUAEa, ed. *Research.* American Urological Association, Inc.; 2010:1–38.
12. Esteves SC, Miyaoka R, Agarwal A. An update on the clinical assessment of the infertile male. [corrected]. *Clinics (Sao Paulo).* 2011;66:691–700.
13. Hamada AJ, Esteves SC, Agarwal A. A comprehensive review of genetics and genetic testing in azoospermia. *Clinics (Sao Paulo).* 2013;68(Suppl. 1):39–60.
14. Kohn TP, Kohn JR, Owen RC, Coward RM. The prevalence of Y-chromosome microdeletions in oligozoospermic men: a systematic review and meta-analysis of European and North American studies. *Eur Urol.* 2019;76:626–636.
15. Bates SE. Classical cytogenetics: karyotyping techniques. *Methods Mol Biol.* 2011;767:177–190.
16. Thirumavalavan N, Gabrielsen JS, Lamb DJ. Where are we going with gene screening for male infertility? *Fertil Steril.* 2019;111:842–850.
17. Donker RB, Vloeberghs V, Groen H, Tournaye H, van Ravenswaaij-Arts CMA, Land JA. Chromosomal abnormalities in 1663 infertile men with azoospermia: the clinical consequences. *Hum Reprod.* 2017;32:2574–2580.
18. ElBardisi H, Majzoub A. Klinefelter syndrome. In: Aziz N, Agarwal A, eds. *The Diagnosis and Treatment of Male Infertility.* Springer; 2017:133–150.
19. Stahl PJ, Schlegel PN. Genetic evaluation of the azoospermic or severely oligozoospermic male. *Curr Opin Obstet Gynecol.* 2012;24:221–228.
20. Hotaling J, Carrell DT. Clinical genetic testing for male factor infertility: current applications and future directions. *Andrology.* 2014;2:339–350.
21. Schiff JD, Palermo GD, Veeck LL, Goldstein M, Rosenwaks Z, Schlegel PN. Success of testicular sperm extraction [corrected] and intracytoplasmic sperm injection in men with Klinefelter syndrome. *J Clin Endocrinol Metab.* 2005;90:6263–6267.
22. Majzoub A, Arafa M, Al Said S, et al. Outcome of testicular sperm extraction in nonmosaic Klinefelter syndrome patients: what is the best approach? *Andrologia.* 2016;48:171–176.

23. Arshad MA, Majzoub A, Esteves SC. Predictors of surgical sperm retrieval in non-obstructive azoospermia: summary of current literature. *Int Urol Nephrol.* 2020;52:2015–2038.

24. Okada H, Goda K, Muto S, Maruyama O, Koshida M, Horie S. Four pregnancies in nonmosaic Klinefelter's syndrome using cryopreserved-thawed testicular spermatozoa. *Fertil Steril.* 2005;84:1508.

25. Bourne H, Stern K, Clarke G, Pertile M, Speirs A, Baker HW. Delivery of normal twins following the intracytoplasmic injection of spermatozoa from a patient with 47,XXY Klinefelter's syndrome. *Hum Reprod.* 1997;12:2447–2450.

26. Vicdan K, Akarsu C, Vicdan A, et al. Birth of a healthy boy using fresh testicular sperm in a patient with Klinefelter syndrome combined with Kartagener syndrome. *Fertil Steril.* 2011;96:577–579.

27. Ferhi K, Avakian R, Griveau JF, Guille F. Age as only predictive factor for successful sperm recovery in patients with Klinefelter's syndrome. *Andrologia.* 2009;41:84–87.

28. Okada H, Goda K, Yamamoto Y, et al. Age as a limiting factor for successful sperm retrieval in patients with nonmosaic Klinefelter's syndrome. *Fertil Steril.* 2005;84:1662–1664.

29. de la Chapelle A. The etiology of maleness in XX men. *Hum Genet.* 1981;58:105–116.

30. Rajender S, Rajani V, Gupta NJ, Chakravarty B, Singh L, Thangaraj K. SRY-negative 46,XX male with normal genitals, complete masculinization and infertility. *Mol Hum Reprod.* 2006;12:341–346.

31. Dauwerse JG, Hansson KB, Brouwers AA, Peters DJ, Breuning MH. An XX male with the sex-determining region Y gene inserted in the long arm of chromosome 16. *Fertil Steril.* 2006;86:463 e1–5.

32. Vorona E, Zitzmann M, Gromoll J, Schuring AN, Nieschlag E. Clinical, endocrinological, and epigenetic features of the 46,XX male syndrome, compared with 47,XXY Klinefelter patients. *J Clin Endocrinol Metab.* 2007;92:3458–3465.

33. Majzoub A, Arafa M, Starks C, Elbardisi H, Al Said S, Sabanegh E. 46 XX karyotype during male fertility evaluation; case series and literature review. *Asian J Androl.* 2017;19:168–172.

34. Peschka B, Leygraaf J, Van der Ven K, et al. Type and frequency of chromosome aberrations in 781 couples undergoing intracytoplasmic sperm injection. *Hum Reprod.* 1999;14:2257–2263.

35. Mau-Holzmann UA. Somatic chromosomal abnormalities in infertile men and women. *Cytogenet Genome Res.* 2005;111:317–336.

36. Morin SJ, Eccles J, Iturriaga A, Zimmerman RS. Translocations, inversions and other chromosome rearrangements. *Fertil Steril.* 2017;107:19–26.

37. Oliver-Bonet M, Ko E, Martin RH. Male infertility in reciprocal translocation carriers: the sex body affair. *Cytogenet Genome Res.* 2005;111:343–346.

38. Suzumori N, Sugiura-Ogasawara M. Genetic factors as a cause of miscarriage. *Curr Med Chem.* 2010;17:3431–3437.

39. Güney AI, Javadova D, Kırac D, et al. Detection of Y chromosome microdeletions and mitochondrial DNA mutations in male infertility patients. *Genet Mol Res.* 2012;11:1039–1048.

40. Noordam MJ, Repping S. The human Y chromosome: a masculine chromosome. *Curr Opin Genet Dev.* 2006;16:225–232.

41. Kaluarachchi NP, Randunu MH, Jainulabdeen M, Thavarajah A, Padeniya P, Galhena P. Complex Y chromosome anomalies in an infertile male. *JBRA Assist Reprod.* 2020;24:510–512.

42. Nuti F, Krausz C. Gene polymorphisms/mutations relevant to abnormal spermatogenesis. *Reprod Biomed Online.* 2008;16:504–513.

43. Krausz C, Casamonti E. Spermatogenic failure and the Y chromosome. *Hum Genet.* 2017;136:637–655.

44. Esteves SC. Clinical management of infertile men with nonobstructive azoospermia. *Asian J Androl.* 2015;17:459–470.

45. Gunes S, Esteves SC. Role of genetics and epigenetics in male infertility. *Andrologia.* 2020:e13586.

46. Goncalves C, Cunha M, Rocha E, et al. Y-chromosome microdeletions in nonobstructive azoospermia and severe oligozoospermia. *Asian J Androl.* 2017;19:338–345.

47. Stahl PJ, Masson P, Mielnik A, Marean MB, Schlegel PN, Paduch DA. A decade of experience emphasizes that testing for Y microdeletions is essential in American men with azoospermia and severe oligozoospermia. *Fertil Steril.* 2010;94:1753–1756.

48. Park SH, Lee HS, Choe JH, Lee JS, Seo JT. Success rate of microsurgical multiple testicular sperm extraction and sperm presence in the ejaculate in Korean men with Y chromosome microdeletions. *Korean J Urol.* 2013;54:536–540.

49. Fraietta R, Zylbersztejn DS, Esteves SC. Hypogonadotropic hypogonadism revisited. *Clinics (Sao Paulo).* 2013;68(Suppl. 1):81–88.

50. Sizar O, Schwartz J. Hypogonadism. In: *StatPearls.* StatPearls Publishing Copyright © 2020, StatPearls Publishing LLC.; 2020.

51. Festa A, Umano GR, Miraglia Del Giudice E, Grandone A. Genetic evaluation of patients with delayed puberty and congenital hypogonadotropic hypogonadism: is it worthy of consideration? *Front Endocrinol (Lausanne).* 2020;11:253.

52. Sonne J, Lopez-Ojeda W. Kallmann syndrome. In: *StatPearls.* StatPearls Publishing Copyright © 2020, StatPearls Publishing LLC.; 2020.

53. Casarini L, Crépieux P, Reiter E, et al. FSH for the treatment of male infertility. *Int J Mol Sci.* 2020;21:2270.

54. Hiort O. Clinical and molecular aspects of androgen insensitivity. *Endocr Dev.* 2013;24:33–40.

55. Xiao F, Lan A, Lin Z, et al. Impact of CAG repeat length in the androgen receptor gene on male infertility: a meta-analysis. *Reprod Biomed Online.* 2016;33:39–49.

56. Singh S, Ilyayeva S. Androgen insensitivity syndrome. In: *StatPearls.* StatPearls Publishing Copyright © 2020, StatPearls Publishing LLC.; 2020.

57. Castellani C, Linnane B, Pranke I, Cresta F, Sermet-Gaudelus I, Peckham D. Cystic fibrosis diagnosis in newborns, children, and adults. *Semin Respir Crit Care Med.* 2019;40:701–714.

58. Quinzii C, Castellani C. The cystic fibrosis transmembrane regulator gene and male infertility. *J Endocrinol Invest.* 2000;23:684–689.

59. Mak V, Zielenski J, Tsui LC, et al. Proportion of cystic fibrosis gene mutations not detected by routine testing in men with obstructive azoospermia. *JAMA.* 1999;281:2217–2224.

60. Kanavakis E, Tzetis M, Antoniadi T, Pistofidis G, Milligos S, Kattamis C. Cystic fibrosis mutation screening in CBAVD patients and men with obstructive azoospermia or severe oligozoospermia. *Mol Hum Reprod.* 1998;4:333–337.

61. Giuliani R, Antonucci I, Torrente I, Grammatico P, Palka G, Stuppia L. Identification of the second CFTR mutation in patients with congenital bilateral absence of vas deferens undergoing ART protocols. *Asian J Androl.* 2010;12:819–826.

62. Esteves SC, Lee W, Benjamin DJ, Seol B, Verza S, Jr., Agarwal A. Reproductive potential of men with obstructive azoospermia undergoing percutaneous sperm retrieval and intracytoplasmic sperm injection according to the cause of obstruction. *J Urol.* 2013;189:232–237.

63. Miyaoka R, Esteves SC. Predictive factors for sperm retrieval and sperm injection outcomes in obstructive azoospermia: do etiology, retrieval techniques and gamete source play a role? *Clinics (Sao Paulo).* 2013;68 (Suppl. 1):111–119.

64. Salwan A, Abdelrahman A. Congenital absence of vas deferens and ectopic kidney. *Int J Surg Case Rep.* 2017;34:90–92.

65. Kolettis PN, Sandlow JI. Clinical and genetic features of patients with congenital unilateral absence of the vas deferens. *Urology.* 2002;60:1073–1076.

66. Mickle J, Milunsky A, Amos JA, Oates RD. Congenital unilateral absence of the vas deferens: a heterogeneous disorder with two distinct subpopulations based upon aetiology and mutational status of the cystic fibrosis gene. *Hum Reprod.* 1995;10:1728–1735.

67. Grover MM, Jenkins TG. Transgenerational epigenetics: a window into paternal health influences on offspring. *Urol Clin North Am.* 2020;47:219–225.

68. Sharma P, Ghanghas P, Kaushal N, Kaur J, Kaur P. Epigenetics and oxidative stress: a twin-edged sword in spermatogenesis. *Andrologia.* 2019;51: e13432.

69. Spadafora C. Transgenerational epigenetic reprogramming of early embryos: a mechanistic model. *Environ Epigenet.* 2020;6:dvaa009.

70. Cioppi F, Casamonti E, Krausz C. Age-dependent de novo mutations during spermatogenesis and their consequences. *Adv Exp Med Biol.* 2019;1166:29–46.

71. Phillips N, Taylor L, Bachmann G. Maternal, infant and childhood risks associated with advanced paternal age: The need for comprehensive counseling for men. *Maturitas.* 2019;125:81–84.

72. Menezo Y, Dale B, Elder K. The negative impact of the environment on methylation/epigenetic marking in gametes and embryos: a plea for action to protect the fertility of future generations. *Mol Reprod Dev.* 2019;86:1273–1282.

73. Darbandi M, Darbandi S, Agarwal A, et al. Reactive oxygen species-induced alterations in H19-Igf2 methylation patterns, seminal plasma metabolites, and semen quality. *J Assist Reprod Genet.* 2019;36:241–253.

74. Santana VP, Miranda-Furtado CL, Pedroso DCC, et al. The relationship among sperm global DNA methylation, telomere length, and DNA fragmentation in varicocele: a cross-sectional study of 20 cases. *Syst Biol Reprod Med.* 2019;65:95–104.

75. Poorang S, Abdollahi S, Anvar Z, et al. The impact of methylenetetrahydrofolate reductase (MTHFR) sperm methylation and variants on semen parameters and the chance of recurrent pregnancy loss in the couple. *Clin Lab.* 2018;64:1121–1128.

76. Yu M, Du G, Xu Q, et al. Integrated analysis of DNA methylome and transcriptome identified CREB5 as a novel risk gene contributing to recurrent pregnancy loss. *EBioMedicine.* 2018;35:334–344.

77. Patel B, Parets S, Akana M, et al. Comprehensive genetic testing for female and male infertility using next-generation sequencing. *J Assist Reprod Genet.* 2018;35:1489–1496.

78. Yuen RK, Merkoulovitch A, MacDonald JR, et al. Development of a high-resolution Y-chromosome microarray for improved male infertility diagnosis. *Fertil Steril.* 2014;101:1079–1085.e3.

79. Jorgez CJ, Weedin JW, Sahin A, et al. Aberrations in pseudoautosomal regions (PARs) found in infertile men with Y-chromosome microdeletions. *J Clin Endocrinol Metab.* 2011;96: E674–E679.

80. Sawyer SL, Mukherjee N, Pakstis AJ, et al. Linkage disequilibrium patterns vary substantially among populations. *Eur J Hum Genet.* 2005;13:677–686.

Section 3 Clinical Evaluation and Treatment of Male Infertility

Chapter 17
Andrological Care of the Patient with Spinal Cord Injury

Christian Fuglesang S. Jensen, Jens Sønksen, and Dana A. Ohl

17.1 Introduction

Spinal cord injury (SCI) has a major impact on male sexual and reproductive health. Most men with SCI will experience erectile dysfunction (ED) as a result of the neurogenic damage that will often also cause anejaculation or retrograde ejaculation depending on the characteristics of the SCI. Further, some men with SCI become hypogonadal and suffer from symptoms of low testosterone. Restoring functions related to sexual and reproductive health is a top priority for men with SCI [1]. Although both ED, ejaculatory dysfunction, and hypogonadism are common andrological problems, there are special concerns and needs to accommodate in the andrological care of the patient with SCI.

17.2 Erectile Dysfunction

Erectile dysfunction occurs in an estimated 54–95% of men with SCI with sexual intercourse possible in 5–75% [2,3]. The broad ranges are in part due to natural variation in erectile function in patients with SCI due to the level of injury. The broad ranges also reflect differences in methodology and definition of ED and sexual intercourse used in different studies. However, ED remains a common and bothersome issue for most men with SCI.

Normal erectile function depends on coordination of sympathetic, parasympathetic, and somatic neural pathways with two main mechanisms responsible for erection namely reflex erections and psychogenic pathways. In men with SCI both mixed and incomplete patterns exist. Reflex erections occur by genital stimulation and are more common in men with an intact sacral reflex arch, typically men with a lesion at or above T10. Tactile stimulation of the genitals creates signals that travel through the dorsal nerve of the penis to the sacral spinal cord (S2–S4). This leads to inhibition of sympathetic outflow and an increased parasympathetic outflow causing erection. Neurogenic pathways responsible for reflex erections are usually intact when the lesion is above the level of L2. On the other hand, these lesions will typically compromise psychogenic erections as these originate from higher cortical centers of the brain and travel through the thoracolumbar fibers to modulate the spinal erection center and depend on intact sympathetic pathways. Consequently, psychogenic erections are more common when the lesion is located below L2 where reflex erections are typically compromised.

An important point in the management of ED in men with SCI is that usual treatment regiments for ED will often work. The first-line therapy is phosphodiesterase-5 inhibitors (PDE-5 inhibitors). A post hoc analysis of a randomized study on 248 men with SCI and ED, solely attributed to SCI, found significant improvements in all International Index of Erectile Function outcomes among the men treated with sildenafil versus placebo [4]. This included both achieving and maintaining erections. Further, the percentage of successful intercourse attempts was higher among the men who were taking sildenafil (53% vs. 12%) and sildenafil also worked in men with complete SCI. The treatment was well tolerated with complications including headache (16%), urinary tract infection (11.6%), flushing (4.1%), and dyspepsia (3.3%) as the most common [4]. Urinary tract infection was likely related to SCI and not to sildenafil whereas headache, flushing, and dyspepsia are common side effects from PDE5 inhibitors. Only 2.1% discontinued treatment due to side effects.

Some men with SCI might experience hypotension from PDE5 inhibitor treatment and it is recommended to begin with the lowest dose. Further, flushing in relation to PDE5 inhibitor treatment could be misinterpreted as autonomic dysreflexia (AD) and the men might get nitrates to treat suspected AD, which is contraindicated when taking PDE5 inhibitors due to the risk of severe hypotensive episodes. Therefore, it is vital to fully counsel the men on possible side effects of PDE5 inhibitors to prevent the above scenario.

In general, more than 80% of men with SCI are expected to respond positively to PDE5 inhibitor treatment [5]. As mentioned, the level of injury is an important factor for success and men with lesions affecting lower motor neurons compromising the reflex arch responsible for reflex erection are less likely to respond to PDE5 inhibitors. Intracavernosal injections with alprostadil, for example, are used as second-line therapy and are highly effective. Based on 713 men with SCI a recent meta-analysis found that 88% achieved successful erections after treatment with intracavernosal injection therapy [6]. Injection therapy bears the risk of priapism and some physicians and men with SCI prefer to try vacuum devices before continuing to intracavernosal injections. However, this therapy is not as efficient as injections. With proper counseling and instructions on how to use injections as well as information on strategies to reduce unwanted erections (application of cold to the penis, sympathomimetic medicine) injection therapy seems the best option for men who fail PDE5 inhibitor treatment. Of note, men with SCI who fail PDE5 inhibitor treatment might benefit from testosterone replacement therapy (TRT) if they are hypogonadal and evaluation for hypogonadism may be performed in nonresponders to PDE5 inhibitors. However, no studies have looked at the effect of TRT on erectile function in men with SCI.

Finally, men who fail intracavernosal injection therapy still have an option to get a penile prosthesis implantation (Figure 17.1). Typically, a three-piece inflatable implant is inserted with the two cylinders placed in the corporal bodies, a pump in the scrotum, and a reservoir placed either in the retropubic space of Retzius or submuscularly under the abdominal wall. In a study investigating long-term results from penile prosthesis implantation 82.6% of men with SCI were satisfied with their erectile function 10 years after implantation [7]. Complications are slightly more frequent among men with SCI compared to other men with ED having a penile implant inserted but are still acceptable with infection rates of around 5%. Rates of erosion are higher when using semirigid implants and inflatable implants are therefore preferred. Finally, when placing the implant care should be taken not to harm the dorsal nerves of the penis as these must be intact for penile vibratory simulation (PVS) to work [8].

17.3 Fertility

Most men with SCI suffer from ejaculatory dysfunction, which is often complicated by poor semen quality characterized by normal sperm concentration but low sperm motility and viability [5]. Only 5–10% of men with SCI can ejaculate by masturbation and 5% will be able to have biological children without treatment [9]. This contrasts with the fact that one-third of men with SCI desire children in the future [10].

Assisted ejaculation through neurostimulation is first-line treatment for patients with anejaculation due to SCI. The two available options are PVS and electroejaculation (EEJ). Both work by initiating the ejaculatory reflex (Figure 17.2) while EEJ in men with low lesions are thought to be a more direct stimulation of the ejaculatory organs (below T10). The reflex involves coordination of input from the dorsal nerve of the penis, spinal sympathetic outflow (T10–L2), and sacral parasympathetic and somatic output (S2–S4). Penile vibratory stimulation should be considered first due to the less invasive nature of the treatment, the possibility of the man to perform the procedure at home, the low cost, and encouraging success rates. Further, it has been suggested that the semen quality is better when using PVS as compared to EEJ [11]. When PVS

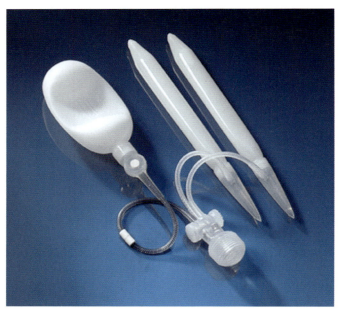

Figure 17.1 A three-piece inflatable penile prosthesis

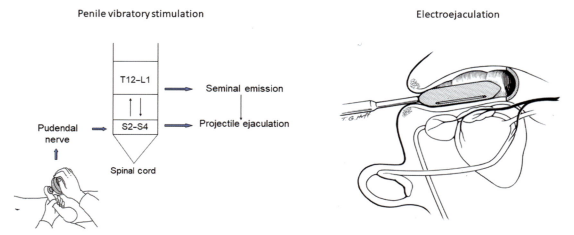

Figure 17.2 Illustration of penile vibratory stimulation and electroejaculation

fails, EEJ should be used and collectively the two procedures will ensure ejaculation in almost all men with SCI [9].

Reflex ejaculation following vibratory stimulation in men with SCI was first described in 1981 [12]. Since then, several studies have reported successful sperm retrieval from PVS [9, 13–15]. Penile vibratory stimulation is performed by placing a medical vibrator on the glans penis to mechanically "hyperstimulate" the penis to initiate a reflex ejaculation. Stimulation is given in intervals of two minutes with a break in between until ejaculation occurs. Tonic muscle contractions often precede ejaculation and the ejaculate after PVS is most often antegrade. Vibratory stimulation depends on intact lower cord reflexes and the level of SCI is an important determining factor for success [13]. The higher the level of the lesion, the higher the likelihood for a successful treatment and, generally, injuries rostral to T10 are preferred for PVS attempts [9]. Intact bulbocavernosal reflex and hip flexor response predicts success with PVS [16]. The vibratory settings also have a major impact on the success of the procedure, and a peak-to-peak amplitude of 2.5 mm and a frequency of 100 Hz is used to optimize the treatment. This was first demonstrated in a cohort of 66 men with SCI infertility where increasing the amplitude from 1 mm to 2.5 mm increased successful sperm retrieval from 32% to 96% [15].

Penile vibratory stimulation is a safe procedure with only minor complications, such as penile skin abrasion, occurring in few men. However, there is a risk for AD, which is also the case for EEJ. Autonomic dysreflexia is an unregulated and uncontrolled response of the sympathetic nervous system that usually occurs after noxious stimuli but can also occur after nonnoxious stimuli in men with SCI. Symptoms of AD include a rise in systolic blood pressure, flushing, headache, sweating, and nasal congestion. The risk of AD is highest in men with SCI with an injury above T6 as the nuclei of the sympathetic system is then separated from descending supraspinal control mechanisms. When understood and respected, AD can be safely managed. Importantly, continuous blood pressure monitoring should be performed during assisted ejaculation and if the systolic blood pressure rises above 165 mmHg the procedure should be stopped. Patients at risk of AD (history of AD, injury above T6) should be pretreated with antihypertensive medication, for example the calcium channel blocker, nifedipine, usually given sublingually 15–20 minutes before the procedure [17]. Nifedipine can also be used orally before sexual activity in men with SCI prone to AD but patients should be carefully counseled on the risk of hypotension from taking nifedipine. If AD develops during assisted ejaculation, or sexual activity, evident by symptoms of AD or a rise in systolic blood pressure, the first step is to stop the stimulation and place the patient in an upright position. If this does not mitigate the symptoms and drop the blood pressure after a few minutes medical management should be cautiously initiated [5]. This includes nitrates; however, these are contraindicated in men with SCI taking PDE5 inhibitors for ED.

Men with failed PVS attempts will often benefit from EEJ. Electroejaculation in men with SCI was first described in 1948 [18] followed by the development of rectal probe electroejaculation equipment for men with SCI in 1987 [19]. Multiple studies have since then demonstrated the effectiveness of the technique with retrieval rates between 75% and 100% [9,20–24]. Electroejaculation is performed with a rectal probe administering an alternative pattern of stimulations to the rectal mucosa close to the prostate and seminal vesicles. The procedure is performed under general anesthesia if the men with SCI has sensory function. The initial stimulation is set to 5 volts with current delivered for 5 seconds. After a break and if no ejaculation has occurred the voltage is increased by 2.5 or 5 volts and stimulation is again performed for 5 seconds. This pattern continues in an on/off fashion with increasing voltage until ejaculation occurs. This usually happens in the breaks between stimulation. This pattern of stimulation was derived from a physiological study on internal and external bladder sphincter pressures during PVS and EEJ in men with SCI. During successful cases of EEJ and PVS the external sphincter pressure first rises to about 180 cm H_2O then decreases followed by a peak in internal sphincter pressure exceeding the external sphincter pressure. This always precedes ejaculation during EEJ and PVS and failed attempts are characterized by lack of the forceful contraction of the external sphincter. However, during EEJ a more rapid return of external sphincter pressure occurs, greater than the internal sphincter pressure, which might be the reason that some of the ejaculate following EEJ is often retrograde. Subsequent catherization of the bladder should therefore be performed to collect the retrograde sample. To ensure the survival of sperm cells in the retrograde ejaculate a pH-buffered medium is instilled in the bladder prior to the procedure.

Success rates are high and vary mainly due to different outcome measures as some studies use cut-offs for sperm number and motility. In a retrospective study of 84 men with SCI 100% of the patients achieved ejaculation by EEJ but with motile sperm cells found in 88.1% of the samples [21]. In a similar study on 198 men, including both SCI and retroperitoneal lymph node dissection as causes for anejaculation, ejaculates with progressively motile sperm counts of >10 million was collected in 75% of men with SCI and 87% of the men with anejaculation after surgery [20].

When performing EEJ an anoscopy should be conducted prior to the procedure to evaluate the intactness of the rectal mucosa to avoid any injuries resulting from electrical stimulation. When this is done, complications from EEJ are rare. In a study reporting results from 915 adult EEJ procedures there were no reports of mechanical or thermal rectal injuries [9].

Although there is a lack of randomized trials investigating the treatment of anejaculation in infertile men, results from observational studies on assisted ejaculation procedures are so convincing that PVS and EEJ should always be considered before continuing with surgical sperm retrieval. Not all centers use assisted ejaculation and, in fact, the original vibratory

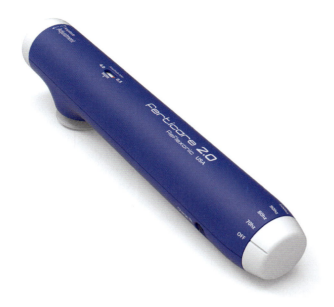

Figure 17.3 The Ferticare 2.0 medical vibrator for penile vibratory stimulation in men with spinal cord injury

device developed for men with SCI (Ferticare Personal) was discontinued in 2017 leaving a void in the ability to obtain a medical vibrator. However, a reengineered device (Ferticare 2.0) (Figure 17.3) has now become available making PVS accessible again. In a recent study comparing the Ferticare 1.0 and the Ferticare 2.0, the latter was found safe and effective for inducing ejaculation in men with SCI [25].

Surgical sperm retrieval is reserved for those men who fail assisted ejaculation, which are few. This is seen in a study where 97% of 500 men with SCI had sperm obtained without surgical sperm retrieval [9]. The procedure used for surgical sperm retrieval should be the least invasive and the most inexpensive method available [26]. This makes testicular sperm aspiration a natural choice as this method can be safely performed in an outpatient clinic setting with few complications and because it is successful in almost all [27].

Once sperm cells are obtained, whether from PVS, EEJ, or surgical sperm retrieval, the path to achieving a pregnancy should be chosen. If no female factors are present the number of motile sperm is a guide for selecting the assisted reproductive technique (ART). The lower the total motile sperm count is, the more advanced ART procedure is needed. Home insemination can be offered to the couple, if the men are able to produce an ejaculate by PVS, without risk of AD, and if the ejaculate has a good number of motile sperm cells. This method is the least expensive, the closest to natural conception, and gives good results. A study on home vaginal self-insemination of partners to 140 men with SCI, who used PVS for ejaculation, demonstrated a pregnancy rate of 43% with delivery of 73 healthy babies [28]. The next step for ART is intrauterine insemination (IUI) followed by the more advanced options including in vitro fertilization (IVF) with or without intracytoplasmic sperm injection (ICSI) [23]. Finally, one must remember that if surgical sperm retrieval is chosen, this commits the couple to the most invasive and costly method of ART, which is IVF with ICSI.

17.4 Hypogonadism and Testosterone Replacement Therapy

The male hormone, testosterone, is important for sexual functioning and several other functions including bone mineralization and muscle size and strength. Hypogonadism is characterized by a decrease in the functional activity of the testes and the clinical condition, male hypogonadism, is diagnosed in men with simultaneous low levels of testosterone and symptoms of low testosterone. These include lack of sexual desire, ED, decreased energy, decreased muscle strength, low mood, and fatigue [29]. In men with SCI it can be difficult to determine if such symptoms are a result of neurological damage or low testosterone, however, low sexual desire has been shown to be an independent predictor of low testosterone in men with SCI [30].

Up to one-third of men with SCI are biochemically hypogonadal and age-related declines in testosterone levels are more severe and are seen at an earlier age when compared to controls [31,32]. The decline in androgen levels among men with SCI is thought to be the result of a chronic alteration in the hypothalamic-pituitary axis regulating testosterone production resulting in hypogonadotropic hypogonadism. However, other causes of low testosterone found in the general population such as obesity, diabetes, and metabolic syndrome may also cause hypogonadism in men with SCI. In fact, these conditions are highly prevalent among men with SCI [33].

Testosterone replacement therapy may be used in men with SCI to alleviate symptoms of sexual dysfunction. Further, TRT is sometimes used in the controversial area of giving androgens to prevent muscle wasting, which is becoming more prevalent in the physical medicine world. However, exogenous testosterone decreases sperm production and might limit the chance of biologic fatherhood, which should be clearly communicated to the patients. The aim of TRT in men with SCI is to reach eugonadal levels of testosterone that may improve sexual drive, energy, muscle strength, body composition, and mood. Improvements in lean tissue mass and resting energy expenditure have been demonstrated to be retained for up to six months after discontinuation of TRT [34]. However, the study only included 22 men with SCI and larger randomized trials are needed to confirm these findings. In general, specific studies investigating TRT in SCI populations are limited and, for example, no studies have looked at the effect of TRT on erectile function in men with SCI.

Follow-up and monitoring during TRT is important and should follow regular guidelines [29].

17.5 Conclusion

Men with SCI often suffer from sexual and reproductive issues including ED, ejaculatory disorders, infertility, and hypogonadism. With proper andrological care and knowledge of the special concerns related to SCI treatments are both safe and effective. Erectile dysfunction is managed by the usual treatment regimens available for the general population including PDE5 inhibitors, intracavernosal injections, and penile implants. Penile vibratory stimulation and EEJ are effective treatments for anejaculation in infertile men with SCI with successful retrievals reported in up to 75–100% of patients. Surgical sperm retrieval is an option for men with failed attempts of assisted ejaculation. Strategies for assisted reproduction depend on the number of available motile sperm and range from home insemination to IVF with ICSI. Hypogonadism is prevalent in men with SCI and TRT may be used to alleviate symptoms of low testosterone. Such treatment with TRT, however, is likely to impair sperm production.

References

1. Simpson LA, et al. The health and life priorities of individuals with spinal cord injury: a systematic review. *J Neurotrauma.* 2012;29(8):1548–1555.
2. Biering-Sørensen F, Sønksen J. Penile erection in men with spinal cord or cauda equina lesions. *Semin Neurol.* 1992;12(2):98–105.
3. Biering-Sørensen F, Sønksen J. Sexual function in spinal cord lesioned men. *Spinal Cord.* 2001;39(9):455–470.
4. Ohl DA, et al. Efficacy and safety of sildenafil in men with sexual dysfunction and spinal cord injury. *Sex Med Rev.* 2017;5(4):521–528.
5. Sinha V, et al. Reproductive health of men with spinal cord injury. *Top Spinal Cord Inj Rehabil.* 2017;23(1):31–41.
6. Chochina L, et al. Intracavernous injections in spinal cord injured men with erectile dysfunction, a systematic review and meta-analysis. *Sex Med Rev.* 2016;4(3):257–269.
7. Zermann DH, et al. Penile prosthetic surgery in neurologically impaired patients: long-term followup. *J Urol.* 2006;175(3 Pt 1):1041–1044; discussion 1044.
8. Wieder JA, et al. Anesthetic block of the dorsal penile nerve inhibits vibratory-induced ejaculation in men with spinal cord injuries. *Urology.* 2000;55(6):915–917.
9. Brackett NL, et al. Treatment for ejaculatory dysfunction in men with spinal cord injury: an 18-year single center experience. *J Urol.* 2010;183(6):2304–2308.
10. Anderson KD, et al. The impact of spinal cord injury on sexual function: concerns of the general population. *Spinal Cord.* 2007;45(5):328–337.
11. Kathiresan AS, et al. Semen quality in ejaculates produced by masturbation in men with spinal cord injury. *Spinal Cord.* 2012;50(12):891–894.
12. Brindley GS. Reflex ejaculation under vibratory stimulation in paraplegic men. *Paraplegia.* 1981;19(5):299–302.
13. Brackett NL, et al. An analysis of 653 trials of penile vibratory stimulation in men with spinal cord injury. *J Urol.* 1998;159(6):1931–1934.
14. Castle SM, et al. Safety and efficacy of a new device for inducing ejaculation in men with spinal cord injuries. *Spinal Cord.* 2014;52(Suppl. 2):S27–S29.
15. Sønksen J, Biering-Sørensen F, Kristensen JK. Ejaculation induced by penile vibratory stimulation in men with spinal cord injuries: the importance of the vibratory amplitude. *Paraplegia.* 1994;32(10):651–660.
16. Bird VG, et al. Reflexes and somatic responses as predictors of ejaculation by penile vibratory stimulation in men with spinal cord injury. *Spinal Cord.* 2001;39(10):514–519.
17. Krassioukov A, et al. A systematic review of the management of autonomic dysreflexia after spinal cord injury. *Arch Phys Med Rehabil.* 2009;90(4):682–695.
18. Horne HW, Paull DP, Munro D. Fertility studies in the human male with traumatic injuries of the spinal cord and cauda equina. *N Engl J Med.* 1948;239(25):959–961.
19. Halstead LS, VerVoort S, Seager SW. Rectal probe electrostimulation in the treatment of anejaculatory spinal cord injured men. *Paraplegia.* 1987;25(2):120–129.
20. Denil J, et al. Treatment of anejaculation with electroejaculation. *Acta Urol Belg.* 1992;60(3):15–25.
21. Heruti RJ, et al. Treatment of male infertility due to spinal cord injury using rectal probe electroejaculation: the Israeli experience. *Spinal Cord.* 2001;39(3):168–175.
22. McGuire C, et al. Electroejaculatory stimulation for male infertility secondary to spinal cord injury: the Irish experience in National Rehabilitation Hospital. *Urology.* 2011;77(1):83–87.
23. Ohl DA, et al. Electroejaculation and assisted reproductive technologies in the treatment of anejaculatory infertility. *Fertil Steril.* 2001;76(6):1249–1255.
24. Soeterik TF, et al. Electroejaculation in patients with spinal cord injuries: a 21-year, single-center experience. *Int J Urol.* 2017;24(2):157–161.
25. Ibrahim E, et al. Evaluation of a re-engineered device for penile vibratory stimulation in men with spinal cord injury. *Spinal Cord.* 2021;59(2):151–158.
26. Fode M, Ohl DA, Sønksen J. A stepwise approach to sperm retrieval in men with neurogenic anejaculation. *Nat Rev Urol.* 2015;12(11):607–616.
27. Jensen CF, et al. Multiple needle-pass percutaneous testicular sperm aspiration as first-line treatment in azoospermic men. *Andrology.* 2016;4(2):257–262.
28. Sønksen J, et al. Vibratory ejaculation in 140 spinal cord injured men and home insemination of their partners. *Spinal Cord.* 2012;50(1):63–66.
29. Salonia A, Carvalho JP, Corona G, et al. EAU Guidelines on Sexual and Reproductive Health. 2020. https://uroweb.org/guideline/sexual-and-reproductive-health/#3. Accessed November 1, 2022.
30. Barbonetti A, et al. Correlates of low testosterone in men with chronic spinal cord injury. *Andrology.* 2014;2(5):721–728.

31. Behnaz M, et al. Prevalence of androgen deficiency in chronic spinal cord injury patients suffering from erectile dysfunction. *Spinal Cord*. 2017;55(12):1061–1065.
32. Sullivan SD, et al. Prevalence and etiology of hypogonadism in young men with chronic spinal cord injury: a cross-sectional analysis from two university-based rehabilitation centers. *PM R*. 2017;9(8):751–760.
33. Lim CAR, et al. Lifestyle modifications and pharmacological approaches to improve sexual function and satisfaction in men with spinal cord injury: a narrative review. *Spinal Cord*. 2020;58(4):391–401.
34. Bauman WA, et al. Lean tissue mass and energy expenditure are retained in hypogonadal men with spinal cord injury after discontinuation of testosterone replacement therapy. *J Spinal Cord Med*. 2015;38(1):38–47.

Section 3 Clinical Evaluation and Treatment of Male Infertility

Chapter 18

Clinical Fertility Preservation Decision-Making for Prepubertal and Postpubertal Individuals with Male Gametes

Jerrine Morris, Heiko Yang, John Lindsey, and James F. Smith

18.1 Introduction

Fertility-threatening medical and surgical treatments for benign and malignant conditions often cause a wide range of deleterious effects on reproductive and sexual function. Many chemotherapeutic agents can induce significant declines in sperm concentration, motility, and morphology. During recovery from these exposures, elevated DNA damage can impair the quality of sperm and is associated with higher rates of miscarriages. Radiation can induce azoospermia or severe oligozoospermia at relatively low testicular exposures, while larger exposures can cause significant hypogonadism. Surgical procedures (e.g., retroperitoneal lymph node dissection for metastatic testicular cancer) can cause dry ejaculation. Nerve damage from rectal and anal radiation or surgery is associated with erectile dysfunction. Hormone therapy to treat gender dysphoria (e.g., leuprolide, estradiol, and spironolactone) can significantly suppress spermatogenesis. While life changing and/or saving, innumerable treatments have known and unknown consequences on the male gametes that underscore the importance of fertility preservation (Figure 18.1). However, the complexities that surround clinical decision-making as the patient and family considers fertility preservation, particularly when factoring in socioeconomic and logistical barriers as well as ethical dilemmas and research advances, are the main focus of this chapter.

The World Health Organization maintains that "infertility is a disease of the reproductive system defined by the failure to achieve a clinical pregnancy after 12 months or more of regular unprotected intercourse" [1, p. 1522]. Not being able to have children is a well-established source of major stress; infertility is comparable to cancer and heart disease [2]. These feelings, coupled with their preexisting diagnosis, lead to increased distress and impaired quality of life among adolescent and young adult survivors of cancer as compared to their counterparts [3]. Infertility is recognized as a byproduct of childhood cancer therapy and affects up to 50% of male survivors [3]. With increased survivorship among this population and demonstrated importance of future family building, fertility preservation discussions are not only recommended but highly desired in a comprehensive manner, prior to treatment initiation given gonadotoxicity is often associated with these life-saving therapies [4,5].

18.2 Epidemiology of Benign and Malignant Conditions

Roughly 70,000 new cases of invasive cancer among adolescents and young adults aged 15–39 occur annually in the United States [9]. Between 2013 and 2017, of those diagnosed with invasive cancer, close to 10% of these cases occur among individuals 15–45 years of age with one-tenth of those occurring in adolescents less than age 20 (Figure 18.2) [9,10]. As compared to rates observed between 1975 and 1979, the prevalence of invasive cancer diagnosed among adolescent and young adults has increased roughly 30% [9,11]. While there are both age-related and sex-specific factors that contribute to cancer prevalence within certain populations, the overall 5-year survival rate has improved from 71% to 86% among adolescents and young adults diagnosed with cancer over the last 20 years [9,12]. Owing to enhanced multimodal treatments and combined chemotherapeutic regimens, close to 80% of those diagnosed will achieve a long-term cure [12].

In a survey by Schover et al., 51% of male patients either recently diagnosed or treated for cancer between the ages of 14 and 40 expressed desire to have a child in the future including 77% of men who were childless at diagnosis [13]. Among adolescents surveyed about their life goals, nearly half ranked having children as a top priority often just after overall health and work (or school) success as life goals [3]. Besides from diagnosis, young survivors have expressed an unmet desire to understand fertility information at the time of diagnosis [14]. When previously surveyed about satisfaction, everyone who attempted cryopreservation felt they made the right decision regardless of the outcome [3]. However, despite the known adverse effects of specific chemotherapeutic agents on one's future fertility and clear importance of fertility to adolescents and young adults diagnosed with cancer, few cryopreserve their gametes for future utilization. Only 28% of adolescents banked sperm prior to undergoing treatment in the United States and Canada between 2006 and 2007 [15]. This result was comparable to reports in 1999 despite continued improvements in mortality seen in this population [13]. There are disparities in fertility preservation counseling and utilization associated with age at diagnosis, race/ethnicity, and gender despite widespread recommendations [16,17].

- Azoospermia
- Oligospermia
- Poor quality sperm, functional infertility
- Inability to ejaculate (spine or pelvic surgery)
- Hypogonadism

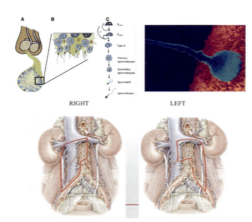

Figure 18.1 Potential sequelae of therapy on male reproductive and sexual function [69]

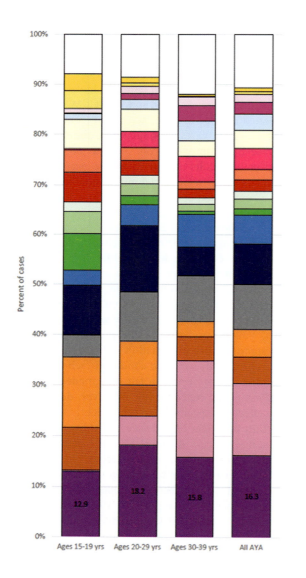

Figure 18.2 Case distribution of selected adolescent and young adult cancer types by age group – data from the Surveillance, Epidemiology, and End Results Program (2011–2015) [10]

Furthermore, indications for utilization of gonadotoxic therapies now include nononcologic indications. From use of cyclophosphamide for treatment of autoimmune conditions, a known gonadotoxic medication, to feminizing hormone therapy with deleterious effects of sperm quality even in the absence of continued use, recognition of the potential need for fertility preservation is important [18]. Benign hematologic and autoimmune diseases, genetic disorders, and gender dysphoria are a few of the nononcologic indications that account for roughly 10% of the demand for fertility preservation [19]. Most of these studies reflect the importance of oocyte or ovarian tissue cryopreservation to preserve fertility. There is an overall dearth of studies examining reproductive toxicity among spermatogonia in those utilizing therapies for benign indications [20].

In the United States, though possibly a significant underestimate, approximately 1 in 200 individuals consider themselves transgender [6]. The World Professional Association for Transgender Health (WPATH) and the American Society of Reproductive Medicine (ASRM) recommend fertility preservation (FP) discussions for these individuals [7,8]; however, accurate data on FP utilization are unknown. Furthermore, data on the effects of utilization of long-term agents for gonadal suppression in transgender patients with gender dysphoria are limited [19,20]; however, both WPATH and ASRM recommend FP discussions for transgender individuals. These limitations likely further lead to decreased access and utilization of FP practices within disparate populations similarly offered gonadotoxic therapies for nononcologic indications.

The Oncofertility Consortium (OC), composed of a multidisciplinary group of medical and pediatric oncologists, urologists, gynecologists, psychologists, and researchers, has been dedicated to improving research and access to fertility preservation services for patients with cancer for over 15 years [9]. Current published guidelines encourage providers to discuss potential threats to fertility early in their course as well as offer options for fertility preservation [5]. While no similar governing body disseminates guidelines for fertility preservation for nononcologic indications, the OC has broadened its approach in recent years [21]. While this chapter will briefly highlight how gonadotoxic therapy affects spermatogonia and modalities of sperm cryopreservation, the focus will be to critically assess the current barriers and limitations in fertility preservation of the male gamete for benign and malignant indications.

18.3 Mechanisms of Toxic Therapies

Spermatogenesis, particularly spermatogonia undergoing differentiation, is highly sensitive to the effects of most cytotoxic chemotherapy and radiation [22,23]. As noted by Meistrich, later germ cells can survive and progress along their differentiation pathway but are infrequently replaced due to the loss of spermatogonia in a process called "maturation depletion" leading to progressive decline of ejaculated sperm counts and eventual azoospermia at roughly 18 weeks postexposure [22]. Both chemotherapy and radiation exhibit dose-dependent effects of spermatocyte number that can be transient or irreversible.

Radiation therapy is used for hematologic malignancies and carcinoma of the male reproductive tract, and colorectal disease. The testicles are extremely radiation sensitive with greatest effects exhibited through germ cell loss in a dose-dependent fashion. Radiation therapies begin to affect spermatogenesis at doses as low as 0.1 Gy even if the testes are not directly irradiated [24]. If radiation therapy is proximal to the testes and the dose is sufficient, testis shielding may not be adequate to quell the effects on sperm production [24]. While the dose limits at which azoospermia is permanent is unknown, the higher the dose as well as use of fractionated, instead of single-dose radiation, can lead to greater delays in spermatogenic recovery [22]. While discernible changes in one's semen analysis may not be seen until 70 days after radiation therapy, it can lead to morphological changes and DNA fragmentation of sperm exposed, underscoring the importance of fertility preservation prior to undergoing treatment [25,26].

Most chemotherapeutic drugs, particularly alkylating medications, are considered to be toxic to the gonads. Similar to radiation exposure, the effects of chemotherapy are related to both the duration of exposure and dose administered (Table 18.1) [22]. It is often challenging to determine the offending agent(s) as chemotherapeutic regimens are usually combinatorial. For example, vinca alkaloids (e.g., vincristine and vinblastine) generally cause only a temporary reduction in sperm concentration; however, they are typically administered in a multidrug setting with high-risk alkylating agents like cyclophosphamide (Table 18.2) [25]. Thus, the aspect of cytotoxic treatment that is responsible for its increased efficacy in oncologic conditions is also what contributes to its greatest impact on male fertility [26]. In nononcologic conditions, there is similar usage of alkylating agents for the management of benign diseases with severe multiorgan dysfunction for which fertility preservation prior to initiation would be indicated [18,19].

While not as toxic to spermatogenesis as many chemotherapeutic agents, patients with gender nonconformity frequently take potentially fertility-toxic medications to affirm their individual gender. Gender nonconformity refers to the extent to which a person's gender identity, role, or expression differs from the cultural norms prescribed for people of a particular sex. Gender dysphoria refers to discomfort or distress that is caused by a discrepancy between a person's gender identity and that person's sex assigned at birth [7]. Those experiencing gender dysphoria may pursue feminizing hormone therapy (FHT) and/or surgery to alleviate this distress [7]. In transwomen, FHT can lead to hypospermatogenesis with eventual progression to azoospermia [27]. Furthermore, the use of FHT at the time of semen collection has been associated with

Table 18.1 Male gamete toxicity by antineoplastic agent and dose [22]

Antineoplastic agents that can cause or add to prolonged azoospermia in humans.

Effect	Agent	Mechanism of action	Dose to produce effect
Prolonged azoospermia	Ionizing radiation	DNA breaks	2.5 Gy
	Chlorambucil	Alkylating	1.4 g/m^2
	Cyclophosphamide	Alkylating	19 g/m^2
	Procarbazine	Alkylating	4 g/m^2
	Melphalan	Alkylating	140 mg/m^2
	Cisplatin	DNA cross-link	500 mg/m^2
Azoospermia in adulthood after treatment prior to puberty	BCNU	Alkylating	1 g/m^2
	CCNU	Alkylating	500 mg/m^2
Likely to cause prolonged azoospermia, but always given with other highly sterilizing agents	Busulfan	Alkylating	600 mg/m^2
	Ifosfamide	Alkylating	42 g/m^2
	Nitrogen mustard	Alkylating	
	Actinomycin D	DNA intercalating	
Reported to be additive with above agents in causing prolonged azoospermia, but cause only temporary reductions in sperm count when not combined with above agents	Adriamycin	DNA intercalating	770 mg/m^2
	Thiotepa	Alkylating	400 mg/m^2
	Cytosine arabinoside	Nucleoside analogue	1 g/m^2
	Vinblastine	Microtubule inhibitor	50 mg/m^2

decreased semen quality [28]. While cessation of gender-affirming medication can lead to an improvement in semen parameters, the degree to which FHT use can lead to azoospermia is not well known and requiring cessation of hormonal medication for even a short period of time may be distressing to the individual (Figure 18.3).

Whether removal of gonads for testicular cancer or gender-affirming surgery, those who undergo an orchiectomy if unilateral will have reduced numbers of germ cells in effect leading to a reduction in the overall testicular reserve. Even nontesticular surgical procedures, including retroperitoneal lymph node dissection, prostatectomy, pelvic exenteration, and other similar deep pelvis surgery can lead to varied effects on the sympathetic and parasympathetic neural pathways important for seminal emission or ejaculation [12,26]. The effects of surgery can then range from direct nerve injury resulting in ejaculatory dysfunction and obstructive azoospermia [12,26]. While improvements in surgical technique have decreased the risk of damage to neural and anatomic pathways leading to increased paternity rates for males undergoing these procedures, infertility is still a prevalent risk factor underscoring the importance of preprocedural fertility preservation.

18.4 Cryopreservation Options

Semen cryopreservation requires masturbation and ejaculation into a sterile cup. Each semen sample can be aliquoted into one or more vials. On average, approximately 50% of sperm will survive the freezing and thawing process. Thawed sperm can be used for intrauterine insemination (IUI) if at least 5 million motile sperm are present, while in vitro fertilization (IVF) can be used for motile sperm more than zero. Vials can be combined when necessary to achieve a patient's fertility treatment goals. While not formalized in guidelines, clinicians providing FP counseling seek to maximize future fertility options for their patients while minimizing cost of freezing samples.

For those who are unable to produce semen through masturbation, penile vibratory stimulation provides a useful alternative with success rates ranging from 65% to 83% [29,30]. Those who do not respond to vibratory stimulation can be offered electroejaculation as an alternative. Electroejaculation stimulates the pelvic tissues via a transrectal probe, which may lead to seminal emission [30]. In a single-center experience and review of the literature, up to 45% of pubertal boys obtained a successful sperm yield through electroejaculation and those with higher testosterone levels were more likely to demonstrate adequacy in yield [31]. For men with erectile dysfunction or retrograde ejaculation, a number of medications including phosphodiesterase inhibitors and alpha agonists, respectively, have been proposed and shown helpful for producing a semen sample when indicated [30,32].

Approximately 12% of men are azoospermic or have severe oligospermia or immotile sperm either attributable to their underlying malignancy or due to preexisting genetic aberrations [33,34]. These individuals may require alternative sperm retrieval approaches namely through testicular sperm extraction. While this is a surgical procedure that takes place in an operating or procedural room, there is a small incision made on the scrotum while the patient is under conscious sedation to expose the seminiferous tubules. A biopsy of tubules is excised and transported to the lab where it is evaluated for the presence of sperm.

Table 18.2 Risk of gonadotoxicity based on antineoplastic agent [70,71]

Lowest Risk

• Vincristine
  Methotrexate
  Dactinomycin
  Mercaptopurine
  Mitoxantrone
  Vinblastine

Intermediate Risk

• Cisplatin
  Carboplatin
  Doxorubicin
  BEP (bleomycin, etoposide, cisplatin)
  ABVD (adriamycin, bleomycin, vinblastine, dacarbazine)

Highest Risk

• Cyclophosphamide
  Busulfan
  Ifosfamide
  thio-TEPA
  Melphalan
  Procarbazine
  Chlorambucil
  MOPP (mechlorethamine, vincristine, procarbazine, prednisone)
  CHOP (cyclophosphamide, doxorubicin, vincristine, and prednisone)

18.5 Fertility Preservation Decision-Making

Imagine a typical 25-year-old patient presenting to your clinic with desire for fertility preservation. Several key questions are critical to identify to help this patient achieve their future fertility goals. These questions can be difficult to answer for some patients but are essential to helping a clinician guide their patients.

18.5.1 Does This Individual Have an Ejaculate with Motile Sperm?

If the patient is unable to produce a semen sample or no motile sperm is found within the semen sample, surgical approaches should be considered. For a patient undergoing orchiectomy, sperm can be found within the testicle or epididymis in cancer

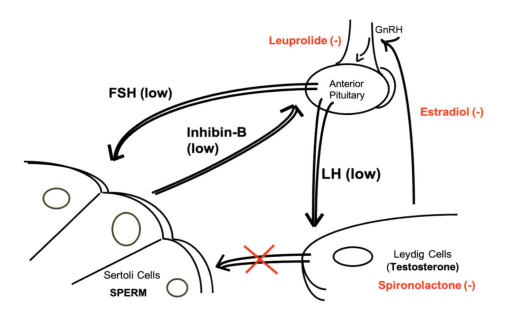

Figure 18.3 Mechanisms of gonadal suppression in transgender females

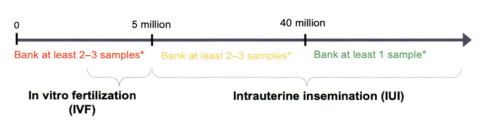

Figure 18.4 Cryopreservation strategies by total motile count

*Divided into multiple aliquots
~50% survives thaw

patients (onco-testicular sperm extraction) or within the testicle for transgender patients undergoing simple orchiectomy [35,36].

18.5.2 What Is the Total Motile Count of the Semen Sample?

The total motile count is an essential piece of data to help guide a patient in how many ejaculates to bank and how many vials should be used for each sample. On average, 50% of a sample does not survive the freeze thaw process, though for some cancer patients, even before therapy, survival may be as low as 10%. In general, banking more samples is best; however, limitations in time before initiating therapy, logistics of producing the sample in context of other therapies, and cost play a role in how many samples are produced (Figure 18.4).

18.5.3 How Much Time Does the Patient Have before Starting Therapy?

Some patients have weeks or months before starting fertility-threatening therapy, while for many cancer patients, they may only have days or hours (Figure 18.5). The logistics of banking semen samples are time consuming and labor intensive. A specific, often quite long, consent form is required that asks patients to acknowledge the inherent uncertainties of the freeze-thaw process and also to document their preferences for disposition of the sample in the event of their death. For adults, three options are possible: discard the sample, use the sample for research, and have their partner determine what should be done with the sample. For children and adolescents, only discarding and using for research options are ethically appropriate. Additionally, FDA labs including Hep B, Hep C, HTLV I/II, RPR, and HIV are essential to obtain so that samples can be utilized in the future for assisted reproductive therapies. Many fertility clinics will not accept semen samples cryopreserved at an outside facility that lacks results of infectious disease testing prior to collection.

18.5.4 Does the Patient Have Insurance Coverage for Cryopreservation?

The cost of cryopreservation can be very prohibitive for patients. A high cost also leads to a dilemma for patients and

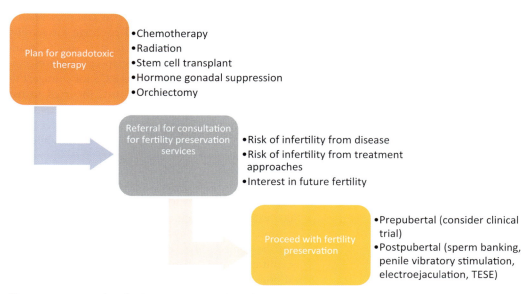

Figure 18.5 Approach to fertility preservation in the male

clinicians. While more samples is almost always better, patients may not be able to afford additional costs of each sample. Details of cost are explored below in greater detail.

18.5.5 Does the Patient Have a Partner with a Uterus and Ovaries? Or if No Current Partner, Does the Individual Imagine Themselves in the Future with a Partner Who Has a Uterus and Ovaries?

Thawed ejaculate can be used for either intrauterine insemination (IUI) or in vitro fertilization (IVF). Generally, at least 5 million motile sperm are necessary for IUI. Under the best circumstances in terms of uterine and ovarian health, per cycle pregnancy rates is approximately 15–20% [37]. Most dyads will pursue at least 3–4 IUI cycles before moving to the more expensive and invasive IVF. IVF is a much more successful technique (50% pregnancy per cycle) and requires many fewer motile sperm (as few as 10–20 depending on the number of eggs retrieved from the female partner). This technique, however, is far more expensive ($10–20,000 per fresh egg retrieval and IVF cycle compared to ~$1,500 per cycle for IUI) [38,39]. For transgender female patients, it is important to ask them whether they imagine having a biological family with a partner who has a uterus and ovaries. If their partner does not have a uterus and ovaries, then identifying an egg donor and also a surrogate to carry the embryo in addition to IVF will be necessary. Informing patients of this process allows each individual to plan effectively for the future.

18.6 Barriers to Accessing Fertility Preservation Therapy

The American Society of Clinical Oncology (ASCO), ASRM, American Academy of Pediatrics, and WPATH are among the few organizations/societies with published guidelines recommending fertility counseling and fertility preservation be offered to all patients with a risk of subfertility due to cytotoxic treatment, surgery, or prolonged FHT [5,7,30,40]. Barriers to undergoing sperm cryopreservation are ubiquitous among individuals with a diagnosis of cancer; similar barriers exist among those without cancer and with a risk for future infertility. These barriers often fit within three main schemata: patient-centered (knowledge, education, socioeconomic, social), physician-centered (knowledge, geography, implicit biases), and system-centered barriers (cost, insurance coverage, lack of referral structure) [41]. The latter are extremely important as the logistical challenges in banking are often very imposing. Developing systems to cryopreserve sperm that provide affordable fertility preservation and eliminate this logistical friction for patients and doctors would likely make a huge positive impact for patients and lower frustration for doctors.

The decision to proceed with sperm cryopreservation is highly individualized. To that end, there are several characteristics that differentially affect one's access and utilization of fertility preservation services. In a small prospective study of male patients aged 13 and above newly diagnosed with cancer and eligible to undergo fertility preservation from 2006 to 2007, only 28.1% banked sperm. Those who proceeded to sperm cryopreservation tended to be older (p = 0.06), have a central nervous system (CNS) or non-CNS solid tumor malignancy as compared to leukemia/lymphoma (p<0.02), and have higher socioeconomic status (p<0.05) [15]. Researchers have evaluated sociodemographic factors that have been shown to be associated with fertility preservation. In a study by Goodman et al., Caucasian race and having medical insurance were both associated with fertility preservation referral [42]. The family unit including the presence of a partner and parity also influences whether patients seek information about fertility preservation services and proceed with sperm cryopreservation [14]. While there is limited information about how religion contributes to decisions regarding fertility preservation, Evangelical patients were found to bank sperm significantly less frequently than others [15]. Moreover, the legitimacy of assisted reproductive therapies is considerably variable among the major world religions [15,43]. Even though patient-centered factors influence the utilization of fertility preservation services, provider influences are paramount. In one study, men who received information about sperm banking were more likely to choose cryopreservation and also displayed more knowledge regarding cancer-related infertility. This underscores the importance of the provider as an intrinsic decision aid [13].

Despite recognition that clinicians should inform patients about their options for fertility preservation prior to initiation of any treatment that may confer subfertility [30], this practice is not ubiquitous among providers. Both pediatric and adult oncologists stated little to no training in discussions surrounding fertility preservation or accompanying resources [44]. There are also pervasive misperceptions and assumptions about affordability, patient interest, acceptability, and uncertainty of use in cases of late-stage disease or the science surrounding cryopreservation techniques that contribute the reticence for providers to discuss fertility preservation with patients and caregivers [44]. In a physician-centric study by Schover et al., 91% of respondents agreed that sperm banking should be offered to all at risk; however, roughly 75% of respondents either never bring it up or mention it in less than a quarter of eligible patients [45]. Barriers cited included lack of time for the discussion, perceived high cost, and lack of convenient facilities. Furthermore, physicians were less likely to offer to men who were homosexual or HIV positive and more likely to offer to men who were married, highlighting the implicit bias that contributes to whether fertility preservation is offered to patients [45]. Lastly, in a systematic review performed by Anazoda, there was profound dissent regarding the role of each individual to initiate the conversation. Whether initiated from the patient, parent, healthcare team, or primary provider, there was no overwhelming consensus for who bears the brunt of the responsibility of broaching the topic of fertility preservation, which contributes to the limited utilization of this technology [46].

The diagnosis of cancer is one that often incurs immediate treatment. For oncologists without a fertility preservation program built into their practice, they may perceive fertility as not a priority at the time of diagnosis [14]. Prior studies have shown that the identification of fertility preservation as an integral part of the treatment plan as well as the presence of an established referral pathway are associated with increased referrals [46]. This suggests that while increasing awareness to the importance of fertility preservation particularly in a population likely to be exposed to gonadotoxic therapy or surgical removal of gonads is important, system-specific factors like a standardized referral process may be advantageous to ensure access to timely consultations for fertility preservation [14]. Letorneau et al. found that socioeconomic status was associated with greater utilization of sperm cryopreservation [47]. This is not surprising as national coverage for fertility preservation is ill-reported and limited to state specific mandates that vary widely. While the cost of sperm cryopreservation is roughly $250 per sample as well as $275 for storage, this does not take into account continued costs incurred to use sperm either through insemination or IVF in which costs are increased 10-fold. Insurance coverage is either employer sponsored or through Medicaid and there is great variability in what constitutes necessary coverage. Some state-sponsored plans only cover patients who have demonstrated infertility and/or are married, which neglects the adolescent population substantially. For adolescents who are Medicaid eligible, there is continued variation in what services are deemed "medically necessary," and, even with physician recommendation, coverage can still be denied [34]. This systemic limitation exacerbates inequalities in fertility preservation acquisition.

In addition to barriers revealed throughout this chapter, there are unique barriers seen within the transgender population that deserve highlighting. Given increased discrimination faced by members of the transgender community, deliberate recognition that gender dysphoria in itself does not constitute a mental disorder is important [7]. Several organizations including the American Medical Association, American Congress of Obstetricians and Gynecologists, and the ASRM all oppose discrimination in health care on the basis of gender identity [8,48]. To that extent, fertility preservation is no exception. In fact, exogenous hormones and gonadectomy have well-recognized impacts on fertility and clinicians are encouraged to counsel both adolescents and adults regarding options for fertility preservation prior to initiating gender affirming therapy [8,48]. Between one- and two-thirds of transgender adolescents and young adults desire to have children at some point in their lifetime; however, discussions on the potential negative impacts of gender-affirming therapy on biological parenthood are often rare unless patients are seen at gender clinics [49]. Barriers to accessing care include poor attitudes and inadequate knowledge of transgender reproductive care on behalf of the healthcare provider [49]. Even worse, patients have reported being denied access to fertility preservation information and services, being misgendered, and treated disrespectfully, which directly challenges tenets by all medical societies regarding transgender care [49].

While barriers in accessing fertility preservation services exist regardless of age, indication, geographic location, and ethnicity, there are some populations with greater barriers than others. Furthermore, studies underscore the immense importance of the provider in navigating these barriers.

18.7 Ethics of Fertility Preservation

Sperm cryopreservation is the only widely accepted modality for fertility preservation of male gametes [50]. In postpubertal males, this often poses few ethical dilemmas; however, this chapter will discuss ethical quandaries that may arise in particular populations. To start, informed consent regarding options for fertility preservation prior to gonadotoxic therapies, as discussed, is widely accepted as standard of care. However, one of the basic ethical tenets in medicine is "do no harm." Studies have shown there is a reluctance among providers to discuss fertility preservation with patients with late-stage disease and/or a poor prognosis [44,45]. Both ASRM and ASCO have firm guidelines that include discussing fertility preservation with all patients of childbearing age; one would be remiss not to sympathize with a provider's perspective of not wanting to add additional stress to the patient or offer patients with a poor prognosis an unrealistic expectation [5,30]. With that being said, medical providers are encouraged to rely on informed consent when discussing fertility preservation even in patients with advanced disease. The ultimate choice to pursue fertility preservation, even in instances when posthumous parenting is likely, is the right of the patient.

In the case of minors, ethical dilemmas become more apparent as informed consent only applies to individuals who have appropriate decisional capacity and legal empowerment. Decision-making involving young patients is typically rendered as the responsibility of both the physician and parent with the intent to act in the best interests of the child. This concept, as alluded to by the American Academy of Pediatrics, is not always easy to define as religious, social, cultural, and philosophical factors all contribute to what is considered to be best [51,52]. For adolescents, there are further complexities as the concept of "assent" enters the equation. Adolescents should be included in the conversation with the intent to assess their understanding of the scenario as well as their expressed views of proposed treatment options [51]. Among pediatric cancer survivors aged 25–47, the most salient theme expressed was regret that compromised fertility had not been addressed at the time of cancer diagnosis [53]. While almost 60% of survivors were uncertain about their personal fertility, most survivors of childhood cancer expressed a desire to have children in the future [54]. Interestingly, when comparing parental and patient congruence regarding reproductive concerns, studies have shown stronger reproductive concerns that are not echoed similarly or even accurately within the parent [3,55]. Specifically, for minors who are undergoing often swift gonadotoxic treatment, there is an obligation to counsel the family unit on the value of fertility preservation with great consideration to including the patient, as appropriate, in this conversation.

Practically speaking, for patients under 18, both an assent from a child aged 12–17, and a consent from a parent or guardian are required. In this consent, disposition of the tissue in the event of the child's death is essential. Families can choose either to discard the tissue or donate the tissue for research. It is not ethically appropriate to allow minors to designate their parents as the recipients of their tissue for family-building purposes in the event of their death.

Beyond the informed consent process in minors, other ethical dilemmas surrounding collection and future use are unique to this population. While post-pubertal males are capable of ejaculating and providing sperm for storage, there is some degree of stress that may accompany this process [30]. For prepubertal males, the hypothalamic-pituitary-gonadal axis has not yet become active and spermatogenesis has not begun [26]. Therefore, the only current option for prepubertal males is testicular tissue cryopreservation, which is experimental [30]. Both considering or withholding this as an option pose ethical dilemmas due its unproven efficacy. Ginsburg et al. found, when offered an experimental protocol for testicular cryopreservation, 16 out of 21 parents consented to the testicular biopsy. All parents who did not consent revealed they were unsure if it was right for their child. Conversely, all parents who consented to the biopsy expressed an understanding of the importance of future fertility and none of the parents regretted the decision postbiopsy even if there was uncertainty regarding the usability of the tissue [56]. Lastly, testicular tissue cryopreservation is limited to a small segment of programs with an IRB approved protocol thus limiting the access of this potential service to those who can obtain it (Figure 18.6) [30].

18.8 Future Fertility Preservation and Restoration Strategies for Cis-Gender Male Prepubertal Patients

Several experimental techniques are being developed to restore fertility using prepubertal testicular tissue or somatic cells. These techniques include autologous testicular cell transplantation (TCT), which can be performed via direct injection into the testis or surgical implantation in subcutaneous adipose tissue [57, 58] and the conversion of somatic cells into germ cells using induced pluripotent stem cell (iPSC) technology [59,60]. The goal of each of these methods is to obtain sperm from tissue not already undergoing active spermatogenesis, and all three methods have been demonstrated to be successful in animal models.

At this time, autologous TCT appears to be closest to human application. Orwig et al. showed in 2012 that an injection of prepubertal testicular cells into the agametic seminiferous tubules of adult rhesus macaques could reconstitute the spermatogenic machinery of the testis [57]. This group subsequently demonstrated in 2019 that prepubertal tissue implanted en bloc in the subcutaneous adipose tissue of adult animals could also successfully undergo spermatogenesis [58]. In both cases, the sperm obtained after transplantation led to successful embryo fertilization via intracytoplasmic sperm injection and healthy offspring. Importantly, these results demonstrate spermatogenesis can be achieved using immature prepubertal testicular tissue despite bypassing the complex hormonal changes during puberty, thus removing a major hypothetical hurdle for fertility restoration in these patients. Now that results have been convincingly demonstrated in animals, the current challenge is to demonstrate safety, efficacy, and a standardized technical approach for clinical use.

The "reprogramming" of human iPSCs into germ cells is a tantalizing alternative as it can be beneficial to any patient who did not have the opportunity to bank tissue prior to loss of fertility, not just prepubertal patients. The generation of iPSC-derived

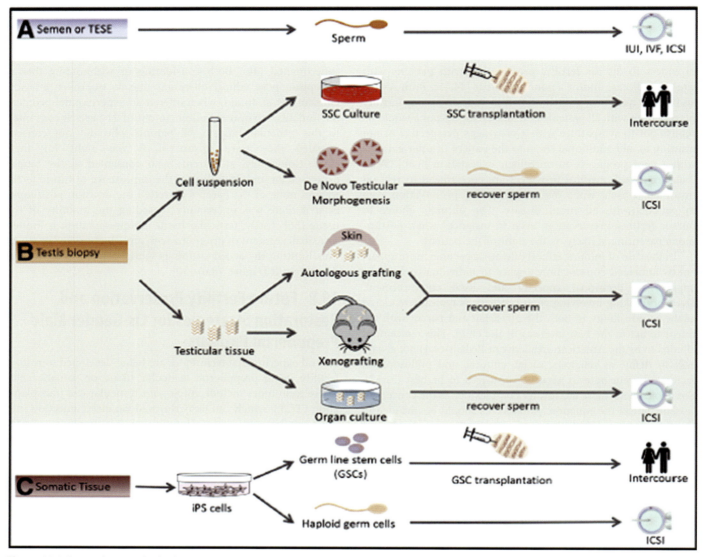

Figure 18.6 Potential options for fertility preservation of the male gamete [69]

germ cells was successfully demonstrated in a mouse model with the production of viable offspring around 2010 [59,60]. However, numerous efforts to apply the same technique to human cells have thus far been thwarted by critical differences in epigenetic modifications and expression patterns between the two species [61,62]. This strategy thus remains purely hypothetical, and much more work needs to be done to understand not just the biology but also the ethics underlying this approach.

18.9 Fertility Preservation Strategies Possible for Transgender Female Patients

In the case of male to female transgender individuals, one of the primary barriers to fertility preservation included the inability to masturbate to produce a semen sample for freezing. Coupled with the mental burden of masturbating, having to do so in a medical setting exacerbated reticence to proceed with fertility preservation [49]. When this is encountered, consideration should be given to sperm collection through penile vibratory stimulation, transrectal electrostimulation, or surgical testicular extraction (testicular sperm extraction), which, similar to tissue cryopreservation, is not always widely available, limiting access of this option [63,64]. However, electrostimulation and surgical sperm extraction require general or local anesthesia and relatively invasive procedures.

If fertility preservation is not conducted prior to initiation of hormonal or surgical gender-affirming therapy, there is a great likelihood of azoospermia or severe oligoasthenospermia [30,63]. Even in the case of hormonal therapy, male to female transgender individuals have expressed hesitation to proceed with fertility preservation if stopping hormonal therapy is a prerequisite, further underscoring the importance of pretherapeutic referrals and counseling [49]. Ethical dilemmas become more apparent in the case of transgender youth as the balance between informed consent, beneficence, nonmaleficence, and justice are all encountered. There is concern that adolescents may lack sufficient capacity to make a decision of this magnitude about their future desires [65]. While few studies have evaluated regret in adolescents who did not undergo fertility preservation prior to gender-affirming therapy, it is reassuring that among adults in a large retrospective cohort in Amsterdam who underwent gender-affirming surgery, less than 1% regretted their decision to proceed with gonadectomy [66]. Furthermore, young adults who underwent pubertal suppression during adolescence were shown to have decreased gender dysphoria and increased psychological functioning, suggesting that well-informed decisions made in adolescents were beneficial into young adulthood [67].

18.10 Concluding and Summarizing Statements

Many benign and malignant conditions are treated with fertility-threatening medical or surgical therapies. Fertility preservation is a recourse critical to discuss prior to initiation of these therapies; however, many barriers exist to their utilization. At the root of most barriers is knowledge. It is incredibly important for physicians to arm patients with information about fertility preservation if at risk for infertility due to potentially gonadotoxic therapy. These discussions are complex as they occur suddenly, during a tenuous time, and often with unimaginable consequences. Secondly, consultation with an expert in providing fertility preservation services is essential to aid patients weighing the pros and cons behind their options. Thirdly, decision aides that have primarily been tested and widely accessible for female oncologic patients interested in pursuing fertility preservation should be expanded to include male oncologic patients as well as individuals undergoing treatment for benign indications [68]. It is only with knowledge that individuals can exercise autonomy in making an informed decision; this has been shown to both increase utilization and decrease long-term decision regret. Lastly, as access to fertility preservation increases, continued research into utilization of these services is paramount to understanding where the deficits lie and how to combat them in future.

References

1. Zegers-Hochschild F, Adamson GD, de Mouzon J, et al. International Committee for Monitoring Assisted Reproductive Technology (ICMART) and the World Health Organization (WHO) revised glossary of ART terminology. *Fertility and Sterility*. 2009;92(5):1520–1524.
2. Anderheim L, Holter H, Bergh C, Moller A. Does psychological stress affect the outcome of in vitro fertilization?. *Hum Reprod*. 2005;20(10):2969–2975.
3. Klosky J, Simmons JL, Russell KM, et al. Fertility as a priority among at-risk adolescent males newly diagnosed with cancer and their parents. *Support Care Cancer*. 2015;23(2):333–341.
4. Barnett M, McDonnell G, DeRosa A, et al. Psychosocial outcomes and interventions among cancer survivors diagnosed during adolescence and young adulthood (AYA): a systematic review. *J Cancer Surviv*. 2016;10(5):814–831.
5. Oktay K, Harvey B, Partridge A, et al. Fertility preservation in patients with cancer: ASCO clinical practice guideline update. *J Clin Oncol*. 2018;36(19):1994–2001.
6. Garcia MM. Genital gender-affirming surgery: patient care, decision making, and surgery options. In: McAninch JW, Lue TF, eds. *Smith & Tanagho's General Urology*. 19th ed. McGraw-Hill; 2020:747–768.
7. Coleman E, Bockting W, Botzer M, et al. Standards of care for the health of transsexual, transgender, and gender-nonconforming people, version 7. *Int J Transgend*. 2012;13(4):165–232.
8. Hembree W, Cohen-Kettenis PT, Gooren L, et al. Endocrine treatment of gender-dysphoric/gender-incongruent persons: an Endocrine Society* clinical practice guideline. *J Clin Endocrinol Metab*. 2017;102(11):3869–3903.
9. Close A, Dreyzin A, Miller KD, Seynnaeve BKN, Rapkin LB. Adolescent and young adult oncology – past, present, and future. *CA Cancer J Clin*. 2019;69(6):485–496.
10. National Cancer Institute. *SEER Cancer Statistics Review 1975–2017*. January 6, 2021. https://seer.cancer.gov/csr/1975_2017/browse_csr.php?sectionSEL=2&pageSEL=sect_02_table.07. Accessed November 1, 2022.
11. Siegel R, Miller KD, Jemal A. Colorectal cancer mortality rates in adults aged 20 to 54 years in the United States, 1970–2014. *JAMA*. 2017;318(6):572–574.
12. Moss J, Choi AW, Keeter MKF, Brannigan RE. Male adolescent fertility preservation. *Fertil Steril*. 2016;105(2):267–273.
13. Schover L, Brey K, Lichtin A, Lipshultz LI, Jeha S. Knowledge and experience regarding cancer, infertility, and sperm banking in younger male survivors. *J Clin Oncol*. 2002;20(7):1880–1889.
14. Flink D, Sheeder J, Kondapalli LA. A review of the oncology patient's challenges for utilizing fertility preservation services. *J Adolesc Young Adult Oncol*. 2017;6(1):31–44.
15. Klosky J, Randolph ME, Navid F, et al. Sperm cryopreservation practices among adolescent cancer patients at risk for infertility. *Pediatr Hematol Oncol*. 2009;26:252–260.
16. Patel P, Kohn TP, Cohen J, Shiff B, Kohn J, Ramasamy R. Evaluation of reported fertility preservation counseling before chemotherapy using the Quality Oncology Practice Initiative Survey. *JAMA Netw Open*. 2020;3(7):e2010806.
17. Lawson A, McGuire JM, Noncent E, Olivieri JF, Smith KN, Marsh EE. Disparities in counseling female cancer patients for fertility preservation. *J Womens Health (Larchmt)*. 2017;26(8):886–891.
18. Yang H, Ramstein J, Smith J. Non-oncologic indications for male fertility preservation. *Curr Urol Rep*. 2019;20(9):51.
19. Condorelli M, Demeestere I. Challenges of fertility preservation in non-

20. Johnson E, Finlayson C, Rowell EE, et al. Fertility preservation for pediatric patients: current state and future possibilities. *J Urol.* 2017;198(1):186–194.
21. Ataman LM, Rodrigues JK, Marinho RM, et al. Creating a global community of practice for oncofertility. *J Glob Oncol.* 2016;2(2):83–96.
22. Meistrich M. Effects of chemotherapy and radiotherapy on spermatogenesis in humans. *Fertil Steril.* 2013;100(5):1180–1186.
23. Frydman R, Grynberg M. Male fertility preservation: innovations and questions. *Fertil Steril.* 2016;105(2):247–248.
24. Okada K, Fujisawa M. Recovery of spermatogenesis following cancer treatment with cytotoxic chemotherapy and radiotherapy. *World J Mens Health.* 2019;37(2):166–174.
25. Stahl P, Stember DS, Hsiao W, Schlegel PN. Indications and strategies for fertility preservation in men. *Clin Obstet Gynecol.* 2010;53(4):815–827.
26. Trost L, Brannigan R. Fertility preservation in males. In: Gracia C, Woodruff TK, eds. *Oncofertility medical practice: clinical issues and implementation.* Springer Science+Business Media; 2012:27–44.
27. T'Sjoen G, Caenegem EV, Wierckx K. Transgenderism and reproduction. *Curr Opin Endocrinol Diabetes Obes.* 2013;20(6):575–579.
28. Adeleye A, Reid G, Kao CN, Mok-Lin E, Smith JF. Semen parameters among transgender women with a history of hormonal treatment. *Urology.* 2019;124:136–141.
29. Mehta A, Sigman M. Management of the dry ejaculate: a systematic review of aspermia and retrograde ejaculation. *Fertil Steril.* 2015;104(5):1074–1081.
30. Practice Committee of the American Society for Reproductive Medicine. Fertility preservation in patients undergoing gonadotoxic therapy or gonadectomy: a committee opinion. *Fertil Steril.* 2019;112(6):1022–1033.
31. Adank M, van Dorp W, Smit M, et al. Electroejaculation as a method of fertility preservation in boys diagnosed with cancer: a single-center experience and review of the literature. *Fertil Steril.* 2014;102(1):199–205.e1.
32. Tur-Kaspa I, Segal S, Moffa F, Massobrio M, Meltzer S. Viagra for temporary erectile dysfunction during treatments with assisted reproductive technologies. *Hum Reprod.* 1999;14(7):1783–1784.
33. Berookhim B, Mulhall JP. Outcomes of operative sperm retrieval strategies for fertility preservation among males scheduled to undergo cancer treatment. *Fertil Steril.* 2014;101(3):805–811.
34. Benoit M, Chiles K, Hsieh M. The landscape of coverage for fertility preservation in male pediatric patients. *Urol Pract.* 2018;5(3):198–204.
35. Jiang D, Swenson E, Mason M, et al. Effects of estrogen on spermatogenesis in transgender women. *Urology.* 2019;132:117–122.
36. Schrader M, Muller M, Sofikitis N, et al. "Onco-Tese": testicular sperm extraction in azospermic cancer patients before chemotherapy – new guidelines? *Urology.* 2003;61(2):421–425.
37. Bhattacharya S, Harrild K, Mollison J, et al. Clomifene citrate or unstimulated intrauterine insemination compared with expectant management for unexplained infertility: pragmatic randomised controlled trial. *BMJ.* 2008;337.
38. Katz P, Showstack J, Smith JF, et al. Costs of infertility treatment: results from an 18-month prospective cohort study. *Fertil Steril.* 2011;95(3):915–921.
39. Wu A, Odisho AY, Washington SL, Katz PP, Smith JF. Out-of-pocket fertility patient expense: data from a multicenter prospective infertility cohort. *J Urol.* 2013;191(2):427–432.
40. Neblett M, Hipp H. Fertility considerations in transgender persons. *Endocrinol Metab Clin North Am.* 2019;48(2):391–402.
41. Mehta A, Nangia AK, Dupree JM, Smith JF. Limitations and barriers in access to care for male factor infertility. *Fertil Steril.* 2016;105(5):1128–1137.
42. Goodman L, Balthazar U, Kim J, Mersereau JE. Trends of socioeconomic disparities in referral patterns for fertility preservation consultation. *Hum Reprod.* 2012;27(7):2076–2981.
43. Schenker J. Assisted reproduction practice: religious perspectives. *Reprod Biomed Online.* 2005;10(3):310–319.
44. Quinn G, Vadaparampil ST, King L, et al. Impact of physicians' personal discomfort and patient prognosis on discussion of fertility preservation with young cancer patients. *Patient Educ Couns.* 2009;77(3):338–343.
45. Schover L, Brey K, Lichtin A, Lipshultz LI, Jeha S. Oncologists' attitudes and practices regarding banking sperm before cancer treatment. *J Clin Oncol.* 2002;20(7):1890–1897.
46. Anazodo A, Laws P, Logan S, et al. How can we improve oncofertility care for patients? A systematic scoping review of current international practice and models of care. *Hum Reprod Update.* 2019;25(2):159–179.
47. Letourneau J, Smith JF, Ebbel EE, et al. Racial, socioeconomic, and demographic disparities in access to fertility preservation in young women diagnosed with cancer. *Cancer.* 2012;118(18):4579–4588.
48. Ethics Committee of the American Society for Reproductive Medicine. Access to fertility services by transgender persons: an Ethics Committee opinion. *Fertil Steril.* 2015;104(5):1111–1115.
49. Baram S, Myers SA, Yee S, Librach CL. Fertility preservation for transgender adolescents and young adults: a systematic review. *Hum Reprod Update.* 2019;25(6):696–716.
50. Martinez F, International Society for Fertility Preservation–ESHRE–ASRM Expert Working Group. Update on fertility preservation from the Barcelona International Society for Fertility Preservation–ESHRE–ASRM 2015 expert meeting: indications, results and future perspectives. *Hum Reprod.* 32(9):1802–1811.
51. Committee on Bioethics, American Academy of Pediatrics. Informed consent, parental permission, and assent in pediatric practice. *Pediatrics,* 1995;95(2):314–317.
52. Ramstein J, Halpern J, Gadzinski AJ, Brannigan RE, Smith JF. Ethical, moral, and theological insights into advances in male pediatric and adolescent fertility preservation. *Andrology.* 2017;5(4):631–639.
53. Stein D, Victorson DE, Choy JT, et al. Fertility preservation preferences and

54. Zebrack B, Casillas J, Nohr L, Adams H, Zeltzer LK. Fertility issues for young adult survivors of childhood cancer. *Psychooncology.* 2004;13:689–699.
55. Quinn G, Knapp C, Murphy D, Sawczyn K, Sender L. Congruence of reproductive concerns among adolescents with cancer and parents: pilot testing an adapted instrument. *Pediatrics.* 2012;129(4):e930–e936.
56. Ginsberg J, Carlson CA, Lin K, et al. An experimental protocol for fertility preservation in prepubertal boys recently diagnosed with cancer: a report of acceptability and safety. *Hum Reprod.* 2010;25(1):37–41.
57. Hermann BP, et al. Spermatogonial stem cell transplantation into rhesus testes regenerates spermatogenesis producing functional sperm. *Cell Stem Cell.* 2012;11(5):715–726.
58. Fayomi AP, Peters K, Suhkwani M, et al. Autologous grafting of cryopreserved prepubertal rhesus testis produces sperm and offspring. *Science.* 2019;363(6433):1314–1319.

perspectives among adult male survivors of pediatric cancer and their parents. *J Adolesc Young Adult Oncol.* 2014;3(2):75–82.

59. Hayashi K, Ohta H, Kurimoto K, et al. Reconstitution of the mouse germ cell specification pathway in culture by pluripotent stem cells. *Cell.* 2011;146(4):519–532.
60. Hayashi K, Ogushi S, Kurimoto K, et al. Offspring from oocytes derived from in vitro primordial germ cell-like cells in mice. *Science.* 2012;338(6109):971–975.
61. Eguizabal C, Montserrat N, Vassena R, et al. Complete meiosis from human induced pluripotent stem cells. *Stem Cells.* 2011;29(8):1186–1195.
62. Easley CA, Philips BT, McGuire MM, et al. Direct differentiation of human pluripotent stem cells into haploid spermatogenic cells. *Cell Rep.* 2012;2(3):440–446.
63. Liu W, Schulster ML, Alukal JP, Najari BB. Fertility preservation in male to female transgender patients. *Urol Clin North Am.* 2019;46(4):487–493.
64. Kafetsoulis A, Brackett NL, Ibrahim E, Attia GR, Lynne CM. Current trends in the treatment of infertility in men with spinal cord injury. *Fertil Steril.* 2006;86(4):781–789.
65. Harris R, Kolaitis IN, Frader JE. Ethical issues involving fertility preservation for transgender youth. *J Assist Reprod Genet.* 2020;37(10):2453–2462.
66. Wiepjes C, Nota NM, Blok CJM, et al. The Amsterdam Cohort of Gender Dysphoria Study (1972e2015): trends in prevalence, treatment, and regrets. *J Sex Med.* 2018;15(4):582–590.
67. de Vries A, McGuire JK, Steensma TD, Wagenaar ECF, Doreleijers TAH, Cohen-Kettenis PT. Young adult psychological outcome after puberty suppression and gender reassignment. *Pediatrics.* 2014;134(4):696–704.
68. Wang Y, Anazodo A, Logan S. Systematic review of fertility preservation patient decision aids for cancer patients. *Psychooncology.* 2018;28(3):459–467.
69. Gassei K, Orwig KE. Experimental methods to preserve male fertility and treat male factor infertility. *Fertil Steril.* 2015;105(2):256–266.
70. Meistrich M, Wilson G, Mathur K, et al. Rapid recovery of spermatogenesis after mitoxantrone, vincristine, vinblastine, and prednisone chemotherapy for Hodgkin's disease. *J Clin Oncol.* 1997;15(12):3488–3495.
71. Sonmezer M, Oktay K. Fertility preservation of female patients. *Hum Reprod Update.* 2004;10(3):251–266.

Chapter 19

Mental Health Considerations in the Infertile Male and Couple

Elizabeth Grill

19.1 Introduction

Sexual dysfunction can significantly affect both partners in a relationship as well as the couple. While there are numerous causes of sexual dysfunction, this chapter will focus on the impact of infertility on sexual dysfunction in the man and the impact of diagnosis and treatment on the couple. Sexual problems related to infertility range from 10% to 60% of couples [1]. For many these difficulties persist long after treatment and regardless of whether the couple conceives [2]. Given the growing body of knowledge relating organic and psychological causes of sexual dysfunction, as well as the growing rate of fertility evaluation and treatment, providing a perspective on the interplay between infertility and sexual dysfunction and appropriate management is necessary. This chapter dissects the relationships between infertility and sexual dysfunction in men as well as in the couple and provides a general framework for understanding the complex struggles that couples face along the family-building journey. This chapter will also provide direction to providers about how to assess and treat these complicated issues.

19.2 Infertility and Distress in the Man and Couple

In general, infertility is defined as the inability to conceive after 1 year of unprotected sex (www.cdc.gov/reproductivehealth/infertility/index.htm) [3] and may affect up to 15% of couples [4,5]. Importantly, male and female factors each can contribute independently to fertility difficulties in up to 50% of cases [6–8]. Sexual function as well as childbearing are considered important aspects of most serious partnerships and deeply impact quality of life. For many couples, the inability to conceive or give birth to a healthy child often forces partners to reevaluate their sense of femininity and masculinity, gender identity, and ultimately the meaning of their relationship.

Individuals and couples experience high levels of stress as they attempt to manage the physical, emotional, social, and financial concerns related to infertility and treatment. Difficulty conceiving is described as an emotional roller coaster and crisis that chips away at one's self esteem, identity, relationships, and ability to cope [9]. On the Life Events Scale, the failure of IVF is rated equally to cancer, death of a family member, and worse than divorce [10].

Couples with fertility difficulties confront many challenges including societal and parental pressures for propagation, physical and psychological burdens, and potential financial burdens if considering artificial reproductive technologies. While trying to conceive, patients no longer feel in control of their bodies or their life plan. Lives are put on hold, attempts to conceive become all consuming, and couples are beholden to treatment [11]. Trying to juggle medical appointments and medicine regimes with job responsibilities can increase pressure and put stress on careers. Not surprisingly, the most common reason why insured patients drop out of treatment is psychological burden resulting from infertility, including treatment [11].

19.3 Infertility and Sexual Dysfunction in the Couple

Infertile couples have reported sexual problems ranging from lack of desire, pleasure, or spontaneity to sexual dysfunction. Keye [12] determined that the three areas of sexual difficulty in infertile couples were: (1) the actual physical condition causing infertility or resulting from treatment; (2) sexual intercourse becoming only a means of reproduction rather than intimacy or pleasure; and (3) the global psychological impact of the infertility experience.

Organic sexual dysfunctions are regarded as a minor cause of infertility, impacting approximately 5% of all infertility cases [13]. Overall, sexual dysfunction alone is common, with 40–45% of adult women and 20–30% of adult men with at least one manifestation of sexual dysfunction [14]. Male sexual disorders such as chronic erectile dysfunction (ED) and anejaculation make natural conception impossible [15].

Loss of libido may be the result of chronic health problems or the invasiveness of medical treatment for infertility. It may be due to the medications and hormones that can interfere with sexual response and/or interest or to the stresses and demands that infertility places on the marriage, social relationships, work life, or financial resources [16]. In some couples, partners blame themselves or each other for infertility or the medical diagnosis, resulting in anger that interferes with sexual desire and functioning.

Sexual impairment in infertile couples is often due to the performance pressure experienced in response to planned sex, pressure to perform on demand, extensive and painful tests, intense feelings of anxiety and the highly personal matter of sexuality being turned over to the external control of a physician, and the psychologic feeling of the medical team in the bedroom [17,18]. As infertility drags on and the focus of sexual activity continues to emphasize procreation, infertile men and women may feel depressed, lose interest in "sex on demand," or find it difficult to feel sexual when they are chronically frustrated and unhappy due to childlessness [19]. Couples in infertility treatment report avoiding sexual intimacy during nonfertile times. Men and women lose pleasure from nonprocreative sexual activity and develop an apathetic attitude about sex [20]. These tensions frequently lead to a reduction in nonsexual intimacy, resulting in feelings of disconnection and exacerbating couple tension [21].

Such stressors can lead to poor marital adjustment and decreased quality of life, as well as to sexual dysfunction. Common feelings in the setting of infertility, such as loss, anger, guilt, despair, depression, shame, and anxiety, often overshadow the usual feelings of warmth, affection, and emotional connection that are the natural prerequisites of sexual intimacy [16,22]. Men may begin to feel as though their partners have lost interest in sex especially when they only express interest mid-cycle when they are fertile. This may add additional pressure for men to perform on demand (e.g., during ovulation, post-coital tests, producing semen samples). Sex lives are quickly taken from the intimacy of the bedroom to the control of the healthcare establishment [23]. Sex is altered and becomes methodical, predictable, and unexciting for many couples struggling with infertility, and couples begin to associate sex with failure to conceive and may avoid it.

Overall, infertility is associated with decreased sexual activity and appears to become worse as the number of childless years increases [24]. Studies have linked the physical, psychological, and financial challenges of assisted reproduction to increased marital conflict, decreased sexual self-esteem, feelings of inadequacy, and frequency of sexual intercourse [25,26]. The interplay between the infertility and sexual dysfunction can affect one's reproductive potential and impact interpersonal relationships and self-image.

19.4 Infertility and Sexual Dysfunction in Men

Sexual disorders may be a cause and/or a consequence of infertility and its treatments for men. The emotional ramifications of a diagnosis of infertility, no matter the etiology, can further impact procreative potential through alteration of physical function, and a vicious cycle can develop where one condition can potentiate the other. Men in infertile relationships have a higher than expected incidence of ED and depressive symptoms, lower self-esteem, higher anxiety, more somatic symptoms, and more dysfunctional sexual relationships [27]. During infertility, many men develop performance anxiety, sexual avoidance, or even aversion to sex, especially if sex is for "procreation purposes only" and their partner is sexually unresponsive. Frequently, infertile men complain of feeling "used," like a "stud service" (that all his partner wants from him is his sperm), or of the "queen bee syndrome" (his sole importance is to fertilize his partner) [28,29]. In a study of infertile men in Germany, a short-lasting partnership and high sexual dissatisfaction prior to the diagnosis of infertility caused more distress in infertile men whereas being in a longer-lasting and sexually satisfying partnership seemed to have a buffering effect with regard to sexual distress and infertility [30].

The male sexual dysfunctions most likely to affect male fertility are those that cause ED and affect sexual desire, arousal, and ejaculation, limiting the ability to effectively inseminate the female partner [14]. Sex on demand and providing an erection and ejaculation that is timely and efficient become the goals of sex when struggling to conceive [12,16].

One of the most common sexual difficulties for men is ED. Berger reported that 63% of the men in his study of azoospermic men experienced ED after they received their diagnosis [31]. Regimenting intercourse can decrease libido in 10% of patients, and ED may occur in up to 20% of men engaging in timed intercourse [32]. The causes of ED are often multifactorial, comprising a mix of organic and psychogenic factors, although a psychogenic factor is a contributor in almost all cases, particularly in younger men [33]. Importantly, depression and other psychological factors are also linked to ED. The Massachusetts Male Aging Study observed an increased risk of ED (OR 1.82) in men with depressive symptoms [34], and other studies have supported this relationship [31]. In a recent study [35], 32% of men seeking treatment for infertility experienced depression and 61% of men experienced anxiety. When considering psychogenic ED, the link with sexual confidence and performance anxiety should not be overlooked, and numerous studies have reinforced a clear association between ED and sexual confidence [36,37].

Ejaculatory disorders are also common. Men report less ability to control ejaculation and less satisfaction with their sexual performance in general [4,38,39]. Men who are the sole contributors to infertility in the relationship have a higher incidence of depression compared with men who were either fertile or shared the problem with their partners [40].

Beyond intercourse, there are other issues related to infertility treatment that make performance difficult for men. Men often express frustration and humiliation related to specimen collection and complain about the lack of privacy, problems with concentration, and lack of sufficient erotic material [9]. Saleh and colleagues (2003) found that among men undergoing infertility evaluation, 11% failed to collect semen by masturbation for a semen analysis after repeated attempts; 20% were able to collect semen using vibration stimulation; and 31% experienced problems with erection or orgasm in addition to severe anxiety during attempts to masturbate and have sexual contact with their partners [41].

Whether the cause is organic or psychogenic, the result is the same, with decreased sexual desire, an inability to achieve and maintain an adequate erection, or the inability to deliver sperm to the optimal location for fertilization. Sexual dysfunction not only limits the man's fertility but can also have a profound negative impact on quality of life, psychosocial health, and relationships.

19.5 Psychosocial Implications

For many men, masculinity and fertility are deeply intertwined. Stereotypes that men are ready, willing, and able to engage in sexual activity at any time or any place have contributed to unrealistic expectations regarding sexual functioning in men, and infertile men in particular [16,42]. Infertility (especially male factor infertility) frequently triggers feelings of failure, sexual inadequacy, diminished masculinity, loss of potency or power, and altered sense of self, which are all contributory factors in male sexual dysfunction [19,43,44].

An inability to impregnate his partner may strike heavily at a man's view of himself as "whole" and as virile and masculine. Women often have difficulty having empathy for their partners and may not understand the shame a man who associates potency with manliness may feel when he can't "make" his partner pregnant, or the anxiety and shame he reports feeling when forced to provide a sperm sample. In a recent study [45], 93% of men stated their well-being had been impacted by infertility and described it as "the most upsetting, dark and emasculating experience of my life." There is also less social acceptability for men to express these feelings as well as those of disappointment and grief to their partner. Their reluctance to share may also be caused by fear that they will only contribute further to the emotional distress that the couple already experiences.

Some studies suggest that infertile men experience less distress than women using various indices of emotional state [46,47]. However, over time, male partners of infertile couples report significantly less desire, more stressful marital relationships, and worse sexual function and satisfaction compared to fertile control couples [48–52]. Having a diagnosis of male factor infertility lasting 3–6 years contributes to decreased relationship stability, sexual activity, and lower sexual satisfaction in both male and female partners from infertile couples, with the decrease in sexual activity increasing as the amount of fruitless years accrue [15,52].

19.6 Treatment of Sexual Dysfunction in the Couple

Couples may be reticent to broach sexual concerns with a healthcare provider for fear that it will interrupt their medical treatment. However, ignoring or minimizing these problems may also serve to worsen psychological and relational distresses, which can negatively impact treatment outcomes [53].

Mental health professionals trained in the field of reproductive medicine as well as a sex therapist can intervene on several different therapeutic levels by providing psychosocial and psychosexual patient education, supportive and grief counseling, and helping patients with treatment decisions. Given the reported levels of distress experienced by infertility couples, medical treatment should be in conjunction with counseling, emphasizing the importance of emotional health and well-being in couples struggling to build their families.

Even couples that never encounter major or disrupting sexual problems often experience episodic or situational diminished sexual desire and satisfaction in response to the emotional distress or physical strains of infertility or a specific treatment. Episodic loss of libido or sexual dysfunction in one or both partners can usually be addressed with minimal education and reassurance. However, consistent and extensive diminished sexual desire or dysfunction in infertile men and women is more problematic and usually multifactorial.

Overall, the management of sexual dysfunction is best provided by a combination approach, which successfully integrates both physical and psychosocial factors [54]. Combination therapy integrating sex therapy and oftentimes sexual pharmaceuticals is frequently the best treatment approach for sexual dysfunction. Contextual factors, including difficulties with a current interpersonal relationship, should also be clarified and sexual history and functioning prior to trying to conceive should be assessed [55].

19.7 Conclusions

The stress, psychological demands, and physically intrusive procedures associated with infertility treatment can affect sexual self-image, desire, and performance. Whether sexual dysfunction is a preexisting condition or an unwelcome side effect of infertility treatment, it can be a devastating and discouraging blow, compounding the disappointment of childlessness and the distress of medical treatment. All too often, the sexual problems of infertile couples are ignored or minimized in a belief that they will dissipate on their own or will have few long-term consequences. Unfortunately, although some sexual problems may disappear when the pressures of infertility treatment end, sexual difficulties typically linger or become more problematic after treatment ends or parenthood is achieved [56,57]. Depending on the comfort level, preference, resources, and availability, the physician may choose to treat the couple or refer them to a sex therapist and/or infertility counselor [16,58].

References

1. Wischmann TH. Sexual disorders in infertile couples. *J Sex Med*. 2010;7(5):1868–1876.
2. Schanz S, Reimer T, Eichner N, et al. Long-term life and partnership satisfaction in infertile patients: a 5-year longitudinal study. *Fertil Steril*. 2011;96(2):416–421.
3. American Urological Association Male Infertility Best Practice Policy Panel. (2010). *The optimal evaluation of the infertile male: AUA best practice statement*; American Society for

Reproductive Medicine. (2012). *Optimizing natural fertility.*

4. Monga M, Alexandrescu B, Katz SE, Stein M, Ganiats T. Impact of infertility on quality of life, marital adjustment, and sexual function. *Urology.* 2004;63 (1):126–130.

5. Mosher WD. Infertility trends among U.S. couples: 1965–1976. *Fam Plann Perspect.* 1982;14(1):22–27.

6. Thonneau P, Marchand S, Tallec A, et al. Incidence and main causes of infertility in a resident population (1,850,000) of three French regions (1988–1989). *Hum Reprod.* 1991;6 (6):811–816.

7. Eisenberg ML, Lathi RB, Baker VL, Westphal LM, Milki AA, Nangia AK. Frequency of the male infertility evaluation: data from the national survey of family growth. *J Urology.* 2013;189(3):1030–1034.

8. Wong WY, Thomas CM, Merkus JM, Zielhuis GA, Steegers-Theunissen RP. Male factor subfertility: possible causes and the impact of nutritional factors. *Fertil Steril.* 2000;73(3):435–442.

9. Andrews FM, Abbey A, Halman LJ. Is fertility-problem stress different? The dynamics of stress in fertile and infertile couples. *Fertil Steril.* 1992;57 (6):1247–1253.

10. Van den Broeck UE, Pasch L, Katz P, Millstein S, D'Hooghe T, Demyttenaere K. Longitudinal follow-up of the intrusiveness of the infertility experience: predictors and gender differences. *Fertil Steril.* 2010;94(4):S65.

11. Pasch LA, Holley SR, Bleil ME, et al. Addressing the needs of fertility treatment patients and their partners: are they informed of and do they receive mental health services. *Fertil Steril.* 2016;106(1):209–215.

12. Keye W. The impact of infertility on psychosexual function. *Fertil Steril.* 1980;34(3):308–309.

13. Wischmann TH. Psychogenic infertility: myths and facts. *J Assist Reprod Genet.* 2003;20(12):485–494.

14. Lewis RW, Fugl-Meyer KS, Bosch R, et al. Epidemiology/risk factors of sexual dysfunction. *J Sex Med.* 2004;1 (1):35–39.

15. Nene UA, Coyaji K, Apte H. Infertility: a label of choice in the case of sexually dysfunctional couples. *Patient Educ Couns.* 2005;59(3):234–238.

16. Burns L. Sexual counseling and infertility. In: Burns LH, Covington SN, eds. *Infertility Counseling: A Comprehensive Handbook for Clinicians.* 2nd ed. Parthenon Publishing; 2006:212–235.

17. Applegarth LD, Grill EA. Psychological issues in reproductive disorders. In: Chan P, Goldstein M, Rosenwaks Z, eds. *Reproductive Medicine Secrets.* Hanley & Belfus; 2004:391–402.

18. Daniluk JC. *Women's Sexuality across the Lifespan: Challenging Myths, Creating Meanings.* Guilford Press; 1998.

19. Kedem P, Mikulincer M, Nathanson YE, Bartoov B. Psychological aspects of male infertility. *Br J Med Psychol.* 1990;63(1):73–80.

20. Leiblum SR. Love, sex and infertility: the impact of infertility on couples. In Leiblum SR, ed. *Infertility: Psychological Issues and Counseling Strategies.* Wiley; 1997:149–166.

21. Perelman MA. The impact of relationship variables on the etiology, diagnosis and treatment of erectile dysfunction. *Adv Primary Care Med: Clin Update.* 2007;3:3–6.

22. Irvine SCE. Male infertility and its effect on male sexuality. *Sex Rel Ther.* 1996;11 (3):273–280.

23. Nachtigall RD, Becker G, Wozny M. The effects of gender-specific diagnosis on men's and women's response to infertility. *Fertil Steril.* 1992;57 (1):113–121.

24. Nene UA, Coyaji K, Apte H. Infertility: a label of choice in the case of sexually dysfunctional couples. *Patient Educ Couns.* 2005;59(3):234–238.

25. Andrews FM, Abbey A, Halman LJ. Is fertility-problem stress different? The dynamics of stress in fertile and infertile couples. *Fertil Steril.* 1992;57 (6):1247–1253.

26. Whiteford LM, Gonzalez L. Stigma: the hidden burden of infertility. *Soc Sci Med.* 1995;40(1):27–36.

27. Shindel AW, Nelson CJ, Naughton CK, Ohebshalom M, Mulhall JP. Sexual function and quality of life in the male partner of infertile couples: prevalence and correlates of dysfunction. *J Urology.* 2008;179(3):1056–1059.

28. Zoldbrod A. *Men, Women, and Infertility: Intervention and Treatment Strategies.* Lexington Books; 1993.

29. Mazor M. Emotional reactions to infertility. In: Mazor M, Simons H, eds. *Infertility: Medical, Emotional and Social Considerations.* Human Science Press; 1984:23–35.

30. Schilling G, Muller MJ, Haidl G. Sexual dissatisfaction and somatic complaints in male infertility. *PPmP: Psychotherapie, Psychosomatik, medizinische Psychologie.* 1999;49 (8):256–263.

31. Perelman MA. Erectile dysfunction and depression: screening and treatment. *Urol Clin North Am.* 2011;38 (2):125–139.

32. Sigg C. Sexuality and sterility. *Therapeutische Umschau Revue therapeutique.* 1994;51(2):115–119.

33. Ralph D, McNicholas T. UK management guidelines for erectile dysfunction. *BMJ.* 2000;321 (7259):499–503.

34. Araujo AB, Durante R, Feldman HA, Goldstein I, McKinlay JB. The relationship between depressive symptoms and male erectile dysfunction: cross-sectional results from the Massachusetts Male Aging Study. *Psychosom Med.* 1998;60 (4):458–465.

35. Pasch LA, Holley SR, Bleil ME, Shehab D, Katz PP, Adler NE. Addressing the needs of fertility treatment patients and their partners: are they informed of and do they receive mental health services? *Fertil Steril.* 2016;106(1):209–215.e2.

36. Althof SE, Wieder M. Psychotherapy for erectile dysfunction: now more relevant than ever. *Endocrine.* 2004;23 (2–3):131–134.

37. Morse WI, Morse JM. Erectile impotence precipitated by organic factors and perpetuated by performance anxiety. *Can Med Assoc J.* 1982; 127 (7):599–601.

38. Abbey A, Andrews FM, Halman LJ. Provision and receipt of social support and disregard: what is their impact on the marital life quality of infertile and fertile couples? *J Pers Soc Psychol.* 1995;68(3):455–469.

39. O'Brien JH, Lazarou S, Deane L, Jarvi K, Zini A. Erectile dysfunction and andropause symptoms in infertile men. *J Urology.* 2005;174(5):1932–1934; discussion 4.

40. Slade P, Raval H, Buck P, Lieberman BE. A 3-year follow-up of emotional,

40. marital, and sexual functioning in couples who were infertile. *J Reprod Infant Psychol.* 1992;10(4):233–243.
41. Saleh RA, Ranga GM, Raina R, Nelson DR, Agarwal A. Sexual dysfunction in men undergoing infertility evaluation: a cohort observational study. *Fertil Steril.* 2003;79(4):909–912.
42. Zilbergeld B. *The New Male Sexuality.* Bantam Books; 1999.
43. Applegarth L, Grill E. Psychological issues in reproductive disorders. In: Chan PTK, Goldstein M, Rosenwaks Z, eds. *Reproductive Medicine Secrets.* Hanley & Belfus; 2004:391–402.
44. Nachtigal RD, Becker G, Wozny M. The effect of gender-specific diagnosis on men's and women's response to infertility. *Fertil Steril.* 1992;57(1):113–121.
45. Hanna E, Gough B. Emoting infertility online: a qualitative analysis of men's forum posts. *Health (London).* 2016;20(4):363–382.
46. Wright J, Duchesne C, Sabourin S, Bissonnette F, Benoit J, Girard Y. Psychosocial distress and infertility: men and women respond differently. *Fertil Steril.* 1991;55(1):100–108.
47. Stanton AL, Tennen H, Affleck G, Mendola R. Cognitive appraisal and adjustment to infertility. *Women Health.* 1991;17(3):1–15.
48. Berg BJ, Wilson JF. Psychological functioning across stages of treatment for infertility. *J Behav Med.* 1991;14(1):11–26.
49. Khademi A, Alleyassin A, Amini M, Ghaemi M. Evaluation of sexual dysfunction prevalence in infertile couples. *J Sex Med.* 2008;5(6):1402–1410.
50. Lotti F, Corona G, Castellini G, et al. Semen quality impairment is associated with sexual dysfunction according to its severity. *Hum Reprod.* 2016;31(12):2668–2680.
51. Purcell-Lévesque C, Brassard A, Carranza-Mamane B, Péloquin K. Attachment and sexual functioning in women and men seeking fertility treatment. *J Psychosom Obstet Gynecol.* 2019;40(3):202–210.
52. Drosdzol A, Skrzypulec V. Evaluation of marital and sexual interactions of Polish infertile couples. *J Sex Med.* 2009;6(12):3335–3346.
53. Grill E, Schattman GL. Female sexual dysfunction and infertility. In: *Management of Sexual Dysfunction in Men and Women: An Interdisciplinary Approach.* Springer; 2016:337–342.
54. Perelman M. Combination therapy for sexual dysfunction: integrating sex therapy and pharmacotherapy. In: Balon R, Segraves R, eds. *Handbook of Sexual Dysfunction.* Taylor & Francis; 2005:13–41.
55. Gagnon JH, Rosen RC, Leiblum SR. Cognitive and social aspects of sexual dysfunction: sexual scripts in sex therapy. *J Sex Marital Ther.* 1982;8(1):44–56.
56. Boxer A. Infertility and sexual dysfunction. *Infertil Reprod Med Clin North Am.* 1996;7:565–575.
57. Burns L. An overview of sexual dysfunction in the infertile couple. *J Fam Psychother.* 1995;6:25–46.
58. Perelman MA. Sex coaching for physicians: combination treatment for patient and partner. *Int J Impot Res.* 2003;15(Suppl. 5):S67–S74.

Section 4 Laboratory Evaluation and Treatment of Male Infertility

Chapter 20

The Modern Semen Analysis
Theory and Techniques of Ejaculate Examination

Lars Björndahl

20.1 Introduction

The examination of the human ejaculate constitutes a complicated branch of medical laboratory science. To understand the complexity of the human ejaculate knowledge about the physiology and pathology is facilitating. It is also essential to understand that the main value of ejaculate examination is the information that can be obtained on the functional capacity of the male reproductive organs. Still the main focus has a long time only been on the prognostic value for the outcome of the fertility of the couple. In this chapter the focus is on how the functional capacity of the male reproductive trace can reflect in the ejaculate examined in the laboratory. Important principles for reliable laboratory techniques for ejaculate volume, sperm concentration and sperm count, sperm motility, sperm vitality and sperm morphology are described with requirements for reliability, assessment of uncertainties, need for staff training, internal quality control and interlaboratory comparisons (external quality control).

20.2 The Development of the Modern Ejaculate Examination

The modern ejaculate examination is based on basic principles of quantitative laboratory medicine. The challenge for an andrology laboratory aiming for modern examination is not primarily to abandon the basic ejaculate examination in exchange for advanced techniques that may be useful for very specific issues. The latter investigations also have their place in the investigations of the reproductive organs of the male partner in an infertile couple. Still, the basic ejaculate examination is a first step to direct the continued investigation of the man. The modern ejaculate examination makes use of the best available techniques – it is cost-efficient and practical to perform but still reliable. Still too many laboratories reduce their investigatory capacity by using techniques with a high degree of uncertainty [1,2]. Also, many studies published in scientific journals can still be based on suboptimal laboratory techniques [3]. The first microscopic examination of human semen was published almost 350 years ago [4]. Reliable laboratory techniques have been well established for decades. The challenge now is to implement such techniques for the benefit of the patients and the development of science [3].

Due to the small size of human spermatozoa direct observation is only possible with the help of optical instruments. The invention of advanced equipment for magnification by the Dutch textile merchant and naturalist Antoni van Leeuwenhoek enabled the first reports in 1677 on "microscopic animals" in human and animal ejaculates [4] based on observations done with a remarkably simple apparatus. Microscope technology has improved a lot since then. The human skills of observations are still unsurpassed when it comes to examination of the human ejaculate, while computer assisted sperm analysis is able to provide much more detailed data from analyses of sperm motility patterns, especially in sperm preparations void of other particular matter like crystals, debris, and other cells.

The need for reliable and robust examination techniques have been known for over 75 years [5]. In a series of studies based on a combination of laboratory examinations and thorough insight into basic male reproductive physiology, John MacLeod (1905–1984) provided important information on semen analysis and male reproductive function [6–19]. Later, Rune Eliasson (1927–2020) continued the line of work by promoting the use of statistical methods to supervise and control results of ejaculate examination [20–23]. Further focus on training and quality control have been given in other publications [3,24–28]. As a part of World Health Organization (WHO) efforts to develop efficient and safe male contraceptive drugs, general recommendations for reliable ejaculate examination were first published in 1980 [29] with following revisions 1987–2021 [30–34].

20.2.1 The Purposes of the Ejaculate Examination

Judging only from the numbers of publications on the possible usefulness of ejaculate examination it is easy to come to the conclusion that ejaculate examination is done only to predict fertility success and support the choice of an optimal treatment modality. Although the ultimate purpose of a spermatozoon certainly is to fertilize an oocyte and thereby initiate embryonic development and pregnancies, ejaculate examination should have a wider scope. To only focus on the prediction of fertility potential, important diagnostic information on male reproductive organ function is neglected or at least disregarded.

Diagnosis of disorders in male reproductive organ function is essential both for infertile couples and for the development of reproductive medicine and andrology. Although assisted reproductive technologies can help many childless couples, there are diseases, disorders, and medical conditions in the male that can be treated and the man should be given appropriate treatment [35]. Even though the in vivo or in vitro potential for fertility success in some cases cannot be improved, the general health, quality of life, and life expectancy of the man can be substantially improved if ejaculate examination is used to understand the functions of the man's reproductive organs [35]. Furthermore, for the follow-up of treatment of such disorders, ejaculate examination is also essential. Another purpose that requires special ejaculate examination is the follow-up of male sterilization (vasectomy), where the aim is to establish with sufficient certainty that the risk for an undesired pregnancy is as low as it possibly can be.

20.2.2 How Exact Must the Ejaculate Examination Be?

The requirements for exactness vary with the purpose of the examination. The degree of uncertainty must therefore be decided in relation to the intended use of the examination result. To determine if a man needs a thorough andrological examination or not, the sperm number may not be determined with extremely high precision, but large random errors due to poor representativity of aliquots examined must be avoided. On the contrary, when a man is given endocrine treatment intended to stimulate sperm production it is essential to detect true increments in sperm output.

The counterquestion to anyone challenging the necessity of modern ejaculate examination techniques is how uncertain is the old, preferred technique? And how much error can be allowed from a medical, ethical, and economical perspective? As an example: Basing clinical decisions on assessments made with too few observations can mean that in two out of three treatment cycles a suboptimal, unintended treatment modality is used [3].

20.2.3 Must the Ejaculate Examination Really Be Standardized?

The answer is unequivocally yes. Without standardization no proper comparisons between centres are valid and treatment options, decision limits, or reference limits obtained in other centers cannot easily be implemented in another center. It is not only that the techniques and procedures must be used in the same way. To achieve true standardization, staff training, internal quality control, and interlaboratory comparisons (external quality assessment) must be undertaken. Standardized training is well known and has been proven it is possible to perform and to be efficient [24–26,36,37]. Still, initial and basic training is only a first step – that should be followed by in-house training [24,25] and internal quality control [38,39]. To be able to claim that a laboratory performs comparable to other laboratories, interlaboratory comparisons are also compulsory [3,40]. Without the latter, implementation of techniques and decision limits developed by other centers is not acceptable.

20.2.4 What Is Normal and What Is Abnormal?

Just looking at sperm counts, it has long been pointed out that there is a relation between testicular size and sperm output, meaning that a low number may be acceptable among men with testicle size in the lower normal range, but not among men with testicle size in the larger range [20,21)].

It is also wrong to believe that there is a sharp limit between "fertile" and "infertile" semen. The reference limits presented in the WHO laboratory manual fifth edition [33] are based only on data from recent fathers volunteering to participate in contraception studies. Although carefully calculated on a large population, the lowest fifth percentile only tells us that 95% of values from this population was above that limit. Since no data from men in barren unions have been included, there is no way to calculate positive and negative predictive values from this distribution. There certainly is value in knowing how low sperm counts can be found among recent fathers, but there are no data to give a sharp limit between fertile and infertile men. It means that men with results above the "limit" may still have disorders needing further investigation and even treatment in some cases [41].

20.3 Ejaculate Physiology

The ejaculate does not exist in the male body. It is produced during sexual stimulation and extremely heterogenous even during the expulsion from the male. The quality and duration of sexual stimulation can increase both volume and sperm count [42].

In this section an overview is given of aspects of the human ejaculate that is important for understanding ejaculate examination results and variability due to physiology and pathology.

20.3.1 Sperm Production and Ejaculate Sperm Content

Basically, sperm production depends on the presence of stem cells (spermatogonia) able to go through repeated mitotic divisions and finally for some daughter cells to continue into a meiotic division to produce the gametes with half of the genetic complement for a new individual. In general, in a fully fertile man the amount of germ cells corresponds to the testicular volume. Furthermore, the total number of mitotic divisions before going into meiosis is also a determinant for the sperm output – genetic variability may thus at least partially explain the huge quantitative variability in sperm production also among fertile men. Other aspects of genetic factors that can cause reduced sperm production includes Y-chromosome microdeletions (damage to genes controlling spermatogenesis) and aneuploidy and translocations (interacting with chromosome pairing in meiosis as well as increasing risk for genetic abnormalities in the embryo).

For men with hypogonadism, endocrine stimulation (FSH, LH) can sometimes improve spermatogenesis. Testosterone supplementation may improve symptoms of hypogonadism but quite often counteracts spermatogenesis by negative feedback to LH. This is also the likely mechanism for the negative action of anabolic steroids on spermatogenesis.

The transport of spermatozoa from the testicle to the expected storage site in the epididymis is passive, dependent on a slow flow of fluid from the ducts of formation to the epididymis. In the body of the epididymis a multitude of parallel tubules join into one single channel, explaining why infection and inflammatory processes or other damage in the single tube in this part of the epididymis can result in a completely blocked passage.

Epididymal sperm storage in humans does not seem to be of great biological importance. For the interpretation of ejaculate examination results it can induce considerable variability. The WHO [33] recommends 2–7 days of abstinence from sexual activity. It should, however, be remembered that studies on daily sperm output show that 2–3 days of daily ejaculations appear to be necessary to deplete the epididymal stores of spermatozoa [43]. However, in the clinical situation it is only practical to record the actual period of sexual abstinence in the days before the day of collection of the ejaculate to be examined. In addition, for the interpretation of results it is important to keep in mind that the sexual activity (or lack of activity) before that abstinence period actually can contribute significantly to variability in results.

The transport of spermatozoa from the cauda epididymis to the urethra is by smooth muscle cell contractions initiated by autonomic nerve impulses acting on α_1-adrenoreceptors. This means that pharmaceutical drugs blocking α_1-receptors (hypertension treatment and antidepressants) may obstruct sperm transport. Such agents can also interact with the emptying of the accessory sex glands.

20.3.2 Contribution of the Accessory Sex Glands

The main part of the ejaculate volume comes from the seminal vesicles and the prostate. Other glands, like the epididymal secretion and the urethral Cowper's glands, also appear to have significance for optimal sperm performance. The limpid urethral secretion from the Cowper's glands usually precedes ejaculation during sexual excitement and may contain significant numbers of sperm.

Emptying of the prostatic glandular acini and the seminal vesicles is, like the sperm transport to the urethra, dependent on autonomic nerve stimulation of smooth muscle cells in the glandular walls, and can therefore be affected by the same agents as the sperm transport.

"Dry ejaculation" – orgasm without antegrade (normal) ejaculation can be due to retrograde ejaculation: All or most of the ejaculate is forced into the urinary bladder. If the ejaculation is retrograde, spermatozoa should be detected in urine after orgasm. Sometimes antegrade ejaculation can be obtained by treatment with an α_1-adrenoreceptor agonist. If no sperm are found in the urine after orgasm stimulation with an α_1-adrenoreceptor antagonist it may not be successful in achieving either retrograde ejaculation or even antegrade ejaculation.

20.3.3 The Sequence of Ejaculation

Normal ejaculation is characterized by sequential events. First, spermatozoa are expelled into the prostatic urethra simultaneously with the start of emptying of the prostatic acini. The mixture of prostatic fluid and spermatozoa dominates the first ejaculate fractions. The last two-thirds of the ejaculate are dominated by seminal vesicular fluid and contain much fewer spermatozoa [6,44]. The latter secretion is likely to resemble the seminal plug found in some other mammals. The seminal vesicular fluid has a negative influence on human sperm motility, survival, and protection of the sperm DNA [44,45]. In vivo, successful spermatozoa are not likely to have any contact with seminal vesicular fluid [10,44,45]. An abnormal contact between spermatozoa and the seminal vesicular fluid can impair sperm motility significantly. An abnormal sequence of ejaculation can be caused by an obstruction of the ejaculatory ducts at the entrance to the urethra. A complete occlusion causes complete lack of spermatozoa in the ejaculate, as well as lack of seminal vesicular fluid. A partial occlusion of the duct opening can delay the emptying of the spermatozoa into the urethra until the seminal vesicles empty their secretion, causing a primary contact between spermatozoa and the seminal vesicular fluid. The diagnosis of abnormal sequence of ejaculation can only be detected by examination of split-ejaculate fractions [44] and by ejaculatory duct obstruction by ejaculatory duct manometry [46].

20.3.4 Semen Characteristics and Age

The most common change in reported results by increased age is impaired sperm motility. At least in part longer abstinence time might contribute to this deterioration. However, a decrease in motility is not directly equivalent to a loss of fertility capability. Almost all studies are based on comparisons of different populations, not where the same individual is assessed at different ages. This complicates the evidence base since bias can be very different between such populations, not the least due to selection of participants both in treatment and in control groups [47].

20.4 Proper Techniques for Reliable Results

Details and step-by-step instructions are available in other sources [28,34]. Here the principles for reliable laboratory procedures will be outlined. All results should be reported together with information on period of sexual abstinence before examination and time between ejaculate collection and start of examination.

20.4.1 Ejaculate Volume

Determination of ejaculate volume by weight is far more exact than using measuring pipettes, cylinders, and centrifuge tubes

[48]. The error due to variation in specific weight of semen is negligible compared to errors due to volume losses in transfer to measuring equipment and errors in ocular readings of uncertain tube graduation.

20.4.2 Sperm Number

The aliquots examined must be satisfactorily representative of the examined ejaculate. This means that the sample must be visibly well mixed. Another aspect is that even macroscopically well-mixed ejaculates may still have small compartments with different contents of spermatozoa. An aliquot of 50 µL usually compensates for most variability but still two independent aliquots of at least 50 µL should be withdrawn and diluted for concentration assessment. Dilution is essential to obtain sufficiently diluted samples to facilitate reliable counting. Furthermore, the dilution should also immobilize the spermatozoa, which makes counting results much less prone to errors.

A suitable counting chamber – preferably a haemocytometer with improved Neubauer ruling to make counting easy – is essential: low error in measurements can be achieved by using a reliable known volume in the assessment. The results of the two assessments for each sample should be compared and results only accepted if the difference between the counts is sufficiently small, reducing the risk for influence of random errors. It is also essential that the total number of counted spermatozoa is at least 400 – the theoretical maximum random error is then only ±10%.

The obtained value for sperm concentration is finally multiplied by the volume to obtain the sperm count in the ejaculate. This number is more informative of sperm production and transport than the concentration that is also highly dependent on the volume contributions from the seminal vesicular glands and the prostate.

The techniques used to obtain the results from sperm counting do not justify the use of decimal places. For results less than one million spermatozoa, other presentations can be recommended. For instance, "ca 50,000 spermatozoa" rather than a decimal number (0.05 million).

20.4.3 Sperm Motility

For sperm motility, a temperature-controlled microscope stage is recommended. Sperm velocity is highly temperature dependent and progressiveness can decrease by lowering temperatures. Ideally, the motility assessment should start approximately 30 minutes after sample collection and complete liquefaction. Motility assessments initiated after more than one hour can show impaired motility due to the extended in vitro storage in the ejaculate.

Sperm preparations for motility assessment should be at least 10 µL, preferably ca. 20 µL, to allow free sperm movements.

Two different aliquots should be assessed, and results compared to reduce risk for random errors.

Categorization in four different velocity categories is recommended (immotile, nonprogressive, slow progressive, and rapid progressive). Distinction between slow and rapid progressive spermatozoa is of clinical importance [27,28,34].

Proportions of the velocity groups should be presented as integer percentages. Also, as a help to referring clinics the progressive (rapid and slow progressive) and motile (nonprogressive and progressive) value proportions can be presented in the report.

20.4.4 Sperm Vitality

Sperm vitality is only of interest when few sperm are motile. When at least 40% of spermatozoa are motile, it means that at least 40% of the spermatozoa are alive.

For diagnostic use a simple EosinY-Nigrosin staining test can be used. The criteria in the fifth edition of the WHO manual [33] are unfortunately erroneous [27,49]. Comparisons of replicate assessments are not necessary [50].

Clinically the interest is to distinguish between samples with many dead spermatozoa and samples with live but immotile spermatozoa. The latter indicate a ciliary dyskinesia where intracytoplasmic sperm injection (ICSI) could be successful. The former indicates presence of microorganisms or other cytotoxic agents like inflammatory cells – clinical investigation of the man is essential to exclude active bacterial infection that requires medical intervention.

20.4.5 Sperm Morphology

For reliable morphology assessment the best staining is the sperm-adapted Papanicolaou staining that gives the best overall staining of all parts of the spermatozoon.

The Tygerberg strict criteria is recommended by WHO [34] to be the best level of validation and evaluations. With this assessment scheme most spermatozoa are "abnormal" in the sense that the morphology is not corresponding to the morphology observed among spermatozoa that have passed through cervical mucus and that bind to human zona pellucida. It is important to evaluate all four aspects of sperm morphology (head, neck–midpiece, tail, cytoplasmic residue). Most studies on sperm morphology have focused on prediction of fertility success, but information about male reproductive organ function can be obtained by registering abnormalities in the four regions. For instance, motility impairment can be explained by tail abnormalities or lack of mitochondria in the midpiece and epididymal problems can cause abnormal cytoplasmic residues.

The training in proper assessment of human sperm morphology according to the Tygerberg strict criteria is the most important aspect for reliable results, combined with participation in external quality assessment. Comparisons of replicate assessment are not necessary [27].

20.5 Assessments of Questionable Value

Some "classical" elements beyond the basic examination of human ejaculates can be called in question based on the clinical usefulness lack of scientific evidence.

20.5.1 Other Cells Than Spermatozoa

All human ejaculates contain lots of particulate matter besides spermatozoa: cells (epithelial cells, germ cells, white blood cells, and occasional erythrocytes), cell parts, crystals, and other debris. Large quantities of pus (massive occurrence of live and dead white blood cells) is indicative of active bacterial infection. Large quantities of erythrocyte indicate haemorrhage somewhere in the tract. To some extent distinction between immature germ cells (indicating testicular damage) and polymorph nuclear granulocytes can be done in smears stained for sperm morphology assessment.

20.5.2 Antisperm Antibodies

The interest in antisperm antibodies (ASA) goes back to the rise of clinical laboratory immunology in the early 1980s. There is only one brand of screening test commercially available, but the clinical usefulness and scientific evidence is very limited indicating that positive or negative tests have very little impact on investigations and treatments. A general problem is that available tests have very low predictive value and no specific causal treatment can be offered in positive cases, only symptomatic treatment of the couple with IVF or ICSI. In some cases, presence of ASA can be suspected in the initial microscopic assessment but further testing with elaborate antibody testing is not likely to change the continued care of the couple.

20.5.3 Microbiological Cultures

This is also an area of great controversy. It is well known that microbiological culture from semen is extremely difficult, not the least due to high pH and presence of bactericidal agents like lysozymes and zinc [25].

20.6 Conclusions

Ejaculate examination represents a complex medical laboratory science. Robust and comprehensive techniques have been described and have spread globally. The challenge for scientists and clinicians interested in promoting development in reproductive medicine and andrology is now to implement those techniques and procedures that can deliver better patient care (diagnosis and treatment) and a base for preclinical and clinical scientific development.

References

1. Barratt CLR, Björndahl L, De Jonge CJ, et al. The diagnosis of male infertility: an analysis of the evidence to support the development of global WHO guidance – challenges and future research opportunities. *Hum Reprod Update*. 2017;23:660–680.
2. Keel BA. How reliable are results from the semen analysis? *Fertil Steril*. 2004;82:41–44.
3. Björndahl L, Barratt CL, Mortimer D, Jouannet P. 'How to count sperm properly': checklist for acceptability of studies based on human semen analysis. *Hum Reprod (Oxford)*. 2016;31:227–232.
4. van Leeuwenhoek A. Observationes D. Anthonii Lewenhoeck, de natis'e semine genitali animalculis. *Philos Trans R Soc Lond B Biol Sci*. 1677;12:1040–1046.
5. Harvey C, Jackson MH. Assessment of male fertility by semen analysis – an attempt to standardise methods. *Lancet*. 1945:99–104.
6. MacLeod J, Hotchkiss RS. The distribution of spermatozoa and of certain chemical constituents in the human ejaculate. *J Urology*. 1942;48:225–229.
7. MacLeod J. The male factor in fertility and infertility; an analysis of ejaculate volume in 800 fertile men and in 600 men in infertile marriage. *Fertil Steril*. 1950;1:347–361.
8. MacLeod J, Gold RZ. The male factor in fertility and infertility. IV. Sperm morphology in fertile and infertile marriage. *Fertil Steril*. 1951;2:394–414.
9. MacLeod J, Gold RZ. The male factor in fertility and infertility. II. Spermatozoon counts in 1000 men of known fertility and in 1000 cases of infertile marriage. *J Urology*. 1951;66:436–449.
10. MacLeod J, Gold RZ. The male factor in fertility and infertility. III. An analysis of motile activity in the spermatozoa of 1000 fertile men and 1000 men in infertile marriage. *Fertil Steril*. 1951;2:187–204.
11. MacLeod J. The biochemistry of the human male genital tract. *Int Rec Med Gen Pract Clin*. 1951;164:671–673.
12. MacLeod J. Effect of chickenpox and of pneumonia on semen quality. *Fertil Steril*. 1951;2:523–533.
13. MacLeod J. Semen quality in 1000 men of known fertility and in 800 cases of infertile marriage. *Fertil Steril*. 1951;2:115–139.
14. MacLeod J. Sulfhydryl groups in relation to the metabolism and motility of human spermatozoa. *J Gen Physiol*. 1951;34:705–714.
15. MacLeod J, Gold RZ. The male factor in fertility and infertility. V. Effect of continence on semen quality. *Fertil Steril*. 1952;3:297–315.
16. MacLeod J, Gold RZ. The male factor in fertility and infertility. VI. Semen quality and certain other factors in relation to ease of conception. *Fertil Steril*. 1953;4:10–33.
17. MacLeod J, Gold RZ. The male factor in fertility and infertility. VII. Semen quality in relation to age and sexual activity. *Fertil Steril*. 1953;4:194–209.
18. Gold RZ, Macleod J. The male factor in fertility and infertility. VIII. A study of variation in semen quality. *Fertil Steril*. 1956;7:387–410.
19. MacLeod J, Gold RZ. The male factor in fertility and infertility. IX. Semen quality in relation to accidents of pregnancy. *Fertil Steril*. 1957;8:36–49.
20. Eliasson R. Analysis of semen. In: Behrman SJ, Kistner RW, eds. *Progress in Infertility*. Little, Brown and Co; 1975:691–713.
21. Eliasson R. Semen analysis and laboratory workup. In: Cockett ATK, Urry RL, eds. *Male Infertility Workup, Treatment and Research*. Grune & Stratton; 1977:169–188.
22. Eliasson R. Analysis of semen. In: Burger HG, De Kretser DM, eds. *The Testis*. Raven Press; 1981:381–399.

23. Arver S, Kvist U, Bjorndahl L. In memoriam: Rune Eliasson MD, PhD. *Andrology*. 2020;8:530–531.
24. Mortimer D. Laboratory standards in routine clinical andrology. *Reprod Med Rev*. 1994;3:97–111.
25. Mortimer D. *Practical Laboratory Andrology*. Oxford University Press; 1994.
26. Björndahl L, Barratt CL, Fraser LR, Kvist U, Mortimer D. ESHRE Basic Semen Analysis Courses 1995–1999: immediate beneficial effects of standardized training. *Hum Reprod (Oxford)*. 2002;17:1299–1305.
27. Barratt CL, Björndahl L, Menkveld R, Mortimer D. ESHRE Special Interest Group For Andrology Basic Semen Analysis Course: a continued focus on accuracy, quality, efficiency and clinical relevance. *Hum Reprod (Oxford)*. 2011;26:3207–3212.
28. Mortimer D, Björndahl L, Barratt CLR, et al. *A Practical Guide to Basic Laboratory Andrology*. 2nd ed. Cambridge University Press; 2022.
29. Belsey M, Eliasson R, Gallegos AJ, Moghissi KS, Paulsen CA, Prassad AMN. *Laboratory Manual for the Examination of Human Semen and Semen-Cervical Mucus Interaction*. Press Concern; 1980.
30. World Health Organization. *WHO Laboratory Manual for the Examination of Human Semen and Semen-Cervical Mucus Interactions*. 2nd ed. Cambridge University Press; 1987.
31. World Health Organization. *WHO Laboratory Manual for the Examination of Human Semen and Sperm-Cervical Mucus Interactions*. 3rd ed. Cambridge University Press; 1992.
32. World Health Organization. *WHO Laboratory Manual for the Examination of Human Semen and Sperm-Cervical Mucus Interactions*. 4th ed. Cambridge University Press; 1999.
33. World Health Organization. *WHO Laboratory Manual for the Examination and Processing of Human Semen*. 5th ed. World Health Organization; 2010.
34. World Health Organization. *WHO Laboratory Manual for the Examination and Processing of Human Semen*. 6th ed. World Health Organization; 2021.
35. Eisenberg ML, Li S, Behr B, et al. Semen quality, infertility and mortality in the USA. *Hum Reprod (Oxford)*. 2014;29:1567–1574.
36. Punjabi U, Spiessens C. Basic Semen Analysis Courses: experience in Belgium. In: Ombelet W, Bosmans E, Vandeput H, Vereecken A, Renier M, Hoomans E, eds. *Modern ART in the 2000s: Andrology in the Nineties*. The Parthenon Publishing Group; 1998:107–113.
37. Vreeburg JTM, Weber RFA. Basic Semen Analysis Courses: experience in the Netherlands. In: Ombelet W, Bosmans E, Vandeput H, Vereecken A, Renier M, Hoomans E, eds. *Modern ART in the 2000s: Andrology in the Nineties*. The Parthenon Publishing Group; 1998:103–106.
38. Mortimer D, Shu MA, Tan R. Standardization and quality control of sperm concentration and sperm motility counts in semen analysis. *Hum Reprod (Oxford)*. 1986;1:299–303.
39. Cooper TG, Neuwinger J, Bahrs S, Nieschlag E. Internal quality control of semen analysis. *Fertil Steril*. 1992;58:172–178.
40. Cooper TG, Björndahl L, Vreeburg J, Nieschlag E. Semen analysis and external quality control schemes for semen analysis need global standardization. *Int J Androl*. 2002;25:306–311.
41. Björndahl L. What is normal semen quality? On the use and abuse of reference limits for the interpretation of semen analysis results. *Hum Fertil (Camb)*. 2011;14:179–186.
42. Pound N, Javed MH, Ruberto C, Shaikh MA, Del Valle AP. Duration of sexual arousal predicts semen parameters for masturbatory ejaculates. *Physiol Behav*. 2002;76:685–689.
43. Amann RP. Considerations in evaluating human spermatogenesis on the basis of total sperm per ejaculate. *J Androl*. 2009;30:626–641.
44. Björndahl L, Kvist U. Sequence of ejaculation affects the spermatozoon as a carrier and its message. *Reprod Biomed Online*. 2003;7:440–448.
45. Björndahl L, Kvist U. A model for the importance of zinc in the dynamics of human sperm chromatin stabilization after ejaculation in relation to sperm DNA vulnerability. *Syst Biol Reprod Med*. 2011;57:86–92.
46. Eisenberg ML, Walsh TJ, Garcia MM, Shinohara K, Turek PJ. Ejaculatory duct manometry in normal men and in patients with ejaculatory duct obstruction. *J Urology*. 2008;180:255–260; discussion 60.
47. Björndahl L. Semen characteristics and aging: technical considerations regarding variability. In: Carrell D, ed. *Paternal Influences on Human Reproductive Success*. Cambridge University Press; 2013:183–190.
48. Cooper TG, Brazil C, Swan SH, Overstreet JW. Ejaculate volume is seriously underestimated when semen is pipetted or decanted into cylinders from the collection vessel. *J Androl*. 2007;28:1–4.
49. Björndahl L, Mortimer D, Barratt CLR, et al. *A Practical Guide to Basic Laboratory Andrology*. Cambridge University Press; 2010.
50. Mortimer D. A technical note on the assessment of human sperm vitality using eosin-nigrosin staining. *Reprod Biomed Online*. 2020;40:851–855.

Section 4: Laboratory Evaluation and Treatment of Male Infertility

Chapter 21: The Future of Computer-Assisted Semen Analysis in the Evaluation of Male Infertility

David Mortimer and Sharon T. Mortimer

21.1 Introduction

The fundamental biological significance of Eutherian sperm motility has been reviewed extensively elsewhere [1] and its assessment is a key component of semen analysis [2]. But it is not just the proportion of the spermatozoa that show flagellar motility that is important, rather it is the quality of their movement that is key. For seven decades we have known that the quality of sperm motility is a prime factor to be considered in semen analysis, that the achievement of intra- and inter-observer standardization is essential in any method used to assess sperm motility, and that observers must be properly trained [3]. While basic subclassifications of progression such as rapid, slow, and nonprogressive motility can be assessed by trained observers [2–5], patterns of sperm movement are described using kinematic measures that cannot be determined objectively by eye. Hence the need for computer-aided (or -assisted) sperm analysis technology, or CASA.

Early methods for determining sperm kinematics used microcinematography, multiple-exposure or timed-exposure photomicrography, and videomicrography [1,4,5]. Modern sperm kinematics (Figures 21.1 and 21.2) derive from microcinematography with manual frame-by-frame tracking of the spermatozoa and manual analysis of the sperm tracks [6]. VSL and VAP indicate the progression of the cells, while ALH is related to the amplitude of the proximal flagellar wave, making it a measure of the vigour of progression.

While CASA has clear research benefits and potential, poor marketing strategies on the part of some early CASA companies advertising systems as "computer-automated semen analyzers" led to extensive criticism of the technology since it was simply unfit for this purpose [7–9]. Consensus guidelines on the application of CASA technology identified limitations in its use for analyzing human semen samples [10]. A core issue was, and still is, the inappropriate use of sperm population-averaged kinematic values (that are often biologically meaningless), which has long undermined attempts to identify clinically significant CASA-based parameters, and prevented CASA from realizing its true potential in human clinical andrology. A lack of functional improvements in the commercial technology since that time (beyond simple developments in computer and imaging capabilities) mean that those guidelines are largely still pertinent today [9,11], and CASA is still viewed with substantial skepticism by many scientists and clinicians alike [12]. Overviews of the various technical factors that affect CASA systems' operations have been published elsewhere [1,4,5].

This chapter reviews the current limitations of CASA in routine clinical andrology and describes a way forward so that it can become a robust valuable technology. Particular

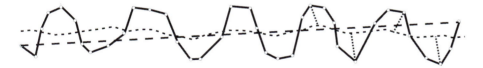

Figure 21.1 The derivation and calculation of kinematics from a sperm track plotted by following the head centroid (white circles). Adapted from [29]. By international consensus, VCL, VAP, VSL, ALH, and BCF are reported to one decimal place, the ratios LIN, STR, and WOB as integers, and D to two decimal places.

Curvilinear velocity (VCL μm/s) ———

Average path velocity (VAP μm/s) - - - - - - -

Straight line velocity (VSL μm/s) — — — —

Ratios:
Linearity (LIN %) = (VSL / VCL) x 100
Straightness (STR %) = (VSL / VAP) x 100
Wobble (WOB %) = (VAP / VCL) x 100

"Risers" : ················
(distance between a point on the smoothed path, however derived, and the corresponding point along the curvilinear path)

ALH = amplitude of lateral head displacement (μm) for the track
 ALHmax = largest riser × 2
 ALHmean = average riser × 2

Beat/cross frequency = number of times the curvilinear path crosses the average path per unit time (BCF Hz)

attention will focus on the need for premarketing validation by manufacturers of CASA systems for semen analysis applications, and on the impact of software differences on the absolute values reported for sperm kinematics.

21.2 Current Status of CASA for Sperm Concentration and Motility

21.2.1 In Semen

Table 21.2 summarizes the main reasons why human semen is such a difficult material to analyze. Indeed, human semen is probably the most difficult type of specimen to analyze by CASA, and many patient samples are "the worst of the worst." Early limitations of CASA technology for identifying human spermatozoa in semen and reliably differentiating them from debris can largely be avoided by using positive-low phase contrast (PL/PC) optics instead of negative-high PC optics [14]. While many systems allow the operator to edit the objects identified within the analysis field to correct for missed or spurious spermatozoa, it is very time consuming and consequently rarely done routinely – causing inaccurate results. Clearly a CASA system that is truly fit-for-purpose should not require human input in such a basic process step.

Because of these issues the CASA-determined sperm concentration in human semen samples is often incorrect – and hence the proportions of motile spermatozoa will also be incorrect. With "clean" semen samples (often a rarity in clinical andrology labs) this issue is greatly reduced, and nonexistent when analyzing washed sperm populations.

Another key issue with human semen is the impossibility of mixing such a viscous fluid to achieve completely random distribution of the cells throughout the sample; there is always a degree of "micro-heterogeneity." The resultant inherent sampling variability when using aliquots of just 2–5 µL to load

Table 21.1 Kinematics values for the 60 Hz sperm track segments shown in Figure 21.2

Kinematics	Seminal sperm tracks		Washed sperm track segments		
	1A	1B	2A	2B	2C
VCL (µm/s)	25.4	131.3	173.7	271.9	228.8
VSL (µm/s)	23.3	96.3	70.2	33.7	30.6
VAP (µm/s)	23.6	101.2	77.3	46.0	32.3
LIN (%)	92	73	40	12	13
STR (%)	99	95	91	73	95
WOB (%)	93	77	44	17	14
ALHmean (µm)	n/a	n/a	4.8	10.5	9.6
ALHmax (µm)	0.8	4.8	6.9	13.6	12.2
D	1.03	1.10	1.24	1.49	1.68

Notes: Values for the seminal spermatozoa were generated by the IVOS-II software whose adaptive smoothing algorithm selected five-point smoothing as optimal for the average path, while values for the washed sperm track were generated using Excel with seven-point smoothing. For ALHmean n/a = not available because the IVOS-II software only provides ALHmax values.

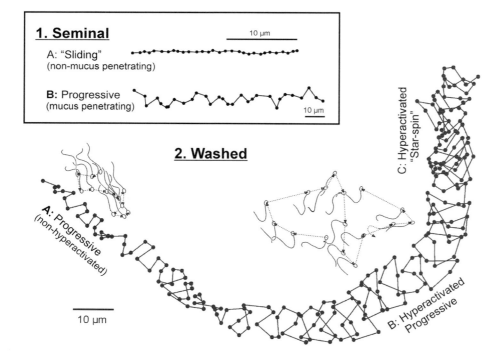

Figure 21.2 Illustration of general types of human sperm tracks seen in semen (tracks 1A and 1B) and washed/capacitating populations (track 2, showing the three phases of movement that the cell switched between spontaneously), all tracked at 60 Hz. The seminal spermatozoa were tracked for 0.5 s (31 points) and analyzed using an IVOS-II system, while the washed spermatozoon was tracked manually for 3.77 s (227 points) and its kinematics analyzed using Excel; for the kinematics values see Table 21.1. Illustrative sperm tail beating patterns are shown for the nonhyperactivated and hyperactivated progressive regions of the washed sperm track; note the much larger amplitude proximal waves in the hyperactivated phase.

Table 21.2 A comparison of biological and technical issues in the analysis of human semen and semen from domesticated mammals using CASA (adapted from [9,11])

Criterion	Domesticated mammals	Humans
General fertility	Selected for high fertility over many generations	A low fecundity species (maximum reported 28%)
Semen cleanliness (presence of other cells, debris, etc.)	Generally "clean"	Typically very "dirty" ejaculates (high background noise)
Semen viscosity	Relatively low in most species	Generally high, with micro-heterogeneity
Possibility for dilution prior to analysis	Ejaculates are typically highly diluted with an "extender" before analysis (many domesticated and wildlife species have $>1000 \times 10^6$ sperm/mL)	Generally $<200 \times 10^6$/mL, often very low ($<25 \times 10^6$/mL); dilution requires homologous seminal plasma to preserve motility kinematics
Proportion of motile spermatozoa	Typically well over 60%, often higher	Typically lower, often <50%; many dead spermatozoa with aggregation
Sperm morphology	Highly consistent in very many species (although in some groups there can be many types of abnormalities, e.g., carnivores)	Highly pleiomorphic

fixed-depth slide preparations such as are used for CASA, or Makler chambers, will be substantial, and confounds replicate analyses [4,9]. Moreover, capillary-loaded shallow chambers are subject to the Segré-Silberberg Effect, causing a viscosity-dependent error in sperm concentration, up to −30% in aqueous specimens [15,16].

Any CASA system should be able to identify moving objects and identify those that are spermatozoa (as opposed to, for example, nonsperm objects showing Brownian motion, or false motion caused by specimen drift, collisions, or "stirring"). Hence CASA should provide accurate results for the *concentrations* of motile spermatozoa, especially those that are defined as progressively motile, when using fixed-depth preparations with appropriate corrections for artifacts such as the Segré-Silberberg Effect. Nonprogressive motility (NPM) remains an issue for most CASA systems since human operators classify these cells based on their flagellar movement with lack of "space gain" whereas CASA tracks sperm head movement. Consequently the NPM subpopulation differs when comparing CASA against motility assessments performed by a trained technician. While this issue will affect software validation, NPM spermatozoa cannot penetrate the cervical mucus in vivo, and hence have no chance of contributing to a conception – they are "biological junk" [17]. CASA software validations should therefore focus on the progressive spermatozoa.

The reference methods for total sperm concentration are flow cytometry and haemocytometry by competent operators [2,18], and although PL/PC-based CASA can come close to such results no system has yet been definitively validated against reference methodology. CASA results are certainly more reproducible, but this is insufficient without evidence of accuracy [9,18]. Various studies have reported perceived agreement between CASA and routine semen analysis but the range of discrepancies between results remains significant [19–23]. Many studies do not reveal the magnitude of differences between CASA and routine semen analysis results [e.g., 21], while others are prepared to consider substantial differences in results as "acceptable" [23]. It is also noted that CASA operators must be well trained [19,22].

But how important is the total sperm concentration? Most clinical situations, for example all forms of assisted reproductive technology, do not rely on this information, and the World Health Organization (WHO) reference limit of 15×10^6/mL has little relevance because it relates to in vivo fertility [24–26]. So, in many clinical situations CASA could be used to analyze the concentration of progressively motile spermatozoa in semen, which any system should be able to do with good accuracy.

In biological terms only those spermatozoa in semen that are capable of penetrating into and migrating within the cervical mucus are of clinical importance for fertility, and these spermatozoa are actually a subpopulation of the "rapid progressive" cells [27], which is why the ESHRE (European Society of Human Reproduction and Endocrinology) Andrology SIG (Special Interest Group) rejected the assessment of the single "progressive" category as per WHO5 [28]. Based on studies of sperm–mucus interaction, adapted for evolving sperm kinematics analysis, over two decades ago we defined a "mucus penetrating" fraction of motile human spermatozoa as part of a more functional approach to routine semen assessment [27,29,30]. The Boolean algorithm defining this subpopulation using Hamilton Thorne IVOS platforms operating at 60 images/s and 37°C (Hamilton Thorne Inc, Beverly, MA, USA; www.hamiltonthorne.com) is:

$$\text{VAP} \geq 25 \text{ μm/s AND STR} \geq 80\% \text{ AND ALH} \geq 2.5 \text{ μm}$$

To avoid including spermatozoa whose kinematics have been compromised by oxidative damage, which can cause a quasi-hyperactivation pattern of movement, a fourth term of ALH <7.0 μm can also be included.

21.2.2 Washed and Capacitating Sperm Populations

Human sperm populations prepared by either density gradient centrifugation or direct swim-up from semen have minimal contamination with dead/immotile spermatozoa or other cells or debris, and very high progressively motility: Reference competence and benchmark values are 90% and $\geq$95% respectively [31]. CASA results for both total and motile sperm concentrations, as well as sperm kinematics, will be accurate for such specimens, and when incubated under capacitating conditions the subpopulation that shows hyperactivated (HA) motility can also be analyzed [1,2,27,30].

Sperm hyperactivation is due to a change in flagellar beat pattern [1,32], and studies on hyperactivating human spermatozoa classified according to such criteria have provided a validated definition for use on the Hamilton Thorne IVOS platforms operating at 60 images/s and 37°C [1,2,27] of:

$VCL \geq 150$ μm/s AND $LIN \leq 50\%$ AND $ALH \geq 7.0$ μm

Hamilton Thorne CASA-II software (IVOS-II and CEROS-II platforms) also includes the fractal dimension kinematic measure (D or FDM), allowing a more robust definition of human sperm hyperactivation that is independent of the track smoothing needed to derive ALH values [11,27]:

$VCL \geq 150$ μm/s AND $D \geq 1.20$

HA motility assessment of washed sperm populations can be used for the prediction of fertilization failure, with reduced levels of HA being associated with reduced fertilizing ability in vivo and in vitro [1,27,33].

21.3 Issues of Noncomparability of Kinematics between CASA Systems

Image capture frequency dramatically affects the observed sperm track (Figure 21.3), with lower sampling rates giving simpler tracks that have reduced VCL and modified ALH values, affecting the proportion of tracks that meet any pre-defined criteria [27,34]. The reason that VCL is affected is relatively straightforward – fewer points along the track means fewer deviations from a straight-line track – but why ALH is affected is more complex.

Having evolved from manual track analysis studies, ALH is an expression of the overall width of the track [6], that is, a "double wave amplitude" value. When CASA derives kinematic values from track point (x,y) coordinates, the local apices along the track are typically identified as local maxima in the lengths of "risers" (the distance between points on the curvilinear path and their corresponding points on the smoothed average path; see Figure 21.1). The most common method used by CASA systems to derive the average path is smoothing using Tukey windows of between 5 and 13 points; the degree of track smoothing achieved affects riser lengths, and hence the derived ALH values (Figure 21.4 and Table 21.3) [5,9,27].

Because different sperm tracks require different degrees of smoothing to derive an optimum average path, applying a fixed-point smoothing algorithm to all tracks in a population will result in many tracks being under- or over-smoothed. Hence a CASA system that employs "adaptive smoothing" algorithms to optimize the smoothing of each track will achieve more robust derivation of ALH values [27]. There are also several techniques for handling the first and last points of a track when performing smoothing, including ignoring these track segments, tapering the smoothing to include the end points, or reflecting the end segments to smooth the full track length. Furthermore, some CASA systems do not conform to the consensus definitions for ALH, and only present the scale-corrected riser value (i.e., a classical wave amplitude value) rather than the full track width (i.e., 2× riser values), while some systems present track-averaged values (ALHmean) and others give the maximum value for the track (ALHmax).

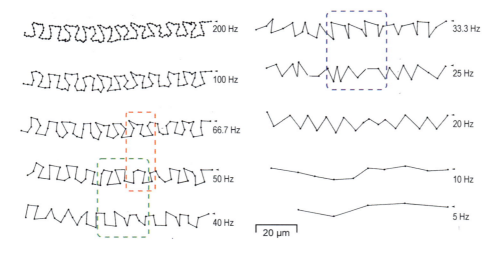

Figure 21.3 The effect of frame rate (image acquisition frequency) on the perceived sperm track. The boxes indicate specific regions of change in the perceived track shape between frame rates. By 50 Hz the track shape is different, making it apparent that around 60 Hz is the minimum frame rate for reliable reconstruction of this particular track. Adapted from [34].

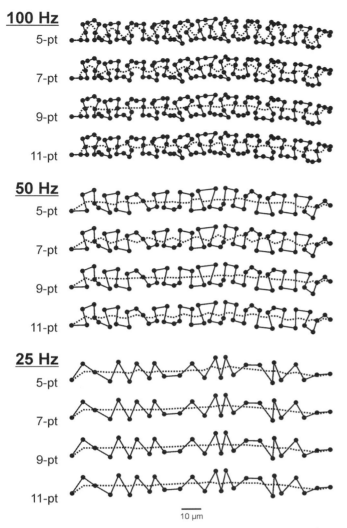

Figure 21.4 Illustration of the influence of smoothing on the perceived average path using the same exemplar track as in Figure 21.3. For each imaging frequency the average path (dotted line) was determined using 5-, 7-, 9- and 11-point Tukey window smoothing. At the ends of the track the size of the smoothing window was tapered according to the number of points available, so that the smoothed path began and ended at the first and last track points respectively; this method is commonly used in CASA software. Kinematics values for each track are shown in Table 21.3. It is clear that 5-point smoothing is inadequate for this sperm track at frame rates over 25 Hz. Note how in under-smoothed tracks (e.g., 100 Hz track, 5- and 7-point smoothing) the average path is pulled toward the apices of the curvilinear path, which will shorten the risers, and hence reduce the derived ALH values(ST Mortimer, unpublished work).

Because all these differences will confound the absolute values of all those kinematic measures that depend on the average path:

- published studies must include, in addition to the CASA instrument model and software version, all necessary information critical to knowing how the average path and ALH were derived, specifically the imaging frequency, track smoothing algorithm, and ALH calculation method, in order to interpret these values – even within a controlled experimental situation;
- conducting meaningful comparisons between published studies using different CASA instruments will not be possible, even knowing the differences in their algorithms, since specific "corrections" cannot be made;
- relationships between sperm kinematics and clinical endpoints, for example threshold or cutoff values, determined using one instrument will not be the same when another system is used (and perhaps might not even exist); and
- a threshold definition, for example for hyperactivated spermatozoa, validated for one instrument's software will not be valid for a different system, and "corrections" will be extremely difficult (*de novo* validation of a system-specific definition will be necessary).

21.4 Clinical Value of Identifying Functional Sperm Subpopulations

The increasing availability of intracytoplasmic sperm injection (ICSI) through the 1990s led to widespread disinterest in identifying or explaining sperm dysfunction. To avoid indiscriminate use of ICSI a concept of "structured management" for infertile couples, using information from simple sperm tests to stream their management, was developed [35]. After initial investigations, couples for whom simple insemination-based treatment would have a good chance of achieving a pregnancy could embark upon such treatment, while couples for whom such treatment would be contraindicated on the grounds of likely impaired gamete approximation would proceed directly to IVF. Cases with severe sperm dysfunction would proceed directly to ICSI. Such a strategy allows prompt application of an appropriate level of intervention with a reasonable chance of a pregnancy, "appropriate" being judged in terms of cost (to both the healthcare system and patients), likelihood of a successful outcome (recognizing the female partner's age), and associated risk factors (e.g., patient morbidity). All too often today recommended treatment seems to be based on financial interests.

A simple andrology lab testing package comprises a semen analysis (including the Teratozoospermia Index, or TZI, rather than simple % normal forms), investigation for sperm surface antisperm antibodies (ASA), a CASA assessment of the "mucus penetrating" sperm fraction, a trial wash using an optimized two-layer density gradient method, and CASA assessment of hyperactivation in the washed sperm population. Detailed methods for all these assessments are available [2,5,25,30], although without Immunobeads a simplified assessment of ASA comparable to that described in the WHO clinical manual for the infertile male [36] is now needed, considering that only a high prevalence of head-directed ASA indicates a need for ICSI.

Table 21.3 Kinematics values for the exemplar sperm track shown in Figure 21.3. Each track was smoothed using 5-, 7-, 9- and 11-point Tukey windows before calculating the kinematics; all values were generated using Excel. Note that at each frame rate the values for VCL, VSL, LIN, and D were unaffected by the smoothing.

Track	100 Hz track				50 Hz track				25 Hz track			
Smoothing	5-pt	7-pt	9-pt	11-pt	5-pt	7-pt	9-pt	11-pt	5-pt	7-pt	9-pt	11-pt
VCL (µm/s)		280.7				246.6				176.9		
VSL (µm/s)		97.1				97.1				97.1		
VAP (µm/s)	151.4	115.4	102.6	107.0	101.5	107.6	100.3	102.7	99.8	98.5	98.5	98.7
LIN (%)		35				39				55		
STR (%)	64	84	95	91	96	90	97	95	97	99	99	98
WOB (%)	54	41	37	38	41	44	41	42	56	56	56	56
ALHmax (µm)	7.2	8.9	10.2	11.1	10.3	11.8	11.3	11.1	10.1	10.6	11.0	10.1
ALHmean (µm)	5.0	6.4	7.6	8.7	7.9	9.1	7.9	7.3	7.5	8.3	8.7	8.4
D		1.23				1.20				1.13		

Combining the two CASA analyses of functional sperm subpopulations ("mucus penetrating" and hyperactivation) with other prognostic markers of sperm dysfunction, especially the TZI, is an effective approach for designing personalized treatment strategies that bypass sperm dysfunction [9]. The proportion of cases treated by ICSI can be limited to only those who need it with good confidence, and failed or low IVF fertilization occurs with very low prevalence, confirming that a "poor" semen analysis, even if several characteristics fall below WHO reference limits, is not adequate justification for using ICSI [37].

21.5 CASA and Sperm Morphology Assessment

Robust sperm morphology assessment requires the analysis of all regions of the cell – head, neck, midpiece, and tail – as well as a sound understanding of the relationships between sperm structure and function at both the cellular and organism (sperm approximation and fertilization) levels [2,38–42].

Compared to assessments of sperm concentration and motility, where good resolution and high frame rate are key but color is not necessary, robust sperm morphology assessment requires the use of high resolution color cameras to take advantage of polychromatic staining methods, combined with sophisticated morphometric and textural analytical techniques.

Early CASA morphology packages analyzed the sperm head but required manual corrections and entry of human observations on the other regions of the spermatozoon [e.g., 43], which made the process of analyzing a morphology slide too laborious and greatly hampered acceptance of the technology. More recently systems have become more robust [e.g., 14] and some can analyze all regions of the cell (e.g., SCA [Sperm Class Analyser] v6, Microptic SL, Barcelona, Spain; www.micropticsl.com), and even derive the TZI. While full validations against expert reference labs remain to be published this is a very promising evolution of the technology.

21.6 CASA and Sperm Vitality Assessment

In routine semen analysis, sperm vitality assessments are performed when the sperm motility is low (typically <40%) to establish whether the immotile spermatozoa are alive or dead [2,5,25,44]. The most common technique uses a combination of eosin as the vital stain with igrosine as a purple background stain to facilitate observation of the unstained live cells. Fluorescence-based methods are also available (e.g., Hoeschst 33258 [45]), but few clinical andrology labs have a fluorescence microscope.

The latest generation Microptic SCA systems are able to analyze eosin-nigrosin preparations [14], and several CASA systems have fluorescence imaging options that permit evaluation of sperm vitality.

21.7 CASA and Assessments of Sperm Function

21.7.1 Sperm DNA Fragmentation

The most common type of sperm DNA fragmentation analysis performed in diagnostic andrology labs is based on sperm chromatin dispersion [2], with the Halosperm G2 Kit being the primary commercial product (HalotechDNA, Madrid, Spain; www.halotechdna.com). Several CASA systems are able to read these slides, removing observer subjectivity in estimating halo size and enabling the test result to be based on a larger number of cells [14,46].

21.7.2 Other Tests of Sperm-Fertilizing Ability

Numerous tests of sperm-fertilizing ability have been described over the past 45 years and many have fallen by the wayside as being either too complex for a routine diagnostic andrology lab or have failed to achieve widespread acceptance [reviews: 2,5,47]. Beyond assessing sperm hyperactivation the only other sperm function test that remains of serious interest is evaluating the acrosome reaction, particularly in response to an ionophore challenge. In these "ARIC" tests (acrosome reaction following ionophore challenge) the acrosome status is determined using fluorescence-labeled lectins, most often peanut agglutinin that binds to the outer acrosomal membrane, ideally in conjunction with a fluorescent vital stain [45,48]. Microptic sells a FluoAcro kit based on this methodology and the SCA platform has a software package to analyze the results.

21.8 Strategies to Validate CASA Technology for Clinical Applications

In the early CASA era (1988–1999) many researchers attempted to validate CASA technology for human semen analysis applications [e.g., 7,8,10,49], but much of this work suffered from fundamental technical issues that undermined the data quality, and hence the possible clinical value of the CASA results. Moreover, few andrology labs performed clinical semen analyses using robust methods performed by properly trained competent staff working within a quality-managed environment [18]. Consequently there was often very poor comparability when CASA results were compared to routine semen analysis results, especially when appropriate statistical methodology such as "discrepancy analysis" Bland & Altman plots [50] were used instead of simple linear regression with no consideration of slope or intercept [e.g., 20,49]. In some studies Bland & Altman plots revealed substantial discrepancies between CASA and routine semen analysis that the authors did not consider problematic [e.g., 22,23].

Not surprisingly, studies comparing poor-quality data against diagnostic or prognostic endpoints were severely compromised or even foredoomed – creating frustration for both CASA users and CASA vendors alike. One vendor even told us he couldn't understand why we were so concerned with "the right answer" when the vendor's CASA system's results were so much more reproducible than those from many andrology labs – failing to grasp the vital importance of accuracy compared to precision in laboratory testing. More recent preliminary clinical endpoint data have been reported [e.g., 22], but studies with real statistical power remain to be pursued.

Within the modern regulatory environment for in vitro diagnostic devices, which covers all automated analyzers used in clinical laboratories, it is now incumbent on the manufacturer to establish that a device performs to an adequate standard, including operational quality control aspects of the device or instrument, prior to marketing it for such a purpose or use; for example, for the US FDA, see: www.fda.gov/MedicalDevices/DeviceRegulationandGuidance/IVDRegulatoryAssistance/s (accessed July 9, 2020).

Accuracy and quality control aspects for semen analyses by andrology laboratories operating within the context of ISO 15189 include the expectation of being able to state the measurement uncertainty (MU) of reported results [51,52]. For semen analysis, MU should not exceed ±10% [18], and achieving this depends on rigorous staff training and the objective establishment of competence, routine verification of the reproducibility of replicate assessments, internal quality control, and external quality assurance. While various books provide recommendations for semen analysis methodology [2,5,25] they are only guidelines, not Standards, and a semen analysis laboratory's methods cannot be certified against them within an ISO 15189 accreditation framework. The imminent publication of the technical standard ISO 23162 on basic semen analysis will provide true reference methodology for use in accredited laboratories – and also when validating alternative methods [53].

21.8.1 Recommended Strategy for Validating a CASA System for Semen Analysis

Applying the fundamental principles discussed in this chapter to validate a CASA system for human semen analysis requires the following:

- Sufficient clinical specimens for a robust statistical comparison (ideally several hundred, but at least 120) must be analyzed in parallel in an expert andrology laboratory whose staff all employ reference methodology within a proper quality-managed operational environment, and by the CASA system.
- All assessments must be performed in at least duplicate, with verification of adequate reproducibility of the replicates before calculating the final result.
- If CASA analyses included human intervention to correct the detection and recognition of spermatozoa within the image analysis process this must be stated, and such intervention must become a required step in the subsequent routine clinical use of the instrument.
- Expression of results to an appropriate degree of precision based on the methodology (i.e., no "false precision").
- The CASA-derived result must have an established MU or error, and needs to fall within ±10% of the reference method's result.

Obviously results can only be reported if an actual measurement was made. If an instrument reports a proportion of spermatozoa with normal morphology based entirely on an algorithm that derives that value indirectly from associated sperm concentration and motility data, it cannot be validated as there is no actual value to compare with a reference result.

Without proper validation, no claims of suitability for purpose (e.g., "automated semen analyzer") should be made. Hopefully the modern regulatory environment will improve the performance of

CASA systems for the future – but this will only happen if robust validation studies are performed. Data must be generated by properly trained personnel working in an expert laboratory against appropriate reference material, and must have been subjected to appropriate statistical analysis. Reports need to include a statement of the MU or error, and be published at least on the vendor's website, but ideally in a respected peer-reviewed journal (e.g., impact factor of at least 2.0) using an open access model.

21.9 Conclusions

(1) Much current CASA technology still has significant optical and imaging issues that limit its widespread application for routine human semen analysis.
(2) Without proper validation, total sperm concentration and the proportions of motile and progressively motile spermatozoa in semen cannot be determined by CASA. Criteria for robust validation have been provided, along with the acceptable measurement error.
(3) Great caution must be exercised when considering kinematic values generated by different CASA systems due to inconsistencies and errors inherent in the derivation of the average path and those kinematics that rely upon it, such as ALH.
(4) Because of coexisting heterogeneous subpopulations of spermatozoa in semen, reporting population-averaged values for kinematic measures is biologically meaningless. Instead, functional subpopulations should be identified and quantified, for example those showing kinematics commensurate with penetrating cervical mucus.
(5) CASA technology is ideally suited for analyzing washed populations of human spermatozoa: reliable values for sperm concentration and the proportions of motile and progressively motile spermatozoa are readily obtainable.
(6) Population-averaged values for kinematic measures of washed human sperm preparations are biologically meaningless due to coexisting heterogeneous subpopulations of spermatozoa. Instead, functional subpopulations should be identified and quantified instead, for example hyperactivating spermatozoa.
(7) While human sperm hyperactivation can be reliably determined from head centroid tracks by current CASA technology, classification criteria validated for one system must not be used with another system unless the systems employ the same image sampling frequency, identical trajectory analysis algorithms, and/or the classification criteria have been specifically revalidated for the other system.
(8) CASA instrument vendors must be responsible for validating their systems for each claimed application according to strict criteria and standards.

References

1. Mortimer ST. A critical review of the physiological importance and analysis of sperm movement in mammals. *Hum Reprod Update*. 1997;3:403–439.
2. Björndahl L, Mortimer D, Barratt CLR, et al. *A Practical Guide to Basic Laboratory Andrology*. Cambridge University Press; 2010.
3. MacLeod J, Gold RZ. The male factor in fertility and infertility. III. An analysis of motile activity in the spermatozoa of 1000 fertile men and 1000 men in infertile marriage. *Fertil Steril*. 1951;2:187–204.
4. Mortimer D. Objective analysis of sperm motility and kinematics. In: Keel BA, Webster BW, eds. *Handbook of the Laboratory Diagnosis and Treatment of Infertility*. CRC Press; 1990:97–133.
5. Mortimer D. *Practical Laboratory Andrology*. Oxford University Press; 1994.
6. David G, Serres C, Jouannet P. Kinematics of human spermatozoa. *Gamete Res*. 1981;4:83–95.
7. Mortimer D, Mortimer ST. Value and reliability of CASA systems. In: Ombelet W, Bosmans E, Vandeput H, Vereecken A, Renier M, Hoomans EH, eds. *Modern ART in the 2000's: Andrology in the Nineties*. Parthenon Publishing, 1998:73–89.
8. Mortimer D, Aitken RJ, Mortimer ST, Pacey AA. Clinical CASA: the quest for consensus. *Reprod Fertil Dev*. 1995;7:951–959.
9. Mortimer D, Mortimer ST. Routine application of CASA in human clinical andrology and ART laboratories. In: Flanagan J, Björndahl L, Kvist U, eds. *Proceedings of the 13th International Symposium on Spermatology*. Springer Nature Switzerland AG, 2018:183–197.
10. ESHRE Andrology Special Interest Group. Guidelines on the application of CASA technology in the analysis of spermatozoa. *Hum Reprod*. 1998;13:142–145.
11. Mortimer ST van der Horst G, Mortimer D. The future of computer-aided sperm analysis. *Asian J Androl*. 2015;17:545–553.
12. Sanders D, Fensome-Rimmer S, Woodward B. Uncertainty of measurement in andrology: UK best practice guideline from the Association of Biomedical Andrologists. *Br J Biomed Sci*. 2017;74:157–162.
13. Yeste M, Bonet S, Rodríguez-Gil JE, Rivera Del Álamo MM. Evaluation of sperm motility with CASA-Mot: which factors may influence our measurements? *Reprod Fertil Dev*. 2018;30:789–798.
14. Schubert B, Badiou M, Force A. Computer-aided sperm analysis, the new key player in routine sperm assessment. *Andrologia*. 2019;51: e13417.
15. Douglas-Hamilton DH, Smith NG, Kuster CE, Vermeiden JP, Althouse GC. Particle distribution in low-volume capillary-loaded chambers. *J Androl*. 2005;26:107–114.
16. Douglas-Hamilton DH, Smith NG, Kuster CE, Vermeiden JP, Althouse GC. Capillary-loaded particle fluid dynamics: effect on estimation of sperm concentration. *J Androl*. 2005;26:115–122.
17. Mortimer D. Sperm transport in the female genital tract. In: Grudzinskas JG, Yovich JL, eds. *Cambridge Reviews in Human Reproduction, Volume 2: Gametes – The Spermatozoon*.

Cambridge University Press; 1995:157–174.

18. Björndahl L, Barratt CLR, Mortimer D, Jouannet P. How to count sperm properly: checklist for acceptability of studies based on human semen analysis. *Hum Reprod.* 2016;31:227–232.

19. Dearing C, Jayasena C, Lindsay K. Can the Sperm Class Analyser (SCA) CASA-Mot system for human sperm motility analysis reduce imprecision and operator subjectivity and improve semen analysis? *Hum Fertil (Camb).* 2021;24(3):208–218.

20. Tomlinson MJ, Naeem A. CASA in the medical laboratory: CASA in diagnostic andrology and assisted conception. *Reprod Fertil Dev.* 2018;30:850–859.

21. Lammers J, Splingart C, Barrière P, Jean M, Fréour T. Double-blind prospective study comparing two automated sperm analyzers versus manual semen assessment. *J Assist Reprod Genet.* 2014;31:35–43.

22. Dearing CG, Kilburn S, Lindsay KS. Validation of the sperm class analyser CASA system for sperm counting in a busy diagnostic semen analysis laboratory. *Hum Fertil.* 2014;17:37–44.

23. Agarwal A, Henkel R, Huang C-C, Lee M-S. Automation of human semen analysis using a novel artificial intelligence optical microscopic technology. *Andrologia.* 2019;51: e13440.

24. Cooper TG, Noonan E, von Eckardstein S, et al. World Health Organization reference values for human semen characteristics. *Hum Reprod Update.* 2010;16:231–245.

25. World Health Organization. *WHO Laboratory Manual for the Examination and Processing of Human Semen.* 5th ed. World Health Organization; 2010.

26. Björndahl L. What is normal semen quality? On the use and abuse of reference limits for the interpretation of semen analysis results. *Hum Fertil.* 2011;14:179–186.

27. Mortimer ST. CASA – practical aspects. *J Androl.* 2000;21:515–524.

28. Barratt CLR, Björndahl L, Menkveld R, Mortimer D. The ESHRE Special Interest Group for Andrology Basic Semen Analysis Course: a continued focus on accuracy, quality, efficiency and clinical relevance. *Hum Reprod.* 2011;26:3207–3212.

29. Mortimer D, Mortimer ST. Laboratory investigation of the infertile male. In: Brinsden PR, ed. *A Textbook of In-Vitro Fertilization and Assisted Reproduction.* 3rd ed. Taylor & Francis Medical Books; 2005:61–91.

30. Mortimer D, Mortimer ST. Computer-aided sperm analysis (CASA) of sperm motility and hyperactivation. In: Carrell DT, Aston KI, eds. *Spermatogenesis and Spermiogenesis: Methods and Protocols. Methods in Molecular Biology 927.* Springer (Humana Press); 2013:77–87.

31. ESHRE Special Interest Group of Embryology and Alpha Scientists in Reproductive Medicine. The Vienna Consensus: report of an expert meeting on the development of ART laboratory performance indicators. *Reprod Biomed Online.* 2017;35:494–510.

32. Mortimer ST, Schoëvaërt D, Swan MA, Mortimer D. Quantitative observations of flagellar motility of capacitating human spermatozoa. *Hum Reprod.* 1997;12:1006–1012.

33. Alasmari W, Barratt CLR, Publicover SJ, et al. The clinical significance of calcium signaling pathways mediating human sperm hyperactivation. *Hum Reprod.* 2013;28:866–876.

34. Mortimer D, Serres C, Mortimer ST, Jouannet P. Influence of image sampling frequency on the perceived movement characteristics of progressively motile human spermatozoa. *Gamete Res.* 1988;20:313–327.

35. Mortimer D. Structured management as a basis for cost-effective infertility care. In: Gagnon C, ed. *The Male Gamete: From Basic Knowledge to Clinical Applications.* Cache River Press; 1999:363–370.

36. Rowe PJ, Comhaire FH, Hargreave TB, Mahmoud AMA. *WHO Clinical Manual for the Standardized Investigation, Diagnosis and Management of the Infertile Male.* Cambridge University Press; 2000.

37. Mortimer D, Mortimer ST. The case against intracytoplasmic sperm injection for all. In: Aitken J, Mortimer D, Kovacs G, eds. *Male and Sperm Factors That Maximize IVF Success.* Cambridge University Press; 2020:130–140.

38. Mortimer D, Menkveld R. Sperm morphology assessment: historical perspectives and current opinions. *J Androl.* 2001;22:192–205.

39. Mortimer D. Sperm form and function: beauty is in the eye of the beholder. In: van der Horst G, Franken D, Bornman R, de Jager T, Dyer S, eds. *Proceedings of 9th International Symposium on Spermatology.* Monduzzi Editore; 2002:257–262.

40. Auger J, Jouannet P, Eustache F. Another look at human sperm morphology. *Hum Reprod.* 2016;31:10–23.

41. Gatimel N, Moreau J, Parinaud J, Léandri RD. Sperm morphology: assessment, pathophysiology, clinical relevance, and state of the art in 2017. *Andrology.* 2017;5:845–862.

42. Mortimer D. The functional anatomy of the human spermatozoon: relating ultrastructure and function. *Mol Hum Reprod.* 2018;24:567–592.

43. Coetzee K, Kruger TF, Lombard CJ. Repeatability and variance analysis on multiple computer-assisted (IVOS) sperm morphology readings. *Andrologia.* 1999;31:163–168.

44. Mortimer D. A technical note on the assessment of human sperm vitality using eosin-nigrosin staining. *Reprod Biomed Online.* 2020;40:851–855.

45. Mortimer D, Curtis EF, Camenzind AR, Tanaka S. The spontaneous acrosome reaction of human spermatozoa incubated in vitro. *Hum Reprod.* 1989;4:57–62.

46. Sadeghi S, García-Molina A, Celma F, Valverde A, Fereidounfar S, Soler C. Morphometric comparison by the ISAS® CASA-DNAf system of two techniques for the evaluation of DNA fragmentation in human spermatozoa. *Asian J Androl.* 2016;18:835–839.

47. ESHRE Andrology Special Interest Group. Consensus workshop on advanced diagnostic andrology techniques. *Hum Reprod.* 1996;11:1463–1479.

48. Mortimer D, Curtis EF, Miller RG. Specific labelling by peanut agglutinin of the outer acrosomal membrane of the human spermatozoon. *J Reprod Fertil.* 1987;81:127–135.

49. Mortimer D, Goel N, Shu MA. Evaluation of the CellSoft automated semen analysis system in a routine laboratory setting. *Fertil Steril.* 1988;50:960–968.

50. Bland JM, Altman DG. Statistical methods for assessing agreement between two methods of clinical measurement. *Lancet.* 1986;1: 307–310.
51. International Standards Organization. *ISO 15189:2012 Medical laboratories – Requirements for quality and competence.* International Standards Organization; 2012.
52. International Standards Organization. *ISO/TS 20914:2019 Medical laboratories – Practical guidance for the estimation of measurement uncertainty.* International Standards Organization; 2019.
53. International Standards Organization. *ISO 23162:2021 Basic semen examination – Specification and test methods.* International Standards Organization; 2021.

Section 4 Laboratory Evaluation and Treatment of Male Infertility

Chapter 22: Reactive Oxygen Species and Sperm DNA Damage

Lesley Haddock, Erica Gardiner, and Sheena E. M. Lewis

Up to 50% of couples facing fertility difficulties are found to have a contributing male factor [1]. Traditionally semen analysis has been relied upon to measure male fertility, but with 30% of couples diagnosed with infertility remaining idiopathic, semen analysis alone is proving insufficient [1]. Around 15% of men with normal semen analysis are found to have high sperm DNA damage [2]. As the male gamete contributes half the DNA of the resultant offspring, the integrity of the sperm DNA is vital to fertility success.

This chapter examines the DNA damage to the sperm caused by reactive oxygen species (ROS) and how this damage can either be reduced or avoided to achieve pregnancy and live birth.

22.1 DNA Damage

Around 15% of couples now experience fertility problems and 30% of these cases remain idiopathic with no clear cause identified [1]. Focus has historically been on the female partner, with the belief that responsibility for fertility success or failure lay almost entirely with her. In more recent times the contribution of the male gamete has been recognized. Sperm DNA damage, comprising a variety of damage types and mechanisms, has been linked to infertility with a reduction in all the classic fertility checkpoints including clinical pregnancy, live birth, and an increase in miscarriage when damage levels are higher.

DNA damage in sperm can occur due to lack of repair of physiological DNA strand nicks required during meiosis, defective spermiogenesis, and failure to exchange histones for protamines leading to inadequate DNA condensation and susceptibility to oxidative attack [3].

22.1.1 Testing for DNA Damage

A number of testing methodologies for sperm DNA fragmentation are currently available, with each taking a unique approach and measuring DNA brakeage in a different way. As a consequence, results from these different tests are not directly comparable and each has its own experimentally determined thresholds for fertility.

22.1.1.1 Single-Celled Gel Electrophoresis Assay (Comet Assay)

The Comet assay decondenses and deproteinizes sperm DNA before electrophoresing it through an agarose gel. This enables movement of fragments of damaged DNA away from the intact "comet head" DNA into a visible "comet tail." After staining, the percentage of DNA which has traveled into the comet tail is taken as a measure of damage in individual sperm [6].

This assay can be used to measure total damage (combined single strand [ss] and double strand [ds] breaks) and also specifically ds damage by using alkaline and neutral pH conditions respectively (Figure 22.1). This is of particular importance due to different modes of damage induction and hence different treatment pathways in response.

22.1.1.2 Terminal Deoxynucleotide Transferase dUTP Nick End Labelling (TUNEL)

TUNEL testing detects DNA fragmentation occurring in the last phase of apoptosis. In this assay, TdT enzymes attach chemical or fluorescently tagged nucleotides to the $3'$ free OH terminus of broken DNA and the corresponding signal is used as a measure to quantify the breaks [6].

22.1.1.3 Sperm Chromatin Structure Assay (SCSA)

The SCSA test uses acid denaturation of chromatin followed by acridine orange staining to differentiate between damaged and undamaged DNA. The dye intercalates into undamaged ds DNA where it fluoresces green, while in damaged ss DNA attached dye fluoresces red. A flow cytometer is then used to determine the overall fluorescence color of each sperm and the percentage of sperm appearing red is used as a measure of damaged sperm in the sample [6].

22.1.1.4 Sperm Chromatin Dispersion (SCD)

The SCD test, sold as Halosperm®, uses the natural ability of sperm DNA to create a distinctive halo of intact dispersed loops if undamaged and the loss or reduction of this halo in damaged DNA to determine whether a sperm is fragmented or not. After staining, any sperm with either no halo or a very small halo are classed as fragmented [6].

Pros and cons of each type of test for DNA damage are displayed in Table 22.1.

22.1.2 Impact of Lifestyle and Male Age on Sperm DNA Fragmentation

22.1.2.1 Lifestyle

Interventions against treatable forms of DNA fragmentation include varicocele repair, detecting and treating underlying

Table 22.1 Pros and cons of four testing methods for sperm DNA fragmentation: Comet, TUNEL, SCSA, and SCD [2,6–8].

Test	Pros	Cons
Comet	- Measures damage at the individual sperm level - Most sensitive and specific - Measures total damage and double strand only damage - Can be used with low sperm count samples - Can be used with surgically retrieved samples - Has proven clinical thresholds for diagnosis and treatment outcomes	- No standardization of protocols between labs - Inter user variability - Requires experienced scientists - Time consuming
TUNEL	- Can be used with low sperm count - Commercial kit available is only for research not fertility diagnostics - Very accurate	- Slow - Specialized equipment required (FCM or light microscope) - All or nothing direct measurement - Measures single parameter - Many protocols and a lack of standardization mean results between labs cannot be compared - Absence of standardized clinical thresholds for diagnosis and treatment outcomes
SCSA	- Single standardized protocol - Can measure thousands of sperm per sample - Measures multiple parameters - Rapid	- Proprietary methodology - Expensive equipment - Requires experienced scientists for FCM - Indirect measurement - Poor association with fertility endpoints
SCD	- Simple to use commercial kit	- Measures absence of damage rather than damage - Commercial kit can be expensive - Inter user variability - Poor associations with fertility outcomes

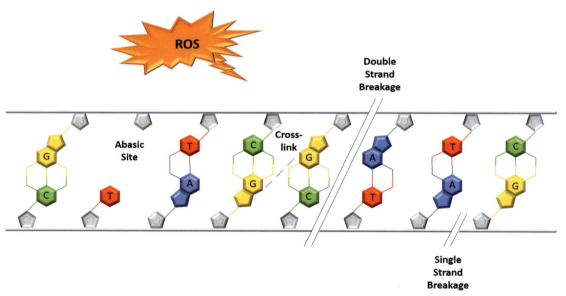

Figure 22.1 Types of DNA damage induced by reactive oxygen species

infections, and improving lifestyle [7]. Consumption of a healthy Mediterranean-style diet and maintaining a healthy weight has been found to improve sperm DNA quality as has lowering alcohol consumption and ceasing smoking and use of recreational drugs. Getting quality sleep and exercising have also been linked to better sperm DNA quality [7,24].

22.1.2.2 Male Age

With societal changes, the prevalence of men with advanced paternal age (APA) is increasing, alongside increasing maternal age [9]. Advancing male age is known to reduce the odds of both achieving a clinical pregnancy and having a successful live birth with each increasing year [10]. As the male partner ages the chance of miscarriage increases and links have been found to obstetric problems and genetic disease in resultant offspring [11].

Male aging has been linked to reductions in all traditional measures of sperm quality assessed by semen analysis, with older sperm also displaying higher levels of DNA fragmentation that has been specifically linked to infertility [9]. The older a man becomes, the greater the number of mitotic divisions his spermatogonial cells will have experienced, reaching more than 800 divisions by age 50. More divisions increases the DNA fragmentation risk, particularly ds fragmentation, and resultant sperm DNA contains more deleterious point mutations [9]. This has led to the recommendation of including DNA fragmentation testing in routine testing for APA men [9].

Paternal age effect disorders include: achondroplasia; Apert, Crouzon, and Pfeiffer syndromes, which are characterized by craniosynostosis; X-linked diseases including hemophilia and Duchenne muscular dystrophy; and potentially autosomal aneuploidies with over 70% of de novo unbalanced chromosomal rearrangements found to be of paternal origin [9]. Multiple studies have now also linked APA with childhood cancers, cleft lip, and also mental health conditions including schizophrenia and bipolar disorder [9].

22.1.3 Sperm DNA Damage Repair

As mature sperm lack the capacity for DNA repair, any damage must be restored by the oocyte post fertilization. The DNA repair capability of the oocyte has not been fully determined to date, but its limited ability to correct damage in the sperm is believed to potentially enable the endurance of DNA lesions and mutated sequence. This could result in increased potential for genetic aberrancy and consequent epigenetic anomalies [6].

Double-stranded DNA breaks, caused by damage to both chains of the double helix, are believed to be the most detrimental to a successful pregnancy due to the separation of the maternal and paternal genomes in the pronucleus stage, resulting in no template for break repair [12]. Nonhomologous end joining, an error-prone process, is the most likely repair mechanism for this damage [13]. As such the male genetic contribution is believed to be the predominant source of chromosome rearrangements and deletions, caused by incorrect rejoining of double-strand broken DNA sequence [14]. This double-strand fragmented sperm DNA does not appear to prevent fertilization, due to the inactivity of the male genome until the postfertilization stages of development [14]. However, when the male contribution becomes transcriptionally active, DNA damage can cause inhibited development of the blastocyst, unequal cleavage, failure to implant or miscarriage [15].

Studies have found increasing maternal age to show a reduction in expression of key genes that are implicated in ability to repair ds DNA damage, potentially increasing resultant consequences of damaged sperm when paired with an older mother [16]. Similarly, repair ability has been determined to be negatively impacted by in vitro culture conditions used in assisted reproductive technologies (ART) [16]. IVF-based research has found DNA damage level to have no effect on fertilization ability; however, embryo development was impacted when sperm with greater damage were used [16].

Currently ds DNA fragmentation can only be measured reliably using the neutral Comet assay. Research is also increasingly focusing on measuring this ds damage as a novel biomarker of testicular and epididymal sperm quality by providing a measure of damage that is occurring during spermiogenesis in contrast to during epididymal maturation [17]. This identifies the levels of damage that would be expected in testicular and caput epididymal sperm without the oxidative stress (OS) of the epididymis and can act as an indicator for likelihood of achieving pregnancy and live birth before deciding on this invasive procedure [17]. In men who consistently present with high levels of total DNA damage measured by alkaline Comet assay, surgical sperm retrieval can be a last opportunity to father a biological child. The likelihood of this invasive procedure leading to a live birth can potentially be predicted by testing for low ds damage production during spermiogenesis. Studies have found testicular sperm to have between two and three times lower DNA fragmentation than the equivalent ejaculated sperm [28]. Intracytoplasmic sperm injection (ICSI) utilizing this testicular sperm in men with high fragmentation in their ejaculates, produces higher pregnancy and live birth rates and lower risk of miscarriage compared to ejaculate ICSI [18,28,29].

22.1.4 Sperm DNA Fragmentation Impact on ART Outcomes

Semen analysis has been shown as insufficient in diagnosis of male infertility with 15% of men who have normal semen analysis results also having high DNA fragmentation [2,19].

Fragmentation assessed by SCSA and TUNEL has been related to failure to achieve pregnancy naturally. Similarly, analysis of 56 studies has shown DNA fragmentation in sperm to reduce the likelihood of achieving pregnancy and also to increase the risk of miscarriage in those who do [20]. Sporadic miscarriage is more than twice as likely in those with high DNA damage levels [21]. Borges et al. found DNA fragmentation above a threshold of 30% to result in a 2.5 times higher miscarriage rate even when the pregnancy rate showed minimal difference [22]. Recurrent pregnancy loss (RPL) is defined as two or more miscarriages before 20 weeks gestation and 40% of couples experiencing RPL have no diagnosed cause or treatment pathway identified [21]. Meta-analysis comparing 517 men whose partners had experienced RPL with 384 fertile controls found the RPL group to have significantly higher sperm DNA fragmentation rates, averaging 10.7% higher [21]. This indicates these undiagnosed couples may benefit from sperm DNA fragmentation testing to identify the cause of their RPL and help to choose the best ART pathway to lead to live birth [2].

Intrauterine insemination (IUI) is often the first option for couples struggling to achieve natural pregnancy, and sperm DNA fragmentation has been identified as a potential cause of

IUI failure by a number of studies and a meta-analysis of 1,135 IUI cycles [7]. DNA damage testing may have predictive value regarding likely success of IUI and could potentially direct couples to a more successful option such as IVF [7]. Meta-analysis has also identified a detrimental effect of DNA damage on pregnancy by both IVF and ICSI, with significantly higher live birth rates for both techniques when used with less damaged sperm [7]. Increasingly it appears that sperm DNA testing can be used diagnostically to choose the ART technique most likely to result in live birth [2,7].

Of particular note is the usefulness of the alkaline Comet assay as a diagnostic tool that can be utilized to improve ART success rates and reduce overtreatment [2]. The alkaline Comet assay provides three measures of DNA fragmentation: the average damage in the semen sample; the proportion of cells with high damage above an experimentally determined threshold; and the proportion of good-quality, low-damage cells below an experimentally determined threshold [2]. These measurements have all been found to be significantly correlated to IVF and ICSI outcomes and by using the specifically determined thresholds for success of the two ART methods the most likely to succeed path can be chosen. This has shown that in men with high fragmentation, pregnancy is more probable when ICSI is chosen [2].

In some studies, confusion remains around the impact of DNA fragmentation on embryo development with conflicting evidence published. However, the fundamental confounding issues in these studies have been the lack of consideration of oocyte quality or subjective morphological assessment and corresponding impact on repair capacity [6]. Future use of artificial intelligence to assess oocyte and embryo quality may enhance studies in this area. Time-lapse studies of ICSI cycles have shown increased times to each stage of embryo development when sperm have fragmented DNA, assessed by alkaline Comet or SCD test [23].

There appears to be increased likelihood of disease in those born after either ART or natural conception when sperm had a high frequency of DNA damage tested by alkaline Comet or SCSA [6]. While not fully understood this is thought to be linked to the consequent epigenetic alterations and there is potentially transgenerational damage being passed down, which will result in subsequent fertility difficulties in offspring [2].

22.1.5 Isolating Sperm with High DNA Integrity

The advent of ICSI in 1995, bypassing natural fertilization, has led to a reduced need to fully investigate the causes of male infertility. However, more recent linking of DNA fragmentation in sperm to reproductive outcomes has placed a spotlight on the paternal contribution, with a 2018 systematic review of 28 studies showing higher fragmentation in the ejaculates of infertile men compared to fertile [6].

When interventions don't produce the desired reduction in DNA damage, other options to isolate high-quality, low-damage sperm can be utilized. These opportunities include sperm sorting techniques and surgically retrieved sperm.

22.1.5.1 Sperm Sorting

Conventional sperm sorting techniques include density gradient centrifugation, swim-up, and sperm washing techniques. These approaches however bypass the natural checkpoints for quality that occur in vivo and may themselves be responsible for inducing damage [25]. Advances are now making use of microfluidic techniques that replicate the journey through the female reproductive tract in a fast and gentle sorting process to collect sperm of the highest quality [25]. The majority of these devices are used to select highly motile sperm and generally give small numbers of quality cells that can be utilized in IVF or ICSI. These devices are however currently somewhat limited by their very nature of being intended for use with tiny volumes of semen and difficulties are encountered in making them clinically relevant for volumes of semen commonly produced [25]. There is also limited evidence of association with DNA quality to date [26,27].

22.2 Reactive Oxygen Species

Sperm DNA damage is an emerging molecular biomarker of male fertility, with its cause often attributed to the production of excessive ROS [2].

22.2.1 What Are Reactive Oxygen Species?

ROS are a group of short-lived reactive intermediate molecules, including free radicals such as O_2- and nonradical molecules such as hydrogen peroxide (H_2O_2) [30]. Free radicals contain one or more unpaired electrons and ROS in particular are highly reactive radicals specifically containing oxygen [31]. ROS are by-products of normal cellular metabolic activity and functionally oxidize lipids, amino acids, and carbohydrates, with lipids being the most readily oxidized [32]. A number of studies have reported high levels of DNA fragmentation in men who have increased concentrations of ROS in their semen, with the damage caused by OS [33–35].

22.2.2 Where Do Reactive Oxygen Species Come From?

ROS can be produced endogenously via the mitochondria, endoplasmic reticulum, or inflammatory cells, or they can also be a result of exogenous sources including environmental pollution and ionizing radiation [32]. The main sources of ROS within the male genital tract (Table 22.2) are other immature or cytoplasm-rich abnormal sperm, which have the capacity to generate higher levels of ROS than mature sperm and also immune cells often in response to infection [32].

22.2.3 Reactive Oxygen Species Are Necessary for Normal Sperm Function

A controlled concentration of ROS is necessary for normal sperm maturation and function including the capacitation process [36]. Capacitation is the first of a series of physiological changes that enable a sperm to fertilize an oocyte.

Capacitation is a maturation process, involving the removal of specific cell surface molecules to reveal cell surface receptors, which sperm undergo within the female genital tract [36]. This process is essential in facilitating sperm binding to the oocyte zona pellucida by enabling the acrosome reaction to occur [37]. This process involves the production of controlled levels of ROS, which act as messengers in many of the signal transduction pathways, facilitating this essential functional development [37]. ROS in sperm, mostly H_2O_2 and O_2-, are maintained within the optimal physiological range by the actions of antioxidants, primarily found in the seminal plasma [38–40].

22.2.4 Consequences of Excess Reactive Oxygen Species

When ROS and antioxidants are imbalanced OS can cause cellular damage, especially to lipid membranes and to DNA, which impact cellular function (Figure 22.2) [30]. Naturally volatile ROS molecules seek stability by appropriating electrons from other surrounding molecules, oxidizing them and initiating a chain reaction of instability [30]. Lipid peroxidation in sperm membranes occurs when free radicals attack unsaturated fatty acid double bonds and generate a lipid peroxide radical. This triggers a positive feedback loop with a cyclical chain of redox reactions, causing damage in neighboring cells that impairs the fluidity of the cell membrane [4,24,41]. This membrane damage has been reported to inhibit individual sperm function by impacting the cellular maturation, motility, and morphology as well as reducing overall sperm concentration in the ejaculate [24,42]. The resulting molecules generated by this lipid peroxidation of membranes are themselves mutagens, which in turn induce damage to the sperm DNA [24,43]. As well as posing a threat to nuclear DNA, mitochondrial DNA is rendered more vulnerable to DNA damage due to its lack of protective histones and protamines and its propensity to replicate rapidly with limited proof reading and repair ability [4,42]. Sperm have a limited capacity for DNA repair in the earlier stages of spermiogenesis

Table 22.2 Pre- and postejaculation causes of oxidative stress in sperm

Pre-ejaculation causes of oxidative stress	Postejaculation causes of oxidative stress
• Advanced male age • Poor diet • Smoking tobacco • Alcohol consumption • Obesity • Recreational drug use • Varicocele • Radiation • Pollution/chemicals • Infection • Immature sperm or abnormal/damaged sperm • Electron leakage from mitochondria	• Activated leukocytes in the ejaculate • Activated leukocytes in the female genital tract • Abnormal/damaged sperm with cytoplasmic retention • Presence of precursor germ cells • Electron leakage from mitochondria

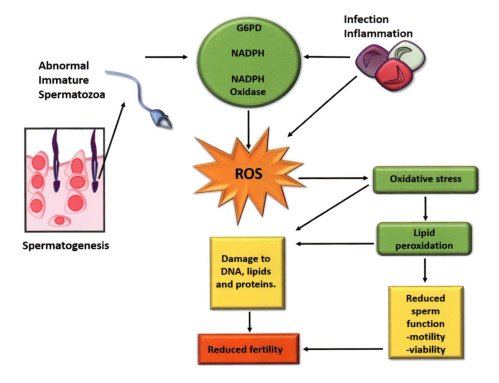

Figure 22.2 Consequences of reactive oxygen species in sperm

that enables the mending of breaks created during the remodeling of chromatin. By the time the sperm have reached the stage of maturation in the epididymis, this repair capability has been lost [24,44]. This is also the stage as the sperm move through the epididymis, in which they become most exposed to oxidative stress and accrue the resultant damage. Any damage incurred during this transit relies on the limited capacity of the oocyte to repair it postfertilization after activation of the paternal genome.

22.2.5 How ROS Damage DNA

The particularly high lipid content of the sperm plasma membrane is notably susceptible to OS-caused lipid peroxidation. The resultant chain of redox reactions lead to genetic damage of the sperm nuclear DNA [4]. This DNA damage can take different forms including ss and ds breaks, creation of abasic sites, and DNA cross-linking (Figure 22.1). This DNA fragmentation, both ss and ds breakage, can alter gene transcription, reduce genomic stability, and produce replication errors in any embryo it goes on to create [4]. In the late stages of spermatogenesis, any DNA repair ability is lost along with the cellular components required for the apoptosis pathway [4]. Sperm that have been marked for apoptosis but have somehow avoided the process either by the system being overwhelmed by large numbers of cells or a malfunctioning of signaling, termed "abortive apoptosis," remain in the ejaculate with fragmented DNA [5].

In cases of natural conception, IUI, and IVF, damage to the plasma membrane caused by OS can disrupt fertilization capability by altering ability to bind to the oocyte. This can be circumvented by use of ICSI, in which the normal fertilization process is bypassed. However, in all cases postfertilization, DNA damage caused by OS can disrupt embryo development due to the impacts of abnormal chromatin packaging and DNA damage per se on epigenetic regulation [4].

22.2.6 Oxidative Stress Impact on ART Outcomes

Among the most common causes of male infertility are hormonal imbalances, genetic factors, systemic disease, varicocele, and lifestyle factors, nearly all of which are associated with excess ROS production [49]. The physiopathological consequences of excessive OS significantly reduces the sperm's fertilizing potential and can result in the generation of genotoxic and mutagenic by-products, with an increased risk of heritable disease in any resultant offspring [49]. With OS being implicated as a major cause of DNA fragmentation and pathology in the male gamete, efforts to reduce ROS are often made when male patients present with subfertility. Varicoceles are the most frequent cause of male infertility, associated with sperm DNA fragmentation due to free radical production and reduced antioxidant activity but can often be successfully surgically repaired [6]. Genital tract infections are also implicated in excessive ROS generation, but simple antibiotic treatment is often effective [6]. Any infection that activates seminal leukocytes can lead to excessive ROS production that may influence ART outcomes; however, vigilant treatment of inflammatory pathologies can reduce OS [6]. Lifestyle changes known to reduce OS include an improved diet, cessation of recreational drugs or smoking, and weight loss to a healthy BMI [6].

With an estimated 190 million people struggling to conceive naturally, the use of ART is becoming more common [49]. However, these therapies themselves expose the gametes to ROS-rich environments during the required laboratory processing steps [31]. Sample preparation for IVF requires washing of sperm, losing the antioxidant activity from the seminal plasma [50]. This renders them more vulnerable to the OS generated during centrifugation, incubation in culture media, and cryopreservation [50]. During ICSI the embryos themselves can create a ROS-rich environment due to high energetic needs and excessive ROS has been linked to poor embryonic cleavage and disruption of embryonic interaction with the uterine lining [50].

With both the sperm-fertilizing potential reduced and the embryonic development dysregulated by OS and resultant DNA damage, much is being done in attempts to limit additional OS during ART [50]. Antioxidant supplementation of in vitro culture media and cryopreservatives has yielded some positive outcomes, increasing fertility parameters and outcomes in mammalian models [31,50].

22.2.7 Antioxidants

During spermiogenesis, sperm differentiate as the majority of the cytoplasm is lost and the head is predominantly made up of the nuclear DNA [31]. As the cytoplasm is lost, the antioxidants it contained are also depleted and the sperm mostly rely on the antioxidants found in the seminal plasma to keep ROS levels in check [31]. The seminal plasma of sperm contains a variety of ROS-scavenging antioxidants, many with catalase activity such as superoxide dismutase and ascorbic acid that break down the damage causing hydrogen peroxide to benign water and oxygen molecules [45]. As the majority of these antioxidant enzymes are lost during the spermiogenesis process, levels of ROS can rise above desired concentrations and induce damage that impairs sperm function [15]. When the delicate equilibrium of ROS and antioxidants is not maintained, the resultant OS reduces the hyperactivation of sperm, which is crucial in enabling travel to the oocyte, reduces the sperm's ability to bind to the zona pellucida, and reduces the acrosome reaction [38,46].

Antioxidant therapy is often used as a fertility treatment in subfertile men, aiming to reduce the elevated levels of ROS and associated pathologies [47]. Oral antioxidant supplements are widely available, representing a large but somewhat unregulated commercial market [47]. Often the supplements contain active ingredients at substantially lower concentrations than those tested and reported in the scientific literature and their overall effectiveness in improving fertility outcomes is still an area of debate [47]. Several studies have reported improvements in sperm quality parameters post treatment, including increased sperm motility and reduced DNA damage; however, most of these studies fail to provide data on outcomes, with key fertility checkpoints such as live birth often missing [31]. Moreover, some studies have reported that overexposure to antioxidants and high doses can be counterproductive, harmful, and associated with other pathologies [31]. Further, the recent Cochrane review [48], a comprehensive meta-analysis combining 61 antioxidant studies, found that only 7 of the studies reported improved birth rates postantioxidant treatment and concluded their overall effectiveness to be inconclusive. The confounding challenges with many of these studies stem from small patient numbers, a lack of proper controls, extensive variety in experimental design, and a lack of concentration-dependent approaches [31]. While antioxidant therapy may be of use in some patients, a more considered and bespoke approach is advised. Further investigation into its usefulness in fertility treatment is crucial.

22.3 Conclusion

The proportion of sperm with high or low levels of DNA damage provides discriminatory information for male infertility diagnosis and prediction of both IVF and ICSI live births. The Comet assay, in particular, provides a pathway for personalized and optimized male fertility diagnosis and treatment in couples with unexplained male infertility and can measure the success of interventions against OS-induced damage.

References

1. Duca Y, Calogero AE, Cannarella R, Condorelli RA, La Vignera S. Current and emerging medical therapeutic agents for idiopathic male infertility. *Expert Opin Pharmacother.* 2019;20(1):55–67.
2. Nicopoullos J, Vicens-Morton A, Lewis S, et al. Novel use of COMET parameters of sperm DNA damage may increase its utility to diagnose male infertility and predict live births following both IVF and ICSI. *Hum Reprod.* 2019;151:1–9.
3. Dada R. Sperm DNA damage diagnostics: when and why. *Transl Androl Urol.* 2017;6(4):S691–S694.
4. Bui AD, Sharma R, Henkel R, Agarwal A. Reactive oxygen species impact on sperm DNA and its role in male infertility. *Andrologia.* 2018;50(8):e13012.
5. Sakkas D, Seli E, Bizzaro D, Tarozzi N, Manicardi GC. Abnormal spermatozoa in the ejaculate: abortive apoptosis and faulty nuclear remodelling during spermatogenesis. *Reprod Biomed Online.* 2003;7(4):428–432.
6. Esteves SC, Santi D, Simoni M. An update on clinical and surgical interventions to reduce sperm DNA fragmentation in infertile men. *Andrology.* 2020;8(1):53–81.
7. Panner Selvam MK, Ambar RF, Agarwal A, Henkel R. Etiologies of sperm DNA damage and its impact on male infertility. *Andrologia.* 2021;53(1):e13706.
8. Cissen M, Van Wely M, Scholten I, et al. Measuring sperm DNA fragmentation and clinical outcomes of medically assisted reproduction: a systematic review and meta analysis. *PLoS ONE.* 2016;11(11):e0165125.
9. Brandt JS, Cruz Ithier MA, Rosen T, Ashkinadze E. Advanced paternal age, infertility, and reproductive risks: a review of the literature. *Prenat Diagn.* 2019;39(2):81–87.
10. Horta F, Vollenhoven B, Healey M, Busija L, Catt S, Temple-Smith P. Male ageing is negatively associated with the chance of live birth in IVF/ICSI cycles for idiopathic infertility. *Hum Reprod.* 2019;34(12):2523–2532.
11. Ramasamy R, Chiba K, Butler P, Lamb DJ. Male biological clock: a critical analysis of advanced paternal age. *Fertil Steril.* 2015;103(6):1402–1406.
12. van Kooij RJ, de Boer P, de Vreeden-Elbertse JMT, Ganga NA, Singh N, te Velde ER. The neutral comet assay detects double strand DNA damage in selected and unselected human spermatozoa of normospermic donors. *Int J Androl.* 2004;27(3):140–146.
13. Hoeijmakers JHJ. Genome maintenance mechanisms for preventing cancer. *Nature.* 2001;411(6835):366–374.
14. Agarwal A, Saleh RA, Bedaiwy MA. Role of reactive oxygen species in the pathophysiology of human reproduction. *Fertil Steril.* 2003;79(4):829–843.
15. Shamsi MB, Kumar R, Dada R. Evaluation of nuclear DNA damage in human spermatozoa in men opting for assisted reproduction. *Indian J Med Res.* 2008;127(2):115–123.
16. Horta F, Catt S, Vollenhoven B, Temple-Smith P. Oocyte DNA repair capacity of controlled sperm DNA damage is affected by female age. *Hum Reprod.* 2018;33(2):529–544.
17. Vyas L, Lewis S, Tharakan T, Jayasena C, Minhas S, Ramsay J. MP75-01 evidence that testicular sperm has improved DNA integrity compared to ejaculated sperm in infertile men. *J Urol.* 2019;201(4).
18. Lopes LS, Esteves SC. Testicular sperm in non-azoospermic infertile men with oxidatively induced high sperm DNA damage. In: Parekattil S, Esteves S, Agarwal A, eds. *Male Infertility.* Springer International Publishing; 2020:735–745.
19. Lewis SEM, Kumar K. The paternal genome and the health of the assisted reproductive technology child. *Asian J Androl.* 2015;17(4):616–622.
20. Simon L, Emery BR, Carrell DT. Review: diagnosis and impact of sperm DNA alterations in assisted reproduction. *Best Pract Res Clin Obstet Gynaecol.* 2017;44:38–56.
21. McQueen DB, Zhang J, Robins JC. Sperm DNA fragmentation and recurrent pregnancy loss: a systematic review and meta-analysis. *Fertil Steril.* 2019;112(1):54–60.e3.
22. Borges E, Zanetti BF, Setti AS, Braga DP de AF, Provenza RR, Iaconelli A. Sperm DNA fragmentation is correlated with poor embryo development, lower implantation rate, and higher miscarriage rate in reproductive cycles of non-male factor infertility. *Fertil Steril.* 2019;112(3):483–490.
23. Wdowiak A, Bakalczuk S, Bakalczuk G. The effect of sperm DNA fragmentation on the dynamics of the embryonic development in intracytoplasmatic

23. sperm injection. *Reprod Biol.* 2015;15(2):94–100.
24. Wright C, Milne S, Leeson H. Sperm DNA damage caused by oxidative stress: modifiable clinical, lifestyle and nutritional factors in male infertility. *Reprod Biomed Online.* 2014;28(6):684-703.
25. Samuel R, Feng H, Jafek A, Despain D, Jenkins T, Gale B. Microfluidic-based sperm sorting & analysis for treatment of male infertility. *Transl Androl Urol.* 2018;7(3):S336–S347.
26. Kishi K, Ogata H, Ogata S, et al. Frequency of sperm DNA fragmentation according to selection method: comparison and relevance of a microfluidic device and a swim-up procedure. *J Clin Diagn Res.* 2015;9(11):QC14–QC16.
27. Yildiz K, Yuksel S. Use of microfluidic sperm extraction chips as an alternative method in patients with recurrent in vitro fertilisation failure. *J Assist Reprod Genet.* 2019;36(7):1423–1429.
28. Esteves SC, Roque M. Extended indications for sperm retrieval: summary of current literature. *F1000Research.* 2019;8.
29. Zhang J, Xue H, Qiu F, Zhong J, Su J. Testicular spermatozoon is superior to ejaculated spermatozoon for intracytoplasmic sperm injection to achieve pregnancy in infertile males with high sperm DNA damage. *Andrologia.* 2019;51(2):e13175.
30. Drevet JR, Aitken RJ. Oxidation of sperm nucleus in mammals: a physiological necessity to some extent with adverse impacts on oocyte and offspring. *Antioxidants.* 2020;9(2):95.
31. Martin-Hidalgo D, Bragado MJ, Batista AR, Oliveira PF, Alves MG. Antioxidants and male fertility: from molecular studies to clinical evidence. *Antioxidants.* 2019;8(4):89.
32. Sanocka D, Kurpisz M. Reactive oxygen species and sperm cells. *Reprod Biol Endocrinol.* 2004;2(1):1–7.
33. Aktan G, Doğru-Abbasoğlu S, Küçükgergin C, Kadıoğlu A, Özdemirler-Erata G, Koçak-Toker N. Mystery of idiopathic male infertility: is oxidative stress an actual risk? *Fertil Steril.* 2013;99(5):1211–1215.
34. Khosravi F, Valojerdi MR, Amanlou M, Karimian L, Abolhassani F. Relationship of seminal reactive nitrogen and oxygen species and total antioxidant capacity with sperm DNA fragmentation in infertile couples with normal and abnormal sperm parameters. *Andrologia.* 2014;46(1):17–23.
35. Shamsi MB, Kumar R, Malhotra N, et al. Chromosomal aberrations, Yq microdeletion, and sperm DNA fragmentation in infertile men opting for assisted reproduction. *Mol Reprod Dev.* 2012;79(9):637–650.
36. Aitken RJ, Jones KT, Robertson SA. Reactive oxygen species and sperm function-in sickness and in health. *J Androl.* 2012;33(6):1096–1106.
37. O'Flaherty C. Reactive oxygen species and male fertility. *Antioxidants.* 2020;9(4):287.
38. Wright C, Milne S, Leeson H. Sperm DNA damage caused by oxidative stress: modifiable clinical, lifestyle and nutritional factors in male infertility. *Reprod Biomed Online.* 2014;28(6):684–703.
39. Lewis SEM, Boyle PM, McKinney KA, Young IS, Thompson W. Total antioxidant capacity of seminal plasma is different in fertile and infertile men. *Fertil Steril.* 1995;64(4):868–870.
40. Lewis SEM, Samantha Sterling EL, Young IS, Thompson W. Comparison of individual antioxidants of sperm and seminal plasma in fertile and infertile men. *Fertil Steril.* 1997;67(1):142–147.
41. Mylonas C, Kouretas D. Lipid peroxidation and tissue damage. *In Vivo (Brooklyn).* 1999;13(3):295–309.
42. Atig F, Raffa M, Ben Ali H, Abdelhamid K, Saad A, Ajina M. Altered antioxidant status and increased lipid per-oxidation in seminal plasma of Tunisian infertile men. *Int J Biol Sci.* 2011;8(1):139–149.
43. Sanocka D, Kurpisz M. Reactive oxygen species and sperm cells. *Reprod Biol Endocrinol.* 2004;2:12.
44. Badouard C, Ménézo Y, Panteix G, et al. Determination of new types of DNA lesions in human sperm. *Zygote.* 2008;16(1):9–13.
45. Lamirande E De, Jiang H, Zini A, Kodama H, Gagnon C. Reactive oxygen species and sperm physiology. *Rev Reprod.* 1997;2(1):48–54.
46. Oehninger S, Blackmore P, Mahony M, Hodgen G. Effects of hydrogen peroxide on human spermatozoa. *J Assist Reprod Genet.* 1995;12(1):41–47.
47. Martins da Silva SJ. Male infertility and antioxidants: one small step for man, no giant leap for andrology? *Reprod Biomed Online.* 2019;39(6):879–883.
48. Smits RM, Mackenzie-Proctor R, Yazdani A, Stankiewicz MT, Jordan V, Showell MG. Antioxidants for male subfertility. *Cochrane Database Syst Rev.* 2019;3(3):CD007411.
49. Agarwal A, Parekh N, Selvam MKP, et al. Male oxidative stress infertility (MOSI): proposed terminology and clinical practice guidelines for management of idiopathic male infertility. *World J Mens Health.* 2019;37(3):296–312.
50. Ritchie C, Ko EY. Oxidative stress in the pathophysiology of male infertility. *Andrologia.* 2020;53(1):e13581.

Section 4 Laboratory Evaluation and Treatment of Male Infertility

Chapter 23

Clinical Value of Sperm DNA Fragmentation Tests

Armand Zini

23.1 Introduction

One of the ongoing challenges in infertility is to identify factors that can influence and/or predict natural and assisted reproduction outcomes. The semen analysis and standard sperm parameters (sperm concentration, motility, and morphology) provide us with information on the function of the testicles and reproductive tract. However, a significant disadvantage of this analysis is that conventional sperm parameters are crude indicators of male fertility potential. Moreover, the reference ranges for these parameters are based on a population of fertile couples who have achieved a natural conception, not on a population of infertile men [1]. In addition, sperm parameters cannot be used to reliably predict reproductive outcomes with assisted reproductive technologies (ARTs). As such, we need to identify markers that may allow us to assess male fertility potential and predict reproductive outcomes with ARTs. To date, one of the most promising markers in the evaluation and management of male infertility is sperm DNA integrity or DNA fragmentation.

The advent of ARTs, particularly intracytoplasmic sperm injection (ICSI), has revolutionized the management of the infertile couple. However, despite the success of this technology, we continue to have concerns regarding the safety of ICSI. These concerns are highly pertinent because advanced ARTs bypass the barriers to natural selection, and we know that infertile men have measurable defects in sperm DNA integrity [2]. As such, the study of sperm DNA damage becomes highly relevant in the era of ARTs.

The full ramifications of successful fertilization and pregnancy with DNA-damaged spermatozoa are unknown but there is some cause for concern given that sperm DNA damage is common in infertile men and, in experimental studies, sperm DNA damage may be detrimental to the health of the offspring [2,3]. Reassuringly, in a clinical study, sperm DNA fragmentation has not been associated with measurable adverse effects on the health of the child [4]. However, studies have found that children of fathers who smoked cigarettes preconceptually (a habit associated with sperm DNA damage) have a higher risk of developing childhood cancers [5]. Moreover, children of fathers with a history of cancer (a condition associated with sperm DNA damage) have a higher risk of developing a birth defect than a population of children whose fathers do not have cancer [6]. Taken together, these studies suggest a possible link between sperm DNA damage and the subsequent development of childhood diseases, but additional studies are required to corroborate these findings.

To date, numerous tests of sperm chromatin and DNA damage have been developed with the hope that these assays may be useful in predicting natural conception and reproductive outcomes with assisted reproduction. These tests have helped advance our understanding of sperm chromatin architecture and function but their use as specialized biomarkers in the evaluation of the infertile man has not been widely adopted.

23.2 Etiology of Sperm DNA Damage

The etiology human sperm DNA damage is multifactorial. Human sperm DNA damage and defective sperm function may be due to a primary defect in spermatogenesis (e.g., developmental abnormalities, advanced age) or to extrinsic factors resulting in sperm injury within the testicle or the posttesticular environment (e.g., hyperthermia, varicocele, gonadotoxins) [7].

At the molecular and cellular level, a number of pathways leading to sperm DNA damage have been proposed. These pathways include protamine deficiency (leading to aberrant spermatid chromatin remodeling), oxidative stress, and abortive apoptosis [7]. De Iuliis et al. [8] have suggested a two-step model to explain the development of sperm DNA damage. Based on the model, spermatozoa with poor chromatin compaction resulting from incomplete replacement of histones by protamines (first step) are susceptible to injury from oxidative stress (second step). This model suggests that primary testicular and posttesticular events may result in sperm DNA damage.

23.2.1 Defective Spermatogenesis

Experimental studies have demonstrated that targeted disruption of spermatogenesis resulting in impaired sperm chromatin compaction can lead to increased levels of sperm DNA fragmentation and impaired male fertility potential [9]. Clinical studies have also demonstrated that defects in spermatogenesis are associated with increased levels of sperm DNA fragmentation [10]. It has been shown that infertile men with poor semen parameters, a marker of defective spermatogenesis, have higher levels of sperm DNA fragmentation than fertile control with normal sperm parameters [11]. Moreover, the severity of the sperm defects is associated with sperm DNA fragmentation. Men with more severe sperm abnormalities have higher levels of DNA fragmentation than men with milder sperm defects [11]. Altogether, these observations indicate that sperm DNA damage is generally accompanied by other sperm parameter defects.

23.2.2 Aging

Advanced paternal age has been associated with a decline in sperm production and Leydig cell dysfunction. Histologic studies have identified a progressive loss of Sertoli cells, as well as a decrease in the number of spermatids and spermatocytes per Sertoli cell with aging [12]. The germ cell loss associated with aging is believed to be a result of increased germ cell apoptosis. Older men often have reduced fertility and poorer semen parameters than younger men, particularly, reduced semen volume, sperm motility, and sperm morphology [13]. A number of studies have demonstrated a correlation between paternal age and sperm DNA fragmentation [14,15]. In addition to having increased levels of DNA fragmentation, spermatozoa of older men have a greater load of chromosomal aberrations and point mutations than do spermatozoa of younger men [16]. These findings may explain the observation that paternal aging is associated with increased genetic risk to offspring. However, the precise age at which a significant genetic risk exists, and the magnitude of the risk, are unknown [16].

23.2.3 Cancer

Several studies have shown that young men with cancer (e.g., Hodgkin's lymphoma and testicular cancer) will frequently have abnormal sperm parameters and poor sperm chromatin and DNA integrity before any cancer-specific therapy has been initiated [17–19]. This is believed to be due to poor overall health caused by factors such as malnutrition, fever, and pain. These men can then experience cumulative dose- and agent-dependent testicular damage following cancer therapy (chemotherapy, radiation) with a small percentage of men remaining azoospermic years after their treatment [20,21]. The gradual recovery of spermatogenesis is generally observed three to six months after cessation of therapy. However, studies indicate that sperm chromatin and DNA damage may persist beyond that period [19,21]. Several studies have shown that sperm DNA fragmentation is increased after radiation therapy [17,18]. In contrast, there are inconsistent reports regarding the effects of chemotherapy on sperm DNA integrity although most studies have shown that this treatment has a detrimental effect on sperm chromatin compaction [17–19,21]. Sperm fluorescent in situ hybridization studies report an increased rate of sperm chromosomal aneuploidy and diploidy in the first two years following chemotherapy [22,23]. Based on these observations, patients who are scheduled to undergo definitive cancer therapy (surgery, chemotherapy, and/or radiation) are strongly encouraged to cryopreserve sperm before their treatments [24].

23.2.4 Hormonal Deficiency

Some evidence points to hormonal deficiency as a possible cause of sperm chromatin and DNA defects. Using an experimental protocol, investigators examined the effects of follicle-stimulating hormone (FSH) immunization on sperm chromatin integrity in men and monkeys. They demonstrated that in both men and monkeys, FSH immunization resulted in low to undetectable levels of serum FSH, reduced sperm chromatin integrity, and sperm DNA fragmentation [25]. FSH receptor knock-out mice have reduced levels of sperm nuclear protamines, lower testosterone, impaired fertility, and increased levels of sperm DNA damage as compared to wild-type mice [26]. Moreover, serum estradiol and free T4 levels are inversely related to sperm DNA damage in infertile men [27].

23.2.5 Genital Tract Infection

Genital tract infection and inflammation, such as epididymo-orchitis or prostatitis, can cause leukocytospermia, and this pathology has been associated with sperm DNA damage [28,29]. Gallegos et al. reported that infertile men with chlamydia trachomatis and mycoplasma have higher levels of sperm DNA fragmentation than a cohort of fertile controls [30]. These investigators also observed that antibiotic therapy was associated with a significant improvement in sperm morphology and DNA fragmentation but not in sperm concentration and motility. Cortés-Gutiérrez et al. (2016) found that although HPV infection is more common infertile than fertile men, it is not associated with high levels of sperm DNA fragmentation [31].

23.2.6 Varicocele

The influence of varicocele on male fertility has long been debated although most studies have shown that varicocele is associated with abnormal sperm parameters and reduced male fertility potential. Recently, an important cross-sectional, multicenter study of 7,035 young men has provided compelling evidence that the presence of a varicocele is associated with poorer sperm parameters and higher semen FSH levels [32]. Moreover, in the same study, increasing varicocele grade was associated with increasingly poor semen quality (sperm count, progressive motility, and morphology). A large body of literature has demonstrated that varicoceles are associated with sperm DNA damage [33,34]. The sperm DNA damage in men with varicocele is believed to be a result of defective spermatogenesis and oxidative stress [35].

23.2.7 Medications

Much of what we know on the adverse effects of drugs on male fertility is anecdotal or based on small observational studies. Indeed, most of the drugs in use today have been approved before adequate United States Food and Drug Administration (FDA) testing on the effects of these drugs on male reproductive potential.

In the United States, it is estimated that 70–80% of men aged 18–60 are taking prescription or over the counter (OTC) medications [36]. Medication use has increased in the USA, in part due to the increased prevalence of obesity and obesity-related metabolic disorders (e.g., diabetes, hypertension). Moreover, the paternal (and maternal) age of couples seeking to have their first child is increasing and with this so is the use of medications [37]. The most commonly utilized prescription drugs in young men are antidepressants, lipid-lowering agents, and analgesics. Other drugs used by this age group include antihypertensives, antidiabetics, and 5-alpha reductase inhibitors.

Studies have reported that the selective serotonin reuptake inhibitors (SSRIs, a class of drugs commonly used to treat depression) may have an adverse effect on conventional sperm parameters [38]. Moreover, several studies have shown that use of SSRI is associated with sperm DNA fragmentation [38,39]. The detrimental impact on sperm DNA integrity was seen with several SSRIs (citalopram, escitalopram, fluoxetine, paroxetine, and sertraline) and is believed to be a posttesticular phenomenon based on the observed effect in relation to the timing of drug intaking.

Studies have shown that most opioid analgesics increase serum prolactin and decrease serum testosterone levels with little known about the effect of these agents on semen parameters. There are no studies on the effects of nonsteroidal anti-inflammatory drugs and acetylsalicylic acid on male fertility potential, but animal studies show that these agents do not have significant effects on semen parameters. However, use of paracetamol (acetaminophen) has been associated with reduced sperm parameters and increased sperm DNA fragmentation in humans.

The limited studies on lipid-lowering agents have shown that use of these drugs is associated with a mild decrease in serum testosterone levels. Although there are no human studies on the effect of these drugs on sperm parameters and/or DNA integrity, animal studies have reported that these agents do not have an adverse effect on semen parameters. Similarly, there are limited studies on the effect of antihypertensives on male reproductive function with no studies on sperm DNA damage.

5-alpha-reductase inhibitors (5ARIs) may cause impaired semen quality, in particular, total sperm count. Younger men taking ARIs for male pattern baldness will use a lower ARI dosage (1 mg) than that used by older men to treat benign prostatic hyperplasia (5 mg). At the 1 mg dosage, finasteride does not appear to affect sperm concentration. However, in infertile men with low sperm concentration, discontinuation of 5ARIs has been associated with a significant increase in sperm concentration [40].

23.2.8 Lifestyle Factors

Cigarette smoking and alcohol consumption are common habits with known detrimental effects on general health. However, the evidence on the impact of these factors on male fertility potential and sperm quality is conflicting. To date, most studies on cigarette smoking and sperm quality suggest that smokers have poorer sperm parameters than nonsmokers [41]. Cigarette smoking has also been associated with increased sperm DNA damage and it is postulated that smoking causes increased leukocyte-derived reactive oxygen species production with subsequent adverse effects on mature sperm [42]. Smoking may also alter the sperm protamine 1 to protamine 2 ratio and the level of sperm DNA methylation, suggesting an intratesticular effect [43,44].

A number of studies have examined the effect of alcohol consumption and generally suggest that heavy alcohol consumption (>2 drinks per day) in infertile men is associated with poor sperm parameters [45]. Moreover, alcohol consumption in these men is also associated with higher levels of sperm DNA fragmentation [45]. Interestingly, low or moderate alcohol consumption has not been associated with adverse effects on sperm quality [45].

23.2.9 Testicular Hyperthermia

Studies have shown that significant testicular hyperthermia (>40°C) can impair spermatogenesis, whereas milder hyperthermia (38°C) results in minimal disruption of spermatogenesis. Experimental studies have clearly shown that sustained testicular hyperthermia (40–42°C) causes sperm DNA damage, as well as an increase in the histone to protamine ratio [46]. In humans, sperm DNA fragmentation is increased at ~20–30 days after a mild-moderate induced hyperthermia (39°C). Clinically, certain behaviors (e.g., hot baths, saunas) and occupations (e.g., welders, bakers, prolonged driving) have been associated with increased scrotal temperatures and an association between hyperthermia and reduced male fertility potential has been demonstrated [47]. However, it is unclear whether common behavioral or occupational testicular hyperthermia (e.g., drivers, tight underwear) can lead to impaired spermatogenesis and sperm DNA damage.

23.2.10 Environmental Factors

Most studies have shown that outdoor air pollution may affect semen quality, primarily motility and morphology [48]. Moreover, these studies have found that air pollution exposure may have a detrimental effect on sperm DNA integrity [48]. Nonetheless, the evidence remains inconclusive largely because the individual estimate of exposure may be inaccurate, studies often include cases that have had a single semen analysis, and there is little known about co-exposure. Exposure to lead and pesticides (organophosphates) has been shown to adversely impact male and female fertility, with couples experiencing a prolonged time to pregnancy [49]. Moreover, there is some evidence to show that exposure to lead, phthalates, and PCBs (polychlorinated biphenyls) is associated with sperm DNA damage. However, the evidence regarding exposure to benzophenones and BPA on male fertility and sperm function remains inconclusive.

23.3 Clinical Aspects of Sperm DNA Tests

23.3.1 Relationship between Sperm DNA Test Results and Reproductive Outcomes

Over the past 20 years, investigators have examined the relationship between sperm DNA damage and reproductive outcomes. These studies have shown that sperm DNA damage is associated with lower rates of natural and intrauterine insemination (IUI) pregnancies. Couples with sperm DNA damage have low potential for natural fertility and a prolonged time to pregnancy [50]. A recent meta-analysis has shown that sperm DNA damage is associated with lower IUI pregnancy rate (relative risk = 3.2, 95% CI: 1.4–6.79; I2 = 13.1%) but the sperm DNA test has a limited capacity in predicting IUI outcome, and therefore, a limited value in the management of these couples [51]. Systematic reviews and meta-analyses of studies relating DNA damage and assisted reproduction outcomes indicate that sperm DNA damage is associated (albeit weakly) with IVF and IVF/ICSI pregnancy rates [52]. Nonetheless, tests of sperm DNA fragmentation have limited capacity to discriminate between couples who have a low chance to conceive and those who have a high chance to conceive after assisted reproduction [53].

One of the most interesting observations regarding sperm DNA damage and assisted reproduction is the association with increased risk of pregnancy loss after both standard IVF and IVF/ICSI [54]. In line with these findings, numerous reports have shown an association between sperm DNA fragmentation and recurrent miscarriages. A meta-analysis of 13 prospective studies suggests that male partners of women with a history of recurrent pregnancy loss have a significantly higher mean sperm DNA fragmentation level compared to partners of fertile control women (mean difference 11.91, 95% CI 4.97–18.86) [55].

23.3.2 Indications for Sperm DNA Testing

Although the use of sperm DNA fragmentation tests in clinical practice appears promising, testing has not gained wide approval and remains controversial. One of the major concerns regarding these tests is the fact that there are multiple assays, with each assay detecting different sites of sperm DNA damage [56]. Moreover, there are no standardized protocols for many of these assays and little is known about the precision of the assays due to a lack of reproducibility studies (intra- and interlaboratory). Another important shortcoming is the fact that the clinical thresholds for many of these tests have not been adequately validated. Finally, most of the clinical studies are retrospective, relatively small (many studies reported on 100–200 ART cycles) with heterogeneous study characteristics, and most fail to demonstrate the predictive value of these tests.

Based on the observed relationship between DNA damage and reproductive outcomes, some investigators have proposed that tests of sperm DNA fragmentation be used as predictors of natural and ART pregnancies and to guide treatment of infertile couples. There is some evidence that sperm DNA tests are used frequently in the clinical management of infertile couples [57], although the routine application of these tests in clinical practice has not been advocated largely due to the shortcomings of these assays [58]. However, there are specific clinical settings where sperm DNA testing may be useful. Sperm DNA testing may be valuable in couples with recurrent pregnancy loss and in those with unexplained recurrent IVF/ICSI failures to determine if a male factor may be responsible and to provide appropriate therapy in these couples [59]. Sperm DNA testing may also be useful in couples with clinical varicocele and borderline normal semen parameters and those with unexplained infertility [59]. Nonetheless, to date, the level of evidence supporting the use of sperm DNA testing in the management of couple infertility and as a predictor of reproductive outcomes remains modest.

23.4 Treatment of Sperm DNA Damage

Much like abnormal semen parameters, sperm DNA damage is a marker of male factor infertility and it has been associated with numerous potentially correctable medical and surgical pathologies. Treatment of sperm DNA damage consists of identifying and correcting male factors. Ultimately, treating a specific male factor may improve fertility potential, as well as sperm DNA integrity. In particular, therapies or procedures that alleviate oxidative stress, a condition known to induce sperm DNA damage, may improve sperm DNA integrity.

23.4.1 Varicocelectomy

Studies of young, healthy men have shown that varicoceles are associated with poor semen quality [32]. Moreover, it has been shown that higher varicocele grade is associated with poorer semen parameters than lower grade varicocele. Several studies of noninfertility populations have also shown that varicoceles are associated with sperm DNA damage. In a number of these reports, the presence of varicocele was specifically associated with oxidative sperm DNA damage suggesting that varicocele may induce sperm DNA damage through increased oxidative stress.

There are now multiple studies showing that varicocelectomy for the management of infertile men with a clinical varicocele and abnormal semen parameters is associated with a reduction in sperm DNA fragmentation levels [33,34]. Moreover, following varicocelectomy, oxidative stress levels are reduced. These findings build on the evidence demonstrating a beneficial effect of varicocele repair on pregnancy rates [60] and provide additional evidence in support of the adverse effect of varicocele on sperm DNA integrity [33,34].

23.4.2 Hormonal Therapy

Based on experimental studies showing that neutralizing circulating anti-FSH antibodies impair sperm quality, clinicians have hoped to treat hormonal deficiency with FSH therapy with the aim of improving semen parameters [25]. A meta-analysis of randomized, double-blind, placebo-controlled studies has found that FSH administration improves natural pregnancy outcomes in couples with idiopathic oligozoospermia [61]. A positive influence of rFSH on sperm chromatin condensation was initially described in a randomized, double-blind, placebo-controlled study involving 67 men [62]. Subsequent studies have also demonstrated an improvement in sperm DNA integrity following three months of FSH therapy [63].

23.4.3 Antioxidant Therapy

Numerous studies have demonstrated a strong relationship between oxidative stress and defective sperm function [8]. Antioxidants have been used in the management of infertile men in view of countering the oxidative stress in the semen of these men and improving couple fertility. A meta-analysis of randomized, double-blind, placebo-controlled studies has shown that the use of antioxidants in infertile men may improve semen parameters and spontaneous pregnancy rate [64]. However, the heterogeneity of these studies is such that a definitive conclusion regarding the effect of AOX therapy in these couples cannot be reached [64].

23.4.4 Short Abstinence

It has been postulated that prolonged epididymal storage may increase sperm oxidative stress leading to sperm dysfunction and DNA damage. This has prompted investigators to evaluate short abstinence time (one-day abstinence) as a way to reduce sperm DNA fragmentation in whole semen. Although a number of studies have reported a reduction in sperm DNA fragmentation with short abstinence, this has not been demonstrated in all studies [65]. As such, this strategy has not been accepted universally as a means of improving sperm DNA fragmentation.

23.4.5 Advanced Sperm Processing Techniques

A number of specialized sperm sorting techniques have been developed in the hope that they may allow for selection of a highly functional sperm fraction. These techniques have generally been effective in selecting a population of sperm with lower levels of DNA fragmentation than neat semen. However, these techniques require technical expertise, as well as additional materials and costs. Moreover, they require lengthier sperm incubation. The specialized separation techniques include hyaluronic acid binding, annexin-V binding, electrophoretic separation, and microfluidic separation.

To date, the application of specialized sperm sorting techniques has not consistently resulted in a significant improvement in ICSI pregnancy rates compared to ICSI with spermatozoa obtained by conventional sperm separation techniques (e.g., density gradient centrifugation and swim-up). A possible explanation as to why these techniques fail to improve pregnancy outcomes is the understanding that most spermatozoa from samples with high sperm DNA fragmentation demonstrate some degree of DNA damage such that the spermatozoa recovered following sperm separation will also possess a measurable degree of DNA damage [66,67].

23.4.6 Use of Testicular Sperm for ICSI in Men with High Levels of Sperm DNA Fragmentation

The advent of ICSI revolutionized the management of male factor infertility, in particular, the treatment of couples with severe male factor infertility. However, it later became evident that ICSI may not overcome significant sperm abnormalities [68]. Moreover, there is some concern that infertile men with abnormal semen parameters could have an underlying sperm genetic defect with a potential adverse impact on ICSI outcomes, including a higher risk of miscarriage [52].

In 2005, Greco et al. reported higher pregnancy rates with ICSI when using testicular rather than ejaculated sperm in couples with sperm DNA damage and observed a lower frequency of sperm showing detectable DNA damage in testicular versus ejaculated sperm [69]. They hypothesized that the DNA damage in ejaculated sperm begins after spermatozoa are released from Sertoli cells and suggested that the poorer outcome with ejaculated sperm was a result of acquired DNA damage during transit through the epididymis or possibly during ejaculation. In the same year, Suganuma et al. [9] conducted experimental studies using an animal model with abnormal spermatogenesis and incomplete sperm nuclear compaction to test the hypothesis proposed by Greco et al. (2005) [69]. They observed that in animals with abnormal spermatogenesis the passage of sperm through the epididymis was associated with a loss of sperm DNA integrity and fertilizing capacity [9]. They proposed that in some men (i.e., those with defective spermatogenesis) the passage of sperm through the epididymis could result in a loss of sperm DNA integrity and fertilizing capacity.

The idea that the posttesticular environment or epididymal transit can induce sperm damage has led clinicians to utilize testicular rather than ejaculated sperm for ICSI in men with abnormal spermatogenesis and poor sperm DNA integrity. To date, several prospective and retrospective studies have supported the findings of Greco et al. (2005) [69] and have demonstrated higher pregnancy rates with ICSI when using testicular rather than ejaculated sperm in couples with sperm DNA damage [70]. Moreover, several studies have observed a lower mean sperm DNA fragmentation in testicular versus ejaculated sperm, in men with sperm DNA fragmentation. However, studies on the use of testicular rather than ejaculated sperm in couples with sperm DNA damage are small and nonrandomized. As such, the evidence in favor of testicular sperm in these men remains modest. Clearly, large, randomized studies are needed before we can demonstrate a true benefit of testicular rather than ejaculated sperm for ICSI in couples with sperm DNA fragmentation.

23.5 Summary

Sperm chromatin and DNA integrity tests have provided us with a better understanding of spermatogenesis, male infertility, and reproductive biology. Studies have shown that the etiology of human sperm DNA damage is multi-factorial.

Genetic and developmental abnormalities, advancing age, gonadotoxins, hyperthermia, varicocele, medications, and endocrine abnormalities have been associated with sperm DNA damage. In experimental studies, sperm DNA fragmentation impairs male fertility potential indicating that sperm genetic integrity is critical for normal reproduction. Clinical studies have also suggested that sperm DNA damage is associated with poorer reproductive outcomes (spontaneous and assisted) and, based on this observation, investigators have proposed that tests of sperm DNA fragmentation be used as predictors of natural and ART pregnancies and to guide treatment of infertile couples. Studies have shown that sperm DNA testing may be particularly valuable in couples with recurrent pregnancy loss and in those with unexplained recurrent IVF/ICSI failures to determine if a male factor may be responsible and to provide appropriate therapy in these cases. Nonetheless, there are some concerns regarding the robustness of sperm DNA assays. Moreover, the level of evidence supporting the use of sperm DNA testing in the management of couple infertility remains modest.

References

1. Cooper TG, Noonan E, von Eckardstein S, et al. World Health Organization reference values for human semen characteristics. *Hum Reprod Update.* 2010;16(3):231–245.
2. Vinnakota C, Cree L, Peek J, Morbeck DE. Incidence of high sperm DNA fragmentation in a targeted population of subfertile men. *Syst Biol Reprod Med.* 2019;65(6):451–457.
3. Fernández-Gonzalez R, Moreira PN, Pérez-Crespo M, et al. Long-term effects of mouse intracytoplasmic sperm injection with DNA-fragmented sperm on health and behavior of adult offspring. *Biol Reprod.* 2008;78(4):761–772.
4. Bungum M, Bungum L, Lynch KF, Wedlund L, Humaidan P, Giwercman A. Spermatozoa DNA damage measured by sperm chromatin structure assay (SCSA) and birth characteristics in children conceived by IVF and ICSI. *Int J Androl.* 2012;35(4):485–490.
5. Ji BT, Shu XO, Linet MS, et al. Paternal cigarette smoking and the risk of childhood cancer among offspring of nonsmoking mothers. *J Natl Cancer Inst.* 1997;89(3):238–244.
6. Al-Jebari Y, Glimelius I, Berglund Nord C, et al. Cancer therapy and risk of congenital malformations in children fathered by men treated for testicular germ-cell cancer: a nationwide register study. *PLoS Med.* 2019;16(6):e1002816.
7. Zini A, Sigman M. Are tests of sperm DNA damage clinically useful? Pros and cons. *J Androl.* 2009;30(3):219–229.
8. De Iuliis GN, Thomson LK, Mitchell LA, et al. DNA damage in human spermatozoa is highly correlated with the efficiency of chromatin remodeling and the formation of 8-hydroxy-2'-deoxyguanosine, a marker of oxidative stress. *Biol Reprod.* 2009;81(3):517–524.
9. Suganuma R, Yanagimachi R, Meistrich ML. Decline in fertility of mouse sperm with abnormal chromatin during epididymal passage as revealed by ICSI. *Hum Reprod.* 2005;20(11):3101–3108.
10. Muratori M, Marchiani S, Tamburrino L, Baldi E. Sperm DNA fragmentation: mechanisms of origin. *Adv Exp Med Biol.* 2019;1166:75–85.
11. Moskovtsev SI, Willis J, White J, Mullen JB. Sperm DNA damage: correlation to severity of semen abnormalities. *Urology.* 2009;74(4):789–793.
12. Johnson L. Spermatogenesis and aging in the human. *J Androl.* 1986;7(6):331–354.
13. Sartorius GA, Nieschlag E. Paternal age and reproduction. *Hum Reprod Update.* 2010;16(1):65–79.
14. Belloc S, Benkhalifa M, Cohen-Bacrie M, Dalleac A, Amar E, Zini A. Sperm DNA damage in normozoospermic men is related to age and sperm progressive motility. *Fertil Steril.* 2014;101(6):1588–1593.
15. Wyrobek AJ, Eskenazi B, Young S, et al. Advancing age has differential effects on DNA damage, chromatin integrity, gene mutations, and aneuploidies in sperm. *Proc Natl Acad Sci U S A.* 2006;103(25):9601–9606.
16. Yatsenko AN, Turek PJ. Reproductive genetics and the aging male. *J Assist Reprod Genet.* 2018;35(6):933–941.
17. Smit M, van Casteren NJ, Wildhagen MF, Romijn JC, Dohle GR. Sperm DNA integrity in cancer patients before and after cytotoxic treatment. *Hum Reprod.* 2010;25(8):1877–1883.
18. Ståhl O, Eberhard J, Cavallin-Ståhl E, et al. Sperm DNA integrity in cancer patients: the effect of disease and treatment. *Int J Androl.* 2009;32(6):695–703.
19. Bujan L, Walschaerts M, Moinard N, et al. Impact of chemotherapy and radiotherapy for testicular germ cell tumors on spermatogenesis and sperm DNA: a multicenter prospective study from the CECOS network. *Fertil Steril.* 2013;100(3):673–680.
20. Brydøy M, Fosså SD, Klepp O, et al. Norwegian Urology Cancer Group (NUCG) III study group. Sperm counts and endocrinological markers of spermatogenesis in long-term survivors of testicular cancer. *Br J Cancer.* 2012;107(11):1833–1839.
21. Paoli D, Gallo M, Rizzo F, et al. Testicular cancer and sperm DNA damage: short- and long-term effects of antineoplastic treatment. *Andrology.* 2015;3(1):122–128.
22. Robbins WA, Meistrich ML, Moore D, et al. Chemotherapy induces transient sex chromosomal and autosomal aneuploidy in human sperm. *Nat Genet.* 1997;16(1):74–78.
23. Martin RH, Ernst S, Rademaker A, et al. Chromosomal abnormalities in sperm from testicular cancer patients before and after chemotherapy. *Hum Genet.* 1997;99(2):214–218.
24. Lee SJ, Schover LR, Partridge AH, et al. American Society of Clinical Oncology recommendations on fertility preservation in cancer patients. *J Clin Oncol.* 2006;24(18):2917–2931.
25. Krishnamurthy H, Kumar KM, Joshi CV, Krishnamurthy HN, Moudgal RN, Sairam MR. Alterations in sperm characteristics of follicle-stimulating hormone (FSH)-immunized men are similar to those of FSH-deprived infertile male bonnet monkeys. *J Androl.* 2000;21(2):316–327.
26. Xing W, Krishnamurthy H, Sairam MR. Role of follitropin receptor signaling in nuclear protein transitions and chromatin condensation during

spermatogenesis. *Biochem Biophys Res Commun.* 2003;312(3):697–701.

27. Meeker JD, Singh NP, Hauser R. Serum concentrations of estradiol and free T4 are inversely correlated with sperm DNA damage in men from an infertility clinic. *J Androl.* 2008;29(4):379–388.

28. Erenpreiss J, Hlevicka S, Zalkalns J, Erenpreisa J. Effect of leukocytospermia on sperm DNA integrity: a negative effect in abnormal semen samples. *J Androl.* 2002;23(5):717–723.

29. La Vignera S, Condorelli R, D'Agata R, Vicari E, Calogero AE. Semen alterations and flow-citometry evaluation in patients with male accessory gland infections. *J Endocrinol Invest.* 2012;35(2):219–223.

30. Gallegos G, Ramos B, Santiso R, Goyanes V, Gosálvez J, Fernández JL. Sperm DNA fragmentation in infertile men with genitourinary infection by chlamydia trachomatis and mycoplasma. *Fertil Steril.* 2008;90(2):328–334.

31. Cortés-Gutiérrez EI, Dávila-Rodríguez MI, Fernández JL, de la O-Pérez LO, Garza-Flores ME, Eguren-Garza R, Gosálvez J. The presence of human papillomavirus in semen does not affect the integrity of sperm DNA. *Andrologia.* 2017;49(10):e12774.

32. Damsgaard J, Joensen UN, Carlsen E, et al. Varicocele is associated with impaired semen quality and reproductive hormone levels: a study of 7035 healthy young men from six European countries. *Eur Urol.* 2016;70(6):1019–1029.

33. Zini A, Dohle G. Are varicoceles associated with increased deoxyribonucleic acid fragmentation? *Fertil Steril.* 2011;96(6):1283–1287.

34. Roque M, Esteves SC. Effect of varicocele repair on sperm DNA fragmentation: a review. *Int Urol Nephrol.* 2018;50(4):583–603.

35. Smith R, Kaune H, Parodi D, et al. Increased sperm DNA damage in patients with varicocele: relationship with seminal oxidative stress. *Hum Reprod.* 2006;21(4):986–993.

36. Kaufman DW, Kelly JP, Rosenberg L, Anderson TE, Mitchell AA. Effect of prescriber education on the use of medications contraindicated in older adults in a managed Medicare population. *JAMA.* 2002;287(3):337–344.

37. Kantor ED, Rehm CD, Haas JS, Chan AT, Giovannucci EL. Trends in prescription drug use among adults in the United States from 1999–2012. *JAMA.* 2015;314(17):1818–1831.

38. Safarinejad MR. Sperm DNA damage and semen quality impairment after treatment with selective serotonin reuptake inhibitors detected using semen analysis and sperm chromatin structure assay. *J Urol.* 2008;180(5):2124–2128.

39. Tanrikut C, Feldman AS, Altemus M, Paduch DA, Schlegel PN. Adverse effect of paroxetine on sperm. *Fertil Steril.* 2010;94(3):1021–1026.

40. Samplaski MK, Lo K, Grober E, Jarvi K. Finasteride use in the male infertility population: effects on semen and hormone parameters. *Fertil Steril.* 2013;100(6):1542–1546.

41. Sharma R, Harlev A, Agarwal A, Esteves SC. Cigarette smoking and semen quality: a new meta-analysis examining the effect of the 2010 World Health Organization Laboratory Methods for the Examination of Human Semen. *Eur Urol.* 2016;70(4):635–645.

42. Fraga CG, Motchnik PA, Wyrobek AJ, Rempel DM, Ames BN. Smoking and low antioxidant levels increase oxidative damage to sperm DNA. *Mutat Res.* 1996;351(2):199–203.

43. Jenkins TG, James ER, Alonso DF, et al. Cigarette smoking significantly alters sperm DNA methylation patterns. *Andrology.* 2017;5(6):1089–1099.

44. Hammadeh ME, Hamad MF, Montenarh M, Fischer-Hammadeh C. Protamine contents and P1/P2 ratio in human spermatozoa from smokers and non-smokers. *Hum Reprod.* 2010;25(11):2708–2720.

45. Boeri L, Capogrosso P, Ventimiglia E, et al. Heavy cigarette smoking and alcohol consumption are associated with impaired sperm parameters in primary infertile men. *Asian J Androl.* 2019;21(5):478–485.

46. Sailer BL, Sarkar LJ, Bjordahl JA, Jost LK, Evenson DP. Effects of heat stress on mouse testicular cells and sperm chromatin structure. *J Androl.* 1997;18(3):294–301.

47. Thonneau P, Bujan L, Multigner L, Mieusset R. Occupational heat exposure and male fertility: a review. *Hum Reprod.* 1998;13(8):2122–2125.

48. Jurewicz J, Dziewirska E, Radwan M, Hanke W. Air pollution from natural and anthropic sources and male fertility. *Reprod Biol Endocrinol.* 2018;16(1):109.

49. Snijder CA, te Velde E, Roeleveld N, Burdorf A. Occupational exposure to chemical substances and time to pregnancy: a systematic review. *Hum Reprod Update.* 2012;18(3):284–300.

50. Spano M, Bonde JP, Hjollund HI, Kolstad HA, Cordelli E, Leter G. Sperm chromatin damage impairs human fertility. The Danish First Pregnancy Planner Study Team. *Fertil Steril.* 2000;73:43–50.

51. Sugihara A, Van Avermaete F, Roelant E, Punjabi U, De Neubourg D. The role of sperm DNA fragmentation testing in predicting intra-uterine insemination outcome: a systematic review and meta-analysis. *Eur J Obstet Gynecol Reprod Biol.* 2020;244:8–15.

52. Simon L, Zini A, Dyachenko A, Ciampi A, Carrell DT. A systematic review and meta-analysis to determine the effect of sperm DNA damage on in vitro fertilization and intracytoplasmic sperm injection outcome. *Asian J Androl.* 2017;19:80–90.

53. Cissen M, Wely MV, Scholten I, et al. Measuring sperm DNA fragmentation and clinical outcomes of medically assisted reproduction: a systematic review and meta-analysis. *PLoS ONE.* 2016;11(11):e0165125.

54. Zini A, Boman J, Belzile E, Ciampi A. Sperm DNA damage is associated with an increased risk of pregnancy loss after IVF and ICSI: systematic review and meta-analysis. *Hum Reprod.* 2008;23:2663–2668.

55. McQueen DB, Zhang J, Robins JC. Sperm DNA fragmentation and recurrent pregnancy loss: a systematic review and meta-analysis. *Fertil Steril.* 2019;112(1):54–60.e3.

56. Gawecka JE, Boaz S, Kasperson K, Nguyen H, Evenson DP, Ward WS. Luminal fluid of epididymis and vas deferens contributes to sperm chromatin fragmentation. *Hum Reprod.* 2015;30(12):2725–2736.

57. Majzoub A, Agarwal A, Cho CL, Esteves SC. Sperm DNA fragmentation testing: a cross sectional survey on current practices of fertility specialists. *Transl Androl Urol.* 2017;6(Suppl. 4):S710–S719.

58. Practice Committee of the American Society for Reproductive Medicine. The clinical utility of sperm DNA integrity testing: a guideline. *Fertil Steril*. 2013;99(3):673–677.
59. Agarwal A, Majzoub A, Esteves SC, Ko E, Ramasamy R, Zini A. Clinical utility of sperm DNA fragmentation testing: practice recommendations based on clinical scenarios. *Transl Androl Urol*. 2016;5(6):935–950.
60. Kroese ACJ, de Lange NM, Collins J, Evers JLH. Surgery or embolization for varicoceles in subfertile men. *Cochrane Database Syst Rev*. 2012;10:CD000479.
61. Attia AM, Abou-Setta AM, Al-Inany HG. Gonadotrophins for idiopathic male factor subfertility. *Cochrane Database Syst Rev*. 2013;23(8):CD005071.
62. Kamischke A, Behre HM, Bergmann M, Simoni M, Schäfer T, Nieschlag E. Recombinant human follicle stimulating hormone for treatment of male idiopathic infertility: a randomized, double-blind, placebo-controlled, clinical trial. *Hum Reprod*. 1998;13(3):596–603.
63. Santi D, Spaggiari G, Simoni M. Sperm DNA fragmentation index as a promising predictive tool for male infertility diagnosis and treatment management: meta-analyses. *Reprod Biomed Online*. 2018;37(3):315–326.
64. Smits RM, Mackenzie-Proctor R, Yazdani A, Stankiewicz MT, Jordan V, Showell MG. Antioxidants for male subfertility. *Cochrane Database Syst Rev*. 2019;3(3):CD007411.
65. Hanson BM, Aston KI, Jenkins TG, Carrell DT, Hotaling JM. The impact of ejaculatory abstinence on semen analysis parameters: a systematic review. *J Assist Reprod Genet*. 2018;35(2):213–220.
66. Ramos L, De Boer P, Meuleman EJ, Braat DD, Wetzels AM. Evaluation of ICSI-selected epididymal sperm samples of obstructive azoospermic males by the CKIA system. *J Androl*. 2004;25(3):406–411.
67. Said TM, Land JA. Effects of advanced selection methods on sperm quality and ART outcome: a systematic review. *Hum Reprod Update*. 2011;17(6):719–733.
68. Strassburger D, Friedler S, Raziel A, Schachter M, Kasterstein E, Ron-el R. Very low sperm count affects the result of intracytoplasmic sperm injection. *J Assist Reprod Genet*. 2000;17(8):431–436.
69. Greco E, Scarselli F, Lacobelli M, et al. Efficient treatment of infertility due to sperm DNA damage by ICSI with testicular spermatozoa. *Hum Reprod*. 2005;20(1):226–230.
70. Esteves SC, Roque M, Bradley CK, Garrido N. Reproductive outcomes of testicular versus ejaculated sperm for intracytoplasmic sperm injection among men with high levels of DNA fragmentation in semen: systematic review and meta-analysis. *Fertil Steril*. 2017;108(3):456–467.

Section 4: Laboratory Evaluation and Treatment of Male Infertility

Chapter 24: The Current Use of Sperm Function Assays

Sara Marchiani and Elisabetta Baldi

24.1 Introduction

When a couple has trouble conceiving, the primary diagnostic tool for assessment of male fertility status is routine semen analysis that evaluates macroscopic (pH, volume, viscosity, aspect, etc.) and microscopic (sperm count, motility, and morphology) semen characteristics. However, semen analysis is poorly predictive of natural and assisted reproduction outcomes, diagnosing less than 50% of male infertility cases [1] and classifying most of them as idiopathic. Hence, there is a growing need to find tests able to evaluate the fertilization competency of spermatozoa. Until some years ago, the research on male reproduction has been little sustained because infertility was considered almost an exclusively female problem. In addition, the advent of assisted reproductive technologies (ART; in particular the increased use of intracytoplasmic sperm injection, ICSI) has been considered a remedy to overcome most problems related to male factor. However, the fact that the reproductive status is now considered an indicator of the general health of an individual [2], the increased use of gamete donation in assisted reproduction, and the relatively little knowledge about possible long-term consequences of IVF/ICSI, has aroused a greater interest in research in sperm biology.

There is still debate about the safety of ART techniques. There is evidence that children born after IVF/ICSI have an increased risk of birth defects compared with those born after natural conception [3]. Whether such defects are due to deficiencies in ART sperm selection, that are not prevalent in natural sperm selection during natural conception [4], problems occurring during laboratory manipulation of gametes and embryo [5], or intrinsic defects present in the gametes, remains to be disclosed. However, the fact that birth defects become evident in ICSI babies after adjustment for female factor [6] and that most defects found in ICSI children at 5 years of age are in the urogenital tract [7] indicates that intrinsic sperm defects or genetic factors present in the male partner may be involved. In addition, evidence suggests that the health of future generations may be influenced epigenetically by the sperm quality of their fathers. Therefore, development and use of tests able to assess the ability of sperm to fertilize and to support a correct embryo growth could provide important benefits, enabling more personalized approaches to achieve pregnancy and to improve male fertility.

After ejaculation, spermatozoa acquire the competence to reach and fertilize the oocyte during transit in the female genital tract, or, in vitro, by incubation in appropriate media. In particular, spermatozoa undergo the process of capacitation, during which they acquire hyperactivated motility (necessary to penetrate oocyte vestments) and the ability to undergo acrosomal exocytosis in response to stimuli present in the proximity of the oocyte. In addition, spermatozoa must be capable to fuse with oolemma and to activate the oocyte by releasing the so-called sperm factor. Finally, to support correct embryo development, the fertilizing spermatozoa must deliver an intact paternal genome. Since each of the above steps/sperm characteristics is crucial to obtain oocyte fertilization and subsequent correct embryo development, it would be ideal to evaluate all these aspects by a single assay. At present, we have available several assays assessing sperm functions necessary for oocyte fertilization. However, although some of these tests are promising, only a few of them have been introduced into clinical practice, mostly because they are difficult to execute or because they require expensive technology.

In this chapter, the most promising current tests assessing sperm function (Figure 24.1) are described, highlighting the data on their validity present so far in the literature, their limitations, and their possible future use in clinical practice.

24.2 Main Assays Evaluating Sperm Function

24.2.1 Assays to Evaluate Sperm Capacitation

Much attention has focused on the capacitation process, which allows the spermatozoon to become competent to fertilize in response to stimuli present in the female reproductive tract [8]. Among the main events that occur during capacitation, the changes in membrane fluidity, the redistribution of specific membrane component, the influx of calcium, and the increase of protein tyrosine phosphorylation have been exploited to develop functional assays. Basal and progesterone-stimulated intracellular calcium levels [9] may be used as an index of occurrence of capacitation. A test based on progesterone-stimulated intracellular calcium levels, developed some years ago [10] and one, more recent, based on the evaluation of sperm membrane potential [11] demonstrated good predictive values of oocyte fertilization in vitro. However, such tests are not easy to perform, require skilled personnel, and necessitate expensive equipment.

Recently a novel test detecting the sperm capacitation status (the Cap-Score Male Fertility Assay) has been developed. Such a test is based on recent findings in murine and bovine

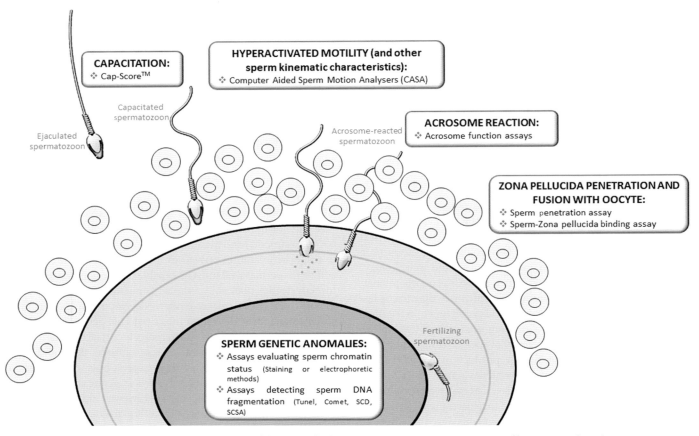

Figure 24.1 Schematic representation of the main steps of the oocyte fertilization process (capacitation, acquisition of hyperactivated motility, acrosome reaction, zona pellucida penetration, fusion with oocyte, and transmission of safe paternal genome). For each step, the most promising assays are indicated, as described in the text.

spermatozoa, demonstrating that the localization of the ganglioside GM1, part of the membrane microdomains, could quantify spermatozoa able to fertilize [12]. In human spermatozoa, GM1 localization is indicative of a capacitated status and identifies also the cells that undergo acrosome exocytosis induced by calcium ionophores [13] or by the physiological stimulus progesterone [14]. The percentage of capacitated spermatozoa determined by the specific pattern of GM1 localization has been used to develop the Cap-Score Male Fertility Assay. In particular, spermatozoa that show an apical GM1 localization in the head identify a capacitated status whereas a posterior GM1 localization indicates a noncapacitated condition. It has been demonstrated that the percentage of capacitated spermatozoa determined by GM1 localization (Cap-Score™) differed between fertile and subfertile men, and retrospectively, between men that achieved a pregnancy after intrauterine insemination (IUI) and those that failed [15]. Interestingly, Cap-Score is not related to conventional semen parameters and it is highly reproducible among ejaculates within a man [15]. All these results have been confirmed in a recent multicenter, prospective observational study [16], where it has been demonstrated also that Cap-Score prospectively predicts IUI outcome and that impaired or reduced capacitation ability was highly prevalent in men questioning their fertility, although with normal semen analysis.

The Cap-Score test is easy to perform, does not require expensive technology, and is commercially available in the USA; however, its results could be influenced by several factors occurring before, during, and after semen sample collection and preparation. Therefore, it must be stressed that this assay should not be used as the sole criterion in the evaluation of male fertility status, but it should be interpreted in the context of both semen analysis and a complete medical workup of both partners. The addition of Cap-Score values in the diagnosis of male fertility could help the clinician in the counseling of a couple on what could be the best intervention to adopt, especially in cases where an IUI is a possible choice for the couple.

24.2.2 Assays to Evaluate Sperm Hyperactivation

In order to penetrate oocyte vestments, spermatozoa must develop a particular type of motility, characterized by disordered movements of the flagellum and the head and vigorous beats. Such type of motility, known as hyperactivated, can be evaluated by computer-aided sperm analysis (CASA).

CASA technology was developed at the end of the 1980s in order to analyse sperm movement and kinematics and it had great success for implementation of research in this field, being user-friendly and producing a large amount of objective data in a short time. The CASA system can be used also to assess sperm concentration and motility parameters in many animal species, allowing its application in animal breeding and reproductive toxicology. In addition, it can provide measures of different sperm parameters that cannot be evaluated by optical microscopy. However, its use in the clinical assessment of human semen quality has had little success, since the current generation of CASA instruments do not provide accurate and reproducible values for sperm concentration and percentage of motile spermatozoa, not distinguishing debris or other cells present in semen from male gametes [17]. Instead, CASA results are quite reliable when selected or washed semen samples, where contamination with other cells or debris is absent or highly reduced, are analysed. Until a few years ago, the technical limit of CASA instruments in evaluating sperm motility was tracking the movement of the sperm head instead of the flagellum [18]. This implied several problems in discriminating motile spermatozoa from immotile or from other nonsperm objects. The implementation of the technology over the years has allowed more parameters to be analyzed and the quality of the sperm sample to be defined more accurately. Moreover, the introduction of detection of the flagellar movement also improved the accuracy of digital image analysis. These new CASA instruments are more reliable for evaluation of hyperactivated motility and integrate the possibility of evaluating other sperm characteristics such as viability, DNA fragmentation, cervical mucus penetration, and acrosome reaction after appropriate staining. In the last decade, the setting of hyperactivation and other kinematic characteristics were better defined allowing an accurate evaluation of these parameters, making it possible to identify sperm subpopulations, such as sperm able to penetrate mucus or sperm developing hyperactivated motility when incubated under capacitating conditions [17]. There are clinical studies demonstrating that assessment of hyperactivation in a capacitated sperm population may be of help in the initial investigation of infertile couples [19,20 reviewed in 17]; however, larger multicentre studies are required in order to better define cut-off values of hyperactivated motility able to predict fertilization outcomes.

In summary, although CASA technology still needs to be improved and validated, it has enormous potential for its future application in the clinical setting of male fertility allowing a rapid (a few seconds) and objective assessment of sperm quality in a large number of cells in comparison with traditional manual semen analysis. Moreover, the CASA system not only will be able to evaluate descriptive semen parameters but also to integrate in its platform tests for assessing sperm functional characteristics, giving insight into new areas in which current analyses are lacking.

24.2.3 Acrosome Function Assays

Acrosome function, in terms of an adequate amount of active acrosome enzymes and the ability to undergo acrosome exocytosis, is a prerequisite for penetration of the oocyte extracellular matrix and zona pellucida, and, finally, for sperm–egg fusion. Being considered a useful diagnostic tool for male infertility, several methods have been set up to assess acrosome enzymes content (including fluorimetry, western blotting, spectrophotometry, substrate assays, and radioimmunoassay) and acrosome reaction (transmission electron microscopy, dyes for bright-field microscopy, and fluorescent labels). Some studies reported a positive correlation between acrosome function, evaluated by different methods, and in vitro fertilization [10,21–23], whereas in others such an association has not been found [24–26]. A recent meta-analysis [27] reported a significant relation between acrosome function scoring and fertilization rate; however, evidencing that the employed assays were moderately specific and sensitive. The meta-analysis concludes that, to improve the accuracy in predicting fertilization, multiple methods may be combined to evaluate sperm acrosome function, thus making it less user-friendly for clinical practice. In addition, also the sperm preparation methods and the assay protocol could affect the diagnostic performance [27].

A subsequent study from the same authors [28] reported that spontaneous acrosome reaction was the only significant predictor of a successful fertilization, whereas another study published later [29] found that progesterone-induced acrosome reaction is a better prognostic predictor for the fertilization rate. Acrosome reaction tests are time-consuming but do not require expensive equipment and could be easily performed in andrology diagnostic laboratories. Clearly, further studies will be needed to understand which is the most accurate method in terms of sensitivity and specificity for the evaluation of the sperm acrosomal status as a potential predictor of fertilization.

24.2.4 Assays to Evaluate Sperm–Zona Pellucida Binding

Sperm ability to bind oocyte zona pellucida is a necessary prerequisite for sperm penetration in the peri-vitelline space. Until a few years ago, it was believed that only acrosome-intact spermatozoa could bind to the zona pellucida. In 2011, Jin et al. [30] demonstrated, by retroactive examination of video recordings of the in vitro fertilization of mouse oocytes with genetically modified fluorescent spermatozoa, that acrosome-reacted spermatozoa have a much greater chance to bind and to penetrate the zona than acrosome-intact ones. Although whether the same occurs also for human spermatozoa is presently unknown, these results, lately confirmed in other studies, opened new perspectives in the research of the molecular mechanisms involved in sperm–zona binding. Several proteins have been indicated as the possible sperm receptor involved in zona binding, yet the ones really involved have remained, remarkably, elusive [31].

The hemizona assay is the most commonly used test to evaluate the ability of spermatozoon to bind the zona pellucida. It employs nonviable, bisected human oocytes, where one half is used to evaluate oocyte competence with spermatozoa of a secure fertile men, and the other half is used for the tested sample. The results are expressed as the hemizona assay index (bound sperm from subfertile male divided by bound sperm from fertile male $\times$ 100, [32]). Abnormal sperm–zona pellucida interaction was frequently observed in the ejaculated spermatozoa of infertile men [33], also despite a normal semen quality. Since hemizona assay results could be influenced by a different oocyte source, oocyte and sperm preparation methods, as well as sperm concentration [34], some protocol modifications have been made over the years. Two meta-analyses [35,36] that examined the association between the use of hemizona assay and IVF outcomes similarly reported that a threshold value of 30–35% of the hemizona assay index is able to predict fertilization with high sensitivity and specificity. These data indicate that hemizona assay is an accurate tool for determining the sperm competence to interact with the oocyte and it could be useful for couple counseling in order to choose the best therapeutic strategy. Moreover, an advantage of this test is that the methodology has undergone small variations among laboratories. The major drawbacks are represented by the limited availability of human oocytes, by the complexity in dissecting the oocytes, and ethical issues complicating the use of the hemizona test in clinical practice. Human oocytes could be potentially replaced by the use of biologically active recombinant human zona pellucida; however, so far, attempts to obtain functional recombinant zona pellucida proteins were mostly unsuccessful.

24.2.5 Assays to Evaluate Sperm–Oocyte Fusion

Sperm oocyte fusion is a complex process that has been elucidated only recently. The process requires expression of a protein located on the midpiece of spermatozoa, known as IZUMO, and one, located on the oolemma, named JUNO [37]. Clearly, genetic mutations in the IZUMO gene may lead to a defective protein that could compromise the fusion process. At present, although some gene polymorphisms have been found in patients with unexplained infertility [38], no IZUMO mutations leading to a nonfunctional protein have been reported in the literature.

The only available assay to evaluate the ability of spermatozoa to fuse with the oolemma is the sperm penetration assay. It foresees the incubation of capacitated spermatozoa with a hamster oocyte, enzymatically devoid of zona pellucida, in order to evaluate the penetration rate. By this assay, the sperm competence to undergo capacitation, acrosome reaction, fusion with oolemma, and chromatin decondensation can be evaluated [39], as all of them are required for penetration. In most studies using this assay, a correlation has been found with IVF outcomes; however, the predictive value is limited due to high false- negative rates [35]. In addition, other studies did not validate sperm penetration assay as a better predictor with regard to CASA or conventional semen analysis [40,41]. The main drawbacks of this test are the great variation in specificity, protocols, capacitation media, and cut-off values [35] as well as the elevated assay time and expensive costs.

24.2.6 Assays to Evaluate Sperm Chromatin Anomalies

DNA integrity is essential to obtain a correct fertilization and a subsequent normal development of the embryo [42] and the spermatozoon is the vehicle designated to deliver the intact haploid paternal genome. Chromosomal (aneuploidies) and nuclear (abnormal chromatin packing or DNA fragmentation) defects are known to affect both natural and assisted reproduction outcomes and are frequently found in infertile men [43]. The possible causes of these anomalies can be endogenous (including errors in meiotic recombination, apotosis, oxidative stress, etc.) and exogenous (infections and xenobiotic exposure). Several tests have been developed to assess sperm chromatin status and sperm DNA fragmentation; however, although some of them showed promising results along with semen analysis, clear conclusions on their clinical use have yet to be drawn. Among the assays proposed to evaluate sperm chromatin structure and packaging, defined by histone-protamine replacement, tests based on staining methods (including Chromomycin A3, Aniline blue, and Toluidine Blue) and those that foresee gel electrophoresis for the measurement of Protamine 1 and 2 as well as histone content, are rapid, easy to perform, inexpensive, and do not require sophisticated instrumentation. However, for those tests using optical or fluorescent microscopy, evaluation is done in a limited number of cells and is affected by interobserver variability [44]. These assays detect different aspects of chromatin structure; in particular, Chromomycin A3 is an index of poor protamination, competing with protamine for binding to DNA, Aniline blue is a measure of histone retention being able to bind histones, and, finally, Toluidine blue is an index of abnormal chromatin structure binding to phosphate groups of DNA when chromatin is loosely accessible. Electrophoretic methods, where the nuclear proteins are extracted and separated by gel electrophoresis according to their molecular weight, stained or immunoblotted, and the intensity of bands relative to protamines or the predominant Histone 2B variant measured using a standard curve, are more sensitive and allow evaluating the concentrations of nuclear proteins but, certainly, more laborious, making their widespread use difficult. Independently from the employed assay, most studies reported an association between sperm chromatin status and assisted reproduction outcomes [44,45]. In a recent paper from our group, we demonstrated that protamine content, indirectly evaluated by Chromomycin A3, when included in a statistical model, predicts the attainment of good-quality embryos in assisted reproduction cycles independently from the presence of other confounding factors [46].

Several assays are available for detection of sperm DNA fragmentation (sDF). In particular, TUNEL, SCD, Comet, and SCSA are those mainly used. These assays are different from each other, since they are able to reveal different types of DNA damage [44] and are differently related to natural and assisted reproduction outcomes [47,48]. Most reviews and meta-analysis seem to agree that Tunel and Comet are good predictors of clinical pregnancy after assisted reproduction, whereas all the tests are good predictors of natural conception. However, although many reproductive societies recognize the contribution of sDF assessment in the management of infertile couples, they do not yet officially recommend routine evaluation of this parameter. Absence of international agreement is mainly due to the lack of standardization for most techniques (except for SCSA), different cut-off values that cannot be compared with each other, and, consequently, a consensus on the definition of the gold standard method has not yet been reached. Hence, large multicenter studies comparing male partners of infertile couples (excluding female factor infertility) with proven fertile subjects, are required in order to define the gold standard method, clear cut-off values, and the categories of patients who most need the sDF test.

24.3 Conclusions

Routine semen analysis is considered the cornerstone in the diagnosis of male infertility, although it discriminates only cases of azoospermia or severe oligozoospermia as definitely infertile. In cases of unexplained male infertility or mild male factor, traditional semen analysis is poorly predictive of fertility status [1]. Indeed, a spermiogram is not able to detect sperm defects at the molecular level. Several tests have been developed based on the requisites of the male gamete to reach and fertilize the oocyte. In particular, tests assessing sperm ability to reach and overcome oocyte barriers, including capacitation, hyperactivated motility, acrosome status, sperm–egg interaction and fusion, as well as tests detecting sperm genetic integrity, have been proposed (Figure 24.1), being of some predictive value of the IVF/ICSI outcomes. However, most of these tests are expensive, time-consuming, require sophisticated equipment and skilled personnel, and, most importantly, are not standardized. In addition, for most of these tests, intrasubject variability has not been assessed. For these reasons, the clinical utility of these methods remains a matter of debate, and, at present, the World Health Organization [49] classified sperm functional assays as research and not diagnostic tests. It should be stressed that the outcome of the fertilization process depends on multiple factors including female characteristics, and that much is still unknown about sperm biology. Further multicenter, large-scale, well-designed, and validated studies will be necessary in order to synthesize multiple sperm functional assays in a simple test, possibly point of care, able to predict natural and assisted reproduction outcomes with good accuracy and cost-effectiveness in order to be adopted in diagnostic and ART laboratories.

References

1. Baskaran S, Finelli R, Agarwal A, Henkel R. Diagnostic value of routine semen analysis in clinical andrology. *Andrologia*. 2020;12:e13614.
2. Eisenberg ML, Li S, Behr B, Pera RR, Cullen MR. Relationship between semen production and medical comorbidity. *Fertil Steril*. 2015;103:66–71.
3. Wen J, Jiang J, Ding C, et al. Birth defects in children conceived by in vitro fertilization and intracytoplasmic sperm injection: a meta-analysis. *Fertil Steril*. 2012;97(6):1331–1337.
4. Sakkas D, Ramalingam M, Garrido N, Barratt CL. Sperm selection in natural conception: what can we learn from Mother Nature to improve assisted reproduction outcomes? *Hum Reprod Update*. 2015;21:711–726.
5. Baldi E, Tamburrino L, Muratori M, Degl'Innocenti S, Marchiani S. Adverse effects of in vitro manipulation of spermatozoa. *Anim Reprod Sci*. 2020;14:106314.
6. Davies MJ, Moore VM, Willson KJ, et al. Reproductive technologies and the risk of birth defects. *N Engl J Med*. 2012;366:1803–1813.
7. Bonduelle M, Wennerholm UB, Loft A, et al. A multi-centre cohort study of the physical health of 5-year-old children conceived after intracytoplasmic sperm injection, in vitro fertilization and natural conception. *Hum Reprod*. 2005;20:413–419.
8. Puga Molina LC, Luque GM, Balestrini PA, Marín-Briggiler CI, Romarowski A, Buffone MG. Molecular basis of human sperm capacitation. *Front Cell Dev Biol*. 2018;6:72.
9. Baldi E, Casano R, Falsetti C, Krausz C, Maggi M, Forti G. Intracellular calcium accumulation and responsiveness to progesterone in capacitating human spermatozoa. *J Androl*. 1991;12:323–330.
10. Krausz C, Bonaccorsi L, Maggio P, et al. Two functional assays of sperm responsiveness to progesterone and their predictive values in in-vitro fertilization. *Hum Reprod*. 1996;11:1661–1667.
11. Baro Graf C, Ritagliati C, Torres-Monserrat V, et al. Membrane potential assessment by fluorimetry as a predictor tool of human sperm fertilizing capacity. *Front Cell Dev Biol*. 2020;7:383.
12. Selvaraj V, Buttke DE, Asano A, et al. GM1 dynamics as a marker for membrane changes associated with the process of capacitation in murine and bovine spermatozoa. *J Androl*. 2007;28:588–599.
13. Moody MA, Cardona C, Simpson AJ, Smith TT, Travis AJ, Ostermeier GC. Validation of a laboratory-developed test of human sperm capacitation. *Mol Reprod Dev*. 2017;84:408–422.
14. Ostermeier GC, Cardona C, Moody MA, et al. Timing of sperm capacitation varies reproducibly among men. *Mol Reprod Dev*. 2018;85:387–396.
15. Cardona C, Neri QV, Simpson AJ, et al. Localization patterns of the ganglioside GM1 in human sperm are indicative of male fertility and independent of traditional semen measures. *Mol Reprod Dev*. 2017;84:423–435.
16. Sharara F, Seaman E, Morris R, et al. Multicentric, prospective observational data show sperm capacitation predicts male fertility, and cohort comparison reveals a high prevalence of impaired capacitation in men questioning their fertility. *Reprod Biomed Online*. 2020;41:69–79.
17. Mortimer ST, van der Horst G, Mortimer D. The future of computer-aided sperm analysis. *Asian J Androl*. 2015;17:545–553.
18. Katz DF, Overstreet JW. Sperm motility assessment by videomicrography. *Fertil Steril*. 1981;35:188–193.
19. Sukcharoen N, Keith J, Irvine DS, Aitken RJ. Definition of the optimal criteria for identifying hyperactivated human spermatozoa at 25 Hz using in-vitro fertilization as a functional end-point. *Hum Reprod*. 1995;10:2928–2937.

20. Mortimer D, Mortimer ST. Computer-aided sperm analysis (CASA) of sperm motility and hyperactivation. *Methods Mol Biol*. 2013;927:77–87.
21. Senn A, Germond M, De Grandi P. Immunofluorescence study of actin, acrosin, dynein, tubulin and hyaluronidase and their impact on in-vitro fertilization. *Hum Reprod*. 1992;7:841–849.
22. Sharma R, Hogg J, Bromham DR. Is spermatozoan acrosin a predictor of fertilization and embryo quality in the human? *Fertil Steril*. 1993;60:881–887.
23. Menkveld R, Rhemrev JP, Franken DR, Vermeiden JP, Kruger TF. Acrosomalmorphology as a novel criterion for male fertility diagnosis: relation with acrosin activity, morphology (strict criteria), and fertilization in vitro. *Fertil Steril*. 1996;65:637–644.
24. Yang YS, Chen SU, Ho HN, et al. Acrosin activity of human sperm did not correlate with IVF. *Arch Androl*. 1994;32:13–19.
25. Liu DY, Baker HWG. Relationships between human sperm acrosin, acrosomes, morphology and fertilization in vitro. *Hum Reprod*. 1990;5:298–303.
26. Parinaud J, Vieitez G, Moutaffian H, Richoilley G, Labal B. Variations in spontaneous and induced acrosome reaction: correlations with semen parameters and in-vitro fertilization results. *Hum Reprod*. 1995;10:2085–2089.
27. Xu F, Guo G, Zhu W, Fan L. Human sperm acrosome function assays are predictive of fertilization rate in vitro: a retrospective cohort study and meta-analysis. *Reprod Biol Endocrinol*. 2018;16:81.
28. Xu F, Zhu H, Zhu W, Fan L. Human sperm acrosomal status, acrosomal responsiveness, and acrosin are predictive of the outcomes of in vitro fertilization: a prospective cohort study. *Reprod Biol*. 2018;18:344–354.
29. Chen X, Zheng Y, Zheng J, Lin J, Zhang L, Jin J. The progesterone-induced sperm acrosome reaction is a good option for the prediction of fertilization in vitro compared with other sperm parameters. *Andrologia*. 2019;51:e13278.
30. Jin M, Fujiwara E, Kakiuchi Y, et al. Most fertilizing mouse spermatozoa begin their acrosome reaction before contact with the zona pellucida during in vitro fertilization. *Proc Natl Acad Sci U S A*. 2011;108:4892–4896.
31. Gahlay GK, Rajput N. The enigmatic sperm proteins in mammalian fertilization: an overview. *Biol Reprod*. 2020;103(6):1171–1185.
32. Burkman LJ, Coddington CC, Franken DR, Krugen TF, Rosenwaks Z, Hogen GD. The hemizona assay (HZA): development of a diagnostic test for the binding of human spermatozoa to the human hemizona pellucida to predict fertilization potential. *Fertil Steril*. 1988;49:688–697.
33. Liu DY, Baker HW. High frequency of defective sperm–zona pellucida interaction in oligozoospermic infertile men. *Hum Reprod*. 2004;19:228–233.
34. Yao YQ, Yeung WS, Ho PC. The factors affecting sperm binding to the zona pellucida in the hemizona binding assay. *Hum Reprod*. 1996;11:1516–1519.
35. Vogiatzi P, Chrelias C, Cahill DJ, et al. Hemizona assay and sperm penetration assay in the prediction of IVF outcome: a systematic review. *Biomed Res Int*. 2013;2013:945825.
36. Oehninger S, Franken DR, Sayed EM, Barroso G, Kohm P. Sperm function assays and their predictive value for fertilization outcome in IVF therapy: a meta analysis. *Hum Reprod Update*. 2000;6:1160–1168.
37. Aydin H, Sultana A, Li S, Thavalingam A, Lee JE. Molecular architecture of the human sperm IZUMO1 and egg JUNO fertilization complex. *Nature*. 2016;534:562–565.
38. Granados-Gonzalez V, Aknin-Seifer I, Touraine RL, Chouteau J, Wolf JP, Levy R. Preliminary study on the role of the human IZUMO gene in oocyte-spermatozoa fusion failure. *Fertil Steril*. 2008;90:1246–1248.
39. Yanagimachi R, Yanagimachi H, Rogers BJ. The use of zona-free animal ova as a test-system for the assessment of the fertilizing capacity of human spermatozoa. *Biol Reprod*. 1976;15:471–476.
40. Ford WC, Williams KM, Harrison S, et al. Value of the hamster oocyte test and computerised measurements of sperm motility in predicting if four or more viable embryos will be obtained in an IVF cycle. *Int J Androl*. 2001;24:109–119.
41. Ho LM, Lim AS, Lim TH, Hum SC, Yu SL, Kruger TF. Correlation between semen parameters and the Hamster Egg Penetration Test (HEPT) among fertile and subfertile men in Singapore. *J Androl*. 2007;28:158–163.
42. Simon L, Murphy K, Shamsi MB, et al. Paternal influence of sperm DNA integrity on early embryonic development. *Hum Reprod*. 2014;29:2402e12.
43. Zini A, Boman JM, Belzile E, et al. Sperm DNA damage is associated with an increased risk of pregnancy loss after IVF and ICSI: systematic review and meta-analysis. *Hum Reprod*. 2008;23:2663e8.
44. Dutta S, Henkel R, Agarwal A. Comparative analysis of tests used to assess sperm chromatin integrity and DNA fragmentation. *Andrologia*. 2020;6:e13718.
45. Marchiani S, Tamburrino L, Muratori M, Baldi E. Spermatozoal chromatin structure: role in sperm functions and fertilization. In: Arafa M, Elbardisi H, Majzoub A, Agarwal A. eds. *Genetics of Male Infertility: A Case-Based Guide for Clinicians*. Springer; 2020:39–57.
46. Marchiani S, Tamburrino L, Benini F, et al. Chromatin protamination and CATSPER expression in spermatozoa predict clinical outcomes after assisted reproduction programs. *Sci Rep*. 2017;7:15122.
47. Simon L, Zini A, Dyachenko A, Ciampi A, Carrell DT. A systematic review and meta-analysis to determine the effect of sperm DNA damage on in vitro fertilization and intracytoplasmic sperm injection outcome. *Asian J Androl*. 2017;19:80–90.
48. Cissen M, Wely MV, Scholten I, et al. Measuring sperm DNA fragmentation and clinical outcomes of medically assisted reproduction: a systematic review and meta-analysis. *PLoS ONE*. 2016;11:e0165125.
49. World Health Organization. *Laboratory Manual for the Examination and Processing of Human Semen*. 5th ed. WHO Press; 2010.

Section 4: Laboratory Evaluation and Treatment of Male Infertility

Chapter 25: Sperm Selection in the Laboratory

Denny Sakkas and Denis A. Vaughan

25.1 Nature

In nature many strategies have evolved to promote, not only the selection of a certain male, but that the sperm is also sorted so that the best sperm arrives at the egg. Charles Darwin originally noted the positive association between the splendor of male plumage and the degree of polygyny in birds and suggested that this was due to sexual selection. Males with brighter/extravagant plumage have a selective advantage in male-male competition or female choice and enjoy greater mating success. When selection strategies are broken down to the cellular level, it is apparent that sperm competition becomes a potent selective force, shaping many male reproductive traits [1]. A simple example is evidenced when mating type and sperm motility is examined. Sperm from polygamous (multipartner) primate species swim with greater force than sperm from monogamous (single-partner) primate species [2].

25.2 In Vitro

The strategies to select the best sperm are very different in the setting of in vitro fertilization [3]. Depending on the assisted reproduction technology (ART) used, different components of the sperm selection process are lost. For example, when intrauterine insemination is performed the selection mechanism that occurs by sperm passage through the cervix is lost. The progressive motility of the spermatozoon is essential for it to pass through the cervical mucus and hence spermatozoa with poor motility and, concomitantly, with abnormal morphology are filtered out in the cervix. Penetrating cervical mucus is a substantial barrier to sperm migration [4,5]. The greatest loss to sperm selection in ART occurs when both testicular biopsy and intracytoplasmic sperm injection (ICSI) are combined. By combining these techniques, one loses all sperm selection mechanisms in both the male and female reproductive tract, as well as through the oocyte vestments.

25.3 Paternal Effects on Reproductive Outcomes

The greatest challenge to identifying a paternal effect on reproduction is that the role of the sperm is always intertwined with that of the egg and, subsequently, the uterus following implantation. One of the largest studies that attempted to parse out these effects examined the Centers for Disease Control and Prevention and the National Center for Health Statistics database, between 2007 and 2016, in the USA [6]. It reported on over 40 million documented live births. After adjustment for maternal age, infants born to fathers aged 45 years or older had 14% higher odds of premature birth (OR [odds ratio] 1.14, 95% CI [confidence interval] 1.13–1.15), independent of gestational age, and 18% higher odds of seizures (1.18, 0.97–1.44) compared with infants of fathers aged 25–34 years. The odds of gestational diabetes was 34% higher (1.34, 1.29–1.38) in mothers with the oldest partners. Moreover, 13.2% (95% CI 12.5–13.9%) of premature births and 18.2% (17.5–18.9%) of gestational diabetes in births associated with older fathers were estimated to be attributable to advanced paternal age. This introduces an interesting dilemma: If sperm create a paternal effect after natural conception then why would in vitro sperm selection strategies work? The answer to this is mostly related to the quality of sperm samples handled in IVF, and in particular when performing true ICSI cases with severe forms of oligo-, astheno-, and/or teratozoospermia.

25.4 Poor Sperm Parameters and Their Characteristics

The relationship between poor sperm parameters and markers of the sperm nuclei and/or membrane are well documented. One of the most studied markers has been sperm DNA fragmentation. Data demonstrating that sperm populations from males with poor sperm numbers, motility, and/or morphology are strongly related to the risk of having poor sperm chromatin, DNA fragmentation, and lower protamination levels are highly convincing. This was originally shown in studies by Evenson in the early 1980s [7,8] and consequently by Bianchi et al. IN 1993 [9,10] and many others in subsequent years. Further studies have also shown this to be true for other markers including abnormal membrane protein expression, abnormal RNA levels, etc. (11–13). Membrane or cytoplasmic protein expression of creatine kinase has been used as an indicator of poor morphology, while lack of the hyaluronan receptor has been correlated to numerous markers of poor sperm quality [14,15]. Krawetz's group have also shown that differential RNA profiles exist in sperm of males with infertility [13,16]. These biological idiosyncrasies have therefore been used to identify sperm selection strategies that can mimic, to some extent, the natural mechanisms of sperm selection (Figure 25.1).

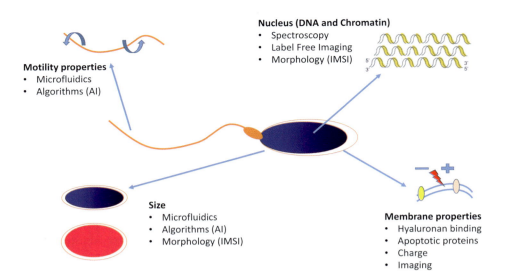

Figure 25.1 A diagrammatic representation of components of the sperm whereby sperm selection strategies are targeted

Notes: AI: artificial intelligence; IMSI: intracytoplasmic morphologically selected sperm injection.

25.5 Sperm Selection

The strategies used to identify the best sperm can be broadly categorized as illustrated in Figure 25.1. Many of the strategies employed have been adapted from diagnostic methods that have been linked to having a positive impact on certain reproductive outcomes.

25.6 Membrane Properties

The most widely tested method of sperm selection has been based on two properties of the sperm membrane. The presence of apoptotic marker proteins on the sperm membrane has been shown to indicate fractions of sperm in the ejaculate that are abnormal. A number of papers have shown the presence of residual apoptotic marker proteins on sperm membranes and these have been linked to abnormalities in sperm, including oligoasthenozoospermia [17–19]. The reason why some ejaculated spermatozoa retain these marker proteins is still disputed, however, and has been thought to be linked to a failure of apoptosis to clear faulty sperm [20,21]. Said and colleagues [22] devised a methodology using magnetic activation cell sorting (MACS) to separate apoptotic from non-apoptotic spermatozoa. They demonstrated that this resulted in a suspension of higher-quality spermatozoa with enhanced sperm-oocyte penetration potential [22]. Lee and colleagues (2010) subsequently reported that the MACS protocol provided spermatozoa with a higher fertilization potential, a finding corroborated by subsequent studies, demonstrating superior reproductive outcomes [23]. However, a recent Cochrane review [24] concluded that the quality of evidence demonstrating an improvement utilizing MACS compared to ICSI alone was poor. One randomized controlled trial (RCT) compared MACS to ICSI for live birth; three reported clinical pregnancy; and two reported miscarriage. They concluded that it is uncertain whether MACS improves live birth (risk ration [RR] 1.95, 95% CI 0.89–4.29, 62 women) or clinical pregnancy (RR 1.05, 95% CI 0.84–1.31, 413 women, $I^2 = 81\%$). In addition, there was no clear indication that MACS reduces miscarriage rates per woman (RR 0.95, 95% CI 0.16–5.63, 150 women, $I^2 = 0\%$) or per clinical pregnancy (RR 0.51, 95% CI 0.09–2.82, 53 women, $I^2 = 0$).

The most rigorously tested sperm selection technique to date has been that using hyaluronic acid binding. Developed in the laboratory of Gabor Huszar [25,26], this simple but intriguing method contrasts with MACS as it allows for the selection of a positive sperm membrane trait, the presence of the hyaluronan (HA) binding receptor. HA-bound sperm have been shown to have numerous positive traits including lower levels of chromosomal abnormalities, better nuclear and cytoplasmic integrity, and lower levels of apoptotic membrane marker proteins [15,25,27,28]. There are now a variety of available commercial products that select sperm on the basis that they express HA receptors, including PICSI® dishes, SpermCatch™, and SpermSlow.™ When HA-bound sperm were specifically selected for treatment as a methodology to improve ICSI outcomes, an initial study by Worrilow et al. showed some promising results [29]. Although this study failed to show a statistically significant difference in implantation rates, it did report a significant reduction in miscarriage rate (3.3% HA-selected vs. 15.1% in controls). Similarly, a recent large randomized clinical trial (the HABSelect trial) [30] found that HA sperm selection did not significantly increase the term livebirth rate compared with standard ICSI, but a significant decrease in miscarriage rates was again observed. One criticism of this trial however was that it included all patients and not those in need of sperm selection because of low binding efficiency of sperm to HA. Ultimately, no difference in live birth has been reported conclusively in the literature [31–33] and a Cochrane review in 2014 [34] found that data was insufficient to conclude that HA-selected sperm improve outcomes in ART. A recent study compared the MACS and HA technique and found that both physiological ICSI (PICSI) (HA) and MACS are efficient techniques for sperm selection in cases with abnormal sperm DNA fragmentation but when tested for clinical outcomes MACS is preferred in younger females (<30 years), while PICSI is preferred in older females [35].

25.7 Microfluidics

The sperm selection technology with the greatest interest at this time is the use of microfluidics. Interestingly, microfluidics and sperm complement each other enormously in the application of selection. Microfluidics-based cell separation techniques offer numerous advantages, including reducing sample volumes, faster sample processing, high sensitivity and spatial resolution, low device cost, and increased portability. It is not therefore surprising that since the publications by Smith and Takayama [36,37] more than 15 years ago, sperm selection has been a focus of microfluidics but has been slow to come to fruition.

In 2017–2020 alone, more than 30 papers were published (microfluidics and sperm selection) on this topic. Many have focused on improving sperm quality based on the intricacies associated with sperm movement. This active rather than passive selection can therefore improve the power of microfluidics to optimize sperm selection. For example, Riordan et al. [38] utilized an approach where they created 2 μm-tall confined selection channels that prohibited rotation of the sperm head and forced them into a planar swimming motion. They found that a planar swimming subpopulation of sperm capable of entering and navigating these channels had improved DNA integrity compared to samples prepared by density gradient. Numerous other studies have also been able to show this improvement in DNA quality of sperm preparations [39,40]. In contrast, however, the microfluidics preparations provide a lower sperm concentration but better motility than standard density gradient and/or swim-up preparations [40,41]. For example, Shirota et al. [40] found that swim-up provided more than 10× the sperm concentration but about 30% lower motility. A further benefit is that some of the microfluidic systems remove the need for centrifugation that has been linked to generation of radical oxygen species by sperm. This was shown by Gode et al. [41] who found that sperm processed through a microfluidic chip also display lower oxidative reduction potential.

Although the benefits of using microfluidics to improve sperm quality are convincing, their translation to a clinical practice in the realm of assisted reproduction is only now being investigated on a larger scale (clinical trials.gov). Numerous smaller-scale studies have been published with varying clinical success. A study by Yidiz and Yuksel [42] showed no difference in first-cycle patients. Fertilization rates were 70% versus 69% and pregnancy rates 51% versus 54%, for the gradient and microfluidic groups respectively. Others however have been more positive. One of the parameters of interest being investigated is the influence of sperm selection by microfluidics on rates of embryo euploidy. Parrella et al. [43] reported that microfluidics may impact the rates of euploid embryos obtained after ICSI. In a small study, four couples underwent 11 ICSI cycles with density gradient sperm preparation and failed to achieve an ongoing pregnancy. In four subsequent ICSI cycles with microfluidic sperm selection, an ongoing clinical pregnancy rate of 50% was achieved. More patients have subsequently been reported with similar improvements in both euploidy rates and pregnancy rates after microfluidic sperm selection [44]. The effect on euploidy rates is supported by other studies that also show modest improvements in euploidy rates. The need for a large clinical trial to ascertain whether microfluidics improves pregnancy rates is imperative. There are currently five trials registered on clinicaltrials.gov that may help to answer this question.

25.8 Charge

Zeta potential is the charge that develops at the interface between a solid surface and its liquid medium. It is used as a measure of cell membrane charge. Semen samples displaying more normal characteristics contain sperm with a more negative charge. A number of studies have found that when spermatozoa were separated on the basis of zeta potential, they exhibited improved strict normal morphology, DNA normal integrity, Chromomycin A3 status, and aniline blue maturity [24,45–47]. In the Kheirollahi-Kouhestani et al. [46] study, ICSI was also performed using Zeta-potential separated sperm. ICSI was performed on 30 couples who had their oocytes split into two groups to receive Zeta versus density gradient prepared sperm. Fertilization rates were improved by Zeta selection while the pregnancy and implantation rates in couples receiving at least one embryo from the Zeta group were 53.57% and 26.18%, respectively, whereas in the control group, they were 33.33% and 15.80%, respectively. In another study, 103 and 102 couples were randomly allocated into the density gradient/Zeta and density gradient groups. When ICSI outcomes were compared between the two groups the Zeta group had significantly improved good-quality blastocyst rates, clinical pregnancy rates (35% vs. 21%), and lower miscarriage rates (8.9% vs. 19.4%).

An advanced electrophoretic sperm separation device is now being developed from an initial prototype first reported by the group of John Aitken [48,49]. The system (Felix: www.memphasys.com.au/separation-technologies.php) separates sperm both by size, through a membrane, and by charge, through application of electric forces to the fluid. An initial pilot study [50] using a split-sample split-cohort study design in 28 couples demonstrated that membrane-based electrophoresis was as effective as density gradients in preparing sperm for IVF and ICSI, although it took only a fraction of the time.

25.9 Artificial Intelligence

The use of artificial intelligence and deep neural networking has begun to play a role in the field of IVF, particularly the analysis of data obtained through time-lapse embryo imaging [51,52]. It is not therefore surprising that the same technology could be applied to selection of sperm. In a recent study Butola et al. [53] reported the analysis of phase maps of 10,163 sperm cells obtained under different stress conditions (2,400 control cells, 2,750 spermatozoa after cryopreservation, 2,515 and 2,498 cells under hydrogen peroxide and ethanol respectively). They applied deep neural networks (DNN) to classify the phase maps for normal and stress-affected sperm cells. When validated against a test dataset, the DNN provided an average sensitivity, specificity, and accuracy of over 85% for the three conditions. In one fascinating study Kandel et al. [54] have combined label-free imaging and artificial intelligence to obtain nondestructive markers for reproductive outcomes. Their phase imaging system revealed nanoscale morphological details from unlabeled sperm cells providing a semantic segmentation map of the head, midpiece, and tail. Using deep learning these annotations were applied to the quantitative phase images to precisely measure the dry mass content of each component. They found that the dry mass ratio represented intrinsic markers with predictive power for zygote cleavage and embryo blastocyst development.

25.10 Microscopy

25.10.1 Morphology

Morphology has been a key, and sometimes controversial, characteristic in assessing spermatozoa during semen analysis [55]. In 2001, Bartoov and colleagues [56] reported a high magnification technique for selecting normal spermatozoa prior to ICSI. The selection of spermatozoa with normal nuclei was shown to improve the pregnancy rate with ICSI. They went on to verify this technique by performing ICSI using morphologically normal sperm, selected at >6,000 times magnification, in couples with repeated ICSI failures. A number of other studies have subsequently shown positive outcomes using a similar selection process. Antinori et al. [57] conducted a prospective randomized study to assess the advantages of ultra-high-magnification (IMSI) sperm selection over the conventional ICSI procedure in the treatment of patients with severe oligoasthenoteratozoospermia. As reported above, IMSI was based on a preliminary motile sperm organellar morphology examination under 6,600× high magnification. A meta-analysis in 2010 [58] however demonstrated no significant difference in fertilization rate between ICSI and IMSI groups, but did report a significantly improved implantation (OR 2.72; 95% CI 1.50–4.95) and pregnancy rate (OR 3.12; 95% CI 1.55–6.26) in IMSI cycles. Moreover, the results showed a significantly decreased miscarriage rate (OR 0.42; 95% CI 0.23–0.78) in IMSI cycles as compared with ICSI cycles. A recently updated Cochrane review [59] was published that included 13 parallel-designed RCTs comparing IMSI and ICSI reported on 2,775 couples (IMSI = 1,256; ICSI = 1,519). It concluded that it was uncertain whether IMSI improved live birth rates (risk ratio [RR] 1.11, 95% CI 0.89–1.39; 5 studies, 929 couples; $I^2 = 1\%$), miscarriage rates per couple (RR 1.07, 95% CI 0.78–1.48; 10 studies, 2,297 couples; $I^2 = 0\%$, very-low-quality evidence), and miscarriage rate per pregnancy (RR 0.90, 95% CI 0.68–1.20; 10 studies, 783 couples; $I^2 = 0\%$, very-low-quality evidence). It concluded the evidence for all outcomes to be of very low quality.

25.10.2 Spectroscopy

Distinct from morphologic assessment using high magnification, the use of other more powerful forms of microscopy may prove more robust. Raman spectroscopy has been suggested for several years now as a methodology to distinguish sperm with improved nuclear integrity [60,61]. Mallidis et al. examined different sperm samples and found that the spectra provided a chemical map delineating each sperm head region. Principal component analysis showed clear separation between spectra from UV-irradiated and untreated samples, delineating two regions of interest indicative of areas susceptible to DNA damage. Similar assessments have also been achieved with different culture media [62]. A recent study has taken this type of assessment to a new level by using a multimodal system to acquire both a quantitative birefringence information and Raman signature simultaneously [63]. The authors showed that this multimodal system could assess the sperm's ability to respond to capacitation stimuli in vitro by exposing sperm from healthy donors to heparin at different time points.

25.11 Alternative Sperm Selection Strategies

It must be remembered that, on the whole, IVF clinics are treating males with possible impairments in the process of producing "normal" sperm. It could therefore be argued that other strategies may assist in providing better-quality sperm for treatment. Two of these are trying to improve the source. One more radical suggestion has been to go back to the source and collect sperm from the testes in order to avoid any exposure to reproductive tract [64]. This theory arose as a number of studies have shown that sperm DNA damage is significantly lower in the seminiferous tubules compared to the cauda epididymis [58] or ejaculated sperm [59]. These reports indicate that the use of testicular sperm in couples with repeated pregnancy failure in ART and high sperm DNA fragmentation in semen result in a significant increase in pregnancy rates in these couples [65]. A systematic review by Awaga et al. in 2018 [66] identified 4 eligible studies out of 757 initially found. They reported that in men with high DNA fragmentation index (DFI) and oligozoospermia, the probability of live birth was significantly higher with testicular compared to ejaculated spermatozoa (RR 1.75, 95% CI 1.14–2.70). They concluded that there is limited, low-quality evidence suggesting that a higher probability of pregnancy might be expected using testicular rather than ejaculated spermatozoa, only in men with high DFI and oligozoospermia. Corollary to this approach, it has also been suggested that a shorter abstinence period may reduce any detrimental influence of the reproductive tract on ejaculated sperm. In fact, a number of studies have now indicated that a short abstinence of less than 24 hours results in sperm with lower rates of DNA fragmentation [67]. An interesting study by Scarselli et al. [68] examined oligoastenoteratozoospermic males who produced two semen samples on the day of oocyte retrieval: the first one after several days of abstinence and the second, one hour after the first one. Oocytes were divided into two ICSI groups (group 1 were injected with spermatozoa from the first ejaculate [N = 121] and group 2 with spermatozoa from the second one [N = 144]). Aneuploidy rates were examined after trophectoderm biopsy and it was found that higher blastocyst euploidy rates resulted in group 2 (43.6%) than in group 1 (27.5%).

25.11.1 Studies Focusing on Sperm Selection: Select the Appropriate Patients

Numerous strategies have been outlined above that attempt to improve the quality of sperm used for an IVF treatment cycle attempt. Although not all sperm selection strategies have been outlined (see reviews by 69–71) a number of common themes arise. Firstly, there are a lack of larger trials in this field and the numerous systematic analysis and Cochrane database reviews have all concluded that data quality is poor, even though some indications exist that a sperm selection strategy shows some benefits. Secondly, a common theme exists when sperm selection strategies are tested that miscarriage rates decline and embryo euploidy rates are improved. This still needs to be reproduced however in larger, more robust studies.

How does one demonstrate irrefutably that sperm selection improves outcomes? As previously mentioned, the challenge to show a true sperm effect is largely burdened by the importance of the oocyte [3]. It is therefore imperative to hone in on the correct population of males to show that improvement. Studies inclusive of all males dilute out any sperm selection event as the good-quality sperm far outweigh the bad-quality sperm and the probability of choosing a bad-quality sperm is far lower (Figure 25.2). Males with higher levels of bad-quality sperm are the patients most in need of sperm selection methods as the odds of choosing the wrong sperm are much greater, especially when performing ICSI. Strategies such as testing sperm selection on males with poor HA binding, high DNA fragmentation, etc. are therefore more likely to show a true difference. If they do not then it is likely that the sperm selection strategies being tested are not sufficient.

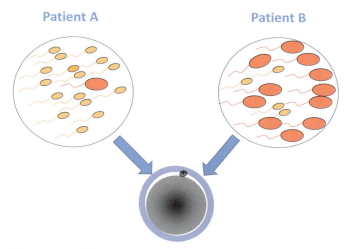

Figure 25.2 Which patients need sperm selection? Trials with patients inclusive of Patient A are less likely to show differences in regard to sperm selection. Patient A has a high proportion of "good quality sperm" (orange) and low proportion of "poor-quality sperm" (red). Hence the likelihood of selecting poor sperm is much lower with or without a sperm selection strategy. Patient B however has a much higher need for sperm selection as the proportion of "poor quality sperm" (red) is far greater

25.12 Conclusions

The preponderance of data indicating that sperm from oligo-, astheno-, and/or teratozoospermic males is compromised in terms of DNA quality and other markers, in addition to the growing number of studies linking older fathers with poor-quality sperm and adverse outcomes, should create concern in the IVF community. These are males that are more likely to be treated in an ART setting. Sperm selection strategies of different types are easy to implement and therefore could be thought of as "do no harm" strategies even though large studies are still needed to show their benefit.

References

1. Lehtonen J, Parker GA. Gamete competition, gamete limitation, and the evolution of the two sexes. *Mol Hum Reprod*. 2014;20(12):1161–1168.
2. Nascimento JM, Shi LZ, Meyers S, et al. The use of optical tweezers to study sperm competition and motility in primates. *J R Soc Interface*. 2008;5(20):297–302.
3. Sakkas D, Ramalingam M, Garrido N, Barratt CL. Sperm selection in natural conception: what can we learn from Mother Nature to improve assisted reproduction outcomes? *Hum Reprod Update*. 2015;21(6):711–726.
4. Katz DF, Drobnis EZ, Overstreet JW. Factors regulating mammalian sperm migration through the female reproductive tract and oocyte vestments. *Gamete Res*. 1989;22(4):443–469.
5. Wolf DP, Blasco L, Khan MA, Litt M. Human cervical mucus. IV. Viscoelasticity and sperm penetrability during the ovulatory menstrual cycle. *Fertil Steril*. 1978;30(2):163–169.
6. Khandwala YS, Baker VL, Shaw GM, Stevenson DK, Lu Y, Eisenberg ML. Association of paternal age with perinatal outcomes between 2007 and 2016 in the United States: population based cohort study. *BMJ*. 2018;363:k4372.
7. Evenson DP, Darzynkiewicz Z, Melamed MR. Relation of mammalian sperm chromatin heterogeneity to fertility. *Science*. 1980;210(4474):1131–1133.
8. Evenson D, Darzynkiewicz Z, Jost L, Janca F, Ballachey B. Changes in accessibility of DNA to various fluorochromes during spermatogenesis. *Cytometry*. 1986;7(1):45–53.
9. Bianchi PG, Manicardi GC, Bizzaro D, Bianchi U, Sakkas D. Effect of deoxyribonucleic acid protamination on fluorochrome staining and in situ nick-translation of murine and human mature spermatozoa. *Biol Reprod*. 1993;49(5):1083–1088.
10. Hughes CM, Lewis SE, McKelvey-Martin VJ, Thompson W. A comparison of baseline and induced

DNA damage in human spermatozoa from fertile and infertile men, using a modified comet assay. *Mol Hum Reprod.* 1996;2(8):613–619.

11. Sakkas D, Seli E, Manicardi GC, Nijs M, Ombelet W, Bizzaro D. The presence of abnormal spermatozoa in the ejaculate: did apoptosis fail? *Hum Fertil (Camb).* 2004;7(2):99–103.

12. Oehninger S, Morshedi M, Weng SL, Taylor S, Duran H, Beebe S. Presence and significance of somatic cell apoptosis markers in human ejaculated spermatozoa. *Reprod Biomed Online.* 2003;7(4):469–476.

13. Jodar M, Selvaraju S, Sendler E, Diamond MP, Krawetz SA. The presence, role and clinical use of spermatozoal RNAs. *Hum Reprod Update.* 2013;19(6):604–624.

14. Cayli S, Jakab A, Ovari L, et al. Biochemical markers of sperm function: male fertility and sperm selection for ICSI. *Reprod Biomed Online.* 2003;7(4):462–468.

15. Yagci A, Murk W, Stronk J, Huszar G. Spermatozoa bound to solid state hyaluronic acid show chromatin structure with high DNA chain integrity: an acridine orange fluorescence study. *J Androl.* 2010;31 (6):566–572.

16. Burl RB, Clough S, Sendler E, Estill M, Krawetz SA. Sperm RNA elements as markers of health. *Syst Biol Reprod Med.* 2018;64(1):25–38.

17. Manicardi GC, Tombacco A, Bizzaro D, Bianchi U, Bianchi PG, Sakkas D. DNA strand breaks in ejaculated human spermatozoa: comparison of susceptibility to the nick translation and terminal transferase assays. *Histochem J.* 1998;30(1):33–39.

18. Manicardi GC, Bianchi PG, Pantano S, et al. Presence of endogenous nicks in DNA of ejaculated human spermatozoa and its relationship to chromomycin A3 accessibility. *Biol Reprod.* 1995;52 (4):864–867.

19. Varghese AC, Bragais FM, Mukhopadhyay D, et al. Human sperm DNA integrity in normal and abnormal semen samples and its correlation with sperm characteristics. *Andrologia.* 2009;41(4):207–215.

20. Aitken RJ, De Iuliis GN. On the possible origins of DNA damage in human spermatozoa. *Mol Hum Reprod.* 2010;16(1):3–13.

21. Sakkas D, Seli E, Bizzaro D, Tarozzi N, Manicardi GC. Abnormal spermatozoa in the ejaculate: abortive apoptosis and faulty nuclear remodelling during spermatogenesis. *Reprod Biomed Online.* 2003;7(4):428–432.

22. Said TM, Agarwal A, Zborowski M, Grunewald S, Glander HJ, Paasch U. Utility of magnetic cell separation as a molecular sperm preparation technique. *J Androl.* 2008;29(2):134–142.

23. Lee TH, Liu CH, Shih YT, et al. Magnetic-activated cell sorting for sperm preparation reduces spermatozoa with apoptotic markers and improves the acrosome reaction in couples with unexplained infertility. *Hum Reprod.* 2010;25 (4):839–846.

24. Lepine S, McDowell S, Searle LM, Kroon B, Glujovsky D, Yazdani A. Advanced sperm selection techniques for assisted reproduction. *Cochrane Database Syst Rev.* 2019;7(7): CD010461.

25. Jakab A, Sakkas D, Delpiano E, et al. Intracytoplasmic sperm injection: a novel selection method for sperm with normal frequency of chromosomal aneuploidies. *Fertil Steril.* 2005;84 (6):1665–1673.

26. Sati L, Huszar G. Methodology of aniline blue staining of chromatin and the assessment of the associated nuclear and cytoplasmic attributes in human sperm. *Methods Mol Biol.* 2013;927:425–436.

27. Huszar G, Ozkavukcu S, Jakab A, Celik-Ozenci C, Sati GL, Cayli S. Hyaluronic acid binding ability of human sperm reflects cellular maturity and fertilizing potential: selection of sperm for intracytoplasmic sperm injection. *Curr Opin Obstet Gynecol.* 2006;18 (3):260–267.

28. Ovári L, Sati L, Stronk J, Borsos A, Ward DC, Huszar G. Double probing individual human spermatozoa: aniline blue staining for persistent histones and fluorescence in situ hybridization for aneuploidies. *Fertil Steril.* 2010;93 (7):2255–2261.

29. Worrilow KC, Eid S, Woodhouse D, et al. Use of hyaluronan in the selection of sperm for intracytoplasmic sperm injection (ICSI): significant improvement in clinical outcomes – multicenter, double-blinded and randomized controlled trial. *Hum Reprod.* 2013;28(2):306–314.

30. Miller D, Pavitt S, Sharma V, et al. Physiological, hyaluronan-selected intracytoplasmic sperm injection for infertility treatment (HABSelect): a parallel, two-group, randomised trial. *Lancet.* 2019;393(10170):416–422.

31. Tarozzi N, Nadalini M, Bizzaro D, et al. Sperm-hyaluronan-binding assay: clinical value in conventional IVF under Italian law. *Reprod Biomed Online.* 2009;19(Suppl. 3):35–43.

32. Parmegiani L, Cognigni GE, Bernardi S, et al. Comparison of two ready-to-use systems designed for sperm-hyaluronic acid binding selection before intracytoplasmic sperm injection: PICSI vs. Sperm Slow: a prospective, randomized trial. *Fertil Steril.* 2012;98 (3):632–637.

33. Majumdar G, Majumdar A. A prospective randomized study to evaluate the effect of hyaluronic acid sperm selection on the intracytoplasmic sperm injection outcome of patients with unexplained infertility having normal semen parameters. *J Assist Reprod Genet.* 2013;30(11):1471–1475.

34. McDowell S, Kroon B, Ford E, Hook Y, Glujovsky D, Yazdani A. Advanced sperm selection techniques for assisted reproduction. *Cochrane Database Syst Rev.* 2014(10):CD010461.

35. Hasanen E, Elqusi K, ElTanbouly S, et al. PICSI vs. MACS for abnormal sperm DNA fragmentation ICSI cases: a prospective randomized trial. *J Assist Reprod Genet.* 2020;37(10):2605–2613.

36. Schuster TG, Cho B, Keller LM, Takayama S, Smith GD. Isolation of motile spermatozoa from semen samples using microfluidics. *Reprod Biomed Online.* 2003;7(1):75–81.

37. Smith GD, Takayama S. Application of microfluidic technologies to human assisted reproduction. *Mol Hum Reprod.* 2017;23(4):257–268.

38. Riordon J, Tarlan F, You JB, et al. Two-dimensional planar swimming selects for high DNA integrity sperm. *Lab Chip.* 2019;19(13):2161–2167.

39. Quinn MM, Jalalian L, Ribeiro S, et al. Microfluidic sorting selects sperm for clinical use with reduced DNA damage compared to density gradient centrifugation with swim-up in split semen samples. *Hum Reprod.* 2018;33 (8):1388–1393.

40. Shirota K, Yotsumoto F, Itoh H, et al. Separation efficiency of a microfluidic

sperm sorter to minimize sperm DNA damage. *Fertil Steril.* 2016;105 (2):315–321 e1.

41. Gode F, Gürbüz AS, Tamer B, Pala I, Isik AZ. The effects of microfluidic sperm sorting, density gradient and swim-up methods on semen oxidation reduction potential. *Urol J.* 2020;17 (4):397–401.

42. Yildiz K, Yuksel S. Use of microfluidic sperm extraction chips as an alternative method in patients with recurrent in vitro fertilisation failure. *J Assist Reprod Genet.* 2019;36(7):1423–1429.

43. Parrella A, Keating D, Cheung S, et al. A treatment approach for couples with disrupted sperm DNA integrity and recurrent ART failure. *J Assist Reprod Genet.* 2019;36(10):2057–2066.

44. Parrella A, Tavares RS, Haddad M, et al. A novel method to attenuate embryo aneuploidy due to paternal inheritance. *Fertil Steril.* 2020;114(3):e424–e425.

45. Chan PJ, Jacobson JD, Corselli JU, Patton WC. A simple zeta method for sperm selection based on membrane charge. *Fertil Steril.* 2006;85 (2):481–486.

46. Kheirollahi-Kouhestani M, Razavi S, Tavalaee M, et al. Selection of sperm based on combined density gradient and Zeta method may improve ICSI outcome. *Hum Reprod.* 2009;24 (10):2409–2416.

47. Simon L, Ge SQ, Carrell DT. Sperm selection based on electrostatic charge. *Methods Mol Biol.* 2013;927:269–278.

48. Ainsworth C, Nixon B, Aitken RJ. Development of a novel electrophoretic system for the isolation of human spermatozoa. *Hum Reprod.* 2005;20 (8):2261–2270.

49. Ainsworth C, Nixon B, Jansen RP, Aitken RJ. First recorded pregnancy and normal birth after ICSI using electrophoretically isolated spermatozoa. *Hum Reprod.* 2007;22 (1):197–220.

50. Fleming SD, Ilad RS, Griffin AM, et al. Prospective controlled trial of an electrophoretic method of sperm preparation for assisted reproduction: comparison with density gradient centrifugation. *Hum Reprod.* 2008;23 (12):2646–2651.

51. Tran D, Cooke S, Illingworth PJ, Gardner DK. Deep learning as a predictive tool for fetal heart pregnancy following time-lapse incubation and blastocyst transfer. *Hum Reprod.* 2019;34(6):1011–1018.

52. Zaninovic N, Rosenwaks Z. Artificial intelligence in human in vitro fertilization and embryology. *Fertil Steril.* 2020;114(5):914–920.

53. Butola A, Popova D, Prasad DK, et al. High spatially sensitive quantitative phase imaging assisted with deep neural network for classification of human spermatozoa under stressed condition. *Sci Rep.* 2020;10(1):13118.

54. Kandel ME, Rubessa M, He YR, et al. Reproductive outcomes predicted by phase imaging with computational specificity of spermatozoon ultrastructure. *Proc Natl Acad Sci U S A.* 2020;117(31):18302–18309.

55. Kovac JR, Smith RP, Cajipe M, Lamb DJ, Lipshultz LI. Men with a complete absence of normal sperm morphology exhibit high rates of success without assisted reproduction. *Asian J Androl.* 2017;19(1):39–42.

56. Bartoov B, Berkovitz A, Eltes F. Selection of spermatozoa with normal nuclei to improve the pregnancy rate with intracytoplasmic sperm injection. *N Engl J Med.* 2001;345(14):1067–1068.

57. Antinori M, Licata E, Dani G, et al. Intracytoplasmic morphologically selected sperm injection: a prospective randomized trial. *Reprod Biomed Online.* 2008;16(6):835–841.

58. Setti SA, Ferreira RC, Braga DPAF, Figueira RCS, Iaconelli A Jr, Borges E Jr. Intracytoplasmic sperm injection outcome versus intracytoplasmic morphologically selected sperm injection outcome: a meta-analysis. *Reprod Biomed Online.* 2010;21 (4):450–455.

59. Teixeira DM, Hadyme Miyague A, Barbosa MA, et al. Regular (ICSI) versus ultra-high magnification (IMSI) sperm selection for assisted reproduction. *Cochrane Database Syst Rev.* 2020;2(2):CD010167.

60. Mallidis C, Sanchez V, Wistuba J, et al. Raman microspectroscopy: shining a new light on reproductive medicine. *Hum Reprod Update.* 2014;20 (3):403–414.

61. Huser T, Orme CA, Hollars CW, Corzett MH, Balhorn R. Raman spectroscopy of DNA packaging in individual human sperm cells distinguishes normal from abnormal cells. *J Biophotonics.* 2009;2(5):322–332.

62. Da Costa R, Amaral S, Redmann K, Kliesch S, Schlatt S. Spectral features of nuclear DNA in human sperm assessed by Raman microspectroscopy: effects of UV-irradiation and hydration. *PLoS ONE.* 2018;13(11):e0207786.

63. De Angelis A, Ferrara MA, Coppola G, et al. Combined Raman and polarization sensitive holographic imaging for a multimodal label-free assessment of human sperm function. *Sci Rep.* 2019;9(1):4823.

64. Sakkas D, Alvarez JG. Sperm DNA fragmentation: mechanisms of origin, impact on reproductive outcome, and analysis. *Fertil Steril.* 2010;93 (4):1027–1036.

65. Esteves SC, Sánchez-Martín F, Sánchez-Martín P, Schneider DT, Gosálvez J. Comparison of reproductive outcome in oligozoospermic men with high sperm DNA fragmentation undergoing intracytoplasmic sperm injection with ejaculated and testicular sperm. *Fertil Steril.* 2015;104(6):1398–1405.

66. Awaga HA, Bosdou JK, Goulis DG, et al. Testicular versus ejaculated spermatozoa for ICSI in patients without azoospermia: a systematic review. *Reprod Biomed Online.* 2018;37 (5):573–580.

67. Gosálvez J, González-Martínez M, López-Fernández C, Fernández JL, Sánchez-Martín P. Shorter abstinence decreases sperm deoxyribonucleic acid fragmentation in ejaculate. *Fertil Steril.* 2011;96(5):1083–1086.

68. Scarselli F, Casciani V, Cursio E, et al. Influence of human sperm origin, testicular or ejaculated, on embryo morphokinetic development. *Andrologia.* 2018;50(8):e13061.

69. Vaughan DA, Sakkas D. Sperm selection methods in the 21st century. *Biol Reprod.* 2019;101(6):1076–1082.

70. Albertini DF. The problem with being choosy when it comes to sperm selection. *J Assist Reprod Genet.* 2019;36 (7):1297–1298.

71. Henkel R. Sperm preparation: state-of-the-art physiological aspects and application of advanced sperm preparation methods. *Asian J Androl.* 2012;14(2):260–269.

Chapter 26: Methods to Select Ejaculated, Epididymal, and Testicular Spermatozoa for Assisted Conception

Sergey I. Moskovtsev, Michal Dviri, and Clifford L. Librach

26.1 Introduction

Since the introduction of in vitro fertilization (IVF) and intracytoplasmic sperm injection (ICSI) almost four decades ago, millions of children have been conceived with the help of these technologies. Despite some progress toward increasing the efficiency of assisted reproductive technology (ART), almost 70% of IVF cycles fail to achieve a live birth. Human fertility is very complex and requires a synchrony of events to achieve a successful pregnancy, either naturally or through ART. Selection of competent spermatozoa in the laboratory is particularly challenging and mostly based on two parameters assessed on live spermatozoa; ability to move and gross morphology. Each semen sample is extremely heterogeneous, containing spermatozoa with different motility, kinetics, viability, maturity, morphology, and a unique genetic and epigenetic makeup. Each of these factors influences the fertility potential of a particular spermatozoa in the sample. In this chapter, conventional, advanced, and emerging ART sperm selection techniques will be reviewed based on up-to-date and reliable evidence-based literature.

26.2 Conventional Sperm Selection

Several sperm preparation techniques have been developed over the years to process fresh or frozen semen samples and that are still employed worldwide in fertility laboratories for both diagnostic and therapeutic purposes. These sperm preparation techniques were first used for intrauterine insemination (IUI) and were later adopted for ART and are referred to as conventional sperm preparation methods [1].

26.2.1 Sperm Wash Method

The simplest method is based on centrifugation of the ejaculate diluted with medium, followed by removal of the supernatant. This procedure allows a technologist to concentrate spermatozoa and remove the seminal fluid. However, it does not remove debris and somatic cells or separate motile from non-motile spermatozoa [1]. The method is advantageous when separation of motile spermatozoa is challenging, specifically for specimens with low sperm concentration (oligozoospermia) or low motility (asthenozoospermia) in preparation for ICSI.

26.2.2 Swim-Up (SU) Method

This procedure does not require centrifugation, is easy to perform, and allows for recovery of a fraction of motile spermatozoa. It is performed by layering culture medium over an ejaculate that is placed on an angle to maximize surface interaction between the sample and medium. Over the course of an hour incubation, motile spermatozoa migrate against gravity into the medium. This method results in a lower yield of motile sperm, compared with other methods. It is suitable for IUI when there is normozoospermia, whereas it can be used for IVF with ICSI of oligoasthenospermic samples, since the low yield of motile spermatozoa is not concerning [2].

26.2.3 Density Gradient Centrifugation (DGC) Method

DGC involves centrifugation of semen over gradients of coated colloidal silica beads for separation of spermatozoa based on size, density, and motility. This technique removes proteins, prostaglandins, pathogens, debris, and somatic cell contaminants, found in seminal fluid. The soft pellet obtained is enriched with mostly motile spermatozoa and must then undergo a second simple centrifugation step to remove silica contamination. This is the most common method currently used, even in cases of diminished sperm quality, as a part of preparation prior to IUI and IVF [1,2].

A combination of DGC with SU (DGC/SU) has been used effectively for conventional IVF, but is unsatisfactory when a poor-quality semen sample is provided. Performing two consecutive (double) DGC, followed by SU, referred as DDGC/SU, was assessed on 500 semen samples with very poor quality and was reported to improve sperm recovery as well as result in similar fertilization rate (FR), embryo development (ED), clinical pregnancy rate (CPR), miscarriage rate (MR), and life birth rate (LBR), as compared to semen samples isolated by DGC/SU [3].

26.2.4 Effect of Conventional Sperm Preparation on IUI Outcomes

There are concerns that certain sperm preparation techniques can cause iatrogenic sperm DNA damage due to mechanical stress, endotoxins, and/or high levels of reactive oxygen species production [2]. Recent randomized controlled trials (RCTs) compared the effect of DGC versus SU on sperm DNA damage in 65 subfertile patients undergoing IUI [4]. While SU has been shown to select spermatozoa with lower DNA damage, CPR was not reported in the study. Moreover, a recent meta-analysis of 10 studies concluded that high sperm DNA fragmentation was associated with lower CPR and LBR in couples undergoing IUI [5]. Another systematic review meta-analysis based on nine studies concluded that sperm DNA damage testing itself has a poor predictive value for CPR in couples undergoing IUI. However, couples with low sperm DNA fragmentation were three times more likely to conceive with IUI [6].

Three sperm preparation techniques (sperm wash, SU, and DGC) were compared in terms of clinical outcome in a recent Cochrane review based on six RCTs [7]. The meta-analysis concluded that due to very low quality of available evidence, it was not possible to determine any differences in CPR or MR between analyzed sperm preparation techniques, and none of the RCTs reported LBR.

26.3 Advanced Sperm Selection Techniques for Ejaculated Spermatozoa

Since ART success rates have not improved appreciably over the past decade, there is growing interest in more advanced sperm selection techniques. These are based on principles of physiological selection of spermatozoa in the female reproductive tract. They attempt to utilize their molecular, chemical, and possibly epigenetic properties, as well as use high-resolution microscopy. Such selection would be particularly beneficial for ICSI, where a single competent spermatozoon is required to fertilize each retrieved mature oocyte.

26.3.1 Molecular Binding Selection Methods
26.3.1.1 Hyaluronic Acid (HA) Binding Selection

The principle of this method is based on spermatozoa exhibiting binding sites to HA, which is the main component of the extracellular matrix surrounding the cumulus-oophorus. The observation that HA-bound spermatozoa are more likely to be mature, morphologically normal, have a lower percentage of chromosomal aneuploidies, and less DNA damage, has led to development of the physiological intracytoplasmic sperm injection (PICSI) method [8]. The PICSI dish, precoated with HA microdroplets, allows for visual selection of HA-bound spermatozoa at the time of ICSI.

Despite this appealing physiological approach and several encouraging retrospective and observational studies, a large-scale RCT involving 16 UK clinics and 2,772 couples undergoing fresh embryo transfer did not observe any differences in CPR or LBR between PICSI and standard ICSI [9]. The most recent Cochrane review, including eight RCTs, concluded that HA-binding sperm selection does not increase the chance of CPR or LBR, although low-quality evidence may suggest reduction of MR with this method [10]. Overall, the current evidence does not support routine use of HA-binding assays in ICSI cycles [9,10].

26.3.1.2 Annexin V (AV) Magnetic Activated Cell Sorting (MACS)

An early sign of apoptosis is the presence of phosphatidylserine on the membrane of spermatozoa, which has high affinity to AV. AV-positive apoptotic spermatozoa can be removed with AV-coated magnetic beads or columns, leaving intact functional spermatozoa. A systematic review with meta-analysis based on five studies concluded that utilization of AV with MACS to select sperm for either IUI or IVF resulted in a significantly increased CPR in comparison to conventional methods [11]. LBR was not reported in any studies included in the meta-analysis. In contrast, another RCT of particular interest is a report of 237 male partners from couples undergoing ovum donation. Applying AV with MACS technology did not improve CPR or LBR when compared to conventional sperm selection method [12]. Moreover, a recent Cochrane review based on three studies could not confirm efficacy of MACS to improve CPR, MR, or LBR due to low quality of evidence [10].

26.3.2 Surface Charge Selection Methods
26.3.2.1 Zeta Potential (ZP)

During epididymal maturation, spermatozoa become negatively charged due to acquisition of lipid-anchored proteins, referred to as the ZP. Isolation of mature spermatozoa by their adherence to the surface of a positively charged tube has been suggested [13]. The only RCT that has reported a significant increase in ED and CPR with ZP sperm selection [14] was also included in a recent Cochrane review that concluded that there is uncertainty regarding the use of ZP sperm selection on CPR, MR, and LBR [10]. A more recent RCT that utilized ZP with ICSI in cases of male infertility found a significantly higher CPR when using the ZP method compared with DGC [15].

26.3.2.2 Electrophoresis

Electrophoresis has been utilized to separate spermatozoa based on electronegative charge and size [16]. This separation technique has been shown to isolate highly motile, morphologically normal spermatozoa with a lower degree of DNA damage. A pilot prospective trial of 28 couples undergoing IVF compared DGC with the electrophoretic method and showed that both methods had comparable sperm recovery, DNA damage, FR, and CPR [17]. To date, no RCT assessing the efficacy of electrophoresis has been performed, making it difficult to justify the use of this method in clinical practice.

26.3.3 Sophisticated Morphological Assessment Methods
26.3.3.1 Intracytoplasmic Morphologically Selected Sperm Injection (IMSI)

Digital magnification with Nomarski interference contrast microscopy can provide evaluation of subcellular organelles (nucleus, acrosome, postacrosomal lamina, neck, mitochondria, and tail) of motile spermatozoa. A recent systematic review with meta-analysis compared clinical outcomes of

IMSI and ICSI. The quantitative analysis of six RCTs showed no differences in MR or LBR between the two methods. However, an analysis of five observational studies showed an increased LBR and decreased MR with IMSI [18]. A recent Cochrane review also assessed the available evidence regarding the efficacy and safety of IMSI in 13 RCTs, concluding that low evidence of published data cannot support or discourage regular use of IMSI [19].

26.3.3.2 Polarization Microscopy

Polarization microscopy implementing birefringence (double refraction) of light has been used to evaluate organelles of live spermatozoa [20]. One RCT reported higher implantation rates when acrosome-reacted spermatozoa, identified by birefringence, was used for ICSI, although results of ICSI with ejaculated and testicular spermatozoa were combined [20]. Another study that quantified birefringence found that spermatozoa with a head retardance between 0.56 and 0.91 nm was associated with a higher CPR [21]. However, a Cochrane review could not include any published studies to a quantitative analysis to determine if birefringence can assist with sperm selection for ART, prompting a request for properly designed RCTs [10].

26.3.4 Microfluidic Sperm Selection (MSS)

Microfluidics is one emerging technology with the potential to provide a rapid, simple, and standardizable method of sperm selection. Motility-based methods using passive flow, laminar flow, or rheotaxis have been used for isolation of spermatozoa with low DNA damage. Active MSS, which uses external forces (hydrostatic pressure, capillary forces, chemotaxis, electric fields) or light-induced dielectrophoresis has been reported and is summarized in the two recent comprehensive reviews of MSS [22,23]. Testicular spermatozoa has also been subjected to MSS [24], as will be addressed later in this chapter.

26.3.5 Artificial Intelligence (AI) and Sperm Selection

Methods involving AI are steadily progressing from being experimental to clinical medicine, including for ART. These methods include machine learning, robotics, and data mining, which can integrate large datasets with a personalized approach (lifestyle and environmental factors), in order to improve the predictive value of diagnostic and treatment options to enhance natural and ART conceptions [25].

Machine learning and automation techniques can provide real-time quantitative data for selection of single sperm for ICSI. For example, differential interference contrast subcellular structure imaging with multisperm tracking software allows noninvasive measurement of single sperm morphology and motility in real time [26]. In addition, automatic selection can be integrated with robotic sperm immobilization in preparation for manual ICSI. This has the potential to be developed into a fully robotic ICSI system in the future [27].

26.4 Preparation and Selection of Surgically Retrieved Spermatozoa

26.4.1 Obstructive Azoospermia (OA) and Epidydimal Spermatozoa

OA is caused by blockage of spermatozoa transport in the male reproductive tract. The latest American Society for Reproductive Medicine (ASRM) summary provides an overview of the surgical treatment of OA, vasovasostomy, and vasoepididymostomy, as well as recommendations of sperm retrieval techniques and cost-effectiveness of surgical reconstruction of sperm transport versus sperm retrieval [28]. The following surgical retrieval methods are reviewed: percutaneous epididymal sperm aspiration (PESA), microsurgical epididymal sperm aspiration (MESA), percutaneous testicular sperm aspiration (TESA), percutaneous testicular biopsy (PercBiopsy), and conventional testicular sperm extraction (cTESE). Utilization of sperm cryopreservation is also discussed, concluding that similar outcomes are expected when fresh or frozen epididymal spermatozoa is used in ART.

There is universal agreement that the quantity of retrieved epididymal spermatozoa is not sufficient for IUI and should be utilized with ICSI. A recent systematic review and meta-analysis compared utilization of epididymal and testicular spermatozoa in patients with OA. Data from eight studies revealed similar CPR and MR between PESA and TESA [29]. No details on the sperm selection was provided in any of the studies.

26.4.2 Nonobstructive Azoospermia (NOA) and Testicular Spermatozoa

Men with NOA produce none or very few spermatozoa, and represent the most severe cases of infertility. The latest summary on the management of men with NOA reviews pharmaceutical optimization and preoperative treatment and sperm retrieval procedures, including TESA, cTESE, and microdissection testicular sperm extraction (mTESE) [30]. While the summary indicates that no RCT has been performed to compare sperm retrieval techniques, two systematic reviews have been included in it, concluding that mTESE is superior to cTESE to successfully retrieve testicular spermatozoa in men with NOA [31,32]. No data on testicular sperm selection methods had been included in this ASRM summary [30]. Another systematic review included an original review by Bernie [31] and four additional studies. They concluded that the overall chance to retrieve spermatozoa from NOA men by mTESE is approximately 65% [33]. In contrast, the largest systematic review and meta-analysis of 117 studies reported sperm recovery of 46% by either cTESE or mTESE [34].

Timing of the sperm retrieval in relation to IVF has been also debated; similar CPR were reported in a meta-analysis of 11 studies with fresh (28.1%) versus frozen (28.7%) testicular spermatozoa [35]. A larger meta-analysis that expanded to

17 studies reconfirmed similar CPR and LBR when fresh or frozen testicular spermatozoa were utilized for ICSI [36]. In contrast, the largest meta-analysis expanding to 38 studies reported significantly higher CPR with fresh testicular spermatozoa as compared with frozen spermatozoa, but comparable cumulative LBR [34].

26.4.3 Laboratory Processing of Testicular Tissue

Although the success of testicular spermatozoa retrieval is dependent on the surgical technique itself, the postoperative laboratory processing of the testicular tissue cannot be underestimated. It has been reported that technical laboratory skills, experience, time, and number of technicians involved influences successful identification and utilization of testicular spermatozoa for ICSI [33].

Mechanical tissue dissection, enzymatic tissue digestion, or a combination of both have been reported to assist with testicular tissue processing [37]. Several methods of mechanical testicular tissue dissection including "tissue shredding" with fine needles or glass slides; a "squeezing method" using the banded site of a Pasteur pipette to squeeze the contents of the seminiferous tubule; a "strainer method" and "grinding method" have been reported. Enzymatic tissue digestion using collagenase type IV has been optimized and successfully used [37]. A study from 11 IVF centers in Germany compared enzymatic versus mechanical sperm preparation, confirming safety of the enzymatic method with no negative impact on FR, ED, or CPR [38]. In addition, it has also been reported that mechanical processing using erythrocyte-lysing buffer, followed by the enzymatic method, improves sperm recovery up to 7% in subjects where no spermatozoa were detected by mechanical dissection [33].

26.4.4 Methods of Testicular Spermatozoa Selection

Most of the available references are focused on identifying testicular spermatozoa in a large amount of somatic cells and debris. However, several methods have been published to assist with the selection of those spermatozoa identified for use in fertilization by ICSI. Since testicular spermatozoa often lack motility, some methods have been developed to stimulate sperm motility to assist the embryologist in identifying viable spermatozoa more easily. Incubation of testicular spermatozoa with pentoxifylline to stimulate sperm motility has been suggested [39]. Theophylline is another chemical that has been used to initiate sperm motility in TESE samples, significantly reducing search time through the samples prior to ICSI [40].

Other methods help to select immotile, but viable, spermatozoa for ICSI. For example, the hypoosmotic swelling test (HOST) can evaluate functional integrity of the sperm membrane and allows selection of spermatozoa by observing the controlled swelling of the tail. An RCT has reported that immotile spermatozoa selected by HOST resulted in higher FR, ED, and CPR in comparison to regular morphological sperm selection [41]. Birefringence characteristics of testicular spermatozoa with presumed complete acrosome reaction have been also used to help improve the outcome of ICSI [20]. A single laser pulse application to the tip of the sperm tail, causing viable spermatozoa tails to coil, has also been suggested as a technique for identification [42]. However, despite several publications on testicular sperm selection, a systematic review concluded that the available data is controversial, inconclusive, and often used in the clinical practice without proper safety validation [43].

Some novel microfluidic methods that have been applied on different cell lines are showing promise for optimization of MSS testicular sperm recovery [44]. A novel MSS method has been reported to isolate immotile spermatozoa from minced testicular samples [24]. Utilization of this device led to rapid isolation of 8.9-fold more spermatozoa from testicular samples, in comparison to the tedious manual process performed by experienced embryologists.

26.4.5 Using Testicular Sperm in Cases without Azoospermia

Testicular sperm retrieval was originally utilized for patients with azoospermia only, but its use has recently been expanded to patients with high sperm DNA damage. A systematic review and meta-analysis, which included seven studies, compared ART outcomes in patients with high DNA damage using testicular versus ejaculated spermatozoa [45]. Sperm DNA damage was significantly lower, while CPR, MR, and LBR were significantly higher from testicular spermatozoa, as compared to ejaculated spermatozoa, in these patients. In contrast, a more recent systematic review that included eight studies that used testicular sperm with ICSI in patients with high DNA damage, concluded that the quality of data was not adequate to perform a quantitative analysis and could not recommend testicular sperm for ICSI in nonazoospermic patients [46].

Testicular sperm extraction has also been suggested for infertile men with severe abnormal sperm quality. The recent systematic review based on four studies could not confirm any benefit of ICSI with testicular sperm in men with severe asthenozoospermia or teratozoospermia [47]. However, the same review cautiously suggested some evidence that men with a history of failed IVF, oligozoospermia, and high DFI might benefit from ICSI with testicular sperm. A recent systematic review and meta-analysis, that included six studies of men with cryptozoospermia, reported significantly higher FR, ED, and CPR when testicular versus ejaculated spermatozoa was used for ICSI [48]. The same group reported that men with cryptozoospermia can achieve lower MR and higher LBR when testicular spermatozoa are used for ICSI [49].

26.5 Summary

The quality of selected spermatozoa is crucial for successful ART. While some studies report that advanced sperm selection techniques have a positive impact on ART outcomes, the evidence is weak and is not supported by the most recent Cochrane reviews and meta-analysis. In addition, the majority of sperm selection methods are conducted manually at the time of ICSI and are based on the judgment, experience, and effort of embryology laboratory personnel.

The only unanimous consensus thus far is that well-designed, large-scale, sufficiently powered RCTs are required to evaluate sperm selection techniques and provide robust evidence to support routine application of single sperm selection techniques. It should be further determined which subgroups of infertile patients may benefit most from these techniques. The clinical safety of these advanced selection methods, in terms of possible effects on the health of children born after utilizing them, must be also property addressed.

Despite vast knowledge of human reproduction, the molecular mechanisms of natural selection of spermatozoa in the female reproductive tract remain poorly understood and might hold the key to more efficient selection of spermatozoa for ART. Concomitantly, personalized approaches of sperm selection have the potential to improve ART treatment outcomes. Moreover, sperm selection cannot be effective without taking into consideration female factors, such as egg quality, hormonal support, and receptivity of the uterus. To improve sperm selection, we need to integrate individual genetic and epigenetic diagnostic approaches, together with our knowledge of preconception health, diet, substance use, and environmental factors on the health of gametes. We can only hope that combining personalized medicine, microfluidic, AI, and robotics in ART clinics in the future will improve the outcomes for infertile patients.

References

1. World Health Organization, ed. *WHO Laboratory Manual for the Examination and Processing of Human Semen*. 5th ed. World Health Organization; 2010.
2. Henkel RR, Schill W-B. Sperm preparation for ART. *Reprod Biol Endocrinol*. 2003;1(1):108.
3. Dai X, Wang Y, Cao F, et al. Sperm enrichment from poor semen samples by double density gradient centrifugation in combination with swim-up for IVF cycles. *Sci Rep*. 2020;10(1):2286.
4. Oguz Y, Guler I, Erdem A, et al. The effect of swim-up and gradient sperm preparation techniques on deoxyribonucleic acid (DNA) fragmentation in subfertile patients. *J Assist Reprod Genet*. 2018;35(6):1083–1089.
5. Chen Q, Zhao J-Y, Xue X, Zhu G-X. The association between sperm DNA fragmentation and reproductive outcomes following intrauterine insemination, a meta analysis. *Reprod Toxicol Elmsford N*. 2019;86:50–55.
6. Sugihara A, Van Avermaete F, Roelant E, Punjabi U, De Neubourg D. The role of sperm DNA fragmentation testing in predicting intra-uterine insemination outcome: a systematic review and meta-analysis. *Eur J Obstet Gynecol Reprod Biol*. 2020;244:8–15.
7. Boomsma CM, Heineman MJ, Cohlen BJ, Farquhar C. Semen preparation techniques for intrauterine insemination. *Cochrane Database Syst Rev*. 2007;4:CD004507.
8. Huszar G, Ozkavukcu S, Jakab A, Celik-Ozenci C, Sati GL, Cayli S. Hyaluronic acid binding ability of human sperm reflects cellular maturity and fertilizing potential: selection of sperm for intracytoplasmic sperm injection: *Curr Opin Obstet Gynecol*. 2006;18(3):260–267.
9. Miller D, Pavitt S, Sharma V, et al. Physiological, hyaluronan-selected intracytoplasmic sperm injection for infertility treatment (HABSelect): a parallel, two-group, randomised trial. *Lancet*. 2019;393(10170):416–422.
10. Lepine S, McDowell S, Searle LM, Kroon B, Glujovsky D, Yazdani A. Advanced sperm selection techniques for assisted reproduction. *Cochrane Database Syst Rev*. 2019;7:CD010461.
11. Gil M, Sar-Shalom V, Melendez Sivira Y, Carreras R, Checa MA. Sperm selection using magnetic activated cell sorting (MACS) in assisted reproduction: a systematic review and meta-analysis. *J Assist Reprod Genet*. 2013;30(4):479–485.
12. Romany L, Garrido N, Motato Y, Aparicio B, Remohí J, Meseguer M. Removal of annexin V-positive sperm cells for intracytoplasmic sperm injection in ovum donation cycles does not improve reproductive outcome: a controlled and randomized trial in unselected males. *Fertil Steril*. 2014;102(6):1567–1575.
13. Chan PJ, Jacobson JD, Corselli JU, Patton WC. A simple zeta method for sperm selection based on membrane charge. *Fertil Steril*. 2006;85(2):481–486.
14. Nasr Esfahani MH, Deemeh MR, Tavalaee M, Sekhavati MH, Gourabi H. Zeta sperm selection improves pregnancy rate and alters sex ratio in male factor infertility patients: a double-blind, randomized clinical trial. *Int J Fertil Steril*. 2016;10(2):253–260.
15. Karimi N, Mohseni Kouchesfahani H, Nasr-Esfahani MH, Tavalaee M, Shahverdi A, Choobineh H. DGC/zeta as a new strategy to improve clinical outcome in male factor infertility patients following intracytoplasmic sperm injection: a randomized, single-blind, clinical trial. *Cell J*. 2020;22(1):55–59.
16. Ainsworth C, Nixon B, Aitken RJ. Development of a novel electrophoretic system for the isolation of human spermatozoa. *Hum Reprod*. 2005;20(8):2261–2270.
17. Fleming SD, Ilad RS, Griffin A-MG, et al. Prospective controlled trial of an electrophoretic method of sperm preparation for assisted reproduction: comparison with density gradient centrifugation. *Hum Reprod*. 2008;23(12):2646–2651.
18. Duran-Retamal M, Morris G, Achilli C, et al. Live birth and miscarriage rate following intracytoplasmic morphologically selected sperm injection vs intracytoplasmic sperm injection: an updated systematic review and meta-analysis. *Acta Obstet Gynecol Scand*. 2020;99(1):24–33.
19. Teixeira DM, Miyague AH, Barbosa MA, et al. Regular (ICSI) versus ultra-high magnification (IMSI) sperm selection for assisted reproduction. *Cochrane Database Syst Rev*. 2020;2:CD010167.
20. Gianaroli L, Magli MC, Ferraretti AP, et al. Birefringence characteristics in

sperm heads allow for the selection of reacted spermatozoa for intracytoplasmic sperm injection. *Fertil Steril.* 2010;93(3):807–813.

21. Vermey BG, Chapman MG, Cooke S, Kilani S. The relationship between sperm head retardance using polarized light microscopy and clinical outcomes. *Reprod Biomed Online.* 2015;30(1):67–73.

22. Nosrati R, Graham PJ, Zhang B, et al. Microfluidics for sperm analysis and selection. *Nat Rev Urol.* 2017;14(12):707–730.

23. Marzano G, Chiriacò MS, Primiceri E, et al. Sperm selection in assisted reproduction: a review of established methods and cutting-edge possibilities. *Biotechnol Adv.* 2020;40:107498.

24. Samuel R, Son J, Jenkins TG, et al. Microfluidic system for rapid isolation of sperm from microdissection TESE specimens. *Urology.* 2020;140:70–76.

25. Wang R, Pan W, Jin L, et al. Artificial intelligence in reproductive medicine. *Reproduction.* 2019;158(4):139–154.

26. Dai C, Zhang Z, Huang J, et al. Automated non-invasive measurement of single sperm's motility and morphology. *IEEE Trans Med Imaging.* 2018;37(10):2257–2265.

27. Zhang Z, Dai C, Huang J, et al. Robotic immobilization of motile sperm for clinical intracytoplasmic sperm injection. *IEEE Trans Biomed Eng.* 2019;66(2):444–452.

28. Practice Committee of the American Society for Reproductive Medicine in collaboration with the Society for Male Reproduction and Urology. The management of obstructive azoospermia: a committee opinion. *Fertil Steril.* 2019;111(5):873–880.

29. Shih K-W, Shen P-Y, Wu C-C, Kang Y-N. Testicular versus percutaneous epididymal sperm aspiration for patients with obstructive azoospermia: a systematic review and meta-analysis. *Transl Androl Urol.* 2019;8(6):631–640.

30. Practice Committee of the American Society for Reproductive Medicine. Management of nonobstructive azoospermia: a committee opinion. *Fertil Steril.* 2018;110(7):1239–1245.

31. Bernie AM, Mata DA, Ramasamy R, Schlegel PN. Comparison of microdissection testicular sperm extraction, conventional testicular sperm extraction, and testicular sperm aspiration for nonobstructive azoospermia: a systematic review and meta-analysis. *Fertil Steril.* 2015;104(5):1099–1103.

32. Deruyver Y, Vanderschueren D, Van der Aa F. Outcome of microdissection TESE compared with conventional TESE in non-obstructive azoospermia: a systematic review. *Andrology.* 2014;2(1):20–24.

33. Flannigan RK, Schlegel PN. Microdissection testicular sperm extraction: preoperative patient optimization, surgical technique, and tissue processing. *Fertil Steril.* 2019;111(3):420–426.

34. Corona G, Minhas S, Giwercman A, et al. Sperm recovery and ICSI outcomes in men with non-obstructive azoospermia: a systematic review and meta-analysis. *Hum Reprod Update.* 2019;25(6):733–757.

35. Ohlander S, Hotaling J, Kirshenbaum E, Niederberger C, Eisenberg ML. Impact of fresh versus cryopreserved testicular sperm upon intracytoplasmic sperm injection pregnancy outcomes in men with azoospermia due to spermatogenic dysfunction: a meta-analysis. *Fertil Steril.* 2014;101(2):344–349.

36. Yu Z, Wei Z, Yang J, et al. Comparison of intracytoplasmic sperm injection outcome with fresh versus frozen-thawed testicular sperm in men with nonobstructive azoospermia: a systematic review and meta-analysis. *J Assist Reprod Genet.* 2018;35(7):1247–1257.

37. Popal W, Nagy ZP. Laboratory processing and intracytoplasmic sperm injection using epididymal and testicular spermatozoa: what can be done to improve outcomes? *Clin Sao Paulo Braz.* 2013;68(Suppl. 1):125–130.

38. Baukloh V, German Society for Human Reproductive Biology. Retrospective multicentre study on mechanical and enzymatic preparation of fresh and cryopreserved testicular biopsies. *Hum Reprod.* 2002;17(7):1788–1794.

39. Kovacic B, Vlaisavljevic V, Reljic M. Clinical use of pentoxifylline for activation of immotile testicular sperm before ICSI in patients with azoospermia. *J Androl.* 2006;27(1):45–52.

40. Ebner T, Tews G, Mayer RB, et al. Pharmacological stimulation of sperm motility in frozen and thawed testicular sperm using the dimethylxanthine theophylline. *Fertil Steril.* 2011;96(6):1331–1336.

41. Sallam HN, Farrag A, Agameya A-F, El-Garem Y, Ezzeldin F. The use of the modified hypo-osmotic swelling test for the selection of immotile testicular spermatozoa in patients treated with ICSI: a randomized controlled study. *Hum Reprod.* 2005;20(12):3435–3440.

42. Nordhoff V, Schüring AN, Krallmann C, et al. Optimizing TESE-ICSI by laser-assisted selection of immotile spermatozoa and polarization microscopy for selection of oocytes. *Andrology.* 2013;1(1):67–74.

43. Rubino P, Viganò P, Luddi A, Piomboni P. The ICSI procedure from past to future: a systematic review of the more controversial aspects. *Hum Reprod Update.* 2015; 22(2):194–227.

44. Mangum CL, Patel DP, Jafek AR, et al. Towards a better testicular sperm extraction: novel sperm sorting technologies for non-motile sperm extracted by microdissection TESE. *Transl Androl Urol.* 2020;9(2):S206–S214.

45. Esteves SC, Roque M, Bradley CK, Garrido N. Reproductive outcomes of testicular versus ejaculated sperm for intracytoplasmic sperm injection among men with high levels of DNA fragmentation in semen: systematic review and meta-analysis. *Fertil Steril.* 2017;108(3):456–467.

46. Ambar RF, Agarwal A, Majzoub A, et al. The use of testicular sperm for intracytoplasmic sperm injection in patients with high sperm DNA damage: a systematic review. *World J Mens Health.* 2020;200084.

47. Awaga HA, Bosdou JK, Goulis DG, et al. Testicular versus ejaculated spermatozoa for ICSI in patients without azoospermia: a systematic review. *Reprod Biomed Online.* 2018;37(5):573–580.

48. Kang Y-N, Hsiao Y-W, Chen C-Y, Wu C-C. Testicular sperm is superior to ejaculated sperm for ICSI in cryptozoospermia: an update systematic review and meta-analysis. *Sci Rep.* 2018;8(1):7874.

49. Ku F-Y, Wu C-C, Hsiao Y-W, Kang Y-N. Association of sperm source with miscarriage and take-home baby after ICSI in cryptozoospermia: a meta-analysis of testicular and ejaculated sperm. *Andrology.* 2018;6(6):882–889.

Section 4 Laboratory Evaluation and Treatment of Male Infertility

Chapter 27: Optimal Sperm Selection in the ICSI Era

Joshua Calvert, Darshan Patel, and James M. Hotaling

27.1 Introduction

After one year of unprotected intercourse 15% of couples fail to conceive, with a male factor implicated in roughly 50% of couples [1]. A thorough medical history, physical examination, hormonal profile, and semen analysis (SA) are essential in the evaluation of azoospermic males. Current American Urological Association guidelines recommend two separate SAs in the initial evaluation of an infertile male [2]. These semen samples can be interpreted based on the World Health Organization (WHO) parameters such as semen volume, vitality (live spermatozoa), sperm morphology, sperm concentration, and absolute sperm count [3].

The prevalence of azoospermia in the general population is 1% and azoospermic men constitute approximately 10–15% of all infertile men [4]. Azoospermia is defined as the absence of spermatozoa in the semen. If no spermatozoa are observed in the wet preparation, WHO recommends an examination of the centrifuged sample (3,000 × g for 15 minutes). If no sperm are observed in the centrifuged pellet, the SA should be repeated [3]. Azoospermia may be due to obstruction of the male reproductive tract (obstructive azoospermia [OA]) or inadequate sperm production (nonobstructive azoospermia [NOA]).

NOA is the most severe form of male factor infertility and is characterized by little or no sperm production in the seminiferous tubules. Up to 30–60% of males with NOA can have surgical sperm identified on microdissection testicular sperm extraction (microTESE) [5,6]. In comparison, OA is caused by ductal system obstruction leading to male factor infertility. OA is characterized by adequate testicular sperm production that may be successfully extracted through testicular sperm aspiration (TESA) or testicular sperm extraction (TESE) [7]. Another cause of OA is congenital bilateral absence of the vas deferens (CBAVD), responsible for 2–6% of cases of OA. CBAVD may present as low semen volume and low pH and fructose levels on SA caused by an obstructed epididymis as well as atrophic or congenital absence of the seminal vesicles, in an azoospermic male with nonpalpable vas deferens on physical examination [8,9].

Sperm extraction from patients with NOA is more difficult and requires additional steps before fertilization can occur using artificial reproductive technologies (ART). Previously, severe cases of NOA required use of donor sperm to result in successful pregnancy. The challenge with sperm retrieval in NOA is that testicular sperm are often nonmotile and extremely rare [10]. The introduction of intracytoplasmic sperm injection (ICSI) has allowed the use of even a single extracted sperm to fertilize an oocyte, which can lead to clinical pregnancy. This has offered an opportunity for men with NOA to become biological fathers [11].

Multiple methods have been developed to extract testicular sperm in NOA. Nonselective, open biopsies have been used; however, multiple nonselective testicular biopsies may risk damage to the testes [12]. TESA is a percutaneous procedure where a needle is advanced through the skin into the testicle while applying suction and the aspirated fluid is then checked for sperm. This technique carries the risk of injuring small vessels causing a hematoma and often fails to recover sperm in patients with NOA [13]. In 1997, Turek et al. used fine needle aspiration with mapping (defined as more than four fine needle aspiration sites per testis following systematic planned aspiration site mapping), which yielded sperm in 33% of patients with NOA [14]. These sperm extraction techniques have led to TESE using a high magnification surgical microscope or microTESE. MicroTESE has higher sperm retrieval rates when compared to both random multiple-biopsy TESE and TESA for retrieving sperm in NOA [12,13].

In contrast to traditional TESE, microTESE is performed using a surgical microscope to distinguish dilated seminiferous tubules while minimizing tissue damage. Dissection is performed at 15–20× magnification to search for and extract large diameter tubules resulting in a selective biopsy, decreased tissue removal, and an increased yield of sperm retrieval [13]. Caroppo et al. showed that the sperm retrieval rate was higher from dilated seminiferous tubules (90%) when compared with non-dilated tubules (7%) [15]. Representative sperm retrieval rates increased from 16–45% using simple TESE to 42–63% using microTESE [16]. While the advent of microTESE substantially improved sperm recovery compared to standard biopsy or other techniques the procedure remains inefficient, costly, and very time consuming, both in retrieval and separation/sorting.

27.2 Limitations of Conventional Sperm Sorting

Three conventional sperm sorting techniques are commonly used in andrology clinics: density gradient centrifugation, sperm washing, and swim-up (SU), all of which have provided reliable solutions to isolate normal sperm from highly concentrated semen samples [17].

Density gradient preparation consists of filtering sperm by centrifugal force through either one or multiple layers of increasingly concentrated silane-coated silica particles. The process can generate a pellet at the bottom of a tube, which contains a higher percentage of clean, motile sperm for intrauterine insemination (IUI) [18].

Physiologic intracytoplasmic sperm injection (PICSI) is a biologically inspired technology that mimics the natural attraction between mature sperm and oocytes. A layer of hyaluronan hydrogel at the bottom of a petri dish acts like an oocyte cell, which induces sperm to swim through its surface. Because this technique depends on motility of sperm, it offers an additional motility test for normal sperm selection along with morphology-based tests [19].

The main concerns of conventional sorting methods are they bypass the natural barriers that sperm would experience in vivo, and many studies have associated the centrifugation steps of the sorting process with sperm DNA damage [20]. Furthermore, conventional clinical methods mentioned above are suitable for highly concentrated samples with plenty of motile sperm. Thus, these methods are not feasibly applied to sperm samples with low concentrations (<100 sperm/mL) that only contain immotile sperm such as microTESE samples.

Currently, sperm detection and separation in samples with low sperm concentrations (microTESE, oligozoospermic samples, etc.) is a time-, cost-, and labor-intensive process. Tissue obtained by microTESE requires careful processing in the laboratory in order to separate and identify sperm within the biopsied tissue. First, mechanical tissue-mincing methods are utilized in order to release spermatocytes from seminiferous tubules and eventually to achieve a tissue suspension. Various mechanical techniques are employed, including passing tissue through angiocaths/syringe needles, tissue shredding with fine needles or glass slides, tubule squeezing, or cell straining [21,22]. Next, and most time-consuming, is the tissue-processing step, which involves manually searching through the testicular tissue specimens for sperm. Testicular sperm are generally nonmotile, making the search for sperm more difficult due to inability to distinguish them from surrounding tissue. Each microscopic field examined under 200–400× magnification contains a combination of red blood cells, white blood cells, Sertoli cells, sperm precursor cells, and debris that must be distinguished from the spermatocytes [21,22]. Depending on the level of spermatogenesis and the number of sperm cells present, this step may take as little as one hour to find a sufficient number of sperm, or as long as 12–14 hours with multiple personnel examining tissue specimens to find just a handful of sperm. There is an inverse relationship between the time spent on searching for sperm and the likelihood of successful sperm retrieval, which ultimately impacts pregnancy rates [23].

Another concern is sperm damage during processing. Sperm is exposed to environmental and chemical processing during and after testicular extraction. Testicular tissues are often degraded by enzymatic digestion including collagenases. Collagenases are a type of matrix metalloproteinase, which can dissolve tissues. Collagenase can hydrolyze the three-dimensional helical structure of collagen to release cells from the extracellular matrix but have also been shown to digest cell surface proteins [24]. This may have consequences on sperm viability for ART. Some clinics use an erythrocyte lysing buffer to reduce the number of red blood cells within the cell suspension, or pentoxyfylline (a methylxanthine derivative, an agent primarily used in the treatment of intermittent claudication and other vascular disorders [25]) to chemically induce motility in testicular sperm; however, these additives, like collagenase, are controversial for their effects on sperm viability [22]. A retrospective study was performed by Baukloh et al. that compared the ICSI pregnancy rate between samples that were either mechanically or enzymatically degraded. No differences were shown in pregnancy or live birth rates, although fertilization rates were higher in motile sperm derived from mechanical mincing versus enzyme degradation [26].

There is a strong interest in improving the processing and sorting of sperm in men with NOA after testicular extraction, which would reduce the rate of human error and fatigue with acceptable sperm retrieval rates. For patients with a paucity of sperm at baseline, failing to identify even a few sperm could mean the difference between infertility and a successful pregnancy. By removing the human factor and moving toward automated cell separation, not only would it be possible for sperm to be identified faster and more accurately, but also sperm could be separated from somatic cells and debris simultaneously, facilitating downstream preparation for ICSI.

There are several novel technologies that may improve sperm retrieval after microTESE. These technologies include microfluidics (including dielectrophoresis (DEP), pinched flow, and spiral microfluidic devices; Figure 27.1) that use small streams of fluid to sort cells, magnetic-activated cell sorting (MACS) that uses a magnetically activated column of water that can sort antibody-cell surface antigen tagged cells, and fluorescence-activated cell sorting (FACS), where fluorescent-labeled cells are sorted based on light scattering from a laser source.

27.3 Microfluidics

The field of microfluidics is the most rapidly developing field for sperm selection related to the field of ART. It is particularly powerful when considering applications in single-cell or low-cell number analyses. Microfluidics devices offer a label-free technique for cell sorting by using their physical characteristics such as cell size, electrical charge, and impedance of the cells of interest [27]. In the field of ART, microfluidic technologies have previously been applied to sperm manipulation for purposes such as analysis, sorting, and separation [28]. Compared to traditional sorting and separation techniques utilized for microTESE, microfluidics offers unique advantages. Specifically, there

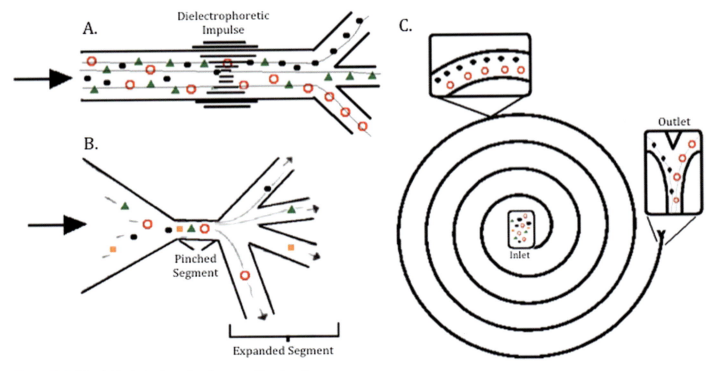

Figure 27.1 Microfluidic device illustrations for nonmotile cell sorting

are two key areas that may benefit from microfluidic technology, namely the identification of sperm in heterogeneous tissue preparations derived from TESE and microTESE procedures, and the identification of "high quality" or "genetically fit" sperm in heterogeneous semen samples [17].

Microfluidics involves the study and control of fluids, ranging from picoliters to microliters, inside micrometer-sized channels [27]. Microfluidic devices use microchannels made from polydimethylsiloxane silicon polymers that are nontoxic and transparent [29]. It is ideally suited to sperm as it can be used to simulate the geometry of microconfined regions within the female reproductive tract, thereby allowing for biomimicry-based selection approaches that are more representative of the in vivo selection environment [30].

Fluid mechanics is a complex physical and mathematical science. A comprehensive technical and mathematical description of microfluidic physics can be found in the reviews from Beebe et al. and Brody et al. [31,32].

Briefly, fluids at the microscale are subject to forces typically not considered on a macroscopic level. Fluids in our normal environment move in an unpredictable pattern. Turbulent flow depends on certain fluid characteristics (viscosity, density, and velocity) and the geometry and size of the channel, leading to calculation of a value known as the Reynold's number. As the scale of the channel reaches micrometer levels, the Reynold's number decreases and becomes increasingly dependent on fluid characteristics. Decrease of the Reynold's number below a threshold value leads to fluid flow in a laminar fashion. Restated, a low Reynold's number indicates laminar flow while a high Reynold's number indicates turbulent flow. Thus at a low Reynold's number, such as within microchannels, flow becomes streamlined and predictable as particles become smaller [33]. This predictably can then be used for sorting.

One of the first attempts to utilize microfluidics for sperm sorting was performed by Smith and Takayama, who published a series of papers showing that microfluidics was a viable approach to improving not only sperm quality but also laboratory efficiency [33]. In their research they used two parallel laminar flow channels where nonmotile spermatozoa and debris would flow along their initial streamlines and exit one outlet, whereas motile spermatozoa had an opportunity to swim into a parallel stream and exit a separate outlet. They found that both motility (98%) and morphology (22%) improved significantly compared to density gradient preparations [33].

In addition, several microfluidic devices manipulate either hydrostatic and/or capillary forces to aid in selection or identification of the most mobile and robust spermatozoa [33].

Some of the potential advantages of utilizing a microfluidics platform include increased automation, scalability, and timesaving. However, to date most of the sperm separation approaches utilizing microfluidics rely on sperm motility for separation with added features through which only highly motile sperm cells can pass, such as chemo-attractants, and physical obstacles.

Other major advantages of microfluidic devices over conventional selection techniques are the ability to work with small sperm sample volume, the short processing times, and the ability to manipulate single cells in a noninvasive manner. Another advantage is the one-step process that eliminates centrifugation and the exposure to reactive oxygen species (ROS) and thereby preserves the DNA integrity. Additionally, DNA fragmentation is significantly decreased in sperm separated with the microfluidic sperm sorting system [34]. The potential for clogging within the microchannels is the biggest limitation and drawback of microfluidics technologies, particularly in the setting of a heterogeneous sample common in NOA patients. Additionally, there is an incomplete understanding of how microfluidic applications impact sperm structural and membrane integrity.

A small handful of microfluidics devices including dielectrophoretic sorting, pinched flow fractionation, and spiraled channels are capable of sorting nonmotile cells and may be applicable for sperm harvested from NOA patients and are discussed below.

DEP cell sorting uses an external energy source, such as an electrical, magnetic, or acoustic field to separate nonmotile cells [35–37]. The cells are suspended in a field gradient, inducing a dipole that can stimulate cell motility up or down the field. In this technique, two laminar streams of media are injected into the microfluidic device and run parallel to each other. The external energy source is then activated and can pull a cell toward or away from the energy field based on the size and charge to separate cells into the adjacent stream of flow, thus effectively sorting the cells from contaminants as other contaminants within the sample are not pulled into the second stream. The force exerted on a cell can be determined based on the conductivity, permittivity, and size of each cell.

De Wagenaar et al. demonstrated the ability to separate boar sperm based on cytoplasmic droplets on the flagella. They also demonstrated separation of sperm cells from 3 μm beads using impedance-controlled cell sorting to show that this method could noninvasively sort sperm. As the sperm and beads passed through the microfluidic channel, they demonstrated a clear impedance change from the population of beads versus the population of sperm. When an impedance change was detected, the DEP electrodes would activate to sort the particle into a separate channel [35].

Ohta et al. utilized optoelectric tweezers (optically induced DEP) to noninvasively identify and sort viable live nonmotile sperm from nonviable sperm without inflicting DNA damage on the cells [36]. Their study was intended to show that DEP does not injure sperm cells and used the absence of Trypan blue dye as a marker for viability. In this study, 100% (200 individual sperm) were Trypan blue negative, and it was concluded that using this method for DEP cell sorting maintains cell viability and could be a reliable method for separating Trypan blue cells. One strength of this study was that in addition to the freshly ejaculated samples, researchers also diluted samples to better mimic the microTESE samples. Thus, these results confirm that optoelectric tweezers can distinguish among and sort live nonmotile spermatozoa from nonviable spermatozoa.

Huang et al. used DEP charges to separate circulating tumor cells from blood based on the capacitance and conductivity of the tumor cells [37]. Tumor cells have more folds on the plasma membrane when compared to other contents in the blood. These folds can increase the capacitance up to 300%, allowing for DEP manipulation of cells against a background of normal blood cells including white blood cells that have a similar size profile as many tumor cells. This study further demonstrates that nonmotile cells can be separated using laminar flow microfluidics with DEP.

In 2019, Shuchat et al. used DEP for sorting sperm cells. Using a quadrupolar electrode array it was shown that the head and tail of the sperm had independent and unique crossover frequencies corresponding to the transition of the DEP force from repulsive (negative) to attractive (positive). Authors were able to show that the head and tail or sperm have their own distinct electrical properties, and that DEP has the potential to automate and improve the processing of semen samples, especially those containing only rare spermatozoa [38].

Although dielectrophoretic cell sorting may be a future candidate for nonmotile sperm separation from a microTESE sample, further research is needed. There is also an incomplete understanding on how dielectrophoretic manipulation impacts sperm viability for ART. Another potential limitation of DEP is identifying the optimal settings for separation of sperm from debris.

Pinched flow fractionation separates cells based on their size as they follow a path of media flow through a pinched and then expanded microdevice. At a low Reynold's number, a particle is presumed to follow a stream of flow in a direction based on size. The sample of cells is injected at the inlet of a device with a "pinched" bottleneck segment. The particles are forced to align against the walls of the narrow segment, regardless of size, with small molecules aligning closer to the walls than larger molecules. Because of the differing radii between different cell types, the centers of cell types lie on different streamlines. After the pinched segment, the stream of media is allowed to expand, which amplifies the slight difference in streamlines from the pinched segment, effectively separating and sorting cells based on size as they follow their streamline. The cells can then be collected in smaller outlets. The flow of media, channel geometry, and outlet location can be altered based on the sample to control the direction of flow of particles by size.

Liu et al. used this technique to separate sperm from epithelial cells for forensic analysis in sexual assault cases. A microfluidic channel with pinched flow separated female epithelial cells from the sperm cells based on size. They were then able to use short tandem repeats to identify male DNA fraction (94% male) indicating a high purification rate of sperm [39]. Importantly, flow dynamics through a pinched flow model does not rely on motility, and may be a viable option for sperm cell sorting for microTESE.

The shape of cells appears to be a very important variable within pinched flow fractionation and may limit the application for nonmotile sperm. Takagi et al. observed that red blood cells, which have a disc-like shape, have disparate trajectories and poor sorting [40]. Given the highly heterogeneous mixture in a microTESE sample, it is possible that some of the larger tissue debris may clog in the pinched section of this device as well. There is also a concern that the passage of viable sperm through the pinched flow fractionation system may induce structural or mechanical damage.

In 2019, Berendsen et al. published their results on a 2.5% sperm spiked sample, further supporting the importance of size when utilizing pinched flow techniques. Researchers used the knowledge that while the width of the sperm is similar to that of an erythrocyte, the length of the spermatozoon is five times larger. They built a microfluidic chip, in which the tumbling behavior of spermatozoa in pinched flow fractionation separated sperm from red blood cells. They were able to separate 95% of the spermatozoa from a sample while removing around 90% of the erythrocytes. Importantly, a 2.5% spiked sperm sample does not mimic the rare nonmotile sperm found in a typical microTESE sample for a man with NOA [41].

27.4 Spiral Microfluidics

Most of the sperm separation approaches utilizing microfluidics rely on sperm motility. Thus, these techniques can separate only progressive motile sperm cells from semen samples. Accordingly, they lose a significant number of sperm cells including viable nonprogressive motile and nonmotile sperm cells, and are not feasible for use with immature and nonmotile sperm cells that may be the only sperm cells produced by some patients. Thus, a system to recover all sperm cells, not just motile sperm cells, is needed. To this end researchers set out to develop spiral channel separation.

In spiral microfluidics, a precisely designed spiral channel is fabricated. The sample is then inserted into the center of the spiral. As the cells are carried forward within the spiral channel, each cell will migrate laterally until an equilibrium position is reached within the spiral. Cells will continue at this lateral position at a constant flow rate until they reach the outlet of the tube. This method bypasses the need for labeling, centrifuging, or radiolabeling. Inertial microfluidic theory relies on the separation of particles in a spiral chamber based on size and shape of the constituents within a sample. The device relies on sperm size compared to the other cells in solution rather than motility, making it a viable option to separate sperm from microTESE samples.

In 2015, Son et al. demonstrated sperm separation from a simulated microTESE sample, which included sperm cells, blood cells, and other debris. They used a passive, purely mechanical, label-free microfluidic approach based on inertial microfluidics that separated sperm cells (regardless of their motility state) from other unwanted cells/debris. The approach did not require any externally applied forces except the movement of the fluid sample through the instrument. The system could recover not only motile sperm cells, but also viable less-motile and nonmotile sperm cells with high recovery rates. This study also suggested that a precisely designed spiral channel could generate some flow focusing of sperm cells, making it a suitable solution for increasing the purity of sperm cells from semen samples with high concentrations of unwanted particles [42].

The same group demonstrated and published their findings on the efficacy of inertial microfluidic technology on separating sperm from leukocytes. Using this approach, it was possible to recover not only motile sperm, but also viable less-motile and nonmotile sperm cells with high recovery rates. When the group performed an input mixture of sperm/white blood cells, the result was that 83% of sperm cells and 93% of white blood cells were collected separately from two distinct outlets [43].

27.5 Magnetically Activated Cell Sorting

MACS is the method of separation of various cell populations based on their surface antigens. By using magnetic nanoparticles coated with antibodies against a particular surface antigen, the cells expressing this antigen attach to the magnetic nanoparticles and remain in the sample while other cells (not expressing the antigen) flow through. This has been utilized for sperm sorting to retain sperm with evidence of apoptosis, and allowing viable sperm to flow through.

Phosphatidylserine is a phospholipid that is present on the inner leaflet of the plasma membrane of a cell and has been used in MACS sperm sorting [44,45]. When a cell is damaged phosphatidylserine moves to the outer surface, thus, externalization of the phosphatidylserine residue is a marker of apoptosis [44]. Annexin V is a phospholipid-binding protein, and has a strong affinity for phosphatidylserine residue. As it cannot pass through the sperm membrane, Annexin V binding to the outer sperm membrane signifies externalization of phosphatidylserine and thus that the sperm integrity has been compromised. Therefore Annexin V is used to label sperm that have a compromised membrane integrity and are less able to fertilize the egg [45]. By using colloidal superparamagnetic microbeads conjugated with Annexin V antibodies, and then applying a strong magnetic field, the sperm that are nonapoptotic pass through, whereas those that are apoptotic are tagged and retained in the magnetic field. This allows the rapid separation and selection of nonapoptotic sperm from apoptotic sperm [46,47].

Additional research suggests that sperm selected by MACS before cryopreservation had a larger number of sperm with intact mitochondrial membranes, a reflection of mitochondrial survival after cryopreservation, than sperm prepared by cryopreservation alone [48]. The clinical significance of using the Annexin V MACS technique is that it allows the selection of sperm with improved motility, viability, and morphology and significantly improved fertilization rates and oocyte penetration [49]. Improved pregnancy rates have been reported compared to sperm prepared by density gradient alone [50].

To date, MACS has not been studied using nonmotile sperm extracted by microTESE, and may not address the separation from other live tissues within the heterogeneous sample. While MACS appears to be a viable option for selecting for sperm without membrane damage, this is limited to a relatively homogenous sperm sample. This may not function as well with microTESE samples for nonmotile sperm.

27.6 Fluorescence-Activated Cell Sorting

FACS, a unique type of flow cytometry, is a biological sorting technique in which a population of live cells is separated into subpopulations based on fluorescent labeling. Cells stained using fluorophore-conjugated antibodies can be separated from one another depending on which fluorophore they have been stained with. It provides fast, objective, and quantitative recording of fluorescent signals from individual cells as well as physical separation of cells of interest.

An antibody specific for a particular cell surface protein is associated to a fluorescent molecule and then added to a mixture of cells. The cell suspension is then placed in the center of a narrow, rapidly flowing stream of liquid. The flow is arranged so that there is a large separation between cells relative to their diameter. A vibrating mechanism causes the stream of cells to break into individual droplets. The system is adjusted so that there is a low probability of more than one cell per droplet. Just before the stream breaks into droplets, the flow passes through a fluorescence measuring station where the fluorescent character of interest of each cell is measured. An electrical charging ring is placed just at the point where the stream breaks into droplets. Droplets containing single cells are given a positive or negative charge, based on whether the cell has the fluorescently tagged antibody or not. Droplets containing a single cell are then deflected by an electric field into collection tubes according to their charge [51]. One disadvantage is the requirement for cellular tagging with fluorescent antibodies or DNA labels; however, this labeling and placement in a fluid cell suspension allows effective sorting even for nonmotile cells [52].

At present there are no peer-reviewed published examples of FACS for nonmotile sperm. However, in one small pilot study, FACS was used to separate nonmotile sperm from microTESE samples [53]. Preparation of the samples required filtration, fixation, and DNA staining with To-Pro-3, a fluorescent dye for nuclear counterstaining. Then, cell sorting was completed using FACS to isolate spermatozoa. Each sorted specimen then underwent standard light microscopy to identify spermatozoa. Of the eight patients undergoing microTESE, three (38%) had spermatozoa recovered using standard tissue processing and four (50%) had spermatozoa recovered using this FACS technique. Notably, in this cohort, both patients with maturation arrest with a prior negative microTESE had successful isolation of spermatozoa using FACS. There is a concern regarding the impact on sperm DNA fragmentation due to this sorting process, which is being actively studied by the group. Ultimately, larger studies will need to be conducted to validate these findings, and to assess pregnancy success following sorting with FACS.

27.7 Further Directions

In addition to the techniques and technologies listed above there has been interest in combining different technologies to improve cell sorting. To this end, Samuel et al. proposed the combination of microfluidics with optics, specifically Raman spectroscopy, for nonmotile NOA microTESE sperm samples [20]. This combination has previously been shown to distinguish sperm with improved nuclear integrity [54,55]. Current Raman microspectroscopy efforts have focused exclusively on dead sperm, fixed to a glass cover slip. Combining Raman microspectroscopy and microfluidics could lead to systems that could sort single live sperm and then measure the quality/quantity of their subcellular components. Such systems could theoretically be used to select sperm from nonmotile NOA samples, thus increasing fertility outcomes, and dramatically reducing processing and preparation time [30,56].

27.8 Conclusion

Sperm retrieval from patients with NOA provides a unique challenge for assisted reproduction because the sperm is not present within the ejaculate and testicular sperm is nonmotile. MicroTESE has improved surgical sperm retrieval rates when compared with older methods but the laboratory retrieval and processing of sperm from the testicular biopsy is still time intensive and often results in a low overall sperm yield. Traditional sperm sorting and processing techniques have been historically applied to highly concentrated sperm. Additionally, these processing methods may contribute to sperm damage by removing antioxidant-rich seminal plasma, and induce oxidative stress and formation of free ROS. There is a need for new cell-sorting devices that retrieve a high yield of sperm and can avoid exposure of the sperm to labels, free radicals, and enzymatic degradation. Several solutions are presented in the preceding chapter. In particular, microfluidic technologies appear to offer a cost-effective and efficient solution to improving sperm processing after microTESE for NOA.

References

1. Agarwal A, Mulgund A, Hamada A, Chyatte MR. A unique view on male infertility around the globe. *Reprod Biol Endocrinol.* 2015;13:37.
2. Jarow JP, Sharlip ID, Belker AM, et al. Best practice policies for male infertility. *J Urol.* 2002;77 (5):873–882.
3. World Health Organization. *Laboratory Manual for the Examination and Processing of Human Semen.* Cambridge University Press; 2010.
4. Gudeloglu A, Parekattil SJ. Update in the evaluation of the azoospermic male. *Clinics (Sao Paolo).* 2013;68(Suppl. 1):27–34.
5. Esteves SC. Clinical management of infertile men with nonobstructive azoospermia. *Asian J Androl.* 2015;17 (3):459–470.
6. Silber SJ. Microsurgical TESE and the distribution of spermatogenesis in non-

7. Craft I, Tsirigotis M, Bennett V, et al. Percutaneous epididymal sperm aspiration and intracytoplasmic sperm injection in the management of infertility due to obstructive azoospermia. *Fertil Steril*. 1995;63(5):1038–1042.

8. Donat R, Mcneill AS, Fitzpatrick DR, Hargreave TB. The incidence of cystic fibrosis gene mutations in patients with congenital bilateral absence of the vas deferens in Scotland. *Br J Urol*. 1997;79(1):74–77.

9. Grangeia A, Niel F, Carvalho F, et al. Characterization of cystic fibrosis conductance transmembrane regulator gene mutations and IVS8 poly (T) variants in Portuguese patients with congenital absence of the vas deferens. *Hum Reprod*. 2004;19(11):2502–2508.

10. Tournaye H. Update on surgical sperm recovery: the European view. *Hum Fertil*. 2010;13(4):242–246.

11. Vloeberghs V, Verheyen G, Haentjens P, Goossens A, Polyzos NP, Tournaye H. How successful is TESE-ICSI in couples with non-obstructive azoospermia? *Hum Reprod*. 2015;30(8):1790–1796.

12. Shah R, Gupta C. Advances in sperm retrieval techniques in azoospermic men: a systematic review. *Arab J Urol*. 2018;16(1):125–131.

13. Flannigan RK, Schlegel PN. Microdissection testicular sperm extraction: preoperative patient optimization, surgical technique, and tissue processing. *Fertil Steril*. 2019;111(3):420–426.

14. Turek PJ, Cha I, Ljung BM. Systematic fine-needle aspiration of the testis: correlation to biopsy and results of organ "mapping" for mature sperm in azoospermic men. *Urology*. 1997;49(5):743–748.

15. Caroppo E, Colpi EM, Gazzano G, et al. The seminiferous tubule caliber pattern as evaluated at high magnification during microdissection testicular sperm extraction predicts sperm retrieval in patients with non-obstructive azoospermia. *Andrology*. 2019;7(1):8–14.

16. Deruyver Y, Vanderschueren D, Van der Aa F. Outcome of microdissection TESE compared with conventional TESE in non-obstructive azoospermia: a systematic review. *Andrology*. 2014;2(1):20–24.

17. Samuel R, Badamjav O, Murphy KE, et al. Microfluidics: the future of microdissection TESE? *Syst Biol Reprod Med*. 2016;62(3):161–170.

18. Peterson CM, Hammoud AO, Lindley E, Carrell DT, Wilson K. Assisted reproductive technology practice management. In: Carrell D, Peterson CM, eds. *Reproductive Endocrinology and Infertility: Integrating Modern Clinical and Laboratory Practice*. Springer; 2010:7–37.

19. Parmegiani L, Cognigni GE, Bernardi S, et al. Comparison of two ready-to-use systems designed for sperm-hyaluronic acid binding selection before intracytoplasmic sperm injection: PICSI vs. Sperm Slow: a prospective, randomized trial. *Fertil Steril*. 2012;98(3):632–637.

20. Samuel R, Feng H, Jafek A, Despain D, Jenkins T, Gale B. Microfluidic-based sperm sorting & analysis for treatment of male infertility. *Transl Androl Urol*. 2018;7(Suppl. 3):S336–S347.

21. Esteves SC, Varghese AC. Laboratory handling of epididymal and testicular spermatozoa: what can be done to improve sperm injections outcome. *J Hum Reprod Sci*. 2012;5(3):233–243.

22. Popal W, Nagy ZP. Laboratory processing and intracytoplasmic sperm injection using epididymal and testicular spermatozoa: what can be done to improve outcomes? *Clinics (Sao Paolo)*. 2013;68(Suppl. 1):125–130.

23. Ramasamy R, Schlegel PN. Microdissection testicular sperm extraction: effect of prior biopsy on success of sperm retrieval. *J Urol*. 2007;177(4):1447–1449.

24. Feng X, Liu L, Yu BQ, Huang JM, Gu LD, Xu DF. Effect of optimized collagenase digestion on isolated and cultured nucleus pulposus cells in degenerated intervertebral discs. *Medicine (Baltimore)*. 2018;97(44):e12977.

25. Ghasemzadeh A, Karkon-Shayan F, Yousefzadeh S, Naghavi-Behzad M, Hamdi K. Study of pentoxifylline effects on motility and viability of spermatozoa from infertile asthenozoospermic males. *Niger Med J*. 2016;57(6):324–328.

26. Baukloh V. Retrospective multicentre study on mechanical and enzymatic preparation of fresh and cryopreserved testicular biopsies. *Hum Reprod*. 2002;17(7):1788–1794.

27. Sackmann EK, Fulton AL, Beebe DJ. The present and future role of microfluidics in biomedical research. *Nature*. 2014;507(7491):181–189.

28. Swain JE, Lai D, Takayama S, Smith GD. Thinking big by thinking small: application of microfluidic technology to improve ART. *Lab Chip*. 2013;13(7):1213–1224.

29. Xia Y, Whitesides GM. Soft lithography. *Angew Chem Int Ed Eng*. 1998;37(5):550–575.

30. Vaughan DA, Sakkas D, Gardner DK. Sperm selection methods in the 21st century. *Biol Reprod*. 2019;101(6):1076–1082.

31. Beebe DJ, Mensing GA, Walker GM. Physics and applications of microfluidics in biology. *Annu Rev Biomed Eng*. 2002;4:261–286.

32. Brody JP, Yager P, Goldstein RE, Austin RH. Biotechnology at low Reynolds numbers. *Biophys J*. 1996;71(6):3430–3441.

33. Suh R, Takayama S, Smith GD. Microfluidic applications for andrology. *J Androl*. 2005;26(6):664–670.

34. Quinn MM, Jalalian L, Ribeiro S, et al. Microfluidic sorting selects sperm for clinical use with reduced DNA damage compared to density gradient centrifugation with swim-up in split semen samples. *Hum Reprod*. 2018;33(8):1388–1393.

35. De Wagenaar B, Dekker S, De Boer HL, et al. Towards microfluidic sperm refinement: impedance-based analysis and sorting of sperm cells. *Lab Chip*. 2016;16(8):1514–1522.

36. Ohta AT, Garcia M, Valley JK, et al. Motile and non-motile sperm diagnostic manipulation using optoelectronic tweezers. *Lab Chip*. 2010;10(23):3213–3217.

37. Huang SB, Wu MH, Lin YH, et al. High-purity and label-free isolation of circulating tumor cells (CTCs) in a microfluidic platform by using optically-induced-dielectrophoretic (ODEP) force. *Lab Chip*. 2013;13(7):1371–1383.

38. Shuchat S, Park S, Kol S, Yossifon G. Distinct and independent dielectrophoretic behavior of the head and tail of sperm and its potential for the safe sorting and isolation of rare

spermatozoa. *Electrophoresis.* 2019;40(11):1606–1614.

39. Liu W, Chen W, Liu R, et al. Separation of sperm and epithelial cells based on the hydrodynamic effect for forensic analysis. *Biomicrofluidics.* 2015; 9(4):044127.

40. Takagi J, Yamada M, Yasuda M, Seki M. Continuous particle separation in a microchannel having asymmetrically arranged multiple branches. *Lab Chip.* 2005;9(11):1638–1639.

41. Berendsen JTW, Eijkel JCT, Wetzels AM, Segerink LI. Separation of spermatozoa from erythrocytes using their tumbling mechanism in a pinch flow fractionation device. *Microsystems Nanoeng.* 2019;5:24.

42. Son J, Murphy K, Samuel R, Gale BK, Carrell DT, Hotaling JM. Non-motile sperm cell separation using a spiral channel. *Anal Methods.* 2015;7:8041–8047.

43. Son J, Samuel R, Gale BK, Carrell DT, Hotaling JM. Separation of sperm cells from samples containing high concentrations of white blood cells using a spiral channel. *Biomicrofluidics.* 2017;11(5):054106.

44. Vermes I, Haanen C, Steffens-Nakken H, Reutellingsperger C. A novel assay for apoptosis flow cytometric detection of phosphatidylserine expression on early apoptotic cells using fluorescein labelled Annexin V. *J Immunol Methods.* 1995;184(1):39–51.

45. Glander HJ, Schaller J. Binding of annexin V to plasma membranes of human spermatozoa: a rapid assay for detection of membrane changes after cryostorage. *Mol Hum Reprod.* 1999;5(2):109–115.

46. Paasch U, Grunewald S, Fitzl G, Glander HJ. Deterioration of plasma membrane is associated with activated caspases in human spermatozoa. *J Androl.* 2003;24(2):246–252.

47. Gil M, Sar-Shalom V, Melendez Sivira Y, Carreras R, Checa MA. Sperm selection using magnetic activated cell sorting (MACS) in assisted reproduction: a systematic review and meta-analysis. *J Assist Reprod Genet.* 2013;30(4):479–485.

48. Said TM, Grunewald S, Paasch U, et al. Advantage of combining magnetic cell separation with sperm preparation techniques. *Reprod Biomed Online.* 2005;10(6):740–746.

49. Grunewald S, Reinhardt M, Blumenauer V, et al. Increased sperm chromatin decondensation in selected nonapoptotic spermatozoa of patients with male infertility. *Fertil Steril.* 2009;92(2):572–577.

50. Dirican EK, Özgün OD, Akarsu S, et al. Clinical outcome of magnetic activated cell sorting of non-apoptotic spermatozoa before density gradient centrifugation for assisted reproduction. *J Assist Reprod Genet.* 2008;25(8):375–381.

51. Picot J, Guerin CL, Le Van Kim C, Boulanger CM. Flow cytometry: retrospective, fundamentals and recent instrumentation. *Cytotechnology.* 2012;64(2):109–130.

52. Komoda T, Matsunaga T. Biotechnological study. In: *Biochemistry for Medical Professionals.* Elsevier; 2015:75–93.

53. Mittal S, Mielnik A, Bolyakov A, Schlegel P, Paduch D. PD68-01 pilot study results using fluorescence activated cell sorting of spermatozoa from testis tissue: a novel method for sperm isolation after TESE. *J Urol.* 2017;197:e139.

54. Štiavnická M, Abril-Parreño L, Nevoral J, Králíčková M, García-Álvarez O. Non-invasive approaches to epigenetic-based sperm selection. *Med Sci Monit.* 2017;23:4677–4683.

55. Amaral S, Da Costa R, Wübbeling F, Redmann K, Schlatt S. Raman microspectroscopy analysis of different sperm regions: a species comparison. *Mol Hum Reprod.* 2018;24(4):185–202.

56. Ramser K. Raman spectroscopy of single cells for biomedical applications. In: Ghomi M, ed. *Applications of Raman Spectroscopy to Biology: From Basic Studies to Disease Diagnosis.* IOS Press; 2012:106–147.

Chapter 28: Microfluidics for Sperm Sample Preparation and Sperm Identification

Raheel Samuel, Haidong Feng, Hayden Brady, and Utpal Saha

28.1 Introduction to Microfluidics

Microfluidics is the science and technology of manipulating a small amount of liquid in microscale-sized channels [1]. It has been studied and used in a wide range of fields such as point of care diagnostic, pharmaceutical and life science research, drug delivery, analytical devices, and micro reaction flow chemistry.

Microfluidic devices are designed and built based on specific applications, in which they have unique advantages over traditional biosample treatment methods. In general, microfluidic devices have the following unique set of advantages [1]:

(1) Microfluidic devices are capable of working with low amounts of samples and reagents. This is beneficial in cases where sample sizes are small and reagents are expensive.
(2) Fundamental physics at the microscale, such as diffusion, electrophoresis, and surface to volume ratio, enable new liquid and particle manipulation approaches. The detection resolution and efficiency are improved utilizing these microscale physics.
(3) The feature size in a microfluidic device can be reduced to the scale of the biosample dimension. This allows for precise control and handling of biosamples in application, such as single-cell analysis [3].

Furthermore, biomimicking structures can be fabricated for organ-on-a-chip microfluidic devices [2].

Currently, microfluidic devices are utilized in multiple fields for the biosample treatment process. For example, the microfluidic device can be used for tissue culture and organ-on-a-chip applications [3]. This is due to advances in micromachining processes, that have enabled the manufacture of complex 3D tissue scaffolds and microenvironments that can be precisely controlled with microfluidics. Microfluidic devices also have advantages in manipulating bioparticle movement. High throughput label-free separation of bioparticles can be realized based on different separation criteria, such as particle size, shape, and deformability [4]. Precise particle manipulation can be achieved utilizing different approaches, such as various external fields (electrical, thermal, magnetic, etc.) and geometric designs of microchannels [5]. Additionally, microfluidic-based single-cell trapping and isolation can be achieved for unique single-cell assays [6]. Droplet microfluidics is a unique area of microfluidics utilizing multiphase flow.

In droplet microfluidic systems thousands of droplets can be created in microchannels in few seconds, and each droplet can serve as an independent reaction chamber for a particular cell. This enables high throughput microscale reaction and analysis process. Furthermore, microfluidic devices have been developed and demonstrated for automatic and high-sensitivity detection of biomolecules based on nanofluidic mechanisms [7]. Readers interested in knowing more information about microfluidics are referred to thoughtful reviews by Convery and Gadegaard [8].

In the field of assisted reproductive technology (ART), microfluidic devices have been used for semen quality evaluation, oocyte preparation, in vitro fertilization, testicular tissue culture, and sperm isolation [9,10]. As compared to conventional methods in ART, microfluidic systems for ART lead to improvement of sample treatment efficiency, such as cell recovery, viability, and detection sensitivity. This is because microfluidic devices, unlike bulk sample treatment process, have the capability of single-cell manipulation, and cell viability can be improved due to the low magnitudes of forces generated in a microfluidic system. Since microfluidic systems can be automated, automating any sample treatment process in microfluidic devices reduces operator skill requirements, and human errors. In this chapter, we will provide a brief review of microfluidic devices for sperm identification and sperm sample preparation. For more comprehensive reviews of the application of microfluidics for male reproductive medicine, readers are referred to thoughtful reviews by Kashaninejad et al. and Samuel et al. [9,11].

28.2 Microfluidics for Sperm Sample Preparation

Recently demonstrated microfluidic techniques for sperm sample preparation have shown great improvement over current methods in reducing time, harmful forces applied to the sample, and retrieving more sperm from original sample.

The first publication of human semen processing in a microfluidic device was in 2003 [12]. The device was designed on the foundations of laminar flow and was driven by a gravity-fed pump created specifically for the project. By flowing semen and media in parallel in microfluidic channels, negligible mixing of the two fluids was experienced. This flow provided the conditions required for motile sperm to travel across the streams by their own motility to be collected on the opposite end of the device. Plasma, nonmotile sperm, and other particles stayed in their respective stream. In testing, the sample (raw semen) was shown to be significantly refined going from 44% motile sperm to 98% motile sperm in media, while the sperm maintained standard morphology. Even when the beginning sample was spiked with significant quantities of nongamete human cells the device still processed the motile sperm into recovery, showing that the device lent itself well to semen samples with both low concentrations of sperm cells and atypical semen compositions. This device proved the feasibility of using microfluidic devices in ART and preceded a now developing field of applied reproductive microfluidics.

Zymot is at the forefront of development in the field of microfluidic sperm preparation and is one of the few products available on the market for purchase [13]. In combination with defined microfluidic channels, the Zymot device employs a filter that results in "space-constrained microfluidic sorting." Functionally, the device is as simple as they come. A sample of either 875 μL or 3 mL is inserted into the chip, the chip is then incubated, and after incubation a sample is collected. The length and the filtering time were optimized to show that a 30-minute incubation period inside the device resulted in a collected sample with 100% progressive motile sperm. More time in the device resulted in the sperm showing adverse signs of exhaustion.

The Simple Periodic ARray for Trapping And isolatioN or SPARTAN is another promising device for sperm gathering and separation. Separation of particles is a significant part of the microfluidics field, and one of the more unique ways to perform this separation is through deterministic lateral displacement (DLD) [14]. In microfluidic systems utilizing DLD, discrete microsized pillars are fabricated inside microchannels to manually control the positioning of the particles within the flow across the microchannel. The pillars make possible the separation of particles based on column diameter. The SPARTAN device does exactly this: The array of pillars are set up to direct the healthy motile sperm toward the collection, while the nonmotile sperm and other fragments are small enough to avoid containment and float freely through the device. Pillar-spacing values of 18 × 26 and 30 × 26 μm lead to a collection of 52% morphologically normal sperm when starting with a raw semen sample containing 13% morphologically normal sperm.

Like other medical innovative medical technologies, microfluidics had a slow uptake from research labs commercial applications. Current clinical procedures for sperm preparation including density gradient centrifugation, swim-up, and washing with centrifugation are all effective techniques to isolate sperm. Nonetheless, since 1993 there have been documented cases of centrifugation deteriorating sperm [15]. As the ART field continues to grow in the coming years it is possible that microfluidic sperm sorting employing passive methods becomes the evolutionary step beyond the centrifugation of sperm, leading to less DNA damage, increased access to infertility treatment, and a higher successful birthrate.

28.3 Microfluidics for Sperm Identification

Techniques that utilize microfluidics for sperm identification or selection can be divided into two categories: sperm motility-based and those that are based on other sperm physiology. These techniques are described in detail in the following sections and the main contributions of selected examples of each technique have been summarized in Table 28.1.

Sperm motility-based microfluidics for sperm identification isolate motile sperm for nonmotile sperm or cells, and do not incorporate any external stimulus to separate sperm based on sperm motility [16]. One of the earliest applications of this technique was performed by Schuster and coworkers [17]. They developed a microfluidic system (about the size of a US quarter) that facilitates motile sperm to swim out of raw semen and into media. The system does not require any instrumentation for fluid flow, which allows for compactness and ease of use. The device isolated motile sperm from nonmotile sperm and other cellular debris, based on motile sperm's ability to swim across two distinct fluid streams (semen stream and media stream). This method showed that it can process raw semen to output a processed sample in media containing about 98% motile sperm. Furthermore, an improvement in sperm morphology was also observed when output samples were compared to input samples.

In recent years, a number of microfluidic systems have been demonstrated to purify motile sperm from semen using the same principle utilized by Schuster et al. [12]. A notable example will be Zhang and coworkers, who developed a microfluidic chip to monitor and sort motile sperm simultaneously by integrated specially designed optics with the microfluidic chip [17]. They have claimed that the unique compactness and portability offered by their system will be useful in selecting the most fertile sperms for fertility clinics as well as allowing male individuals to check their fertility at home.

Asghar and coworkers also developed a microfluidic system that separates motile sperm from raw semen by utilizing a polycarbonate membrane filter. The microfluidic system is basically composed of two chambers separated by a membrane filter. Motile sperm pass through the filter while immotile sperm or those with low motility stay behind. The authors claimed that their system yielded more viable sperm and very few reactive oxygen species (free oxygen radicals that are one of the main causes of male infertility) in comparison to the conventional swim-up method via centrifugation. By doing so, they were able to sort out the most motile sperm and with lower DNA damage [18].

Utilizing the progressive motility of sperm, a chip containing 500 parallel microchannels has also been reported [19]. This chip leverages the surface accumulation behavior (tendency of spermatozoa to swim near surfaces) of sperm for

Table 28.1 Summary of selected microfluidic techniques for sperm identification

Type of sperm identification		Working principle	Major findings	Reference
Based on sperm motility	Microscale-integrated sperm sorter	Utilizes ability of motile sperm to swim across streamlines whereas nonmotile cells maintain their position within streamline	Selected subpopulation had 100% motility and 22.4%±3.3% normal morphological properties	Cho and coworkers [30]
	Microfluidic sperm sorter (MFSS)	Analysis of flow cytometric measurement and chromatin structure assay using an MFSS developed by Menicon Co. and approved by the FDA	95% motile sperm selection with only 1% DNA fragmentation index	Shirota and coworkers [31]
	Flowing upstream sperm sorter	Triangular flow region to create a gradient in the main flow stream	High throughput (13-40 KHz rate of sperm processing), with 80% enrichment of viable sperm	Wu and coworkers [32]
	Geometrically confined sperm selector	The device utilizes the natural swimming abilities of sperm such as surface accumulation behavior [20] and boundary-following navigation [21] within a confined geometry	High throughput: collected sperm populations have higher DNA integration (80%) compared to the original population	Nosrati and coworkers [19]
Based on size, shape, and speed of sperm	Sorter of sperm-epithelial (EP) mixture	Sorting of sperm based on size; dependent on the hydrodynamic interaction of fluid flow and cells	41.1% of sperm were recovered from the sperm-EPs mixture	Liu and coworkers [25]
	Spiral sorter using inertial microfluidics	Utilizes inertial microfluidic physics to create two counter-rotating vortices that would create different equilibrium positions for various sized cells. These equilibrium positions are contained in different fluid laminas that can be separately collected downstream for particle separation	Isolating 82% of sperm from a mixture of WBCs and sperm	Son and coworkers [27]
	Microchip-based sperm sorter	Stiction and stabilization of epithelial cells in a glass microfluidic chip	Recovery of 25% sperm from sperm-EPs mixture within 1.16 hours	Horsman et al. [33]
	Insulator-based dielectrophoresis (IDEP) sorter	Variation of electric polarization due to particle shape difference and using IDEP to accumulate sperm cells	High viability of mature sperm cells after sorting them from spermatogenic cells	Rosales-Cruzaley et al. [28]
	Impedance-analyzer-based sperm sorter	Analysis of impedance of morphologically normal and abnormal sperm and sorting them using DEP force triggered by difference in impedance	Sorting speed of 5 cells/s but could be increased to 1,000 cells/s with improved hardware settings for sorting	De Wagenaar et al. [29]
	Sperm sorter and LCR-based sperm counter	Use of conventional swim-up method to sort motile sperm from nonmotile ones and count the sorted sperm using an LCR-based impedance signal generated by microelectrodes integrated with the microchannel	96% of the sorted sperm were motile with 10 μL minimum volume of sample analysis	Phiphattanaphiphop et al. [34]
	Impedance-based sperm concentration analyzer	Integration of planar microelectrodes in a microfluidic chip to measure the impedance of sperm and quantify sperm's concentration in semen	First report of on-chip analysis of sperm concentration in semen	Segerink et al. [35]

sperm selection [20]. Taking 1 mL raw semen as the input, this chip is capable to select sperm based on their motility, in a single step, and in less than 20 minutes. Furthermore, the authors report an improvement in DNA integration of the selected sperm by 80% compared to conventional sperm sorting protocols [19].

Recently, a microfluidic device with three interconnecting channels was designed to separate and automatically count sperm that can overcome a field of fluid flow; a field created by flow of fluid along microchannels [21]. Using this device, the strength of field can be regulated to select and count sperm with a particular range of motility.

Sperm selection based chemotaxis has also been demonstrated in microfluidic systems [22]. In a notable example, Xie and coworkers developed a simple microfluidic system that contained in vitro cultured cumulus cells that generated a chemoattractant gradient in the system. The sperm were injected into this system and responded to the gradient by moving toward the source. This method allowed for a measure of sperm motility and chemotaxis. Similarly, a microfluidic platform for performing each IVF step, including oocyte positioning, fertilization, embryo culture, and sperm screening, has been presented [23]. Oocytes were positioned individually in a 4×4 matrix of cylindrical units at the intersection of two perpendicular microchannels, allowing effective motile sperm separation via chemoattraction and rapid suspension-medium replacement. Researchers report increase in sperm motility from 61% at the input (61% of the sperm were motile in the original/raw sample) to 96% in the oocyte region (96% of the collected sperm were motile). Furthermore, the rates of embryo growth and the formation of microfluidic blastocysts in the platform were comparable with that of conventional protocols. Through basic pipetting for clinical embryo transfer, the healthy blastocysts from the microfluidic platform could be conveniently retrieved. In summary, the authors reported a lab-on-a-chip device that could handle the multistep procedures of IVF impacting the ART significantly.

The behavior or movement of cells or organisms with respect to a temperature gradient is known as thermotaxis. Thermotaxis of sperm has not been significantly studied. However, Li et al. have reported a microfluidic system to identify human sperm based on thermotaxis [24]. They used a temperature gradient control unit to produce a thermal gradient between two microchannels. The microchannel with the higher temperature functioned as the outlet for sperm having more response with thermal gradient, whereas the nonresponsive sperm tended to flow toward both microchannels. Valves enabling air–liquid interface were used to control the trapping of the sperm. Around 6–11% of the motile sperm were responsive to this temperature gradient, which was tested for four different increasing temperatures with small increments.

The identification or selection of sperm based on sperm motility has been the mostly commonly used technique in microfluidic systems. However, there are applications where other physiological aspects of sperm are important, and in some cases more feasible. For example, in the case of criminal investigations involving a sexual assault separation of sperm from epithelial cells will be valuable. Current techniques for separation of epithelial cells from sperm are tedious, time consuming, and can lead to cell losses. With this focus, a microfluidic system was developed by Weiran and coworkers to sort sperm from epithelial cells based on cell size [25]. A mixture of epithelial cells and sperm are injected into the system where due to the cells' difference in size and shape and laminar fluid flow, sperm and epithelial cells flow along different streamlines. This allows for collection of each cell at different outlets of the system. The authors reported that around 94% of the sorted sperm had good DNA integration and the time required to process a 50 µL sample was only 30 minutes. Another size-based separation was reported by Son and coworkers using a spiral channel to sort sperm from white blood cells (WBCs) and red blood cells (RBCs) for treatment of samples in some severe cases of male infertility [26,27]. Son and coworkers used the concept of inertial microfluidics that allows particles to focus on different spatial positions in a curved channel and thereby exiting through separate outlets in the microchannel. As per their report, they were able to sort sperm at rapid speeds 0.52 mL/min with high recovery of sperm (>80%), which is currently not possible in conventional clinical procedures (density gradient centrifugation) for sperm purification.

Microfluidic systems can also be coupled with electrical systems to identify and separate sperm based on their electrical impedance, a property that is sensitive to sperm shape and size. In this regard, a microfluidic system containing integrated microelectrodes was developed by Rosales and coworkers [28]. They report the ability to identify mature and immature sperm and separate them. Another study was reported by de Wagenaar and coworkers [29] to sort morphologically normal sperm from abnormal sperm (poor DNA integration) combining the electrical impedance analysis and dielectrophoretic (DEP) force. The presence of cytoplasmic droplets in sperm flagella (abnormal sperm) gives rise to difference in electrical impedance compared to the normal sperm and this difference of impedance is used to trigger the DEP force. In this system, sperm pass through a microchannel containing two distinct series of electrodes. The first set of electrodes is used to measure their impedance, and the second set of electrodes exposes them to a DEP force that sorts them in two separate collections downstream based on their unique impedance signals.

28.4 Conclusion

Based on the technologies reviewed here, it can be inferred that there are myriad applications of microfluidics relevant to ART and male infertility. Since achieving commercialization has been elusive, the potential of microfluidics has not yet been fully realized for human sperm manipulation. This can be attributed to the difficulty of commercializing microfluidic systems due to the design challenges discussed earlier [36], and acceptance of the technology by the reproductive medicine community. Clinical use of this technology could be achieved by developing microfluidic systems that select the best sperm, lower the cost of male infertility treatment, lower risks of laboratory errors via automation, minimize sample deterioration, and recover a majority of sperm from the initial sample. Recent works by a few research groups show promise that microfluidics can deliver these valuable outcomes in reproductive medicine [37–39].

Acknowledgments:
Funding to support contributions by Raheel Samuel were supported by the Eunice Kennedy Shriver National Institute of Child Health and Human Development of the National Institutes of Health under Award Number R44HD095355. The content is solely the responsibility of the authors and does not necessarily represent the official views of the National Institutes of Health.

Conflicts of Interest:
Raheel Samuel holds equity in Advanced Conceptions Inc. Advanced Conceptions Inc. is developing innovative solutions for reproductive medicine by utilizing microfluidics technology. The other authors have no conflicts of interest to declare.

References

1. Whitesides G. The origins and the future of microfluidics. *Nature.* 2006;442(7101):368–373. doi:10.1038/nature05058
2. Hu C, Chen Y, Tan MJA, Ren K, Wu H. Microfluidic technologies for vasculature biomimicry. *Analyst.* 2019;144(15):4461–4471. doi:10.1039/c9an00421a
3. Kaushik G, Leijten J, Khademhosseini A. Concise review: organ engineering: design, technology, and integration. *Stem Cells.* 2017;35(1):55–60. doi:10.1002/stem.2502
4. Pamme N. Continuous flow separations in microfluidic devices. *Lab Chip.* 2007;7:1644–1659. doi:10.1039/b712784g
5. Feng H, Magda JJ, Gale BK. Viscoelastic second normal stress difference dominated multiple-stream particle focusing in microfluidic channels. *Appl Phys Lett.* 2019;115(26). doi:10.1063/1.5129281
6. Jin D, Deng B, Li JX, et al. A microfluidic device enabling high-efficiency single cell trapping. *Biomicrofluidics.* 2015;9(1):014101. doi:10.1063/1.4905428
7. Schibel AEP, Ervin EN. Decreasing the limits of detection and analysis time of ion current rectification biosensing measurements via a mechanically applied pressure differential. *Anal Chem.* 2015;87(13):6646–6653. doi:10.1021/acs.analchem.5b00757
8. Convery N, Gadegaard N. 30 years of microfluidics. *Micro Nano Eng.* 2019;2:76–91. doi:10.1016/j.mne.2019.01.003
9. Kashaninejad N, Shiddiky MJA, Nguyen N-T, Kashaninejad N, Nguyen N-T, Shiddiky MJA. Advances in microfluidics-based assisted reproductive technology: from sperm sorter to reproductive system-on-a-chip. *Adv Biosyst.* 2018;2(3):1700197. doi:10.1002/adbi.201700197
10. Smith GD, Takayama S. Application of microfluidic technologies to human assisted reproduction. *Mol Hum Reprod.* 2017;23(4):257–268. doi:10.1093/molehr/gaw076
11. Samuel R, Badamjav O, Murphy KE, et al. Microfluidics: the future of microdissection TESE? *Syst Biol Reprod Med.* 2016;62(3). doi:10.3109/19396368.2016.1159748
12. Schuster TG, Cho B, Keller LM, Takayama S, Smith GD. Isolation of motile spermatozoa from semen samples using microfluidics. *Reprod Biomed Online.* 2003;7(1):75–81. doi:10.1016/S1472-6483(10)61732-4
13. Oseguera-López I, Ruiz-Díaz S, Ramos-Ibeas P, Pérez-Cerezales S. Novel techniques of sperm selection for improving IVF and ICSI outcomes. *Front Cell Dev Biol.* 2019;7. doi:10.3389/fcell.2019.00298
14. Chinnasamy T, Kingsley JL, Inci F, et al. Guidance and self-sorting of active swimmers: 3D periodic arrays increase persistence length of human sperm selecting for the fittest. *Adv Sci.* 2018;5(2):1700531. doi:10.1002/advs.201700531
15. Quinn MM, Jalalian L, Ribeiro S, et al. Microfluidic sorting selects sperm for clinical use with reduced DNA damage compared to density gradient centrifugation with swim-up in split semen samples. *Hum Reprod.* 2018;33(8):1388–1393. doi:10.1093/humrep/dey239
16. Knowlton SM, Sadasivam M, Tasoglu S. Microfluidics for sperm research. *Trends Biotechnol.* 2015;33(4):221–229. doi:10.1016/j.tibtech.2015.01.005
17. Zhang X, Khimji I, Gurkan UA, et al. Lensless imaging for simultaneous microfluidic sperm monitoring and sorting. *Lab Chip.* 2011;11(15):2535–2540. doi:10.1039/c1lc20236g
18. Asghar W, Velasco V, Kingsley JL, et al. Selection of functional human sperm with higher DNA integrity and fewer reactive oxygen species. *Adv Healthc Mater.* 2014;3(10):1671–1679. doi:10.1002/adhm.201400058
19. Nosrati R, Vollmer M, Eamer L, et al. Rapid selection of sperm with high DNA integrity. *Lab Chip.* 2014;14(6):1142–1150. doi:10.1039/c3lc51254a
20. Gaffney EA, Gadêlha H, Smith DJ, Blake JR, Kirkman-Brown JC. Mammalian sperm motility: observation and theory. *Annu Rev Fluid Mech.* 2011;43(1):501–528. doi:10.1146/annurev-fluid-121108-145442
21. Chen Y-A, Huang Z-W, Tsai F-S, Chen C-Y, Lin C-M, Wo AM. Analysis of sperm concentration and motility in a microfluidic device. *Microfluid Nanofluidics.* 2011;10(1):59–67. doi:10.1007/s10404-010-0646-8
22. Xie L, Ma R, Han C, et al. Integration of sperm motility and chemotaxis screening with a microchannel-based device. *Clin Chem.* 2010;56(8):1270–1278. doi:10.1373/clinchem.2010.146902
23. Ma R, Xie L, Han C, et al. In vitro fertilization on a single-oocyte positioning system integrated with motile sperm selection and early embryo development. *Anal Chem.*

2011;83(8):2964–2970. doi:10.1021/ac103063g

24. Li Z, Liu W, Qiu T, et al. The construction of an interfacial valve-based microfluidic chip for thermotaxis evaluation of human sperm. *Biomicrofluidics*. 2014;8(2):024102. doi:10.1063/1.4866851

25. Liu W, Chen W, Liu R, et al. Separation of sperm and epithelial cells based on the hydrodynamic effect for forensic analysis. *Biomicrofluidics*. 2015;9(4):044127. doi:10.1063/1.4928453

26. Son J, Murphy K, Samuel R, Gale BK, Carrell DT, Hotaling JM. Non-motile sperm cell separation using a spiral channel. *Anal Methods*. 2015;7:1–7. doi:10.1039/C5AY02205C

27. Son J, Samuel R, Gale BK, Carrell DT, Hotaling JM. Separation of sperm cells from samples containing high concentrations of white blood cells using a spiral channel. *Biomicrofluidics*. 2017;11(5):054106. doi:10.1063/1.4994548

28. Rosales-Cruzaley E, Cota-Elizondo PA, Sánchez D, Lapizco-Encinas BH. Sperm cells manipulation employing dielectrophoresis. *Bioprocess Biosyst Eng*. 2013;36(10):1353–1362. doi:10.1007/s00449-012-0838-6

29. de Wagenaar B, Dekker S, de Boer HL, et al. Towards microfluidic sperm refinement: impedance-based analysis and sorting of sperm cells. *Lab Chip*. 2016;16(8):1514–1522. doi:10.1039/C6LC00256K

30. Cho BS, Schuster TG, Zhu X, Chang D, Smith GD, Takayama S. Passively driven integrated microfluidic system for separation of motile sperm. *Anal Chem*. 2003;75(7):1671–1675. doi:10.1021/ac020579e

31. Shirota K, Yotsumoto F, Itoh H, et al. Separation efficiency of a microfluidic sperm sorter to minimize sperm DNA damage. *Fertil Steril*. 2016;105(2):315–321. doi:10.1016/j.fertnstert.2015.10.023

32. Wu J-K, Chen P-C, Lin Y-N, Wang C-W, Pan L-C, Tseng F-G. High-throughput flowing upstream sperm sorting in a retarding flow field for human semen analysis. *Analyst*. 2017;142(6):938–944. doi:10.1039/C6AN02420C

33. Horsman KM, Barker SLR, Ferrance JP, Forrest KA, Koen KA, Landers JP. Separation of sperm and epithelial cells in a microfabricated device: potential application to forensic analysis of sexual assault evidence. *Anal Chem*. 2005;77(3):742–749. doi:10.1021/ac0486239

34. Phiphattanaphiphop C, Leksakul K, Phatthanakun R, Suthummapiwat A. Real-time single cell monitoring: measurement and counting of motile sperm using LCR impedance-integrated microfluidic device. *Micromachines*. 2019;10(10):647. doi:10.3390/mi10100647

35. Segerink LI, Sprenkels AJ, ter Braak PM, Vermes I, van den Berg A. On-chip determination of spermatozoa concentration using electrical impedance measurements. *Lab Chip*. 2010;10(8):1018–1024. doi:10.1039/b923970g

36. Samuel R, Feng H, Jafek A, Despain D, Jenkins T, Gale B. Microfluidic-based sperm sorting & analysis for treatment of male infertility. *Transl Androl Urol*. 2018;7(S3):S336–S347. doi:10.21037/tau.2018.05.08

37. Gode F, Bodur T, Gunturkun F, et al. Comparison of microfluid sperm sorting chip and density gradient methods for use in intrauterine insemination cycles. *Fertil Steril*. 2019;112(5):842–848.e1. doi:10.1016/j.fertnstert.2019.06.037

38. Jafek A, Feng H, Brady H, et al. An automated instrument for intrauterine insemination sperm preparation. *Sci Rep*. 2020;10(1):21385. doi:10.1038/s41598-020-78390-3

39. Jenkins T, Samuel R, Jafek A, et al. Rapid microfluidic sperm isolation from microtese samples in men with non-obstructive azoospermia. *Fertil Steril*. 2017;108(3):e244. doi:10.1016/j.fertnstert.2017.07.733

Section 4 Laboratory Evaluation and Treatment of Male Infertility

Chapter 29

Practical Concerns for Patient Semen Banking

Grace M. Centola

29.1 Overview of Sperm Banking

Sperm banking has been a routine procedure for male fertility preservation since initial reports in the 1950s by Sherman and colleagues [1,2]. In fact, the earliest report of sperm cryopreservation is by Spallanzani and Mantegazza in 1866 [1,2], with the first reported pregnancy from frozen sperm in 1953 [3]. Since these early reports, sperm cryopreservation has been a standard clinical procedure for fertility preservation.

The reasons for male fertility preservation include, but are not limited to, sperm banking prior to vasectomy, prior to hormonal treatment and gender reassignment surgery [4], medical treatments for malignant or nonmalignant diseases, military deployment, and prior to assisted reproduction [5,6]. Sperm cryopreservation in many cases may provide the only chance for some couples to have children. Cancer treatment, surgery, traumatic injury, and even toxic exposures may result in permanent sterility in these men. Even nonmalignant diseases such as autoimmune disorders and diabetes could lead to testicular damage and decreased fertility [7]. With current widespread use of assisted reproductive technology (ART), sperm cryopreservation fills a niche in cases where the male partner may not be available at the time of oocyte retrieval, or may have difficulty providing a specimen under stressful situations. Sperm cryopreservation also provides as a backup, that is, more sperm, in cases where the sperm concentration is very low. Furthermore, azoospermic men who undergo diagnostic testicular extraction or epididymal aspiration are encouraged to cryopreserve these specimens to avoid repeated testicular biopsies or extractions [7]. These specimens could then be used in ART procedures.

Concerns of decreasing male fertility and increased risks of genetic, psychological, or medical conditions in offspring of older men, have also resulted in an increase in referral for sperm banking in younger men with no underlying medical conditions [8–10]. There has been increased incidence of schizophrenia and autism, as well as other psychological conditions, as well as de novo mutations in offspring of older fathers [8,11].

Even though sperm cryopreservation might be thought of as "routine," many males are not referred for this service, either because the possibility of sterility was not identified prior to surgery or medical treatment, or time constraints precluded referral for that service [12]. One cannot ignore the fact that younger adult males are themselves not aware of the availability of, or the need for, fertility preservation even in the absence of any medical condition that might affect their fertility [6,9].

Presently, there are several fertility preservation companies offering at-home semen collection kits, with transport to the sperm bank. With significant advertising budgets, these companies have been able to inform the younger generation of the availability and need for semen preservation and the ease of banking on their future. Thus, there has been an increase in young adult men using these services, and a subsequent surge in companies or reproductive facilities offering transport of specimens to cryopreservation facilities from domestic and international locales.

29.2 State and Federal Regulatory Issues Surrounding Male Fertility Preservation

Semen cryopreservation, quarantine and retesting prior to release of the semen, along with extensive testing has been required by state and federal regulations for both anonymous and nonsexually intimate known sperm donors since the early 1990s. In the late 1980s, with increasing concerns over the risks of sexual transmission of HIV/AIDS, the New York State Department of Health published strict regulations for use of donated frozen semen, particularly from anonymous sperm donors [13]. Thereafter, the Food and Drug Administration (FDA) refined the federal regulations for tissue banking to specifically include reproductive cells and tissues [14], the California Department of Public Health established regulations for donated reproductive cells and tissues, pretty much mimicking that of New York State [15], and private organizations such as the American Society for Reproductive Medicine [16] also followed suit. The American Association of Tissue Banks standards have also evolved to include the FDA and state statutes over the last two decades [17]. Other states require licensing if donated sperm specimens are shipped into that state (i.e., Maryland), and still others (Oregon and Illinois) require the facility to register with the department of health. States with no state-specific regulations require in-state facilities to follow the FDA regulations, and those with state regulations require that the facilities follow the stricter of the regulations (state vs. FDA). Both state and federal regulatory agencies will perform routine on site inspection of these facilities to ensure that the regulations are followed and detailed records are maintained by the facility documenting the screening and testing of the donors.

These state and federal regulations, and professional guidelines, require that sperm donors undergo rigorous screening and testing in order for acceptance as a sperm donor [6,13–15]. They are then repeatedly rescreened with a shortened risk questionnaire each day of donation, with complete screening and testing every six months. Anonymous donor semen is required to be frozen for a minimum of 180 days, followed by retesting with negative results prior to release of the semen for use in assisted reproduction. These regulations apply to both anonymous and directed (known) sperm donors. However, the FDA and some states allow a waiver of the six-month quarantine for negative screened and tested directed, that is, "known" sperm donors. These regulations also apply to both oocyte and embryo donors with specific points addressing these reproductive cells and tissues.

29.3 Practical Concerns: Consent for Cryopreservation

The consenting process whereby the patient agrees to the cryopreservation and storage process as well as potential future use of the thawed specimens is complex and detailed and can be overwhelming especially in cases of an urgent need to sperm bank prior to treatment. Therefore it is important that the consent is discussed with the patient prior to beginning the cryopreservation process. The informed consent reviews the potential future use of the thawed sperm, long-term storage, and the disposition or advanced directives in case of death of the sperm banker or if he becomes incapable of making such decisions [5,18,19]. The costs for sperm cryopreservation and yearly storage vary among the many facilities. The cost breakdown is usually included in the consent and definitely discussed in person with the client. Additional fees include the fee for shipping frozen specimens to a facility or physician's office for use in assisted reproduction. The patient is given the opportunity to ask questions and, following execution of the consent, is provided with hard copies of the signed consent and written information.

It is important for the healthcare practitioner and/or a representative of the cryopreservation facility to discuss all of these issues surrounding sperm cryopreservation, storage, and future use with the patients. Such discussion should include the reason to freeze sperm, how many ejaculates should be frozen, fresh, or washed sperm, and, most importantly, freezing of severely oligozoospermic specimens. Additionally, there are no guarantees for survival of the frozen sperm, successful pregnancy, or a take-home baby as a result of insemination with frozen-thawed sperm. This is very important and needs to be stressed, not overlooked in the process.

If a patient at some point wishes to discard any frozen specimens, a separate discard consent must be reviewed and signed before a notary before a laboratory will discard any vials of frozen sperm [5,18,19]. Some facilities may charge a fee for discarding of the specimens.

29.4 Practical Concerns: Process of Cryopreservation

Successful semen cryopreservation requires a facility with trained laboratory staff, proper equipment, and well-maintained storage tanks [5,7]. The freezing process for fresh ejaculated sperm is relatively simple. Following semen liquefaction, an appropriate cryopreservative, most often glycerol either alone or with extenders such as a buffer or egg yolk, is added to the raw semen in a gradual drop-wise manner to avoid osmotic shock to the cells. Following mixing, the specimen is placed into labeled cryovials, which are then slowly frozen using a programmable freezer or manually cooled in a refrigerator followed by freezing in liquid nitrogen vapor [5]. The vials of frozen semen are then stored directly in liquid nitrogen tanks. Other methods include attaching the vials onto a metal holding cane, following by placing the cane directly into a LN dry shipper for approximately 30 minutes followed by plunging into and storing in the liquid phase.

A test vial of the frozen sperm is usually thawed after 24–48 hours storage in LN to test cryosurvival of the sperm. By preparing a slide for measurement of the postthaw sperm count and motility, one can determine the cryosurvival rate based on the fresh sperm count and motility. This also provides a postthaw motile sperm concentration per vial, which of course is helpful for the facility using the specimen in ART.

Semen can be frozen as fresh semen, or prepared by washing the seminal fluid away from the sperm cells prior to freezing. Seminal fluid contains contaminants such as bacteria and prostaglandins, for example, which may affect sperm motility and function as well as cause severe cramping if inseminated directly into the uterus. The prefreeze washing procedure allows the thawed specimen to be used directly upon thaw for an intrauterine insemination (IUI). Otherwise, if the raw semen is cryopreserved, upon thaw, the specimen can only be inseminated by placing the thawed semen onto the female's cervix. Alternately, the thawed semen must be washed in order to remove the seminal fluid and contaminants prior to an insemination. Processing of thawed semen more often results in further loss of sperm numbers and motility, making this method less efficient for use in regular IUI.

With facilities that store and distribute donor sperm specimens, there is an acceptable minimum sperm concentration in the fresh ejaculate as well as in the postthaw vial. However, in men freezing their own sperm for any of the aforementioned reasons, it is important to discuss the potential for use of specimens with few sperm. Additionally, there appears to be different cryosurvival rates among specimens from the same man as well as between different men [20,21].

With the advent of ART, primarily intracytoplasmic sperm injection (ICSI), theoretically, only enough sperm are required for the number of oocytes that are retrieved from the partner. It is for this very reason that all specimens, even those presumably "azoospermic," could and should be cryopreserved for potential future use [7,20,22]. ART laboratory staff have been known to search for hours for the elusive sperm for use in ICSI, and have been successful in that task [20]. Clearly, even those specimens with severely low numbers of sperm, or the supposed azoospermic specimen, should be cryopreserved for later use in ART. The patients are appropriately counseled to consider donor sperm back-up in the event that no useful sperm are found, but at least this has provided the couple with the potential for using their own sperm and having a biological child.

In cases of surgical sperm retrieval (i.e., testicular biopsy or epididymal aspiration) very few sperm may be retrieved, and those that are retrieved usually do not exhibit progressive motility. With these types of specimens and the severely oligozoospermic specimens, novel methods have been proposed to freeze individual sperm, or small volumes with several sperm [7]. These methods include use of an empty zona pellucida to contain the sperm [22], use of an ICSI pipette to hold the individual sperm [23], a cryoloop apparatus [24], and mini-straws [25] for cryopreservation and storage. Clearly, such specimens are used solely for IVF/ICSI procedures.

It is generally acceptable for a 40–60% loss of sperm motility with cryopreservation in most specimens. More often, those specimens presenting with high sperm counts will result in less loss than those with a lower sperm count and motility. Generally, in specimens with normal sperm parameters prior to freezing, a recovery of at least 50% is expected. However, in many men who bank sperm due to underlying illness or infertility, there may be a lower recovery of sperm motility and higher loss of sperm numbers. In fact, even with "normal" sperm parameters, there will be varying degrees of sperm cryosurvival [5,20,21,26]. This loss has very little impact on ICSI or conventional ART inseminations.

29.5 Practical Concerns: Fresh versus Frozen Sperm

ICSI revolutionized the treatment for severe male factor infertility, allowing men with severe oligozoospermia and azoospermia to potentially have their own biological children. Contributing to this is our ability to successfully cryopreserve even the poorest specimens, including testicular biopsies and epididymal aspirates for use in ART. Several have reported that similar pregnancy rates were obtained using fresh or frozen ejaculated sperm, or fresh or frozen testicular or epididymal sperm [27,28]. Kucznynski et al. compared 118 ICSI cycles with fresh sperm and 122 ICSI cycles with frozen-thawed sperm from men with low concentration, low motility, and low percent normal morphology and showed no statistically significant difference between use of the fresh or the frozen sperm [29]. Interestingly, data also showed that the fertilization rate, implantation rate, and pregnancy rate was not different when fresh or frozen sperm were used [29–32], although one group demonstrated a higher ongoing pregnancy rate in the group of patients using frozen-thawed sperm [29]. Some have suggested that the freezing-thaw process selected for the most normal and vigorous sperm for use in ART [32].

Large-scale donor sperm insemination cycles have shown similar pregnancy outcomes between frozen donor sperm and nondonor fresh cycles [33]. Similarly, between 2012 and 2013, no differences were seen in miscarriage rate, gestational age at delivery, or birth rate between donor sperm and partner sperm ART or insemination cycles [34,35]. Similar results have been reported using frozen surgically retrieved sperm [36–39].

29.6 The Future of Sperm Banking

Studies continue to investigate optimal sperm cryopreservation methodology and, most importantly, the effects of cryopreservation on sperm DNA and molecular processes. There has been shown to be minimal impact of the freeze-thaw process on functionality of most specimens, especially the normal parameter specimen [29,32]. We are still faced with the challenge of optimal cryopreservation and storage processes for those specimens with severe impairment. In those cases, it is often difficult to retrieve usable individual sperm upon thaw. Some have even reported the use of freeze drying methods for sperm preservation [40,41].

Currently, there are increasing numbers of private companies, sperm banks, and ART facilities offering transport kits where patients can collect a specimen at home, add preservative or nutrient media, and ship specimens to the facility for cryopreservation. With significant advertising budgets, many of these facilities have been able to inform a younger generation of males of the availability and need for semen preservation and the ease of banking on their future. This type of process is certainly appealing to those men who might live a significant distance from a hospital or sperm bank. Furthermore, the ability to collect a semen specimen in the privacy of their own home is attractive for many men, who might be uncomfortable in appearing at a sperm banking facility and interacting with facility staff.

One of the most interesting and promising advances in this field is the preservation of spermatogonial stem cells from prepubertal boys and young adolescents [42,43]. The seminiferous tubules in the adult testes contain a small population of spermatogonial stem cells (SSCs) that undergo self-renewing mitotic divisions that maintain the SSC population as well as divisions that ensure sperm production [44]. Over the past few decades, several technologies have emerged including SSC transplantation and in vitro culture of SSCs in the adult as well as the prepubertal male [44–47]. Whereas adult men can provide a semen specimen for cryopreservation prior to cancer treatment or surgery, prepubertal boys, who are not producing sperm, are thus not able to provide a semen specimen for cryopreservation prior to their treatment or surgery.

Several centers currently offer testicular biopsy with SSC cryopreservation for prepubertal boys and young adult men prior to potential sterilizing treatment [44–48]. The intent is for future autologous isolated SSC or testicular transplantation or in vitro maturation of the SSCs and in vitro growth of testicular tissue both resulting in sperm production for use in ART [42,46–48]. Use of experimental SSC-based therapies is not currently approved by the FDA since these procedures require more than minimal manipulation. However, research results have been promising and accepted treatments are anticipated in the not so distant future.

References

1. Shehata F, Chian RC. Cryopreservation of sperm: an overview. In: Chian RC, Quinn P, eds. *Fertility Cryopreservation.* Cambridge University Press; 2010:39–45.
2. Sherman JK. Synopsis of the use of frozen human semen since 1964: state of the art of human semen banking. *Fertil Steril.* 1973;24:397–412.
3. Bunge RG, Sherman JK. Fertilizing capacity of frozen human spermatozoa. *Nature.* 1953;172:767–768.
4. Li K, Rodriguez D, Gabrielsen JS, Centola, GM, Tanrikut C. Transgender sperm cryopreservation: trends and findings in the past decade. *Andrology.* 2018;6(6):860–864.
5. Alouf CA, Celia G, Centola GM. Sperm cryopreservation – a practical guide. In: Allahbadia GN, Ata B, Lindheim SR, Woodward BJ, Bhagavath B, eds. *Textbook of Assisted Reproduction.* Springer; 2019:497–504.
6. Centola GM, Sperm banking, donation, and transport in the age of assisted reproduction: federal and state regulation. In: Carrell DT, Peterson CM, eds. *Reproductive Endocrinology and Infertility: Integrating Modern Clinical and Laboratory Practice.* Springer; 2010:509–516.
7. Di Santo M, Tarozzi N, Nadalini M, Borini A. Human sperm cryopreservation: update on techniques, effect on DNA integrity, and implications for ART. *Adv Urol.* 2012;2012:854837.
8. Kong A, Frigge ML, Masson G, et al. Rate of de novo mutations and the importance of father's age to disease risk. *Nature.* 2012;488(7412):471–475.
9. Centola GM, Blanchard A, Demick J, Li S, Eisenberg M. Decline in sperm count and motility in young adult men from 2003–2013: observations from a U.S. sperm bank. *Andrology.* 2016;4(3):270–276.
10. Sharma R, Agarwal A, Rohra VK, Assidi M, Abu-Elmagd M, Turki RF. Effects of increased paternal age on sperm quality, reproductive outcome and associated genetic risks to offspring. *Reprod Biol Endoc.* 2015;13:35.
11. D'Onofrio BM, Rickert ME, Frans E, et al. Paternal age at childbearing and offspring psychiatric and academic morbidity. *JAMA Psychiatry.* 2014;71(4):432–438.
12. Pacey AA. Referring patients for sperm banking. In: Pacey AA, Tomlinson MJ, eds. *Sperm Banking: Theory and Practice.* Cambridge University Press; 2009:30–40.
13. New York State, Part 52, Tissue Banks and Non Transplant Anatomic Banks, Public Health Section 4365; Subpart 52–58; www.wadsworth.org/regulatory/btrp/laws. Accessed November 9, 2022.
14. US Food and Drug Administration, 21 CFR 1271; www.accessdata.fda.gov/scripts/cdrh/cfdocs/cfcfr/CFRSearch.cfm?CFRPart=1271. Accessed November 9, 2022.
15. California Department of Public Health (CDPH) Tissue Bank Regulation, Article 2. 1639–1641.1. https://leginfo.legislature.ca.gov/faces/codes_displayText.xhtml?lawCode=HSC&division=2.&title=&part=&chapter=4.1.&article=2. Accessed November 9, 2022.
16. Practice Committee of American Society for Reproductive Medicine and the Practice Committee of Society for Assisted Reproductive Technology. Recommendations for gamete and embryo donation: a committee opinion. *Fertil Steril.* 2013;99(1):47–62.
17. American Association of Tissue Bank. *Standards for Tissue Banking*, 14th ed., January 31, 2020. https://static1.squarespace.com/static/5f2dc76b6a743f2147b29a37/t/5f3334d90f2540201689051c/1597191396553/AATB+Standards+for+Tissue+Banking+-14th+Edition+-+-Posted+8-3-16-.pdf. Accessed November 9, 2022.
18. Shuster TG, Hickner-Cruz K, Ohl DA, Goldman E, Smith G. Legal considerations for cryopreservation of sperm and embryos. *Fertil Steril.* 2003;80:61–66.
19. Joint Commission. *Informed consent: more than getting a signature.* www.jointcommission.org/-/media/tjc/documents/newsletters/quick_safety_issue_twenty-one_february_2016pdf.pdf
20. Centola GM. Sperm or no sperm, that is the question! Finding the elusive spermatozoa. *Fertil Steril.* 2012;98:822.
21. Centola GM, Raubertas RF, Mattox JH. Cryopreservation of human semen: comparison of cryopreservatives, sources of variability and prediction of post-thaw survival. *J Androl.* 1992;13(3):283–288.
22. Cohen J, Garrisi GJ, Congedo-Ferrara TA, Kieck, KA, Sehimmel TW, Scott RT. Cryopreservation of single human spermatozoa. *Hum Reprod.* 1997;12:994–1001.
23. Gvakharia M, Adamson, G. A method of successful cryopreservation of small numbers of human spermatozoa. *Fertil Steril.* 2001;76:S101.
24. Desai NN, Culler C, Goldfarb J. Cryopreservation of single sperm from epidermal and testicular samples on cryoloops: preliminary case report. *Fertil Steril.* 2004;82:S264.
25. Isachemko V, Isachenko E, Montag M, et al. Clean technique for cryoprotectant-free vitrification of human spermatozoa. *RBMO.* 2005;10:350–354.
26. Centola GM, Allen J. The ability of sperm to survive cryopreservation is not related to initial sperm concentration. Paper presented at the American Society of Andrology Annual Meeting, April 1993.
27. Nagy Z, Liu J, Cecile J, Silber S, Devroey P, Van Steirteghem A. Using ejaculated, fresh, and frozen-thawed epididymal and testicular spermatozoa gives rise to comparable results after intracytoplasmic sperm injection. *Fertil Steril.* 1995;63(4):808–815.
28. Yu Z, Wei Z, Yang J, et al. Comparison of intracytoplasmic sperm injection outcome with fresh versus frozen-thawed testicular sperm in men with nonobstructive azoospermia: a systematic review and meta-analysis.

29. Kuczyński W, Dhont M, Grygoruk C, Grochowski D, Wołczyński S, Szamatowicz M. The outcome of intracytoplasmic injection of fresh and cryopreserved ejaculated spermatozoa: a prospective randomized study. *Hum Reprod*. 2001;16(10):2109–2113.
30. Ragni G, Caccamo AM, Dalla Serra A, Guercilena S. Computerized slow-staged freezing of semen from men with testicular tumors or Hodgkin's disease preserves sperm better than standard vapor freezing. *Fertil Steril*. 1990;53(6):1072–1075.
31. Ragni G, Somigliana E, Restelli L, Salvi R, Arnoldi M, Paffoni A. Sperm banking and rate of assisted reproduction treatment: insights from a 15 year cryopreservation program for male cancer patients. *Cancer*. 2003;97(7):1624–1629.
32. Borges E, Jr., Rossi LM, Locambo de Freitas CV, et al. Fertilization and pregnancy outcome after intracytoplasmic injection with fresh or cryopreserved ejaculated spermatozoa. *Fertil Steril*. 2007;87(2):316–320.
33. Gerkowicz SA, Crawford S, Hipp H, Boulet S, Kissin DM, Kawwass JF. Assisted reproductive technology with donor sperm: national trends and perinatal outcomes. *Fertil Steril*. 2017;108(3):e72.
34. Fritz R, Jindal S, Yu B, Vega M, Buyuk E. Does donor sperm affect birth weight, preterm birth, and miscarriage rates in fresh autologous in vitro fertilization cycles? Analysis of 46.061 cycles reported to SART. *Fertil Steril*. 2017;107(3):e30.
35. Malchau SS, Loft A, Henningsen A-K, Andersen AN, Pinborg A. Perinatal outcomes in 6338 singletons born after intrauterine insemination in Denmark, 2007 to 2012: the influence of ovarian stimulation. *Fertil Steril*. 2014;102:1110–1116.
36. Shin DH, Turek PJ. Sperm retrieval techniques. *Nature Rev Urology*. 2013;10:723–730.
37. Devroey P, Silber S, Nagy Z, et al. Ongoing pregnancies and births after intracytoplasmic sperm injection with frozen-thawed epididymal spermatozoa. *Hum Reprod*. 1995;10:903–906.
38. Fischer R, Baukloh V, Naether OGJ, Schulze W, Salzbrunn A, Benson DM. Pregnancy after intracytoplasmic sperm injection of spermatozoa extracted from frozen-thawed testicular biopsy. *Hum Reprod*. 1996;11:2197–2199.
39. Gil-Slamon M, Romeo J, Mingues Y. Pregnancies after intracytoplasmic sperm injection with cryopreserved testicular sperm. *Hum Reprod*. 1996;11:1309–1313.
40. Patrizio P, Natan Y, Barak Y, Levi Setti P. A simple new method for the freeze-drying and storage of human sperm. *Fertil Steril*. 2016;106(3):e307.
41. Frydman R, Grynberg M. Male fertility preservation: innovations and questions. *Fertil Steril*. 2015;105:247–248.
42. Moss JL, Choi A, Keeter MKF, Brannigan RE. Male adolescent fertility preservation. *Fertil Steril*. 2015;105(2):267–273.
43. Gies I, Oates R, De Schepper J, Tournaye H. Testicular biopsy and cryopreservation for fertility preservation of prepubertal boys with Klinefelter syndrome: a pro/con debate. *Fertil Steril*. 2016;105(2):249–255.
44. Gassei K, Orwig KE. Experimental methods to preserve male fertility and treat male factor infertility. *Fertil Steril*. 2016;105(2):256–266.
45. Sinha N, Whelan EC, Brinster RL. Isolation, cryopreservation, and transplantation of spermatogonial stem cells. *Methods Mol Biol*. 2019;2005:205–220.
46. Valli H, Phillips BT, Shetty G, et al. Germline stem cells: toward the regeneration of spermatogenesis. *Fertil Steril*. 2014;101(1):3–13.
47. Goossens E, Van Saen D, Tournaye H. Spermatogonial stem cell preservation and transplantation: from research to clinic. *Hum Reprod*. 2013;28:897–907.
48. Fertility preservation program of Magee-Womens Hospital in Pittsburgh. https://mageewomens.org/for-researchers/research-centers/fertility-preservation-program-fpp#:~:text=The%20Fertility%20Preservation%20Program%20in%20Pittsburgh%20is%20committed%20to%3A,preserve%20fertility%20and%20treat%20infertility.

Section 4 Laboratory Evaluation and Treatment of Male Infertility

Chapter 30: The Potential Future Applications of In Vitro Spermatogenesis in the Clinical Laboratory

Swati Sharma and Stefan Schlatt

30.1 Clinical Need for In Vitro Gamete Production for ART Treatment

Around 50% of the subfertility cases reported in couples are due to male factor infertility and reproductive dysfunction [1]. An increase in the rate of male infertility (poor sperm and semen parameters) in the past 50 years has been reported with reasons attributed to various risk factors, including either epigenetic or genetic causes, socioeconomic and lifestyle changes, environmental exposure, or life-saving therapies for cancer treatment [2,3]. As described in Table 30.1, these infertile patient groups include patients from all age groups, who suffer reproductive dysfunction due to distinct known and unknown causes. Young patients include those affected by sex/genitalia developmental disorders like mixed gonadal dysgenesis, ovo-testicular disorder, Klinefelter syndrome, and XX male [4,5]. The second patient group includes infant, prepubertal, adolescent, and adult cancer survivors, at risk of losing their fertility due to chemotherapeutic treatment [6]. Last but not least, adult infertile patients constitute a huge number including those suffering from sexual disorders, defective sperm production and transportation function, and endocrine-related dysfunction [1,4].

Depending on the specific infertility disorder, surgical and nonsurgical treatment strategies can be employed to restore fertility in infertile men from different patient groups (Table 30.1). Surgical treatment for male infertility includes treatments for varicocele and azoospermia, microsurgical vasovasostomy, vasoepididymostomy, and transurethral resection of the ejaculation duct. Alternate treatment options for patients with unknown causes of male infertility include assisted reproductive technology (ART), intrauterine insemination, IVF, intracytoplasmic sperm injection, sperm retrieval for ART, testicular sperm extraction, testicular fine needle aspiration, pericutaneous epididymal sperm aspiration, and microsurgical epididymal sperm aspiration [7]. Nonsurgical treatment for specific male infertility conditions will include anejaculation, history of surgical treatments, diseases like diabetes, multiple sclerosis, birth defects, congenital adrenal hyperplasia, genital tract infection, hyperprolactinemia, hypogonadotropic hypogonadism, immunologic infertility, reactive oxygen species, and retrograde ejaculation. Besides these known therapeutic options, there is an urgent clinical need to identify strategies for functional gamete production for ART treatment for remaining infertile patient groups, to fulfill their fatherhood desires. For developing fertility preservation and restoration strategies, it is necessary to better understand the differences or abnormalities in the functional regulation of the testis in infertile patients compared to their age-matched controls. There is also limited knowledge and understanding of the age-dependent testicular differences, for instance key developmental processes in young and old infertile patient groups and those suffering with distinct fertility disorders. Rigorous experimental research is therefore required in this direction to gain more in-depth understanding of the physiological, molecular, and germline signaling mechanisms leading to the dysfunctional regulation of the testis resulting in specific infertility-related disease etiologies.

For instance, data from retrospective studies indicate 10–15% of infertile adult men are azoospermic and produce no sperm in the ejaculate, with the majority (80%) suffering from nonobstructive azoospermia (NOA) and the rest (20%) from obstructive azoospermia. Some of the NOA patients also consist of "Sertoli cell only" or suffer from "early maturation arrest" with no meiotic cells in their seminiferous tubules, with negligible or low probability of sperm retrieval from these patients. Understanding the defective regulatory or signaling mechanisms in specific patient groups like patients with genetic mutations leading to NOA phenotype may enable researchers to identify customized patient-specific therapeutic strategies to treat such infertile patients [8]. Other patient groups worth noting are those suffering from testicular germ cell tumors in adulthood. These tumor cells are known to be derived from fetal cells (primordial germ cells) during germ cell lineage development [9]. Understanding regulatory mechanisms (involved in upregulation and downregulation of genes) influencing germline development and controlling pluripotency and proliferation is significant for both biological and clinical purposes, like devising fertility preservation strategies and to acquire a comprehensive understanding of germ cell cancer pathogenesis. Therefore, it is significant to elucidate the epidemiological risk factors, genetic aberrations, and susceptibility genes leading to disruptive/altered germline development [10,11]. Another notable example where age-dependent

Table 30.1 Clinical pathologies diagnosed from prenatal to adult age groups

Clinical pathologies	Age group affected (prenatal, neonatal, prepubertal, adult)	Causes/symptoms	Clinical treatment option/possibility
Hormonal deficiencies/male hypogonadism	Any age	Insufficient hormone production	Hormone replacement therapy (HRT)
Primary hypogonadism			
Klinefelter's syndrome	Birth defect (genetic condition by birth)	Characterized by presence of a 47,XXY cell line and clinical features include tall stature, small testes, gynecomastia, primary gonadal failure, progressive germ cell loss, infertility	Assisted reproductive technology (ART) treatment possible for some men
Cryptorchidism or undescended testicles	Birth defect	Failure of testicle to drop to normal area in scrotum	Surgery and hormone treatment in some cases
Mumps orchitis	Postpubertal and adult men	Mumps/bacterial infection may lead to testicle shrinkage	Nonsteroidal antibiotic treatment
Haemochromatosis infertility	Adult	Endocrine cause of subfertility	Therapeutic treatment
Testicular trauma	Neonatal to adult	Injury to testicles	Cryopreservation, medication, ART treatment
Cancer treatment/chemotherapy	Neonatal to adult	Chemotherapy may cause germ cell depletion	Cryopreservation of testicular tissue and semen
Secondary hypogonadism (Kallman's syndrome, pituitary disorders, inflammatory disease, HIV/AIDS, medications, obesity, normal aging)	Adult	Low gonadotropin levels	HRT treatment
Genetic disorders			
Cystic fibrosis, associated congenital bilateral absence of the vas deferens	Adult	Failure in development of vas deferens	Fertilization possible by ART treatment
Autosomal dominant polycystic kidney diseases	Adult	Inherited disorder	ART may be effective
Hypospadias	Adult	Comorbidities may lead to infertility	Surgical repair may be required in some cases
Blockage in tubes	Adult	By injury or vasectomy	Surgery
Sperm abnormalities	Adult		
Oligospermia	Adult	Low sperm count	ART, or combined hormonal therapy
Asthenospermia	Adult	Poor sperm motility due to infections, varoceles, antisperm antibodies, genetic abnormalities	ART
Teratospermia	Adult	Abnormal sperm morphology	Intracytoplasmic sperm injection
Retrograde ejaculation	Adult	Due to medication side effect or severe nerve or muscle damage	May be reversible or irreversible
Medical conditions (tumors)	Adult		
Lifestyle/environment/risk factors	Adult		

fertility restoration strategies will be required are male cancer patients undergoing chemotherapeutic treatment. Adult cancer patients who produce sperm have an option to cryopreserve their semen samples before undergoing cancer therapy. In contrast, young boys do not produce semen samples as their testicular tissue is immature; therefore the clinics cryobank their testicular biopsies prior to treatment, with a potential futuristic possibility for fertility restoration in adulthood [6]. For patients who do not produce sperm, currently there are no *ex vivo* strategies to generate sperm. Therefore, different *ex vivo* strategies are required for fertility restoration in immature and adult patient groups due to their distinct testicular maturation status [8,11]. Thus, more intensive research efforts are required to develop our understanding of the biological mechanisms leading to or resulting in infertility-related clinical pathologies. This will enable researchers to develop specific strategies for targeted clinical applications to address the needs of these patients, including in vitro gamete production or fertility restoration.

Several international, transnational, and regional clinical research efforts have been initiated in the past few years in this field [6]; for instance, formation of task forces focusing on male fertility preservation research from leading reproductive biology and scientific societies like the European Society for Human Reproduction and Embryology, and publication of consensus and opinion papers by expert groups on fertility preservation strategies [6,12]. The formation of the American Oncofertility consortium focusing on research and clinical aspects in the field of fertility preservation is another global initiative in this direction [13]. Various major funding initiatives have been provided that focus on the development of strategies for in vitro spermatogenesis and also create training options for young researchers. A good example of such an action from the European Union is the Marie Curie International Training Network "GROWSPERM" (www.growsperm.eu).

30.2 Challenges for Artificial In Vitro Systems to Recapitulate Testis Function: From Biology to Technology

The male reproductive system primarily includes the testis (the site of spermatogenesis and androgen production), the epididymis (the site of sperm transport and storage), seminal vesicles and prostate gland (glands that produce seminal fluid), the vas deferens (the muscular tube that transports sperm from the epididymis), and the penis (the male sexual organ). The male gonad testis is a dual-functional organ with biological and physiological peculiarities across different species. It has a complex epithelial arrangement and subcompartmental physiology with regulatory pathways controlling both spermatogenic and steroidogenic function [14]. At the physiological and biological level, there is a need to model and deconstruct the testicular developmental process and elucidate the role and specific function of various entities at the cellular, molecular, physiological, and subcompartmental level, including the complex orchestration of the various signaling pathways and regulation of the endocrine axis. As already noted, male germline development is species-specific and a highly synchronized process. Testis development and function initiates with lineage specification and initiation of the male sex-specific developmental pathway, somatic cells self-organize for future niche formation, primordial germ cells colonize the gonads, and endocrine secretion and signaling provides the requisite impetus and environment for testicular maturation further. Germ cell development is dependent on the somatic environment and regulated by the factors secreted by various testicular somatic cell types. Multiple regulatory checkpoints during prenatal male germline development regulate normal testicular development and function during postnatal life. Any aberration or abnormality during the crucial phases may trigger germline developmental errors, which may later lead to impaired testicular function or may result in disorders like germ cell tumors. Both spermatogenic and steroidogenic functions in a testis are controlled by GnRH master regulators modulating the LH–testosterone and FSH–inhibin pathways, respectively [14]. The turning on and off of the GnRH master switch controls the continuous pulsatile secretion of testosterone in males and is responsible for the triphasic testicular development during the neonatal, prepubertal, and adult developmental stages across primate species (Figure 30.1). The surge in testosterone secretion occurs during the neonatal period, the drop in testosterone levels leads to testicular quiescence during the prepubertal period, and a multifold rise in testosterone levels marks the onset of puberty leading to testicular maturation.

Crucial regulatory mechanisms control spermatogonial expansion and differentiation; however, postpubertal differentiation processes are independent of hormonal influence and dependent on species-specific functional requirements (Table 30.2). For instance, in contrast to rodents the germline maturation process in primates is driven by a progenitor-buffered stem cell system. The complex structural and functional organization of the primate testis makes it challenging to recapitulate testicular organ function in vitro [11,14]. Several attempts to mimic the biological function of the primate testis using 2D culture systems reported limited progress (Figure 30.1). Thus, research efforts are continuously ongoing to develop experimental strategies employing 3D models, using both single-cell suspensions as a source for sperm development by using either cell-based culture, by generating "testicular organoid-like structures," or by using "tissue-based" strategies for achieving in vitro spermatogenesis in cultured tissue fragments or tubules (Figure 30.2) [11,78]. However, most of these approaches have specific biological and technological limitations in mimicking in vivo testicular function in in vitro settings and achieving in vitro meiotic differentiation using testicular samples from humans or any nonhuman primate models [79]. For instance, lack of vasculature, lack of

Table 30.2 In vitro culture strategies: advantages and disadvantages

Strategy	Advantages	Disadvantages/challenges
2D cell culture	Easy to establish. Manipulation of cells easy to perform.	Cannot mimic features of tubulogenesis and spermatogenesis in vitro.
3D cell or organoid culture	Possibility of specific cell manipulation during culture.	Random distribution and organization of single cells in organoids.
Tubule culture	Follow-up of specific stages of germ cells possible by transillumination. Eliminates effects of interstitial cells and tissues. Effect of culture condition, medium composition, or physical environment can be easily evaluated.	Manipulation of specific cell type not feasible.
Tissue culture: interphase culture	Preservation of tissue architecture, complex cellular interactions, and structural integrity of the tissue.	Spermatogenic efficiency lower with adult mouse tissue. Exposure of the cells and tissue to oxygen reportedly higher than the in vivo physiological levels. Approach not successful with other species like rats.
Tissue culture: hanging drop method	Preservation of tissue architecture, complex cellular interactions, and structural integrity of the tissue.	Inefficient molecular diffusion and delivery of nutrients in the cultured samples.
Microfluidic system	Improved molecular diffusion, stable maintenance of spermatogenesis over extended time period. Testosterone production and LH stimulation effective. Large-scale production easy and cheap.	Device designing and fabrication requires multistep optimization.
Multi-organ-on-chip culture	Effect on different organ/cells can be simultaneously evaluated.	Limited number of biological replicates due to limited availability of individual donor testis and the labor-intensive nature of multi-organ-chip cocultures.
Transplantation	Vascular support, in vivo physiological environment	Risks related to transplantation of residual malignant cells limit their application.

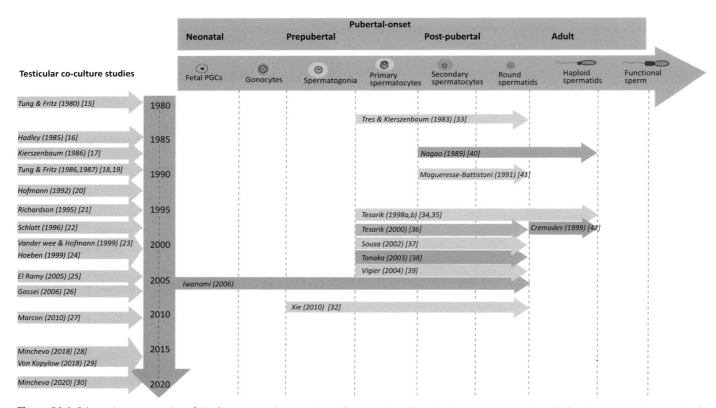

Figure 30.1 Schematic representation of timeline representing experimental progress to achieve in vitro spermatogenesis with 2D cultures using dissociated cells

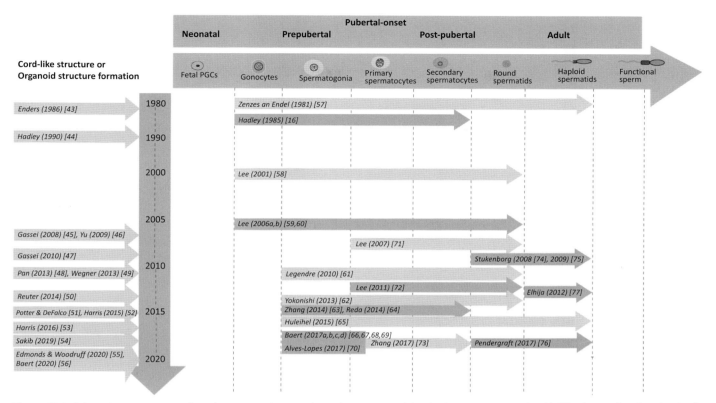

Figure 30.2 Schematic representation of timeline representing experimental progress to achieve in vitro spermatogenesis with 3D cultures using dissociated cells

hormonal support from absent endocrine axis in vitro, and absence of immune-privileged environment in vitro are some of the known barriers, which are challenging to overcome. Emergence of advanced biotechnologies like organ-on-a-chip and biofabrication approaches employing biomaterials like hydrogels, decellularized or recellularized extracellular matrix (ECM), scaffold-free organoids, or microfluidic systems offer promising potential for reengineering the complex testicular environment and restoring testicular organ function in vitro (Figure 30.3) [79,80,81,82].

In addition, we know that for normal spermatogenesis to occur, it is a prerequisite that the intricate system of spermatogonia and their niches should remain intact. These testicular niche factors require structural support to perform their biological function. The findings from experimental studies (using intact and digested testicular tissue) demonstrate the significance of physiological and structural support of the testicular microenvironment in activating niche factors to perform their biological function. This also signifies that individual niche factors may have specific biological function, but they are limited in exerting it autonomously; instead, they act in synergy with other components of the niche to influence germ cell development. Thus, niche factors work in concert with structural, physiological, and biochemical support and stimulation from the niche components to perform their biological function holistically and regulate homeostasis and germ cell maintenance and differentiation. Two-dimensional cell culture experiments provide evidence that complex growth factor supplemented culture conditions do not significantly influence differentiation of primate testicular germ cells in vitro. Thus, providing growth factors exogenously in culture does not resemble and suffice for stimulating their physiological function in vivo. However, using ECM support, creating 3D organoid structures, using structurally intact testicular tissue by employing organ culture, or providing vascularized environment by transplantation approach have shown more promising results in supporting primate germ cell survival and development.

30.3 In Vitro Spermatogenesis

In this section, we will broadly discuss whether "culture strategies" or "culture conditions" influence in vitro spermatogenesis. The current state of the art and research progress made with different "cellular" and "tissue based" approaches to develop testicular organoid-like structures and organ cultures will be discussed, with their specific advantages and limitations (Table 30.2). The role of culture conditions and media composition, and whether supplementation of specific growth factors or hormones influence spermatogenic processes in vitro, are described and reveal the extreme complexity of models and culture systems, and the variability of experimental conditions and outcomes (Table 30.3).

The early attempts to establish testicular organ cultures for in vitro spermatogenesis using rabbit [86] and mouse testis tissues [87] by employing serum plasma clot resulted in

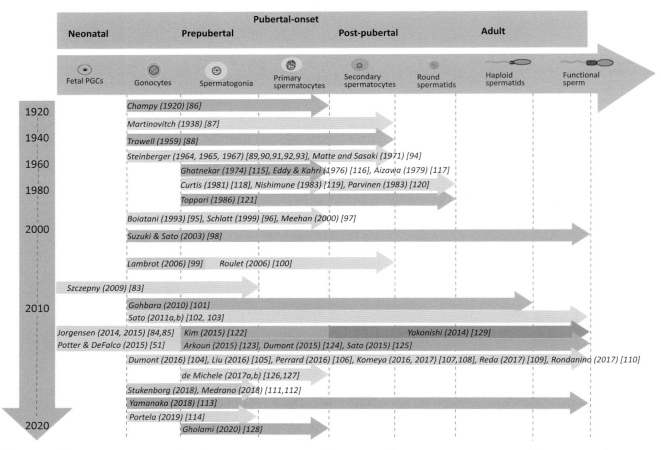

Figure 30.3 Schematic representation of timeline representing experimental progress to achieve in vitro spermatogenesis with intact tissue cultures using isolated testicular fragments or seminiferous tubules

differentiation up to spermatocyte stages. The most remarkable development was the establishment of gas–liquid interphase culture, also known as the Trowell's method [88]. This included a metal grid immersed in media, with a thin agarose layer on top of the grid with the tissue sample. This system supported the in vitro spermatogenic progression in cultured testicular fragments up to the stage of secondary spermatocytes from a wide range of species, including rats, guinea pigs, rabbits, monkeys, and humans [89,91–93,137,138]. Studies to assess the effects of physical and chemical culture parameters, such as pH, temperature, gas, and culture media composition (synthetic or chemically defined media, serum, hormones, vitamins, and amino acids), provided tremendous knowledge to further optimize efficient culture conditions for in vitro spermatogenesis [89–93,137,138]. Intact seminiferous tubule cultures to investigate spermatogenic development in combination with transillumination microscopy also demonstrated promising outcome in supporting spermatogenic survival [120,139]. Several groups investigated the effects of exogenous hormones and growth factor supplementation to in vitro cell and tissue cultures; these studies provided significant information on the role of specific factors on germ cell maintenance, as summarized in Table 30.3.

The most significant breakthrough was achieved with the generation of functional sperm by in vitro culture of mouse testicular tissue using a modified Trowell's method (using an agarose block) [102,103]. However, this approach suffered from several limitations such as lower spermatogenic efficiency with adult mouse samples and failure with other species like rat and human [125]. Alternate tissue culture systems like hanging drop and porous membrane inserts showed no significant effect on spermatogenic development. Conventional 2D culture approaches reportedly had several limitations in mimicking tubulogenesis and spermatogenesis in vitro, compared to more advanced 3D systems. Novel 3D strategies allowed better simulation and mimicking of specific testicular features (like cell adhesion, migration, and morphogenetic development) in vitro using biomaterials (like Matrigel, collagen, and hydrogel) with substances present in the testicular extracellular matrix. Subcompartmental cellular organization was improved and better mimicked and maintained using 3D culture strategies. Alternate technological approaches like 3D organoids [140] and microfluidic-based organ-on-chip technology have been successfully employed for maintenance of spermatogenesis and functional sperm production in rodent models [107,108,113]. However, these approaches are still being developed and are at a

Table 30.3 Reported effects of different factors tested on various species, on germ cell survival and development

Factors	Effect	Culture strategy/species	References
Temperature			
Temperature 31–33°C	>33°C less optimal for survival and differentiation of germ cells		89 (Steinberger et al., 1964)
Temperature close to 35°C	Better for in vitro spermatogenesis	(Rhesus monkey)	65 (Huleihel et al., 2015)
34°C or 37°C	34°C more efficient		112 (Medrano et al., 2018)
10% calf serum	Effective for maintaining viability of seminiferous epithelium		93 (Steinberger & Steinberger, 1967)
FSH and HCG	Induces maturation of Sertoli cells		93 (Steinberger & Steinberger, 1967)
Vitamin A, C, E	Promote differentiation up to leptotene and zygotene		93 (Steinberger & Steinberger, 1967)
Eagle's minimum essential medium (with pyruvate and six nonessential amino acids)	Effective in inducing maturation up to spermatocytes till four weeks		93 (Steinberger & Steinberger, 1967), 90 (Steinberger et al., 1964b), 91 (Steinberger et al., 1964c)
5% CO_2 with 95% air	Better germ cell survival		130 (Steinberger & Steinberger, 1966)
Glutamine ≥4 mmol/l	Significantly induced spermatocyte production (more than vitamins) until three weeks		93 (Steinberger & Steinberger, 1967)
Sera or tissue extract supplementation, pituitary hormones	Not necessary for supplementation for initiation of spermatogenesis		93 (Steinberger & Steinberger, 1967)
Serum supplemented medium	Effective for maturation of undifferentiated spermatogonia to leptotene and pachytene spermatocytes	Mouse	119 (Nishimune et al., 1983)
FSH	Stimulated proliferation of type A spermatogonia Essential for maturation of type A spermatogonia up to pachytene spermatocytes		119 (Nishimune et al., 1983) 95 (Boitani et al., 1993)
FSH	Up to 5 IU/l supplementation allow meiotic induction 50 IU/l (>20 IU/mL) supplementation did not allow GC differentiation 5 IU/l sufficient for meiotic induction, insufficient for efficient testosterone production in vitro		127 (De Michele et al., 2017a)
Higher FSH supplementation	Results in 10-fold higher concentration of testosterone		126, 127 (De Michele et al., 2017a, 2017b)
FSH supplementation	Enhanced meiotic progression	Cell culture (human)	34, 35, 36 (Tesarik et al., 1998a, 1998b, 2000)
Retinoids	Induced spermatogenesis from type A into intermediate or type B		117, 119 (Aizawa & Nishimune, 1979; Nishimune & Osaka, 1983)

Table 30.3 (cont.)

Factors	Effect	Culture strategy/species	References
Retinol	Differentiation inducing factor		117, 1119 (Aizawa & Nishimune, 1979; Nishimune & Osaka, 1983)
Insulin-like growth factor-1 (IGF1)	Stimulating effects on differentiation of type A spermatogonia		117, 119 (Aizawa & Nishimune, 1979; Nishimune & Osaka, 1983)
Transforming growth factor-α (TGF-α)	No effect on germ cell differentiation through meiotic stage		117, 119 (Aizawa & Nishimune, 1979; Nishimune & Osaka, 1983)
Vitamins A, C, E, LH, testosterone	No effect on differentiation		95 (Boitani et al., 1993)
DMEM with (0.1 mmol/l) alanine, aspartic acid, glutamic acid, glycine, proline, serine, with (1 mmol/l) sodium pyruvate, 10% FBS, glutamine	Round spermatid development		98 (Suzuki & Sato, 2003)
DMEM with 10% FBS; or 0.1% BSA (bovine serum albumin)	Germ cell proliferation up to 14 days, no maturation reported		83 (Szczepny et al., 1999)
Coculture with Sertoli cells	Essential for survival and differentiation of germ cells	Cell culture (rodents)	33 (Tres & Kierszenbaum, 1983)
1:1 mix of Ham's F12 medium and Leibovitz's L15 medium, 10% FBS with epinephrine or norepinephrine	Production of haploid cells from meiotic cells of rat	Cell culture (rodents)	40 (Nagao, 1989)
Coculture with Sertoli cells, at 32°C in F-12 DMEM with insulin, transferrin, retinoic acid (RA), transforming growth factor (TGFα), FSH, testosterone	Pachytene spermatocytes, complete meiosis	Cell culture (rodents)	100 (Roulet et al., 2006)
Hormone supplementation	No effect on meiotic maturation. Positive effect on maintaining cell integrity and viability	Cell culture (rodents)	100 (Roulet et al., 2006)
DMEM with 10% FBS, coculture with Sertoli cell feeder layer	Round spermatid generation in mice	Cell culture (rodents)	131 (Rassoulzadegan et al., 1993)
Coculture of cell lines of peritubular, Leydig and Sertoli cell with germ cells, at 37°C	Differentiation up to haploid cells	Cell culture (rodents)	133 (Hofmann et al., 1994)
DMEM F12, 0.2% FCS (fetal calf serum), testosterone, FSH, coculture with Sertoli cells	Round spermatid generation, 1C cells maintained for three weeks. Testosterone and FSH supplementation increased the number of round spermatids produced	Cell culture (rodents)	39, 106 (Vigier et al., 2004; Perrard et al., 2016)
Serum-free medium (TKM), which includes insulin, insulin-growth factor 1, growth hormone, epidermal growth factor, retinol, testosterone, dihydrotestosterone, coculture with Sertoli cells	Round spermatids and offspring production	Cell culture (rodents)	132 (Marh et al., 2003)
DMEM, 10% FBS, testosterone, FSH, epinephrine, coculture with Sertoli cells	Round spermatids mature to elongated spermatids	Cell culture (rodents)	134 (Hasegawa et al., 2010)

Table 30.3 (cont.)

Factors	Effect	Culture strategy/species	References
Vero cell feeder, 10% synthetic serum	Progression of round spermatids up to elongated spermatids	Cell culture (human)	37, 42 (Sousa et al.,2002; Cremades et al., 1999)
Culturing in a drop of Vero cell conditioned medium with FSH and testosterone	Differentiation of round spermatids into elongated spermatids	Cell culture (human)	37, 42 (Sousa et al.,2002; Cremades et al., 1999)
Vero cell feeder	Differentiation of pachytene spermatocytes to round spermatids	Cell culture (human)	38 (Tanaka et al., 2003)
MEM (minimum essential medium) with 50% boar rete testicular fluid or human synthetic oviduct fluid, 10% human serum	Increased production rate of spermatids (by 10%)	Cell culture (human)	38 (Tanaka et al., 2003)
DMEM or DMEM F12, 10% FBS, with or without testosterone, FSH	Undifferentiated spermatogonia differentiate into differentiating spermatogonia, and after three months appear like elongated cells	(Bovine)	135 (Izadyar et al., 2003)
Medium supplemented with FBS, testosterone, retinol	Spermatogonial differentiated into spermatid-like cells	(Buffalo)	32 (Xie et al., 2010)
SACS (soft-agar culture system, two layers) with gel-agar medium (0.35%) and incubated on a solid-agar base (0.5%) mixed with high glucose DMEM solution, coculture with somatic cells, methylcellulose matrix, hCG, FSH, RPMI, 20% FBS	Meiotic differentiation in mice	(Mice)	74 (Stukenborg et al., 2008)
hCG (1 IU/mL) stimulation of Leydig cells	Stimulated testosterone production and has an anti-apoptotic effect	(Mice, Rhesus monkey)	65, 74, 77 (Huleihel et al., 2015; Stukenborg et al., 2008; Elhiza et al., 2012)
hCG, FSH (5 IU/mL)	Important for complete maturation and maintenance of spermatogenesis	(Mice, Rhesus monkey)	65, 74, 77 (Huleihel et al., 2015; Stukenborg et al., 2008; Elhiza et al., 2012)
Absence of hormones	Supports postmeiotic differentiation, not complete maturation	(Mice, Rhesus monkey)	65, 74, 77 (Huleihel et al., 2015; Stukenborg et al., 2008; Elhiza et al., 2012)
Activin	Stimulatory effect on spermatogonial differentiation		27 (Marcon et al., 2010)
GDNF	Opposite effect or inhibitory effect on differentiation		
Bicameral chamber, DMEM F12, FSH, testosterone, 5% FBS	Pachytene/zygotene spermatocytes differentiate into haploid cells		61 (Legendre et al., 2010)
Retinoic acid	Presence of RA does not allow germ cell differentiation		126 (De Michele et al., 2017a)
HCG supplementation influences FSH function	HCG influences Leydig cell function and role of FSH in induction of testosterone production		126 (De Michele et al., 2017a)
GDNF supplementation	No influence on SSC pool renewal		127 (De Michele et al., 2017b)

Table 30.3 (cont.)

Factors	Effect	Culture strategy/species	References
MEMα, 10% FBS or 10% KOS, with or without 5 IU/l FSH and LH	KOS supplementation superior, KOS shows higher number of conserved tubular cross-sections, expression of germ cell markers better Sertoli cell survival and testosterone secretion. No effect of KOS on maturation of spermatogonia into later spermatogenic stages.		136 (Grinspon et al., 2019)
FSH/LH supplementation	Higher number of undifferentiated spermatogonia, increased number of premeiotic cells, no postmeiotic maturation		136 (Grinspon et al., 2019)
0.5µM-1.5µM MEHP	Active metabolite of commonly used plasticizer di-(2-ethyl hexyl) pthalate (DEHP) implicated in reproductive toxicity		54 (Sakib et al., 2019)
Primary cilia ablation	Antenna-like organelle extending from cell surface is involved in several signal transduction pathways, such as Wnt/β-Catenin, Notch, Hippo, Hedgehog signaling present on somatic cells in testis. Chemical ablation of primary cilia (using 5µM CiliobrevinD) a small molecule inhibitor of primary cilium, organoid development was arrested		54 (Sakib et al., 2019)
RA stimulation	Organoids or testis specific cell associations resist RA stimulation. 2D cultures/germ cells in 2D cultures comparatively less resistant to RA stimulation		54 (Sakib et al., 2019)
Memα with 10% FBS	Maturation up to round spermatids (four weeks)	Tissue Culture (Rodents)	101 (Gohbara et al., 2010)
Memα with 10% KSR (knock-out replacement) or AlbuMax or chromatography purified BSA	Haploid cells, sperm offspring production		125 (Sato et al., 2015)
Kit-ligand and colony-stimulating factor-1 (CSF1) supplementation	Efficient maturation up to sperm production, offspring production		125 (Sato et al., 2015)
VAD-treated testis (adult)	Complete spermatogenesis observed, efficiency much lower than normal		125 (Sato et al., 2015)

nascent stage for culturing primate testicular samples in vitro. Keeping species-specific spermatogenic differences in consideration it is important to develop and optimize species- and age-specific culture conditions.

30.4 Future Scenarios: In Vitro Spermatogenesis for Research and Clinical Applications

We transit into a new era driven by technological advances. In this review we reflect on the many attempts highlighting key achievements in the field of in vitro spermatogenesis made so far. The research in this field is at a crucial juncture. The evolving technologies (like biofabricated 3D organoids, 3D bioprinting, microfluidics, or organ-on-a-chip) may offer excellent tools and in vitro testicular model systems to advance our understanding and bridge the existing knowledge gaps. Each of these culture systems offers unique advantages and may complement each other to address the common goal of achieving primate spermatogenesis in vitro. There are various possibilities and future scenarios for applying in vitro spermatogenesis as a tool for research and clinical applications in the future.

As limited human testicular samples are available for research, either nonhuman primate animal models can be employed as a preclinical research model or human testicular tissue samples can be used in limited quantities. The principles of the 3Rs (Replacement, Reduction, and Refinement) to reduce and avoid animal use should be considered to explore and validate various in vitro experimental approaches further.

As age-dependent effects are evident during in vitro testicular culture studies, it is necessary to develop age-specific and species-specific culture protocols and strategies. Appropriate culture strategies will allow mimicking of testicular development during the various postnatal phases and explore the role and developmental pattern of the specific cell type involved in influencing germ cell development. For instance, the role of factors secreted by testis-specific somatic cell type, that is, Sertoli cells, peritubular myoid cells, other interstitial cells including Leydig cells, endothelial cells, macrophages, fibroblasts, and other blood–testis barrier components. An alternate approach is to create 3D organoid models and manipulate specific cell types, and explore the role and function of these cells in vitro. Technologies like 3D printing allow bioprinting of specific cell types; for example, vascular cell beds in these devices may allow in vitro vascular support. The role of the endocrine environment can be investigated by using stimulatory conditions or perfusion systems to periodically stimulate the cultured samples in vitro and monitor their endocrine profiles.

The many trained scientists and the new technology create an outstanding area of research. It is almost certain that the recently established knowledge and approaches will soon be efficiently applied for achieving in vitro spermatogenesis. An application for fertility restoration in infertile patients is likely to be established in the next decade. The exact nature of such an application has to be decided on safety and efficiency grounds. Unwanted germline manipulation and deterioration has to be strictly avoided by any new approach. Therefore, these approaches need to be carefully evaluated and should be developed in the context of ethically approved human study protocols.

References

1. Anawalt BD. Approach to male infertility and induction of spermatogenesis. *J Clin Endocrinol Metab*. 2013;98(9):3532–3542.
2. Levine H, Jorgensen N, Martino-Andrade A, et al. Temporal trends in sperm count: a systematic review and meta regression analysis. *Hum Reprod Update*. 2017;23:646–659.
3. Sharpe RM, Franks S. Environment, lifestyle, and infertility: an inter-generational issue. *Nat Cell Biol*. 2002; s33–s40.
4. Van Batavia JP, Kolon TF. Fertility in disorders of sex development. *J Pediatr Urol*. 2016;12(6):418–425.
5. Gomes NL, Chetty T, Jorgensen A, Mitchell RT. Disorders of sex development: novel regulators, impacts on fertility, and options for fertility preservation. *Int J Mol Sci*. 2020;21 (7):2282.
6. Picton HM, Wyns C, Anderson RA, et al. ESHRE task force on fertility preservation in severe diseases: a European perspective on testicular tissue cryopreservation for fertility preservation in prepubertal and adolescent boys. *Hum Reprod*. 2015;30 (11):2463–2475.
7. Weblink: www.urologyhealth.org/urologic-conditions/male-infertility
8. Gassei K, Orwig KE. Experimental methods to preserve male fertility and treat male infertility. *Fertil Steril*. 2016;105(2):256–266.
9. Horwich A, Shipley J, Huddart R. Testicular germ-cell cancer. *Lancet*. 2006;367:754–765.
10. Rajpert-De Meyts E, McGlynn KA, Okamoto K, Jewett MAS, Bokemeyer C. Testicular germ cell tumours. *Lancet*. 2016;387:1762–1774.
11. Sharma S, Wistuba J, Pock T, Schlatt S, Neuhaus N. Spermatogonial stem cells: updates from specification to clinical relevance. *Hum Reprod Update*. 2019;25 (3):275–297.
12. Goossens E, Jahnukainen K, Mitchell RT, et al. Fertility preservation in boys: recent developments and new insights. *Hum Reprod Open*. 2020;2020(3): hoaa016.
13. Oncofertility Consortium. Homepage. https://oncofertility.northwestern.edu/
14. Schlatt S, Ehmcke J. Regulation of spermatogenesis: an evolutionary biologist's perspective. *Semin Cell Dev Biol*. 2014;29:2–16.
15. Tung PS, Fritz IB. Interactions of Sertoli cells with myoid cells in vitro. *Biol Reprod*. 1980;23:207–217.
16. Hadley MA, Byers SW, Suárez-Quian CA, Kleinman HK, Dym M. Extracellular matrix regulates Sertoli cell differentiation, testicular cord formation, and germ cell development in vitro. *J Cell Biol*. 1985;101:1511–1522.
17. Kierszenbaum AL, Crowell JA, Shabanowitz RB, DePhilip RM, Tres LL. Protein secretory patterns of rat Sertoli and peritubular cells are influenced by culture conditions. *Biol Reprod*. 1986;35:239–251.
18. Tung PS, Fritz IB. Extracellular matrix components and testicular peritubular cells influence the rate and pattern of Sertoli cell migration in vitro. *Dev Biol*. 1986; 113:119–134.
19. Tung PS, Fritz IB. Morphogenetic restructuring and formation of basement membranes by Sertoli cells and testis peritubular cells in co-culture: inhibition of the morphogenetic cascade by cyclic AMP derivatives and by blocking direct cell contact. *Dev Biol*. 1987;120:139–153.
20. Hofmann MC, Narisawa S, Hess RA, Millan JL. Immortalization of germ cells and somatic testicular cells using the SV40 large T antigen. *Exp Cell Res*. 1992;201:417–435.
21. Richardson LL, Kleinman HK, Dym M. Basement membrane gene expression by Sertoli and peritubular myoid cells in vitro in the rat. *Biol Reprod*. 1995;52:320–330.
22. Schlatt S, de Kretser DM, Loveland KL. Discriminative analysis of rat Sertoli and peritubular cells and their proliferation in vitro: evidence for follicle-stimulating hormonemediated contact inhibition of Sertoli cell mitosis. *Biol Reprod*. 1996;55:227–235.
23. van der Wee K, Hofmann MC. An in vitro tubule assay identifies HGF as a morphogen for the formation of seminiferous tubules in the postnatal mouse testis. *Exp Cell Res*. 1999;252:175–185.

24. Hoeben E, Swinnen JV, Heyns W, Verhoeven G. Heregulins or neu differentiation factors and the interactions between peritubular myoid cells and Sertoli cells. *Endocrinology*. 1999;140:2216–2223.

25. El Ramy R, Verot A, Mazaud S, Odet F, Magre S, Le Magueresse-Battistoni B. Fibroblast growth factor (FGF) 2 and FGF9 mediate mesenchymal–epithelial interactions of peritubular and Sertoli cells in the rat testis. *J Endocrinol*. 2005;187:135–147.

26. Gassei K, Schlatt S, Ehmcke J. De novo morphogenesis of seminiferous tubules from dissociated immature rat testicular cells in xenografts. *J Androl*. 2006;27:611–618.

27. Marcon L, Zhang X, Hales BF, Nagano MC, Robaire B. Development of a short term fluorescence-based assay to assess the toxicity of anticancer drugs on rat stem/progenitor spermatogonia in vitro. *Biol Reprod*. 2010;83:228–237.

28. Mincheva M, Sandhowe-Klaverkamp R, Wistuba J, et al. Reassembly of adult human testicular cells: can testis cord-like structures be created in vitro? *Mol Hum Reprod*. 2018;24(2):55–63.

29. von Kopylow K, Schulze W, Salzbrunn A, et al. *Mol Hum Reprod*. 2018; 24(3):123–134.

30. Mincheva M, Wistuba J, Brenker C, Schlatt S. Challenging human somatic testicular cell reassembly by protein kinase inhibtion: setting up a functional in vitro test system. *Sci Rep*. 2020;10(1):8935.

31. Iwanami Y, Kobayashi T, Kato M, Hirabayashi M, Hochi S. Characteristics of rat round spermatids differentiated from spermatogonial cells during co-culture with Sertoli cells, assessed by flow cytometry, microinsemination and RT-PCR. *Theriogenology*. 2006;65:288–298.

32. Xie B, Qin Z, Huang B, et al. In vitro culture and differentiation of buffalo (Bubalus bubalis) spermatogonia. *Reprod Domest Anim*. 2010;45:275–282

33. Tres LL, Kierszenbaum AL. Viability of rat spermatogenic cells in vitro is facilitated by their coculture with Sertoli cells in serum-free hormone-supplemented medium. *Proc Natl Acad Sci USA*. 1983;80:3377–3381.

34. Tesarik J, Greco E, Rienzi L, et al. Differentiation of spermatogenic cells during in-vitro culture of testicular biopsy samples from patients with obstructive azoospermia: effect of recombinant follicle stimulating hormone. *Hum Reprod*. 1998a;13:2772–2781.

35. Tesarik J, Guido M, Mendoza C, Greco E. Human spermatogenesis in vitro: respective effects of follicle-stimulating hormone and testosterone on meiosis, spermiogenesis, and Sertoli cell apoptosis. *J Clin Endocrinol Metab*. 1998b;83:4467–4473.

36. Tesarik J, Balaban B, Isiklar A, et al. In-vitro spermatogenesis resumption in men with maturation arrest: relationship with in-vivo blocking stage and serum FSH. *Hum Reprod*. 2000;15:1350–1354.

37. Sousa M, Cremades N, Alves C, Silva J, Barros A. Developmental potential of human spermatogenic cells co-cultured with Sertoli cells. *Hum Reprod*. 2002;17:161–172.

38. Tanaka A, Nagayoshi M, Awata S, Mawatari Y, Tanaka I, Kusunoki H. Completion of meiosis in human primary spermatocytes through in vitro coculture with Vero cells. *Fertil Steril*. 2003;79:795–801.

39. Vigier M, Weiss M, Perrard MH, Godet M, Durand P. The effects of FSH and of testosterone on the completion of meiosis and the very early steps of spermiogenesis of the rat: an in vitro study. *J Mol Endocrinol*. 2004;33:729–742.

40. Nagao Y. Viability of meiotic prophase spermatocytes of rats is facilitated in primary culture of dispersed testicular cells on collagen gel by supplementing epinephrine or norepinephrine: evidence that meiotic prophase spermatocytes complete meiotic divisions in vitro. *In Vitro Cell Dev Biol*. 1989;25:1088–1098.

41. Magueresse-Battistoni BL, Gérard N, Jégou B. Pachytene spermatocytes can achieve meiotic process in vitro. *Biochem Biophys Res Commun*. 1991;179(2):1115–1121.

42. Cremades N, Bernabeu R, Barros A, Sousa M. In-vitro maturation of round spermatids using co-culture on Vero cells. *Hum Reprod*. 1999;14:1287–1293.

43. Enders GC, Henson JH, Millette CF. Sertoli cell binding to isolated testicular basement membrane. *J Cell Biol*. 1986;103:1109–1119.

44. Hadley MA, Weeks BS, Kleinman HK, Dym M. Laminin promotes formation of cord-like structures by Sertoli cells in vitro. *Dev Biol*. 1990;140:318–327.

45. Gassei K, Ehmcke J, Schlatt S. Initiation of testicular tubulogenesis is controlled by neurotrophic tyrosine receptor kinases in a three-dimensional Sertoli cell aggregation assay. *Reproduction*. 2008;136:459–469.

46. Yu X, Hong S, Moreira EG, Faustman EM. Improving in vitro Sertoli cell/gonocyte co-culture model for assessing male reproductive toxicity: lessons learned from comparisons of cytotoxicity versus genomic responses to phthalates. *Toxicol Appl Pharmacol*. 2009;239:325–336.

47. Gassei K, Ehmcke J, Wood MA, Walker WH, Schlatt S. Immature rat seminiferous tubules reconstructed in vitro express markers of Sertoli cell maturation after xenografting into nude mouse hosts. *Mol Hum Reprod*. 2010;16:97–110.

48. Pan F, Chi LF, Schlatt S. Effects of nanostructures and mouse embryonic stem cells on in vitro morphogenesis of rat testicular cords. *PLoS ONE*. 2013;8: e60054.

49. Wegner S, Hong S, Yu X, Faustman EM. Preparation of rodent testis co-cultures. *Curr Protoc Toxicol*. 2013; Chapter 16:Unit 16.10.

50. Reuter K, Ehmcke J, Stukenborg JB, et al. Reassembly of somatic cells and testicular organogenesis in vitro. *Tissue Cell*. 2014;46:86–96.

51. Potter SJ, DeFalco T. Using ex vivo upright droplet cultures of whole fetal organs to study developmental processes during mouse organogenesis. *J Vis Exp*. 2015;e53262.

52. Harris S, Hermsen SAB, Yu XZ, Hong SW, Faustman EM. Comparison of toxicogenomic responses to phthalate ester exposure in an organotypic testis co-culture model and responses observed in vivo. *Reprod Toxicol*. 2015;58:149–159.

53. Harris S, Shubin SP, Wegner S, et al. The presence of macrophages and inflammatory responses in an in vitro testicular co-culture model of male reproductive development enhance relevance to in vivo conditions. *Toxicol In Vitro*. 2016;36:210–215.

54. Sakib S, Uchida A, Valenzuela-Leon P, et al. Formation of organotypic testicular organoids in microwell culture. *Biol Reprod*. 2019;100(6):1648–1660.

55. Edmonds ME, Woodruff TK. Testicular organoid formation is a property of immature somatic cells, which self-assemble and exhibit long-term hormone-responsive endocrine function. *Biofabrication*. 2020;12(4):045002.

56. Baert Y, Ruetschle I, Cools W, et al. A multi-organ chip co-culture of liver and testis equivalents: a first step toward a systemic male reprotoxicity model. *Hum Reprod*. 2020;35(5):1029–1044.

57. Zenzes MT, Engel W. The capacity of testicular cells of the postnatal rat to reorganize into histotypic structures. *Differentiation*. 1981;20:157–161.

58. Lee DR, Kaproth MT, Parks JE. In vitro production of haploid germ cells from fresh or frozen-thawed testicular cells of neonatal bulls. *Biol Reprod*. 2001;65:873–878.

59. Lee DR, Kim K-S, Yang YH, et al. Isolation of male germ stem cell-like cells from testicular tissue of non-obstructive azoospermic patients and differentiation into haploid male germ cells in vitro. *Hum Reprod*. 2006a;21:471–476.

60. Lee JH, Kim HJ, Kim H, Lee SJ, Gye MC. In vitro spermatogenesis by threedimensional culture of rat testicular cells in collagen gel matrix. *Biomaterials*. 2006b;27:2845–2853.

61. Legendre A, Froment P, Desmots S, Lecomte A, Habert R, Lemazurier E. An engineered 3D blood-testis barrier model for the assessment of reproductive toxicity potential. *Biomaterials*. 2010;31:4492–4505.

62. Yokonishi T, Sato T, Katagiri K, Komeya M, Kubota Y, Ogawa T. In vitro reconstruction of mouse seminiferous tubules supporting germ cell differentiation. *Biol Reprod*. 2013;89:11–16.

63. Zhang J, Hatakeyama J, Eto K, Abe S. Reconstruction of a seminiferous tubule-like structure in a 3 dimensional culture system of re-aggregated mouse neonatal testicular cells within a collagen matrix. *Gen Comp Endocrinol*. 2014;205:121–132.

64. Reda A, Hou M, Landreh L, et al. In vitro spermatogenesis: optimal culture conditions for testicular cell survival, germ cell differentiation, and steroidogenesis in rats. *Front Endocrinol (Lausanne)*. 2014;5:21.

65. Huleihel M, Nourashrafeddin S, Plant TM. Application of three-dimensional culture systems to study mammalian spermatogenesis, with an emphasis on the rhesus monkey (*Macaca mulatta*). *Asian J Androl*. 2015;17:972–980.

66. Baert Y, De Kock J, Alves-Lopes JP, Söder O, Stukenborg J-B, Goossens E. Primary human testicular cells self-organize into organoids with testicular properties. *Stem Cell Reports*. 2017;1:30–38.

67. Baert Y, Goossens E. Preparation of scaffolds from decellularized testicular matrix. *Methods Mol Biol*. 2018;1577:121–127.

68. Baert Y, Rombaut C, Goossens E. Scaffold-based and scaffold-free testicular organoids from primary human testicular cells. *Methods Mol Biol*. 2019;1576:283–290.

69. Baert Y, Stukenborg JB, Landreh M, et al. Derivation and characterization of a cytocompatible scaffold from human testis. *Hum Reprod*. 2015;30:256–267.

70. Alves-Lopes JP, Soder O, Stukenborg JB. Testicular organoid generation by a novel in vitro three-layer gradient system. *Biomaterials*. 2017;130:76–89.

71. Lee J-H, Gye MC, Choi KW, et al. In vitro differentiation of germ cells from nonobstructive azoospermic patients using three-dimensional culture in a collagen gel matrix. *Fertil Steril*. 2007;87:824–833.

72. Lee JH, Oh JH, Lee JH, Kim MR, Min CK. Evaluation of in vitro spermatogenesis using poly(D,L-lactic-co-glycolic acid) (PLGA)-based macroporous biodegradable scaffolds. *J Tissue Eng Regen Med*. 2011;5:130–137.

73. Zhang X, Wang L, Zhang X, et al. The use of KnockOut serum replacement (KSR) in three dimensional rat testicular cells coculture model: an improved male reproductive toxicity testing system. *Food Chem Toxicol*. 2017;106:487–495.

74. Stukenborg JB, Wistuba J, Luetjens CM, et al. Coculture of spermatogonia with somatic cells in a novel three-dimensional soft-agar-culture-system. *J Androl*. 2008;29:312–329.

75. Stukenborg J-B, Schlatt S, Simoni M, et al. New horizons for in vitro spermatogenesis? An update on novel three-dimensional culture systems as tools for meiotic and post-meiotic differentiation of testicular germ cells. *Mol Hum Reprod*. 2009;15:521–529.

76. Pendergraft SS, Sadri-Ardekani H, Atala A, Bishop CE. Three-dimensional testicular organoid: a novel tool for the study of human spermatogenesis and gonadotoxicity in vitro dagger. *Biol Reprod*. 2017;96:720–732.

77. Elhija MA, Lunenfeld E, Schlatt S, Huleihel M. Differentiation of murine male germ cells to spermatozoa in a soft agar culture system. *Asian J Androl*. 2012;14:285–293.

78. Alves-Lopes JP, Stukenborg JB. Testicular organoids: a new model to study the testicular microenvironment in vitro? *Hum Reprod Update*. 2018;24(2):176–191.

79. Sharma S, Venzac B, Burgers T, Le Gac S, Schlatt S. Microfluidics in male reproduction: is ex vivo culture of primate testis tissue a future strategy for ART or toxicology research? *Mol Hum Reprod*. 2020;26(3):179–192.

80. Sakib S, Goldsmith T, Voigt A, Dobrinski I. Testicular organoids to study cell-cell interactions in the mammalian testis. *Andrology*. 2019; 8(4):835–841.

81. Komeya M, Sato T, Ogawa T. In vitro spermatogenesis: a century-long research journey, still half way around. *Reprod Med Biol*. 2018;17(4):407–420.

82. Gargus ES, Rogers HB, McKinnon KE, Edmonds ME, Woodruff TK. Engineered reproductive tissues. *Nat Biomed Eng*. 2020;4(4):381–393.

83. Szczepny A, Hogarth CA, Young J, Loveland KL. Identification of Hedgehog signaling outcomes in mouse testis development using a hanging drop-culture system. *Biol Reprod*. 1999;80:258–263.

84. Jørgensen A, Young J, Nielsen JE, et al. Hanging drop cultures of human testis and testis cancer samples: a model used to investigate activin treatment effects in a preserved niche. *Br J Cancer*. 2014;110:2604–2614.

85. Jørgensen A, Nielsen JE, Perlman S, et al. Ex vivo culture of human fetal gonads: manipulation of meiosis signalling by retinoic acid treatment disrupts testis development. *Hum Reprod*. 2015;30:2351–2363.

86. Champy CH. De la méthode de culture des tissus. VI. Le testicule. *Arch Zool Exptl Gen*. 1920;60:461–500.

87. Martinovitch PN. The development in vitro of the mammalian gonad. Ovary and ovogenesis. *Proc R Soc B Biol Sci.* 1938;125:232–249.

88. Trowell OA. The culture of mature organs in a synthetic medium. *Exp Cell Res.* 1959;16:118–147.

89. Steinberger E, Steinberger A, Perloff WH. Studies on growth in organ culture of testicular tissue from rats of various ages. *Anat Rec.* 1964a;148:581–589.

90. Steinberger E, Steinberger A, Perloff WH. Initiation of spermatogenesis in vitro. *Endocrinology.* 1964b;74:788–792.

91. Steinberger A, Steinberger E, Perloff WH. Mammalian testis in organ culture. *Exp Cell Res.* 1964c;36:19–27.

92. Steinberger A, Steinberger E. Differentiation of rat seminiferous epithelium in organ culture. *J Reprod Fertil.* 1965;9:243–248.

93. Steinberger A, Steinberger E. Factors affecting spermatogenesis in organ cultures of mammalian testes. *J Reprod Fertil.* 1967;Suppl. 2:117–124.

94. Matte R, Sasaki M. Autoradiographic evidence of human male germ-cell differentiation in vitro. *Cytologia.* 1971;36:298–303.

95. Boitani C, Politi MG, Menna T. Spermatogonial cell proliferation in organ culture of immature rat testis. *Biol Reprod.* 1993;48:761–767.

96. Schlatt S, Zhengwei Y, Meehan T, de Kretser DM, Loveland KL. Application of morphometric techniques to postnatal rat testes in organ culture: insights into testis growth. *Cell Tissue Res.* 1999;298:335–343.

97. Meehan T, Schlatt S, O'Bryan M, de Kretser DM, Loveland KL. Regulation of germ cell and Sertoli cells development by activin, follistatin and FSH. *Dev Biol.* 2000;220:225–237.

98. Suzuki S, Sato K. The fertilising ability of spermatogenic cells derived from cultured mouse immature testicular tissue. *Zygote.* 2003;11:307–316.

99. Lambrot R, Coffigny H, Pairault C, et al. Use of organ culture to study the human fetal testis development: effect of retinoic acid. *J Clin Endocrinol Metab.* 2006;91:2696–2703.

100. Roulet V, Denis H, Staub C, et al. Human testis in organotypic culture: application for basic or clinical research. *Hum Reprod.* 2006;21:1564–1575.

101. Gohbara A, Katagiri K, Sato T, et al. In vitro murine spermatogenesis in an organ culture system. *Biol Reprod.* 2010;83:261–267.

102. Sato T, Katagiri K, Gohbara A, et al. In vitro production of functional sperm in cultured neonatal mouse testes. *Nature.* 2011a;471:504–507.

103. Sato T, Katagiri K, Yokonishi T, et al. In vitro production of fertile sperm from murine spermatogonial stem cell lines. *Nat Commun.* 2011b;2:472.

104. Dumont L, Oblette A, Rondanino C, et al. Vitamin A prevents round spermatid nuclear damage and promotes the production of motile sperm during in vitro maturation of vitrified prepubertal mouse testicular tissue. *Mol Hum Reprod.* 2016;22:819–832.

105. Liu F, Cai C, Wu X, et al. Effect of KnockOut serum replacement on germ cell development of immature testis tissue culture. *Theriogenology.* 2016;85:193–199.

106. Perrard MH, Sereni N, Schluth-Bolard C, et al. Complete human and rat ex vivo spermatogenesis from fresh or frozen testicular tissue. *Biol Reprod.* 2016;95:89.

107. Komeya M, Kimura H, Nakamura H, et al. Long-term ex vivo maintenance of testis tissues producing fertile sperm in a microfluidic device. *Sci Rep.* 2016;6:21472.

108. Komeya M, Hayashi K, Nakamura H, et al. Pumpless microfluidic system driven by hydrostatic pressure induces and maintains mouse spermatogenesis in vitro. *Sci Rep.* 2017;7(1):15459.

109. Reda A, Albalushi H, Montalvo SC, et al. Knock-out serum replacement and melatonin effects on germ cell differentiation in murine testicular explant cultures. *Ann Biomed Eng.* 2017;45:1783–1794.

110. Rondanino C, Maouche A, Dumont L, Oblette A, Rives N. Establishment, maintenance and functional integrity of the blood-testis barrier in organotypic cultures of fresh and frozen/thawed prepubertal mouse testes. *Mol Hum Reprod.* 2017;23:304–320.

111. Stukenborg J-B, Alves-Lopes JP, Kurek M, et al. Spermatogonial quantity in human prepubertal testicular tissue collected for fertility preservation prior to potentially sterilizing therapy. *Hum Reprod.* 2018;33(9):1677–1683.

112. Medrano JV, Vilanova-Pérez T, Fornés-Ferrer V, et al. Influence of temperature, serum, and gonadotropin supplementation in short- and long-term organotypic culture of human immature testicular tissue. *Fertil Steril.* 2018;110(6):1045–1057.

113. Yamanaka H, Komeya M, Nakamura H, et al. A monolayer microfluidic device supporting mouse spermatogenesis with improved visibility. *Biochem BioPhys Res Commun.* 2018;500(4):885–891.

114. Portela JMD, de Winter-Korver CM, van Daalen SKM, et al. Assessment of fresh and cryopreserved testicular tissues from (pre)pubertal boys during organ culture as a strategy for in vitro spermatogenesis. *Hum Reprod.* 2019;34(12):2443–2455.

115. Ghatnekar R, Lima-De-faria A, Rubin S, Menander K. Development of human male meiosis in vitro. *Hereditas.* 1974;78:265–271.

116. Eddy EM, Kahri AI. Cell associations and surface features in cultures of juvenile rat seminiferous tubules. *Anat Rec.* 1976;185:333–357.

117. Aizawa S, Nishimune Y. In-vitro differentiation of type A spermatogonia in mouse cryptorchid testis. *J Reprod Fertil.* 1979;56:99–104.

118. Curtis D. In vitro differentiation of diakinesis figures in human testis. *Hum Genet.* 1981;59:406–411.

119. Nishimune YM, Osaka M. In vitro differentiation mouse cryptorchid of type a spermatogonia from testes in serum-free. *Biol Reprod.* 1983;28:1217–1223.

120. Parvinen M, Wright WW, Phillips DM, Mather NA, Musto NA, Bardin CW. Spermatogenesis in vitro: completion of meiosis and early spermiogenesis. *Endocrinology.* 1983;112:1150–1152.

121. Toppari J, Mali P, Eerola E. Rat spermatogenesis in vitro traced by quantitative flow cytometry. *J Histochem Cytochem.* 1986;34:1029–1035.

122. Kim KJ, Kim BG, Kim YH, et al. In vitro spermatogenesis using bovine testis tissue culture techniques. *Tissue Eng Regener Med.* 2015;12:314–323.

123. Arkoun B, Dumont L, Milazzo JP, et al. Retinol improves in vitro differentiation of pre-pubertal mouse spermatogonial stem cells into sperm during the first wave of spermatogenesis. *PLoS ONE*. 2015;10:e0116660.

124. Dumont L, Arkoun B, Jumeau F, Milazzo J-F, Bironneau A, Liot D, Wils J, Rondanino C, Rives N. Assessment of the optimal vitrification protocol for pre-pubertal mice testes leading to successful in vitro production of flagellated spermatozoa. *Andrology*. 2015; 3(3):611–625.

125. Sato T, Katagiri K, Kojima K, Komeya M, Yao M, Ogawa T. In vitro spermatogenesis in explanted adult mouse testis tissues. *PLoS ONE*. 2015;10:e0130171.

126. de Michele F, Poels J, Weerens L, et al. Preserved seminiferous tubule integrity with spermatogonial survival and induction of Sertoli and Leydig cell maturation after long-term organotypic culture of prepubertal human testicular tissue. *Hum Reprod*. 2017a;32:32–45.

127. de Michele F, Vermeulen M, Wyns C. Fertility restoration with spermatogonial stem cells. *Curr Opin Endocrinol Diabetes Obes*. 2017b;24:424–431.

128. Gholami K, Vermeulen M, Del Vento F, de Michele F, Giudice MG, Wyns C. The air-liquid interface culture of the mechanically isolated seminiferous tubules embedded in agarose or alginate improves in vitro spermatogenesis at the expense of attenuating their integrity. *In Vitro Cell Dev Biol Anim*. 2020;56(3):261–270.

129. Yokonishi T, Sato T, Komeya M, et al. Offspring production with sperm grown in vitro from cryopreserved testis tissues. *Nat Commun*. 2014;5:4320.

130. Steinberger A, Steinberger E. In vitro culture of rat testicular cells. *Exptl Cell Res*. 1966;44:443–452.

131. Rassoulzadegan M, Paquis-Flucklinger V, Bertino B, et al. Transmeiotic differentiation of male germ cells in culture. *Cell*. 1993; 75(5):997–1006.

132. Marh J, Tres LL, Yamazaki Y, Yanagimachi R, Kierszenbaum AL. Mouse round spermatids developed in vitro from preexisting spermatocytes can produce normal offspring by nuclear injection into in vivo-developed mature oocytes. *Biol Reprod*. 2003;69:169–176.

133. Hofmann MC, Hess RA, Goldberg E, Millán JL. Immortalized germ cells undergo meiosis in vitro. *PNAS*, 1994; 91(12): 5533–5537.

134. Hasegawa H, Terada Y, Ugajin T, Yaegashi N, Sato K. A novel culture system for mouse spermatid maturation which produces elongating spermatids capable of inducing calcium oscillation during fertilization and embryonic development. *J Assist Reprod Genet*. 2010;27(9–10):565–570.

135. Izadyar F, Den Ouden K, Creemers LB, Posthuma G, Parvinen M, De Rooij DG. Proliferation and differentiation of bovine type A spermatogonia during long-term culture. *Biol Reprod*. 2003;68 (1):272–281.

136. Grinspon RP, Rey RA. Molecular characterization of XX maleness. *Int J Mol Sci*. 2019;20:6089.

137. Steinberger A, Steinberger E, Perloff WH. Growth of rat testes fragments in organ culture. *Fed Proc*. 1963;22:372.

138. Steinberger A, Steinberger E. Stimulatory effect of vitamins and glutamine on the differentiation of germ cells in rat testes organ culture grown in chemically defined media. *Exp Cell Res*. 1966;44:429–435.

139. Parvinen M, Vanha-Perttula T. Identification and enzyme quantification of the stages of the seminiferous epithelial wave in the rat. *Anat Rec*. 1972;174:435–449.

140. Alves-Lopes JP, Söder O, Stukenborg JB. Use of a three-layer gradient system of cells for rat testicular organoid generation. *Nat Protoc*. 2018;13:248–259.

Spermatogonial Stem Cell Culture and the Future of Germline Gene Editing

Xichen Nie, Jan-Bernd Stukenborg, and Jingtao Guo

31.1 Clinical Significance of Studying Human Spermatogonial Stem Cells

To date, it is estimated that infertility can affect up to 15% of couples globally, amounting to 48.5 million couples, and male factors are found to be responsible for half of those infertile cases [1]. Azoospermia, which means that there is no sperm present in a man's ejaculate, is one of the main causes for male infertility, accounting for 10–15% of all male infertile cases. This disease is classified as obstructive azoospermia or nonobstructive azoospermia (NOA), according to whether it is caused by obstructive or nonobstructive sources. NOA accounts for 80% of azoospermia with human spermatogonial stem cell (hSSC) maturation failure as one of the major causes for NOA [2]. hSSC maturation failures can be caused by either intrinsic or extrinsic reasons. Common intrinsic reasons include chromosomal abnormality. For example, Klinefelter syndrome, in which both somatic and germ cells at least partially contain an extra X chromosome, can be found in about 10% of azoospermic men [3]. It is reported that in this disease hSSC development arrests at the primary spermatocyte or even later stage [4]. Another equally common genetic cause of male infertility is Y chromosome microdeletion. Only one or a few gene deletions on the Y chromosome can lead to failures of the spermatogenic maturation process, when hSSCs develop into haploid cells [5].

One extrinsic and relatively common reason leading to azoospermia is cancer treatments. Each year, approximately 16,000 children are diagnosed with cancer in the United States, irrespective of their ethnic, gender, or socioeconomic background. Remarkably, thanks to advancements in technology and health care, approximately 85% of childhood cancer patients survive. However, this success comes at a cost, as an increasing number of recovered male patients will face subfertility or infertility as a late effect of the disease itself or due to the anticancer treatments. Male childhood cancer patients treated with highly gonadotoxic therapies have a significantly reduced chance of fathering their own biological children later in life. For boys at risk of becoming infertile, infertility has a major impact on their psychosocial well-being, and some survivors even experience problems finding partners because of their infertility, creating additional psychosocial stresses.

Therefore, future medical care needs to focus on hSSC therapy, either by culturing hSSCs in vitro to expand the number of cells and then lead to spermatogenesis through transplantation, or developing improved anticancer treatment with much reduced gonadotoxicity [6].

Abnormal development of hSSCs can cause not only male infertility, but also testicular germ cell tumors (TGCTs). hSSCs originate from primordial germ cells (PGCs) in the fetal stage. The abnormal development of all germline stem cells, including PGCs and hSSCs, may lead to TGCTs due to genetic events, epigenetic events, and environmental factors. For example, spermatocytic tumor is a type of germline tumor that occurs in the testes of older men (average of 53.5 years). It is believed to emerge from expanding spermatogonia [7]. One of the strong correlations of this disease is the amplification of DMRT1 [8] that also plays a role in normal testicular development. Although TGCT is highly sensitive to cancer treatment and therefore relatively easy to cure as a cancer type, its treatment may affect the patient's quality of life for a lifelong time. Combined with the aforementioned hSSCs-related infertile issues, a deep understanding of hSSCs is very important.

31.2 Current Understanding of hSSCs

31.2.1 Models of Human Spermatogonia

The initial classification of hSSCs is based on morphological and histological evidence. hSSCs are located inside the seminiferous tubules, attaching to the basement membrane. Hematoxylin and eosin staining showed that the nuclear staining of these cells could be dark or light, which were therefore named as A_{dark} or A_{pale}, respectively [9,10] (Figure 31.1). Clermont further performed the 3 H-thymidine label experiment and found that in monkeys A_{dark} could not be labeled while A_{pale} could, suggesting that A_{dark} is a type of reserved cell with low proliferation ability, and A_{pale} is active stem cells with relatively higher cell cycle activity [11]. In the prevailing A_{dark}/A_{pale} model, A_{pale} can self-renew to maintain the stem cell pool and further differentiate into mitotic active B type spermatogonia, and then differentiate into primary spermatocytes [11]. Researchers also sought to study the molecular features of hSSCs, as well as examine their functionality. Multiple markers for hSSCs have been proposed, such as

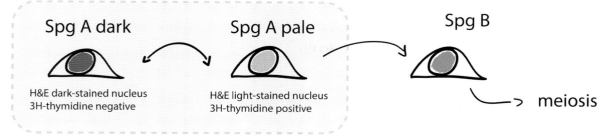
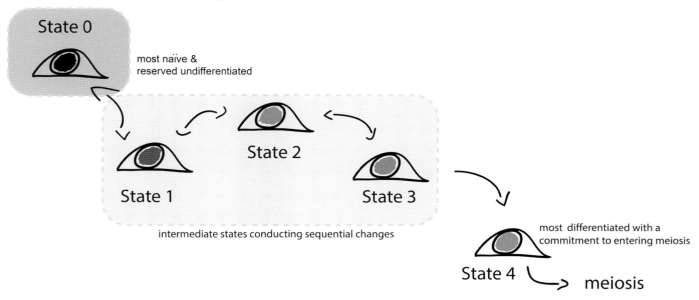

Figure 31.1 Schematic overview of two classification models for human spermatogonia based on morphology or single-cell RNA-sequencing data
Notes: Spg: spermatogonia; H&E: haematoxylin and esosin.

GFRA1 and SSEA4 [12,13]. Glial cell line-derived neurotrophic factor was reported to play a very critical role in maintaining mouse SSC self-renewal in vivo, and is the essential cytokine for the in vitro culture of rodent SSCs [14]. Therefore, its receptor, GFRA1, exhibits high expression in SSCs in both mice and humans. In the meantime, functional assay has been used as the gold standard to evaluate the stemness of SSCs. In mice, SSCs' capacity to self-renew or differentiate can be tested by transplantation, through which collected cells from donor mice are transplanted to the testis of recipient mice whose germ cells are depleted by chemical or genetic approaches. Since SSCs are supposed to home to the receipt niche and establish spermatogenesis, cells with higher transplantation efficiency should contain SSCs with higher purity [15]. However, with regard to primates, animal experiments can be costly and time-consuming. The research on human SSCs is even more challenging. Therefore, xenotransplantation assays have been used to test the functionality of hSSCs. It turns out that hSSCs could colonize in the seminiferous tubules of recipient mice after transplantation, but could not develop into any further stage [16]. In the previous studies, however, the A_{dark}/A_{pale} model has not been fully correlated with molecular research or functional research. Many studies show that A_{dark}/A_{pale} do not have distinct markers or functions, suggesting the morphological difference may not indicate two different cell states and could be caused by other internal factors such as cell cycles.

The recent advantage of single-cell approaches revolutionized our understanding of hSSC and germ cell development. As single-cell technology requires a small amount of materials and profiles global expression at single-cell resolution, it overcomes the obstacles for hSSC studies, such as the lack of precious human samples and cellular heterogeneity. As an example, Guo et al. recently derived a transcriptional cell atlas of the young adult testes by profiling transcriptomes of single testicular cells from young adult testes (17–25 years old), which provided a foundation for further analysis and comparison [17]. Importantly, five distinct molecular states of human spermatogonia in the young adult human testes were identified, termed States 0–4, with State 0 identified as likely the most naïve and reserved undifferentiated stem cell state – as adult State 0 cells highly resemble the sole germ cell state present in infants (Figure 31.1). State 4 was identified as the most differentiated spermatogonial state (with markers that strongly indicate a commitment to entering meiosis), with intermediate states (States 1–3) conducting sequential changes in proliferation, signaling, and metabolic states to confer expansion and preparation for meiosis. Those studies represent one of the first efforts to systematically investigate hSSCs using molecular and genomics approaches.

31.2.2 Human and Mouse SSC Comparison

As there is no robust in vitro culture system for hSSCs, our knowledge on hSSCs was relatively limited and based largely on extrapolation from rodent and primate research. However, as mentioned earlier, in xenotransplantation assay, mouse testis cannot provide conditions for hSSCs to complete spermatogenesis, indicating differences in SSC development between humans and mice. Accumulating evidence shows hSSCs are vastly different from mouse SSCs (mSSCs). First, mice begin to produce a synchronized first-wave spermatogenesis just three days after birth. These differentiated germ cells are generated from gonocytes, the germline stem cells in the fetal period, which directly make differentiating spermatogonia by skipping the self-renewing SSC stage, and complete the first spermatogenesis wave around 35 days postpartum [18]. In contrast, hSSCs stay in a quiescent stage from birth for almost a decade, and begin to differentiate at around puberty. Second, the estimated proportion of mSSCs in all germ cells (around 0.03%) is much lower than that in humans (around 1%) [19]. It is believed that mSSCs need to undergo more cell cycles and rounds of amplication before entering meiosis. In fact, in mice, type A spermatogonia can be classified into several groups: A_{single} is undifferentiated and contains the SSCs that can divide continuously to become A_{pair} and A_{align}, where A_{align} can be syncytia composed of 4, 8, 16, or even 32 cells [20]. Whether hSSCs form syncytia has not been reported and thus remains unknown. As the clonal size increases, these cells have a decline in their regenerative ability [21]. While they are all undifferentiated spermatogonia that can randomly revert back to A_{single}, they also have the ability to become differentiating spermatogonia A1 [20], which then undergo mitosis to become A2, A3, A4, B spermatogonia, and then spermatocytes. However, in the human A_{dark}/A_{pale} model, the dynamic changes and development of hSSCs are largely unknown and should be further explored.

31.3 Approaches to Culture hSSCs: Different Approaches Available and Their Strengths/Limitations

It has been of interest for generations of researchers to establish robust and reliable culture conditions that enable us to monitor details of testis physiology and male germ cell maintenance or differentiation *ex vivo*. Although successful conditions have been reported for several animal models, the development of a robust condition elucidating the details of the multifaceted process of spermatogenesis in humans is still missing. Different *ex vivo* strategies employing various types of cells have been investigated so far; however, due to the challenges in accessibility to healthy and normal testicular tissues at different developmental stages, it still remains unknown how to design a functional system. Current experimental attempts are based on three approaches: SSC propagation combined with auto-transplantation, testicular tissue autografting, and in vitro spermatogenesis. The following chapter will discuss the latest progress for all three strategies in a short summary.

31.3.1 Testicular Tissue Grafting: SSCs Transplanted within Their Natural Niche

Successful transplantation of testicular tissue fragments was first reported in 2002 in mice [22] and since then has been applied as xeno- or autologous tissue transplantation to different animal models including nonhuman primates [23]. The transplantation of an intact tissue piece allows the maintenance of the SSCs within their natural stem cell niche. Thereby this method supports paracrine interaction between germ cells and somatic cells, once the tissue has been transplanted and has been vascularized after transplantation in the host. Although attempts to generate sperm in xenografts from marmoset [24] or human [25] failed, the recent success of autologous transplantation ectopically or into the scrotum in nonhuman primates resulted in the live birth of healthy macaques [26], highlighting the potential of testicular tissue transplantation as a realistic option for clinical fertility preservation techniques in boys at the risk of infertility caused by their cancer treatment or as an effect of certain diseases, if no malignant cells are present in the transplanted tissues.

31.3.2 SSC In Vitro Expansion and Transplantation Back into Their Natural Niche

Transplantation of isolated in vitro propagated SSCs back into the seminiferous tubules can be considered as another strategy, which has a potential to help restore fertility in infertile men. The advantage of this methodology, which has been used as a gold standard to define functionality of SSC populations since its first report in 1994 by Brinster and Zimmermann [16], is the reestablishment of the spermatogenic process in the testis of the host. This method enables natural fertilization without the use of assisted reproductive techniques (e.g., intracytoplasmic sperm injection). However, this method cannot be used for fertility preservation treatments in patients with a malignant disease. Although first reports have described strategies to eliminate malignant cells (e.g., leukemic cells) from SSCs [27], other studies reported the risk of cancer cell contamination in testicular cell suspensions, and even very few malignant cells reintroducing cancer in the host [28]. Until the establishment of a robust protocol to eliminate all malignant cells from SSC suspensions, SSC transplant can be only considered for patients with nonmalignant diseases.

Another crucial step needed to be established before applying germ cell transplantation as a potential clinical option, is to optimize SSC propagation in vitro, in order to obtain sufficient cell number required for successful reestablishment of the spermatogenic process in the host. Long-term propagation of SSCs was established for the first time in 2003 in a mouse model [29] and first studies using SSCs from adult or prepubertal human testes were reported in 2009 [30] and 2011 [31]. Since then additional culture conditions for human SSC propagation have been reported [32]. However, additional studies are needed to evaluate the efficiency of those studies before applying this technique for clinical use.

31.3.3 In Vitro Spermatogenesis: Generating a Functional Niche to Support SSC Maturation

The generation of reliable in vitro conditions to study human male germ cell differentiation is important for the fertility preservation tools previously mentioned. In addition to serving as fertility preservation techniques, in vitro conditions can be used for other important aspects of reproductive sciences, for example toxicology testing for new drugs or testing effects of environmental pollutions on reproductive functions.

The first in vitro studies can date back to the early 1910s (for review see [29]); however the first successful approach to differentiate SSCs into sperm resulting in healthy offspring was reported in mice in 2011 by Sato and colleagues [33]. Since then several groups have used the explant tissue culture to study male germ cell differentiation in different animal models [34]. Although studies to obtain meiotic and postmeiotic cells from human tissue samples have been reported, further studies are needed to prove functionality of those in vitro generated haploid cells [35].

Germ cell differentiation relies on functional paracrine interactions between testicular somatic and germ cells. One crucial aspect to achieve in vitro spermatogenesis is to reconstruct a functional testicular niche. Several studies highlighted the supportive role of 3D culture conditions that create suitable microenvironment for different cell types and organs. Examples of 3D systems include the use of extracellular matrices (e.g., collagen gels or Matrigel), agarose, alginate, or matrices obtained from testicular tissue fragments [36]. Today 3D conditions such as organoids have become promising strategies for establishing a robust model to study male germ cell differentiation. Those organoids are generated from dissociated cell suspensions and, therefore, have a unique potential to study specific paracrine and endocrine pathways. However, despite the tremendous amount of new information obtained over past years, the remaining lack of reliable functional approaches and experimental conditions that mimic the native testicular niche highlights the need for more research to establish robust in vitro conditions for studying male germ cell differentiation.

31.4 Future Perspectives and Conclusion
31.4.1 hSSC Gene Editing

The potential of gene editing by molecular techniques, such as, for example, the clustered regulatory interspaced short palindromic repeats – associated protein 9 (CRISPR-Cas9) system or transcription activator-like effector nucleases (TALENs), has been extensively explored over the past years and has been suggested to be a useful tool to correct genetic mutations in animals and humans. By taking advantage of those techniques, transplantation of genetic-modified SSCs was studied recently (for review see [37]). Studies have shown the potential of using CRISPR-Cas9 to correct mutations in mouse SSCs or using TALENs to correct point mutations of spermatogenic important genes in PGCs, which restored fertility and resulted in fertile offspring. Evaluation of potential epigenetic or off-target genetic changes, with genome-wide screens, showed no obvious influence in mice after transplantation of modified SSCs. Although gene editing techniques have been applied to different human cell types, applying the techniques to human germ cells is limited and ethical issues have been raised constantly.

31.4.2 Transformation of hPSCs into SSCs

Approaches based on human pluripotent stem cells (hPSCs), such as human embryonic stem cells (hESCs) or human-induced pluripotent stem cells (hiPSCs), provide excellent conditions to model in vivo developmental processes, as they can be differentiated into various cell types. Furthermore, the possibility to derive patient-specific cell lines by reprogramming the patient's own somatic cells into hiPSCs highlights the potential use in regenerative medicine. Regarding male fertility, the generation of disease-specific hiPSCs, for example Klinefelter syndrome [38], or NOA [39], may help understand the fundamental aspects of these diseases and offer new treatment strategies.

As concluded from animal studies, specification of PGCs from the epiblast induced by bone morphogenetic protein (BMP) signaling is the first step in germ cell development [40]. Although progress has been made during the past years, the exact mechanism of PGC proliferation in humans is not yet known. Yet, extrapolation from the results of in vivo mouse studies and in vitro differentiation studies has shown that factors, such as BMP4, leukemia inhibitory factor, basic fibroblast growth factor, epidermal growth factor, and platelet derived growth factor play major roles and can support or inhibit in a species-specific manner important pathways [41,42]. Knowledge explaining human in vivo PGC specification and differentiation is mostly extrapolated from animal studies. Since the first report of in vitro germ cell differentiation from hESCs [43], follow-up studies have provided us more insights into human germ cell development [44–46]. Nevertheless, in vitro differentiation approaches are highly variable [47], which can cause reduced reproducibility of described findings. Therefore standardized protocols are needed. The lack of treatment options for men suffering germ cell loss–caused infertility increases the interest in in vitro derivation of germ cells from hPSCs.

31.5 Conclusion

The past decade has witnessed the emergence and wide spread of new technology, such as single-cell genomics profiling techniques and new gene editing tools, which can revolutionize the way to study and manipulate the human germline. By taking advantage of these new techniques, researchers are able to make discoveries in the human germline biology in an unprecedented manner, which can be applied to guide the establishment of a robust in vitro culture system for human SSCs. The application of new gene editing tools offer the possibility to effectively correct deleterious mutations in the human germline, which may help restore fertility for infertile patients, or save the offspring from inheriting genetic disorders. However, we should also be aware of the potential technical limitations and ethical issues, and regulation policy is needed to ensure strict oversight. Ultimately, with the help of scientific and technological development, researchers and clinicians are on the way toward making real advances in reproductive medicine.

References

1. Agarwal A, Mulgund A, Hamada A, Chyatte MR. A unique view on male infertility around the globe. *Reprod Biol Endocrinol*. 2015;13:37.
2. Esteves SC. Clinical management of infertile men with nonobstructive azoospermia. *Asian J Androl*. 2015;17(3):459–470.
3. Foresta C, Garolla A, Bartoloni L, Bettella A, Ferlin A. Genetic abnormalities among severely oligospermic men who are candidates for intracytoplasmic sperm injection. *J Clin Endocrinol Metab*. 2005;90(1):152–156.
4. Georgiou I, Syrrou M, Pardalidis N, et al. Genetic and epigenetic risks of intracytoplasmic sperm injection method. *Asian J Androl*. 2006;8(6):643–673.
5. O'Flynn O'Brien KL, Varghese AC, Agarwal A. The genetic causes of male factor infertility: a review. *Fertil Steril*. 2010;93(1):1–12.
6. Gassei K, Orwig KE. Experimental methods to preserve male fertility and treat male infertility. *Fertil Steril*. 2016;105(2):256–266.
7. Lim J, Goriely A, Turner GD, et al. OCT2, SSX and SAGE1 reveal the phenotypic heterogeneity of spermatocytic seminoma reflecting distinct subpopulations of spermatogonia. *J Pathol*. 2011;224(4):473–483.
8. Looijenga LHJ, Hersmus R, Gillis AJM, et al. Genomic and expression profiling of human spermatocytic seminomas: primary spermatocyte as tumorigenic precursor and DMRT1 as candidate chromosome 9 gene. *Cancer Res*. 2006;66(1):290–302.
9. Clermont Y. Renewal of spermatogonia in man. *Am J Anat*. 1966;118(2):509–524.
10. Clermont Y. Spermatogenesis in man: a study of the spermatogonial population. *Fertil Steril*. 1966;17(6):705–721.
11. Clermont Y. Two classes of spermatogonial stem cells in the monkey (*Cercopithecus aethiops*). *Am J Anat*. 1969;126(1):57–71.
12. Grisanti L, Falciatori I, Grasso M, et al. Identification of spermatogonial stem cell subsets by morphological analysis and prospective isolation. *Stem Cells*. 2009;27(12):3043–3052.
13. Altman E, Yango P, Moustafa R, Smith JF, Klatsky PC, Tran ND. Characterization of human spermatogonial stem cell markers in fetal, pediatric, and adult testicular tissues. *Reproduction*. 2014;148(4):417–427.
14. Kubota H, Avarbock MR, Brinster RL. Growth factors essential for self-renewal and expansion of mouse spermatogonial stem cells. *Proc Natl Acad Sci U S A*. 2004;101(47):16489–16494.
15. Brinster RL, Avarbock MR. Germline transmission of donor haplotype following spermatogonial transplantation. *Proc Natl Acad Sci U S A*. 1994;91(24):11303–11307.
16. Brinster RL, Zimmermann JW. Spermatogenesis following male germ-cell transplantation. *Proc Natl Acad Sci U S A*. 1994;91(24):11298–11302.
17. Guo J, Grow EJ, Mlcochova H, et al. The adult human testis transcriptional cell atlas. *Cell Res*. 2018;28(12):1141.
18. Yoshida S, Sukeno M, Nakagawa T, et al. The first round of mouse spermatogenesis is a distinctive program that lacks the self-renewing spermatogonia stage. *Development*. 2006;133(8):1495–1505.
19. Tegelenbosch RA, de Rooij DG. A quantitative study of spermatogonial multiplication and stem cell renewal in the C3H/101 F1 hybrid mouse. *Mutat Res*. 1993;290(2):193–200.
20. Hara K, Nakagawa T, Enomoto H, et al. Mouse spermatogenic stem cells continually interconvert between equipotent singly isolated and syncytial states. *Cell Stem Cell*. 2014;14(5):658–672.
21. Helsel AR, Yang Q-E, Oatley MJ, Lord T, Sablitzky F, Oatley JM. ID4 levels dictate the stem cell state in mouse spermatogonia. *Dev Camb Engl*. 2017;144(4):624–634.
22. Honaramooz A, Snedaker A, Boiani M, Schöler H, Dobrinski I, Schlatt S. Sperm from neonatal mammalian testes grafted in mice. *Nature*. 2002;418(6899):778–781.
23. Liu Z, Nie Y-H, Zhang C-C, et al. Generation of macaques with sperm derived from juvenile monkey testicular xenografts. *Cell Res*. 2016;26(1):139–142.
24. Wistuba J, Mundry M, Luetjens CM, Schlatt S. Cografting of hamster (Phodopus sungorus) and marmoset (Callithrix jacchus) testicular tissues into nude mice does not overcome blockade of early spermatogenic differentiation in primate grafts. *Biol Reprod*. 2004;71(6):2087–2091.
25. Goossens E, Geens M, De Block G, Tournaye H. Spermatogonial survival in long-term human prepubertal xenografts. *Fertil Steril*. 2008;90(5):2019–2022.

26. Fayomi AP, Peters K, Sukhwani M, et al. Autologous grafting of cryopreserved prepubertal rhesus testis produces sperm and offspring. *Science*. 2019;363(6433):1314–1319.

27. Dovey SL, Valli H, Hermann BP, et al. Eliminating malignant contamination from therapeutic human spermatogonial stem cells. *J Clin Invest*. 2013;123(4):1833–1843.

28. Hou M, Andersson M, Zheng C, Sundblad A, Söder O, Jahnukainen K. Immunomagnetic separation of normal rat testicular cells from Roser's T-cell leukaemia cells is ineffective. *Int J Androl*. 2009;32(1):66–73.

29. Kanatsu-Shinohara M, Ogonuki N, Inoue K, et al. Long-term proliferation in culture and germline transmission of mouse male germline stem cells. *Biol Reprod*. 2003;69(2):612–616.

30. Sadri-Ardekani H, Mizrak SC, van Daalen SKM, et al. Propagation of human spermatogonial stem cells in vitro. *JAMA*. 2009;302(19):2127–2134.

31. Sadri-Ardekani H, Akhondi MA, van der Veen F, Repping S, van Pelt AMM. In vitro propagation of human prepubertal spermatogonial stem cells. *JAMA*. 2011;305(23):2416–2418.

32. Dong L, Kristensen SG, Hildorf S, et al. Propagation of spermatogonial stem cell-like cells from infant boys. *Front Physiol*. 2019;10:1155.

33. Sato T, Katagiri K, Gohbara A, et al. In vitro production of functional sperm in cultured neonatal mouse testes. *Nature*. 2011;471(7339):504–507.

34. Medrano JV, Vilanova-Pérez T, Fornés-Ferrer V, et al. Influence of temperature, serum, and gonadotropin supplementation in short- and long-term organotypic culture of human immature testicular tissue. *Fertil Steril*. 2018;110(6):1045–1057.e3.

35. de Michele F, Poels J, Vermeulen M, et al. Haploid germ cells generated in organotypic culture of testicular tissue from prepubertal boys. *Front Physiol*. 2018;9:1413.

36. Alves-Lopes JP, Söder O, Stukenborg J-B. Testicular organoid generation by a novel in vitro three-layer gradient system. *Biomaterials*. 2017;130:76–89.

37. Mulder CL, Zheng Y, Jan SZ, et al. Spermatogonial stem cell autotransplantation and germline genomic editing: a future cure for spermatogenic failure and prevention of transmission of genomic diseases. *Hum Reprod Update*. 2016;22(5):561–573.

38. Shimizu T, Shiohara M, Tai T, Nagao K, Nakajima K, Kobayashi H. Derivation of integration-free iPSCs from a Klinefelter syndrome patient. *Reprod Med Biol*. 2015;15(1):35–43.

39. Zhao Y, Ye S, Liang D, et al. In vitro modeling of human germ cell development using pluripotent stem cells. *Stem Cell Rep*. 2018;10(2):509–523.

40. Fujimoto T, Miyayama Y, Fuyuta M. The origin, migration and fine morphology of human primordial germ cells. *Anat Rec*. 1977;188(3):315–330.

41. Hiller M, Liu C, Blumenthal PD, Gearhart JD, Kerr CL. Bone morphogenetic protein 4 mediates human embryonic germ cell derivation. *Stem Cells Dev*. 2011;20(2):351–361.

42. Sasaki K, Yokobayashi S, Nakamura T, et al. Robust in vitro induction of human germ cell fate from pluripotent stem cells. *Cell Stem Cell*. 2015;17(2):178–194.

43. Clark AT, Bodnar MS, Fox M, et al. Spontaneous differentiation of germ cells from human embryonic stem cells in vitro. *Hum Mol Genet*. 2004;13(7):727–739.

44. Fox N, Damjanov I, Martinez-Hernandez A, Knowles BB, Solter D. Immunohistochemical localization of the early embryonic antigen (SSEA-1) in postimplantation mouse embryos and fetal and adult tissues. *Dev Biol*. 1981;83(2):391–398.

45. Mouka A, Tachdjian G, Dupont J, Drévillon L, Tosca L. In vitro gamete differentiation from pluripotent stem cells as a promising therapy for infertility. *Stem Cells Dev*. 2016;25(7):509–521.

46. Koopman P, Münsterberg A, Capel B, Vivian N, Lovell-Badge R. Expression of a candidate sex-determining gene during mouse testis differentiation. *Nature*. 1990;348(6300):450–452.

47. Geens M, Sermon KD, Van de Velde H, Tournaye H. Sertoli cell-conditioned medium induces germ cell differentiation in human embryonic stem cells. *J Assist Reprod Genet*. 2011;28(5):471–480.

Section 5 **Medical and Surgical Management of Issues of Male Health**

Chapter 32

Hypogonadism in the Male
Evaluation and Treatment

Parviz K. Kavoussi and G. Luke Machen

32.1 Introduction

In 1889, neurologist and physiologist Charles-Edouard Brown-Sequard first reported improvements in his physical strength and intellectual capacity by self-injecting "liquid testiculaire," a formulation of guinea pig and canine testicles. Treatments have been refined since then; however, there are still gaps in knowledge. Isolation of testosterone by Drs. Butenandt and Ruzicka in 1939 won them the Nobel Prize. Since its discovery, there has been a lack of consensus on the definition of low testosterone, the diagnostic criteria, the appropriate treatment population, and the target treatment serum testosterone levels. The generalized, vague symptomatology of hypogonadism is an additional obstacle in diagnosis and treatment, as are its abuse potential and controversy in risks of treatment. This chapter discusses the anatomy, physiology, diagnostic categories, and treatment options of hypogonadism with associated benefits and risks.

32.2 Anatomy and Physiology of the Hypothalamic-Pituitary-Gonadal axis

The cornerstone of androgen regulation in men is the hypothalamic-pituitary-gonadal (HPG) axis. Pulsatile gonadotropin releasing hormone (GnRH) releases at approximately one pulse per hour from the arcuate nucleus of the hypothalamus to signal the anterior pituitary gland to secrete follicle stimulating hormone (FSH) and luteinizing hormone (LH) [1]. FSH and LH reach the testicles through the blood to stimulate Sertoli cells to facilitate the maturation of sperm and Leydig cells to produce testosterone, respectively [2,3]. A negative feedback loop from gonadal steroids regulates LH secretion at the level of the hypothalamus and the pituitary. Some testosterone is converted peripherally to estradiol by aromatase in adipocytes, the brain, the testes, the liver, skin, and the pituitary gland. Testosterone and estradiol regulate LH secretion by this negative feedback loop [4,5]. When testosterone reaches physiologic levels, the hypothalamus is signaled to decrease secretion of GnRH in turn decreasing gonadotropin secretion [6]. Testosterone has a direct negative feedback on the pituitary decreasing LH secretion [7]. Estradiol can slow GnRH pulses by direct effect on the hypothalamus thereby decreasing the amplitude of LH pulses from the pituitary [4]. Inhibin and steroid hormones regulate FSH secretion from the pituitary. Inhibin is produced by the Sertoli cells and inhibits FSH secretion [8,9] (Figure 32.1).

Cholesterol is the steroid precursor and is derived from serum low-density lipoproteins as well as being synthesized by Leydig cells. Cholesterol is converted to testosterone through a five-step steroidogenesis pathway by the following enzymatic steps: cholesterol side chain cleavage (CYP11A1); 3-beta-hydroxysteroid dehydrogenase (3-B-HSD); 17-alpha hydroxylase (CYP17); 17,20 lyase (CYP17); and 17-beta-hydroxysteroid dehydrogenase 3 (17-beta-HSD3). While conversion of cholesterol to pregnenolone is the first and first rate-limiting step in steroidogenesis, the rate is commonly determined by delivery of cholesterol to cholesterol side-chain cleavage enzyme in the inner mitochondrial membrane steroidogenic acute regulatory protein controlled by LH [10]. Following the initial enzymatic steps in the mitochondria, the remaining steps occur in the endoplasmic reticulum.

With stimulation of Leydig cells by LH, 5–10 mg of testosterone are secreted daily in a pulsatile fashion.[11] Ninety-five per cent of serum testosterone is secreted by the testicles and 5% by the adrenal glands. Serum testosterone levels peak in the mornings in men in the third and fourth decades and the diurnal variation decreases in the fifth decade and shows the least variability by the eighth decade. As peak levels tend to be the most reproducible clinically and least variable from day to day, the recommendation for diagnosing hypogonadism is to obtain serum testosterone levels between 7 and 10 in the morning [11–13]. Intratesticular testosterone concentration is approximately 100 times greater than circulating testosterone in the serum [14]. Peripherally, testosterone can be converted to 5-alpha dihydrotestosterone (5-alpha DHT) by 5-alpha reductase, which mediates differentiation, growth promotion, and functional aspects of androgens in men. Testosterone can be converted peripherally to estradiol and have effects independent of, opposite to, or synergistic to androgens [15]. The typical ratio of testosterone to 5-alpha DHT is 10–15:1, with 5-alpha DHT accounting for 6–8% of testosterone metabolism [16]. Estrogen synergistically inhibits gonadotropins with androgens, and is important for bone density [5]. Men produce approximately 50 mcg of estradiol daily, 85% of which is

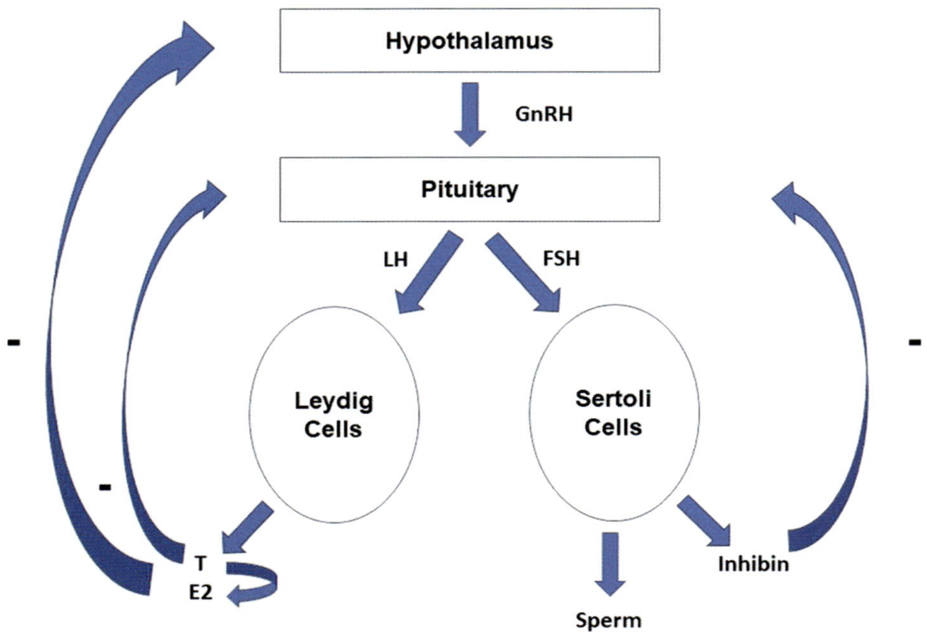

Figure 32.1 Physiology of the hypothalamic-pituitary-gonadal axis

synthesized by adipocytes. Androgens are converted into estrogens by aromatase [17]. Gonadal steroids in the serum are mainly bound to sex hormone-binding globulin (SHBG) and albumin. Two percent of testosterone in the serum is free, 44% is bound to SHBG that has a high affinity for testosterone and does not release it, and 54% is bound to albumin that is releasable for tissue uptake [18]. The sum of free and albumin bound testosterone is considered the bioavailable testosterone.

Androgens in men are important for regulation of gonadotropin release by the HPG axis as described, initiation and maintenance of spermatogenesis, embryologic development of the male phenotype, sexual maturation during puberty, and maintenance of bone mineral density and muscle mass in adults.

32.3 Definition and Diagnosis of Hypogonadism

The diagnosis of hypogonadism relies on patient history, physical examination, and laboratory values. The 2018 American Urological Association (AUA) guidelines on evaluation and management of testosterone deficiency recommend using a cutoff serum testosterone level of 300 ng/dL or less obtained twice in the morning, combined with signs and symptoms, to support the diagnosis. A validated questionnaire is not recommended to support the diagnosis [10]. Hypogonadal symptoms are nonspecific, but the most common symptom is low libido, which is commonly associated with diminished erectile function [20]. Other nonspecific symptoms that should raise suspicion for the diagnosis include hot flashes, reduced energy levels and vitality, decreased muscle mass and strength, depressed mood, infertility, and possibly impaired cognition [21]. The history should include information about current and previous systemic illnesses, and recreational and prescription drug use, especially opioids, testosterone, and anabolic steroids [20].

The physical exam during the hypogonadal evaluation should focus on BMI and abdominal obesity, distribution of body hair, testicular volumes, presence of a varicocele, secondary sexual characteristics, facial and genital hair, pitch of the voice, decreased muscle mass, digital rectal examination, and for the presence of gynecomastia [20].

AUA guidelines recommend obtaining a testosterone level on men with unexplained anemia, bone density loss, diabetes, history of chemotherapy, history of testicular radiation therapy, HIV/AIDS, chronic opioid use, male infertility, pituitary dysfunction, and chronic corticosteroid use. This is recommended even in men without signs or symptoms of low testosterone. When men are found to have a low testosterone level, it is recommended to obtain an LH level, which should prompt obtaining a prolactin level if the LH is low or borderline low. Elevated prolactin levels should prompt further endocrine evaluation such as a pituitary MRI. In hypogonadal men with gynecomastia or breast symptoms, estradiol levels should be obtained. Men considering treatment for hypogonadism should have hemoglobin and hematocrit checked prior to initiating treatment, and in men over the age of 40, prostate-specific antigen (PSA) levels should be obtained [19].

There is controversy regarding what testosterone levels are considered low, and there is evidence suggesting that the same testosterone levels may result in different effects in different individuals [22]. Endocrine Society Guidelines rely on total testosterone primarily and utilize free testosterone when there is diagnostic uncertainty [23]. Two morning testosterone levels are recommended [24]. There is no testosterone level that is universally considered the cut-off for normal; however, a level above 350 ng/dL is typically considered normal and levels below 230 ng/dL are considered hypogonadal. Levels between these values require clinical judgment [25–27]. It is common to offer men in this borderline range a trial of therapy for several months to assess their response to decide to continue or discontinue treatment [20]. No study has defined a testosterone level that consistently separates men who will respond to treatment from those who will not. Any hypogonadal symptom may be caused by other factors. The testosterone level at which symptoms develop may vary by symptom and individual. Clinical judgment is needed for the diagnosis of hypogonadism considering laboratory results along with clinical manifestations including decreased bone mineral density, decreased muscle mass and strength, gynecomastia, anemia, frailty, increased body fat, fatigue, depressed mood, diminished energy and vitality, impaired cognition and memory, diminished libido, erectile dysfunction, and difficulty achieving orgasm [28, 29].

32.4 Testosterone and Sexual Function

Sexual dysfunction is a common complaint of hypogonadal men. There is a well-delineated association between low testosterone and impaired sexual function. The exact effect of low endogenous testosterone and response to treatments of erectile function, libido, and ejaculatory function, is variable and poorly understood.

Anatomic studies have established the presence of androgen receptors in the male reproductive tract and central nervous system [30]. Animal models identified a role for testosterone in achieving and maintaining erections via regulation of the nitric oxide pathway and phosphodiesterase type 5 (PDE5) [31]. Testosterone contributes to prolonged corpus cavernosal smooth muscle relaxation through downregulation of RhoA-ROCK and by decreasing responsiveness to alpha adrenergic agonists [32]. Androgens likely play a role in maintenance of corporal integrity via these same mechanisms, as castrated rats demonstrated decreased corporal smooth muscle and increased venous leak [33,34].

Androgen receptors have been identified in areas of the brain associated with release of stimulatory neurotransmitters playing a role in arousal, specifically the medial preoptic area, amygdala, paraventricular nucleus of the hypothalamus, and periaqueductal gray matter [35]. Among men on testosterone replacement therapy (TRT), blood flow increased in their midbrain and superior frontal gyrus [36]. Neurotransmitters including dopamine and nitric oxide play a role in control of sexual development in adolescence, as well as erection and arousal.

Most data describing the location of androgen receptors and pathophysiology of hypogonadism on sexual function is derived from animal studies. While there is a paucity of such data in humans, some characterization may be derived from men undergoing androgen deprivation therapy (ADT) for prostate cancer (PCa). Approximately 80% of men on ADT experienced erectile dysfunction (ED) within one year of initiating treatment, compared to approximately 30% of those on watchful waiting [37,38]. Similarly, ADT appears to negatively affect libido, with one study indicating among sexually active men at baseline that only 20% remained sexually active after nine months of ADT [39].

Numerous studies have examined the effects of TRT on sexual function, including multiple meta-analyses. One analysis in 2014 by Corona et al. including over 1,400 patients described an 18% risk reduction in ED among men treated with TRT, with a more profound effect when analyzing only studies in which the men were hypogonadal [40]. The inverse relationship between baseline testosterone levels and libido was described and was most significant among hypogonadal men. They also examined the effects of combined testosterone and PDE5-inhibitors treatment for ED, and revealed a positive effect although there were significant limitations to the evidence [40]. These results detailing a potential benefit to libido and erectile function, particularly among men with low pretreatment testosterone levels, have been confirmed by other meta-analyses [41,42].

There is a paucity of data specifically examining testosterone and ejaculatory function, but there appears to be an association between TRT and improved orgasmic scores on the IIEF (International Index of Erectile Function) by 1.62 [40]. A randomized controlled trial found that hypogonadal men on transdermal TRT had improved ejaculatory function scores (MSHQ-EjD-SF [Male Sexual Health Questionnaire-Ejaculatory Dysfunction-Short Form]) compared to placebo [43].

32.5 Testosterone Replacement Therapy for the Treatment of Hypogonadism

TRT modalities are individualized for each patient. Each formulation has its own risks and benefits along with its individual pharmacokinetic profile. This discussion will be limited to FDA-approved treatments, which are approved for treatment of primary and secondary hypogonadism.

32.5.1 Oral Testosterone Undecanoate

In the 1970s several formulations of oral methyltestosterone were approved, but fell out of favor due to hepatotoxicity [44]. Currently, a testosterone undecanoate oral formulation (Jatenzo®) is available in a capsule. It is a lipophilic prodrug taken twice daily with food. It is highly lipophilic, and recognized by the small intestine as fat and self-emulsifies to absorb through the gut and into the intestinal lymphatic system, bypassing first-pass hepatic metabolism. Once in systemic circulation, testosterone undecanoate is released from the lipoprotein particle, and endogenous esterases release active testosterone from it. No hepatic toxicity-related events were observed in clinical trials. The inTUne phase 3 clinical trial started men on a dose of 237 mg twice daily and titrated based on responses, reporting that 87.3% of these men reached eugonadal levels with a mean treatment level of 489 ng/dL ± 155 ng/dL [45].

32.5.2 Buccal Testosterone Tablet

First-pass hepatic metabolism of testosterone can also be bypassed with a 30 mg buccal testosterone tablet (Striant®). Testosterone levels peak 30 minutes after administration of the twice-daily tablet [46]. It is directly applied to the gums and must be removed after 12 hours. It softens and molds to the gums and allows for slow release of testosterone. Approximately 10–20% of men who used the buccal tablet reported gum irritation and altered taste [23].

32.5.3 Transdermal Testosterone Patch

Testosterone patches are either applied on the scrotum (Testosderm®) or elsewhere (Androderm®) and have poor compliance rates due to the frequency of skin reactions. Scrotal patches deliver approximately 5 mg of testosterone daily, with a serum testosterone rise at 2–4 hours after application, which quickly declines after patch removal. For patch adherence shaving the scrotum is recommended. Nonscrotal patches can be applied anywhere on the back, abdomen, upper arms, and thighs, and should be replaced every 24 hours. Removal of the patch will result in a rapid decline in testosterone levels.

32.5.4 Transdermal Testosterone Gels

Transdermal gel formulations (Androgel®, Testim®, Axiron®, Fortesta®) are applied directly to the skin daily, and testosterone is absorbed into the stratum corneum, forming a reservoir providing continuous delivery of testosterone into the serum over a 24-hour period [23]. The gel is applied in the morning at the approved site per formulation, such as the shoulders, the axilla, or the thighs; followed by washing hands and covering the application site with clothing when dry, to minimize transference risk to others with skin-to-skin contact. During absorption time for maximum concentration, the man should avoid sweating too much, showering, or swimming to prevent incomplete dose administration. There are a percentage of men that do not absorb the gel adequately to achieve eugonadal levels.

32.5.5 Intranasal Testosterone Gel

The nasal mucosa provides a rich vascular plexus for absorption of an intranasal testosterone 4.5% gel (Natesto®) that crosses the mucous membrane barrier [47]. Each pump contains 5.5 mg of testosterone. The FDA-approved dosing is one pump to each nostril three times daily, a total of 33 mg daily. Many clinicians start patients at twice-daily dosing off-label for a total of 22 mg daily. Seventy-one percent will achieve eugonadal levels on a twice-daily regimen, whereas 90% of men will achieve eugonadal levels on a three-time daily regimen [48]. Estradiol levels and DHT levels remained within the normal ranges on three-time daily dosing, when baseline estradiol and DHT levels were normal [48].

32.5.6 Intramuscular Testosterone Injections

In ascending order of half-lives, the intramuscular injectable testosterone formulations include testosterone propionate, testosterone cypionate, testosterone enanthate, and testosterone undecanoate (Aveed®) [49]. Testosterone cypionate and enanthate are the most commonly prescribed. They have similar half-lives with a recommended starting dose of 200 mg every 14 days. Following injection, testosterone levels typically reach supratherapeutic levels in 24 hours, with a decline over the following two weeks. This results in fluctuating symptomatology along with the fluctuating levels. Lower doses at more frequent intervals can help minimize the peak to trough ratio. Testosterone undecanoate is a long-lasting testosterone ester with a dosing regimen of 750 mg followed by another 750 mg 4 weeks later, followed by 750 mg every 10 weeks thereafter, which is injected deep into the gluteal muscle. Although rare, this formulation is the only FDA-approved TRT modality with the potential side effect of a pulmonary oil microembolism that has been reported to cause cough [50].

32.5.7 Testosterone Enanthate Subcutaneous Autoinjector

The most recent injectable modality for TRT is a testosterone enanthate subcutaneous autoinjector (Xyosted®). The autoinjector administers testosterone through a 27-gauge needle, which takes approximately 10 seconds to deliver a dose weekly. In the phase 3 study, 98.5% of men reached eugonadal levels by week 12 with dose titration. It has a narrow peak to trough ratio of 1.8, resulting in fewer symptomatic fluctuations. The starting dose of 75 mg can be titrated up to 100 mg or down to 50 mg. The mean trough levels prior to the next injection were 435.6 ng/dL. The peak concentration is reached 22.8 hours after injection with a half-life of 15 days, and 99.4% of 1,519 injections were reported to be pain free, with 0.6% reporting a pain level of 1–2 out of 10 [51].

32.5.8 Subcutaneous Testosterone Pellets

The longest-lasting form of TRT is a crystallized subcutaneous pellet (Testopel®). Individual pellets contain 75 mg of testosterone with approved dosing starting at six pellets. Dose uptitration can achieve eugondal levels with durations of three to six months. The most common insertion site is the upper, outer buttock, but other sites include the lower abdominal wall and upper thigh. The pellet insertion is performed in-office under local anesthesia and takes several minutes. After preparing and draping the site in a sterile fashion, the skin is infiltrated with local anesthesia, followed by a 0.5 cm skin incision to accommodate the trocar. The desired number of pellets are loaded into the trocar, the trocar is tunneled subcutaneously along individual tracts, and an obturator pushes the pellets into the subcutaneous space 5–10 cm from the incision to minimize risk of extrusion. After all the pellets have been inserted, the incision is closed with steri-strip dressing. Testosterone absorbs from the pellets via erosion.

32.5.9 Benefits and Risks of TRT

The majority of TRT trials have not been adequately powered to assess potential benefits or risks. Benefits of TRT have been age stratified. In young men, TRT results in improvement in energy, body composition, bone density, hematocrit, libido, and erectile and ejaculatory function [52–56]. TRT in older men results in improvements in bone density, lean body mass, dyslipidemia, sexual function including libido, with heterogeneous effects on muscle strength [54–57]. Men with baseline testosterone levels <300 ng/dL demonstrated more improvement in libido than men with baselines >300 ng/dL [53]. TRT was reported to improve muscle strength, physical function, body composition, and quality of life in frail, elderly men [58,59]. Depression scores improved in men on TRT versus placebo [60]. There is conflict in the literature regarding improvement in cognitive functions, verbal fluency, and memory in elderly men on TRT [61,62]. Although there is some data indicating benefits of TRT in middle-aged or older men, the level of data does not allow for definitive evidence.

Side effects of TRT can include acne, worsening male pattern balding, gynecomastia, and diminishment of spermatogenesis. Discontinuing TRT typically reverses these side effects. More concerning adverse effects include hepatotoxicity, erythrocytosis, worsening obstructive sleep apnea, exacerbation of heart failure, and controversy on dyslipidemia [61]. TRT increases hematocrit in a dose-dependent manner, with older men demonstrating a greater rise in hematocrit than in younger men [63]. Hematocrit >50% is a relative contraindication to TRT and TRT should not be administered to men with hematocrit >54%. TRT is contraindicated in men with obstructive sleep apnea, but a literature review concluded that the association between TRT and obstructive sleep apnea is weak [64]. TRT and cardiovascular risk, benign prostatic hyperplasia (BPH), and PCa will be discussed in separate sections. Healthcare providers should individualize treatment for hypogonadism while risk stratifying men based on individual comorbidities.

32.6 Treatment of Hypogonadism in a Fertility-Preserving Manner

32.6.1 Selective Estrogen Receptor Modulators

Selective estrogen receptor modulators (SERMs) such as clomiphene citrate (CC) and tamoxifen are off-label treatments for male hypogonadism and infertility. They were designed and approved for ovulation induction and treatment of breast cancer in women, respectively. CC is the most commonly used SERM for hypogonadism in the male in a fertility-preserving manner, by competing with estradiol feedback at the pituitary and hypothalamic levels, resulting in increased FSH and LH secretion and downstream steroidogenesis (Figure 32.2). There is a paucity of prospective studies evaluating the use of CC in this setting. The dosing of CC for hypogonadal men varies between 25 mg every other day to 50 mg every day, with titration to eugondal testosterone levels. Guay et al. demonstrated a significant increase in serum testosterone, LH, and FSH after four months of CC, in 17 men with secondary hypogonadism in a double-blind placebo-controlled study [65]. A prospective study by Katz et al. reported significant increases in LH, FSH, estradiol, and testosterone in 86 primary hypogonadal men treated with CC [66]. Krzastek et al. reported long-term safety and efficacy of CC used for hypogonadism with durations up to eight years [67,68]. Tamoxifen is another SERM with a similar mechanism of action to CC.

32.6.2 Human Chorionic Gonadotropin

Subcutaneous injection of human chorionic gonadotropin (hCG) can also be used to stimulate Leydig cell production of testosterone in a fertility-preserving manner. hCG shares the same beta subunit as LH and thereby directly stimulates androgen production from the testes (Figure 32.2). hCG is dosed between 1,500 and 3,000 IU two to three times weekly, with dose titration to eugonadal levels [69].

32.6.3 Pulsatile GnRH

Pulsatile GnRH is administered by a subcutaneous portable pump, connected to butterfly needle in the abdominal wall, which is changed out every 48 hours [49]. Five to 20 µg of GnRH are administered every 90–120 minutes, with treatment durations of four months on average, although durations up to a year have been reported [69,70].

32.6.4 Aromatase Inhibitors

Hypogonadal men who have elevated estradiol levels >50 pg/mL, or a testosterone to estrogen ratio of <10, may benefit from treatment with an aromatase inhibitor (AI). AIs include anastrozole, testolactone, and letrozole. AIs directly inhibit the peripheral conversion of testosterone to estradiol, thereby increasing testosterone levels [71].

32.6.5 Intranasal Testosterone Gel

CC is the most commonly used medication for increasing testosterone levels in a fertility-preserving manner due to its ease of use, cost, and biochemical effectiveness. Patients often report a less robust symptomatic response to CC than TRT, and some reported worsening of libido on CC from baseline [72]. The challenge has been that TRT suppresses the HPG axis

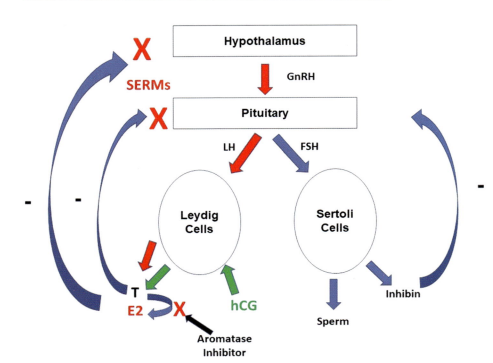

Figure 32.2 The actions of hypothalamic-pituitary-gonadal axis manipulating medications on hormonal function

with an adverse impact on spermatogenesis. The intranasal testosterone gel (Natesto®) appears to be the exception. Ramasamy et al. performed a clinical trial showing that the majority of men maintain gonadotropins and spermatogenesis while being treated for hypogonadism with the intranasal testosterone gel, with a six-month follow up. This is thought to be due to the short-acting nature of this formulation requiring more frequent administration that mimics the circadian and ultradian rhythms of physiologic HPG axis pulsatility [73]. Early data, which needs to be expanded, is showing that although men reach eugonadal levels on both CC and the intranasal gel, CC nearly doubled estradiol levels from baseline, and converting men treated with CC to the intranasal gel returned estradiol levels to baseline, had no detrimental effect on semen parameters, and men subjectively reported improved libido with this medication change [74].

32.7 Varicocele and Hypogonadism

While there is a large body of evidence that varicoceles impact male fertility by impairing sperm production, increasing oxidative stress, and increasing sperm DNA fragmentation, there is evidence indicating that varicoceles may result in global testicular dysfunction, adversely effecting Leydig cells in addition to Sertoli cells. Multiple studies have examined the correlation between varicoceles and Leydig cell dysfunction including one by Tanrikut et al. revealing that men with varicoceles had significantly lower testosterone levels than controls (412.2 ng/dL vs. 462.2 ng/dL) [75].

Numerous studies have demonstrated increases in serum testosterone levels following varicocele repair. A meta-analysis in 2012 assessed 814 men and found a mean improvement in testosterone levels of 97.5 ng/dL following varicocele repair [76]. Another analysis using more stringent inclusion criteria only found improvements in testosterone levels by 34.3 ng/dL (95% CI 22.57–46.04), although larger improvements (123 ng/dL) were identified in men who were hypogonadal preoperatively [77].

A limitation of most existing data is that the studies were performed on men who underwent varicocele repair for infertility and not primarily for hypogonadism. Investigations of varicocele repair purely as a treatment for hypogonadism are limited. Two prospective studies examined hypogonadal men undergoing varicocele repair and found limited testosterone improvements. The baseline testosterone levels were 331 ng/dL and 347 ng/dL, and improved by 26 ng/dL and 45 ng/dL respectively, following varicocele repair (Figure 32.3) [78,79]. Although these studies demonstrate modest testosterone level improvements with varicocele repair, multiple studies have shown improvements in IIEF and MSHQ among hypogonadal men following varicocele repair [80,81].

32.8 Hypogonadism and Prostate Cancer

The hypothesis and dogma that testosterone directly potentiated PCa originated with the discovery of castration resulting in regression of metastatic PCa for some time [82]. This theory was further propagated by a study published in 1981, in which

Hypogonadism in the Male: Evaluation and Treatment

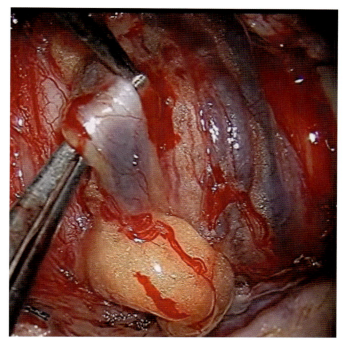

Figure 32.3 Microsurgical view of a varicocele during a subinguinal varicocele repair

testosterone was given to men with advanced PCa, leading to an unfavorable response in close to 90% of their cohort [83].

In the late twentieth and early twenty-first centuries, this paradigm shifted. In 2008, Roddam et al. published prospective data on over 10,000 men, including 3,886 with PCa, and found no increased risk of PCa progression with higher testosterone or DHT levels [84]. It was also discovered that androgen concentrations and histology of prostate tissue were unchanged in patients on TRT despite increases in serum PSA [85]. Khera et al. observed that PSA increased with testosterone levels until a threshold of 231 ng/dL, at which point the PSA level seemed to plateau [86].

These findings led to the saturation model, addressing the paradox of PCa regression with ADT at castrate levels but no progression with TRT. The saturation model proposes that although prostate growth is very sensitive to variations in androgen concentrations at very low concentrations, it is quite insensitive to variations in androgen concentrations at higher androgen concentrations. Maximum androgen receptor binding by androgens is achieved at testosterone levels well below the physiologic range. Changes in testosterone levels below the maximum androgen receptor binding by androgens results in substantial changes in PCa growth, as is the case with castration or when TRT is administered to a previously castrated man. However, once maximum androgen receptor saturation is reached, administering additional androgen results in little further effect [87,88]. While there have been no randomized prospective clinical trials to assess testosterone and PCa risk, the evidence available suggests there is not a significant correlation. Thompson et al. found that hypogonadal men had an increased risk of being diagnosed with PCa diagnosis via biopsy. In a large cohort study, Wallis et al. found that PCa incidence was lower in men receiving TRT (2.8% vs. 3.2%) [89,90]. Other studies describe a correlation between low testosterone and higher grade PCa [90–93].

With the lack of evidence suggesting TRT causes PCa, there was renewed clinical interest in use of TRT among men treated for PCa. In one series, Pastuszak et al. identified a 3.9% biochemical PCa recurrence rate in a cohort of patients on TRT after primary therapy. Ahlering et al. published data finding a lower biochemical recurrence rate in men on TRT after radical prostatectomy (7.2%) when compared to men not on therapy (12.6%) [94]. Results have been comparable when analyzing TRT in other primary treatment modalities, such as radiation therapy [95–98].

The use of TRT on men undergoing active surveillance for PCa has been examined. Multiple studies suggest that PCa progression rates were equivalent or lower among the TRT cohort in comparison to the group in whom hypogonadism was left untreated [98,99]. Limitations to these studies include retrospective designs and relatively small sample sizes, but there is a growing body of evidence that TRT may be safe in this patient population with close monitoring. The AUA guidelines state there is an absence of evidence linking TRT to the development of PCa and, for patients with a history of PCa, there is inadequate evidence to quantify the risk-benefit ratio of TRT [19].

32.9 Hypogonadism and BPH

Dogma similar to that of TRT and PCa exists regarding testosterone and BPH. While testosterone plays a role in both prostate differentiation and proliferation, existing data does not support TRT inducing the development or worsening of BPH and/or lower urinary tract symptoms (LUTS). In contrast, observational data has found that lower testosterone levels may actually be associated with worsened LUTS [100]. A meta-analysis of randomized controlled trials in 2016 by Kohn et al. found TRT was associated with no significant change in LUTS, and a slight improvement in LUTS was even reported when the studies were restricted to injectable testosterone formulations [101].

32.10 Hypogonadism/TRT and Cardiovascular Disease

There is conflicting data regarding TRT and cardiovascular disease. Concern for TRT resulting in adverse effects on cardiovascular health began with the testosterone in older men trial [102], which was discontinued when 23 men in the TRT group versus 5 men in the placebo group experienced cardiovascular-related events. However, this study had a small sample size of an elderly population with a high prevalence of cardiovascular comorbidities and with cardiovascular events having very diverse definitions [103]. Concern grew further in 2013 after a publication by Vigen et al. that retrospectively reviewed records from 8,709 men who underwent coronary angiography and had low testosterone levels, and reported an absolute rate of stroke, myocardial infarction (MI), and death of 25.7% in men who received a testosterone prescription compared with 19.9% in the untreated group within three years after angiography [104]. However, the correct absolute rate of events (number of adverse events divided by the number of individuals) was lower by half in the TRT group compared to the untreated group (10.1% vs. 21.2%) [105]. Following the original publication, *JAMA* published two new versions of the study including corrections of several data errors involving more than 1,000 individuals, and that the all-male study population was comprised of nearly 10% women [106]. Finkle et al. published an analysis of an insurance dataset that reported increased rates of nonfatal MI within a short period after receiving a testosterone prescription compared with the previous 12 months [107]. The methodology of this study has been criticized as well.

A systematic review of the testosterone-related cardiovascular literature revealed four studies showing risk versus dozens showing safety or potentially improvement in cardiovascular risks such as the following: lower testosterone levels associated with increased mortality, atherosclerosis, and coronary artery disease; mortality reduction by one-half in hypogonadal men treated with TRT compared to untreated men; exercise capacity increased with TRT versus placebo in men with known heart disease; and the uniform improvement in cardiovascular risk factors such as fat mass, waist circumference, and insulin resistance with TRT versus placebo [108].

Although no long-term, large controlled studies have definitively determined the cardiovascular risk or safety with TRT, the available evidence tends to favor the cardiovascular benefits of a normal serum testosterone level naturally or with TRT over being hypogonadal. However, studies such as that by Ohlsson et al. found that higher serum testosterone levels were associated with a reduced five-year risk of cardiovascular events in elderly men [109]. A meta-analysis revealed that low testosterone was associated with increased risk of all-cause mortality (11 studies, 35%) and cardiovascular mortality (7 studies, 25%) [110]. However, as the potential association between TRT and cardiovascular risk cannot be definitively denied, it is recommended that TRT not be administered to men with a recent history of acute coronary event, revascularization, or unstable angina.

32.11 Hypogonadism and Specific Etiologies of Endocrinopathy

32.11.1 Primary Hypogonadism

Hypogonadism is categorized as primary and secondary etiologies. Primary hypogonadism stems from testicular failure and may be either acquired or congenital. Among congenital

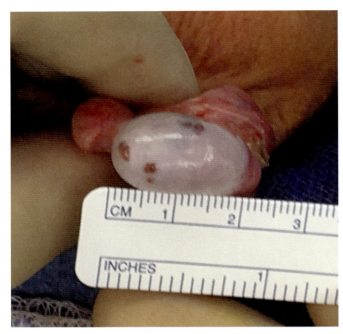

Figure 32.4 Intraoperative demonstration of an atrophic testicle in a man with Klinefelter syndrome undergoing a microdissection testicular sperm extraction

etiologies, the most common chromosomal abnormality resulting in impaired testosterone production is Klinefelter's syndrome (KS). Men with KS have a 47,XXY karyotype due to a meiotic nondisjunction, which is reported in approximately 1/500 males [111]. KS men classically present with atrophic, firm testicles (Figure 32.4), low testosterone levels, elevated gonadotropins, eunuchoid proportions, infertility (typically azoospermic, rarely severely oligospermic), and/or gynecomastia, although in reality there is a diverse phenotypic variability. Approximately 20% of KS men are mosaics with a 46,XY/47,XXY karyotype associated with a milder presentation [112]. Other congenital causes of hypogonadism include 47,XYY and 46,XX males, genetic aneuploidies with prevalence of 1/2000 and 1/10,000–20,000 respectively [113]. Disorders of sexual differentiation, such as Leydig cell hypoplasia, congenital adrenal hyperplasia, adrenal insensitivity syndrome, and/or 5a reductase deficiency may result in lack of virilization and testicular maldevelopment [114]. Another cause of primary hypogonadism is cryptorchidism. Even when corrected with orchiopexies, a history of bilateral cryptorchidism is associated with decreased semen quality indicating persistent testicular dysfunction [115].

Acquired causes of primary hypogonadism include trauma, testicular torsion, genital infections, and systemic diseases. Mumps orchitis after puberty may induce persistent testicular dysfunction. Mumps infections have become less prevalent with the widespread adoption of the vaccine [114]. There is a strong association of chronic, systemic illnesses, such as HIV/AIDS, end stage renal disease, and cirrhosis with primary hypogonadism [116]. Cancer treatments, including chemotherapy (particularly alkylating and platinum agents), radiation therapy, and orchiectomy specifically in the case of testicular cancer may lead to long-term deficiencies of both Sertoli and Leydig cells [117].

32.11.2 Secondary Hypogonadism

Secondary hypogonadism results from inadequate production of gonadotropins resulting in insufficient stimulation of Leydig cells to produce adequate testosterone levels. This may be secondary to insufficient production of GnRH or LH/FSH by the hypothalamus or pituitary gland, respectively. Idiopathic hypogonadotropic hypogonadism (IHH) may be associated with or without anosmia. With anosmia, it is referred to as Kallmann syndrome, which affects between one in 8,000–10,000 males [118,119]. Multiple genetic mutations can lead to IHH and Kallmann syndrome, most commonly manifesting through the mechanism of GnRH-secreting neurons failing to migrate to the hypothalamus [120]. Lack of these neurons in the hypothalamus results in a lack of GnRH secretion, resulting in deficient gonadotropins, and ultimately hypogonadism. The phenotypes of men with IHH are variable, and they may present with absence or delay of puberty or infertility with hypogonadism.

Other rare genetic etiologies include Prader-Willi syndrome, caused by mutations on paternal chromosome 15. Prader-Willi syndrome is associated with varying degrees of mental impairment, hypotonia, and obesity [121]. There are a myriad of other less common genetic mutations that may result in IHH, including alterations in DAX1, leptin, and FGFR1 [114].

Acquired secondary hypogonadism can be caused by processes that result in suppression of GnRH secretion, including illnesses, physiologic stressors, and pharmacologic agents. Chronic opioid use is a common etiology of low testosterone. One meta-analysis reported over 60% of men on chronic opioids were hypogonadal, with larger effects corresponding with higher doses and longer-acting opioids [122]. Prolonged anabolic androgenic steroid (AAS) use is a cause of hypogonadism. It commonly takes an extended period of time for the HPG axis to recover following cessation of AAS. A case-control study found that previous AAS abusers had lower testosterone than controls for 3.7 years following cessation of AAS [123].

Hyperprolactinemia is another etiology of secondary hypogonadism. Symptoms of hypogonadism, especially ED and loss of libido, are the most common presenting symptoms in males with hyperprolactinemia, although galactorrhea and gynecomastia may also be present [124]. Elevated prolactin levels may be secondary to various etiologies, the most common being a prolactinoma. Men with prolactin-producing pituitary adenomas may present with hypogonadal symptoms, as well as peripheral visual disturbances and headaches due to mass effect [125]. Prolactin elevation may be associated with common medical conditions, such as renal failure, hypothyroidism, and cirrhosis. Prolactin levels may also be elevated in certain systemic diseases such as systemic lupus erythematosus, rheumatoid arthritis, celiac disease, and systemic sclerosis. Medications may elevate prolactin levels, especially those that inhibit dopamine, such as some antipsychotics [126].

32.12 Hypogonadism and Comorbidities

Hypogonadism has been associated with components of metabolic syndrome including obesity, dyslipidemia, hypertension, and insulin resistance [29,127]. Among these, data suggests obesity has the closest association to low testosterone levels, perhaps due to increased aromatization of testosterone to estradiol by adipocytes [128]. The HIM (hypogonadism in men) trial reported a prevalence of as high as 50% of hypogonadism in diabetic men [29].

Increased age is associated with decreasing testosterone levels, with some reports indicating testosterone levels may decline by as much as 2.0% per year after age 40 [129]. There is robust data associating hypogonadism with increased incidence of osteoporosis in older men [130]. Despite this, not all men with low testosterone will experience hypogonadal symptoms, which has resulted in controversy regarding the ideal management of men with age-related hypogonadism, and whether elderly men benefit from treatment. The American College of Physicians issued guidelines stating that TRT should only be used to address sexual function complaints in elderly patients, citing inconclusive evidence with regards to improvement of physical function and cognition [131].

References

1. Krsmanovic LZ, Hu L, Leung PK, Feng H, Catt KJ. The hypothalamic GnRH pulse generator: multiple regulatory mechanisms. *Trends Endocrinol Metab.* 2009;20(8):402–408.
2. Dufau ML, Catt KJ. Gonadotropin receptors and regulation of steroidogenesis in the testis and ovary. *Vitam Horm.* 1978;36:461–592.
3. Wahlstrom T, Huhtaniemi I, Hovatta O, Seppala M. Localization of luteinizing hormone, follicle-stimulating hormone, prolactin, and their receptors in human and rat testis using immunohistochemistry and radioreceptor assay. *J Clin Endocrinol Metab.* 1983;57(4):825–830.
4. Hayes FJ, Seminara SB, Decruz S, Boepple PA, Crowley WF, Jr. Aromatase inhibition in the human male reveals a hypothalamic site of estrogen feedback. *J Clin Endocrinol Metab.* 2000;85(9):3027–3035.
5. Morishima A, Grumbach MM, Simpson ER, Fisher C, Qin K. Aromatase deficiency in male and female siblings caused by a novel mutation and the physiological role of estrogens. *J Clin Endocrinol Metab.* 1995;80(12):3689–3698.
6. Matsumoto AM, Bremner WJ. Modulation of pulsatile gonadotropin secretion by testosterone in man. *J Clin Endocrinol Metab.* 1984;58(4):609–614.

7. Sheckter CB, Matsumoto AM, Bremner WJ. Testosterone administration inhibits gonadotropin secretion by an effect directly on the human pituitary. *J Clin Endocrinol Metab.* 1989;68(2):397–401.

8. Anawalt BD, Bebb RA, Matsumoto AM, et al. Serum inhibin B levels reflect Sertoli cell function in normal men and men with testicular dysfunction. *J Clin Endocrinol Metab.* 1996;81(9):3341–3345.

9. O'Connor AE, De Kretser DM. Inhibins in normal male physiology. *Semin Reprod Med.* 2004;22(3):177–185.

10. Stocco DM, Clark BJ. The role of the steroidogenic acute regulatory protein in steroidogenesis. *Steroids.* 1997;62(1):29–36.

11. Winters SJ, Troen P. Testosterone and estradiol are co-secreted episodically by the human testis. *J Clin Invest.* 1986;78(4):870–873.

12. Axelsson J, Ingre M, Akerstedt T, Holmback U. Effects of acutely displaced sleep on testosterone. *J Clin Endocrinol Metab.* 2005;90(8):4530–4535.

13. Saez JM. Leydig cells: endocrine, paracrine, and autocrine regulation. *Endocr Rev.* 1994;15(5):574–626.

14. Jarow JP, Zirkin BR. The androgen microenvironment of the human testis and hormonal control of spermatogenesis. *Ann N Y Acad Sci.* 2005;1061:208–220.

15. Federman DD. The biology of human sex differences. *N Engl J Med.* 2006;354(14):1507–1514.

16. Russell DW, Wilson JD. Steroid 5 alpha-reductase: two genes/two enzymes. *Annu Rev Biochem.* 1994;63:25–61.

17. Mahendroo MS, Mendelson CR, Simpson ER. Tissue-specific and hormonally controlled alternative promoters regulate aromatase cytochrome P450 gene expression in human adipose tissue. *J Biol Chem.* 1993;268(26):19463–19470.

18. Dunn JF, Nisula BC, Rodbard D. Transport of steroid hormones: binding of 21 endogenous steroids to both testosterone-binding globulin and corticosteroid-binding globulin in human plasma. *J Clin Endocrinol Metab.* 1981;53(1):58–68.

19. Mulhall JP TL, Brannigan RE, Kurtz EG, et al. Evaluation and management of testosterone deficiency: AUA guideline. *J Urol.* 2018;200:423–432.

20. Wang C, Nieschlag E, Swerdloff R, et al. Investigation, treatment, and monitoring of late-onset hypogonadism in males: ISA, ISSAM, EAU, EAA, and ASA recommendations. *J Androl.* 2009;30(1):1–9.

21. Emmelot-Vonk MH, Verhaar HJ, Nakhai-Pour HR, Grobbee DE, van der Schouw YT. Low testosterone concentrations and the symptoms of testosterone deficiency according to the Androgen Deficiency in Ageing Males (ADAM) and Ageing Males' Symptoms rating scale (AMS) questionnaires. *Clin Endocrinol (Oxf).* 2011;74(4):488–494.

22. Zitzmann M. Pharmacogenetics of testosterone replacement therapy. *Pharmacogenomics.* 2009;10(8):1341–1349.

23. Corona G, Rastrelli G, Forti G, Maggi M. Update in testosterone therapy for men. *J Sex Med.* 2011;8(3):639–654; quiz 655.

24. Diver MJ, Imtiaz KE, Ahmad AM, Vora JP, Fraser WD. Diurnal rhythms of serum total, free and bioavailable testosterone and of SHBG in middle-aged men compared with those in young men. *Clin Endocrinol (Oxf).* 2003;58(6):710–717.

25. Wu FC, Tajar A, Beynon JM, et al. Identification of late-onset hypogonadism in middle-aged and elderly men. *N Engl J Med.* 2010;363(2):123–135.

26. Bhasin S, Pencina M, Jasuja GK, et al. Reference ranges for testosterone in men generated using liquid chromatography tandem mass spectrometry in a community-based sample of healthy nonobese young men in the Framingham Heart Study and applied to three geographically distinct cohorts. *J Clin Endocrinol Metab.* 2011;96(8):2430–2439.

27. Vesper HW, Bhasin S, Wang C, et al. Interlaboratory comparison study of serum total testosterone [corrected] measurements performed by mass spectrometry methods. *Steroids.* 2009;74(6):498–503.

28. Petak SM, Nankin HR, Spark RF, et al. American Association of Clinical Endocrinologists Medical Guidelines for clinical practice for the evaluation and treatment of hypogonadism in adult male patients – 2002 update. *Endocr Pract.* 2002;8(6):440–456.

29. Mulligan T, Frick MF, Zuraw QC, Stemhagen A, McWhirter C. Prevalence of hypogonadism in males aged at least 45 years: the HIM study. *Int J Clin Pract.* 2006;60(7):762–769.

30. Lewis RW, Mills TM. Effect of androgens on penile tissue. *Endocrine.* 2004;23(2–3):101–105.

31. Morelli A, Filippi S, Mancina R, et al. Androgens regulate phosphodiesterase type 5 expression and functional activity in corpora cavernosa. *Endocrinology.* 2004;145(5):2253–2263.

32. Podlasek CA, Mulhall J, Davies K, et al. Translational perspective on the role of testosterone in sexual function and dysfunction. *J Sex Med.* 2016;13(8):1183–1198.

33. Traish AM, Park K, Dhir V, Kim NN, Moreland RB, Goldstein I. Effects of castration and androgen replacement on erectile function in a rabbit model. *Endocrinology.* 1999;140(4):1861–1868.

34. Davila HH, Rajfer J, Gonzalez-Cadavid NF. Corporal veno-occlusive dysfunction in aging rats: evaluation by cavernosometry and cavernosography. *Urology.* 2004;64(6):1261–1266.

35. Swaab DF. Sexual differentiation of the brain and behavior. *Best Pract Res Clin Endocrinol Metab.* 2007;21(3):431–444.

36. Azad N, Pitale S, Barnes WE, Friedman N. Testosterone treatment enhances regional brain perfusion in hypogonadal men. *J Clin Endocrinol Metab.* 2003;88(7):3064–3068.

37. Hoffman RM, Hunt WC, Gilliland FD, Stephenson RA, Potosky AL. Patient satisfaction with treatment decisions for clinically localized prostate carcinoma: results from the Prostate Cancer Outcomes Study. *Cancer.* 2003;97(7):1653–1662.

38. Potosky AL, Reeve BB, Clegg LX, et al. Quality of life following localized prostate cancer treated initially with androgen deprivation therapy or no therapy. *J Natl Cancer Inst.* 2002;94(6):430–437.

39. Ng E, Woo HH, Turner S, Leong E, Jackson M, Spry N. The influence of testosterone suppression and recovery on sexual function in men with prostate cancer: observations from a prospective study in men undergoing intermittent

androgen suppression. *J Urol.* 2012;187(6):2162–2166.

40. Corona G, Isidori AM, Buvat J, et al. Testosterone supplementation and sexual function: a meta-analysis study. *J Sex Med.* 2014;11(6):1577–1592.

41. Corona G, Rastrelli G, Morgentaler A, Sforza A, Vannucci E, Maggi M. Meta-analysis of results of testosterone therapy on sexual function based on international index of erectile function scores. *Eur Urol.* 2017;72(6):1000–1011.

42. Rastrelli G, Guaraldi F, Reismann Y, et al. Testosterone replacement therapy for sexual symptoms. *Sex Med Rev.* 2019;7(3):464–475.

43. Maggi M, Heiselman D, Knorr J, Iyengar S, Paduch DA, Donatucci CF. Impact of testosterone solution 2% on ejaculatory dysfunction in hypogonadal men. *J Sex Med.* 2016;13(8):1220–1226.

44. Nieschlag E, Nieschlag S. ENDOCRINE HISTORY: The history of discovery, synthesis and development of testosterone for clinical use. *Eur J Endocrinol.* 2019;180(6):R201–R212.

45. Swerdloff RS, Dudley RE. A new oral testosterone undecanoate therapy comes of age for the treatment of hypogonadal men. *Ther Adv Urol.* 2020;12:1756287220937232.

46. Giagulli VA, Triggiani V, Corona G, et al. Evidence-based medicine update on testosterone replacement therapy (TRT) in male hypogonadism: focus on new formulations. *Curr Pharm Des.* 2011;17(15):1500–1511.

47. Banks WA, Morley JE, Niehoff ML, Mattern C. Delivery of testosterone to the brain by intranasal administration: comparison to intravenous testosterone. *J Drug Target.* 2009;17(2):91–97.

48. Rogol AD, Tkachenko N, Badorrek P, Hohlfeld JM, Bryson N. Phase 1 pharmacokinetics and phase 3 efficacy of testosterone nasal gel in subjects with seasonal allergies. *Can Urol Assoc J.* 2018;12(7):E349–E356.

49. Zitzmann M, Nieschlag E. Hormone substitution in male hypogonadism. *Mol Cell Endocrinol.* 2000;161(1–2):73–88.

50. Wang C, Harnett M, Dobs AS, Swerdloff RS. Pharmacokinetics and safety of long-acting testosterone undecanoate injections in hypogonadal men: an 84-week phase III clinical trial. *J Androl.* 2010;31(5):457–465.

51. Kaminetsky JC, McCullough A, Hwang K, Jaffe JS, Wang C, Swerdloff RS. A 52-week study of dose adjusted subcutaneous testosterone enanthate in oil self-administered via disposable auto-injector. *J Urol.* 2019;201(3):587–594.

52. Snyder PJ, Peachey H, Berlin JA, et al. Effects of testosterone replacement in hypogonadal men. *J Clin Endocrinol Metab.* 2000;85(8):2670–2677.

53. Bhasin S, Basaria S. Diagnosis and treatment of hypogonadism in men. *Best Pract Res Clin Endocrinol Metab.* 2011;25(2):251–270.

54. Wang C, Swerdloff RS, Iranmanesh A, et al. Transdermal testosterone gel improves sexual function, mood, muscle strength, and body composition parameters in hypogonadal men. *J Clin Endocrinol Metab.* 2000;85(8):2839–2853.

55. Carani C, Scuteri A, Marrama P, Bancroft J. The effects of testosterone administration and visual erotic stimuli on nocturnal penile tumescence in normal men. *Horm Behav.* 1990;24(3):435–441.

56. Cunningham GR, Hirshkowitz M, Korenman SG, Karacan I. Testosterone replacement therapy and sleep-related erections in hypogonadal men. *J Clin Endocrinol Metab.* 1990;70(3):792–797.

57. Isidori AM, Giannetta E, Greco EA, et al. Effects of testosterone on body composition, bone metabolism and serum lipid profile in middle-aged men: a meta-analysis. *Clin Endocrinol (Oxf).* 2005;63(3):280–293.

58. Srinivas-Shankar U, Roberts SA, Connolly MJ, et al. Effects of testosterone on muscle strength, physical function, body composition, and quality of life in intermediate-frail and frail elderly men: a randomized, double-blind, placebo-controlled study. *J Clin Endocrinol Metab.* 2010;95(2):639–650.

59. Basaria S, Coviello AD, Travison TG, et al. Adverse events associated with testosterone administration. *N Engl J Med.* 2010;363(2):109–122.

60. Zarrouf FA, Artz S, Griffith J, Sirbu C, Kommor M. Testosterone and depression: systematic review and meta-analysis. *J Psychiatr Pract.* 2009;15(4):289–305.

61. Cunningham GR, Toma SM. Clinical review: Why is androgen replacement in males controversial? *J Clin Endocrinol Metab.* 2011;96(1):38–52.

62. Sih R, Morley JE, Kaiser FE, Perry HM, 3rd, Patrick P, Ross C. Testosterone replacement in older hypogonadal men: a 12-month randomized controlled trial. *J Clin Endocrinol Metab.* 1997;82(6):1661–1667.

63. Coviello AD, Kaplan B, Lakshman KM, Chen T, Singh AB, Bhasin S. Effects of graded doses of testosterone on erythropoiesis in healthy young and older men. *J Clin Endocrinol Metab.* 2008;93(3):914–919.

64. Hanafy HM. Testosterone therapy and obstructive sleep apnea: is there a real connection? *J Sex Med.* 2007;4(5):1241–1246.

65. Guay AT, Jacobson J, Perez JB, Hodge MB, Velasquez E. Clomiphene increases free testosterone levels in men with both secondary hypogonadism and erectile dysfunction: who does and does not benefit? *Int J Impot Res.* 2003;15(3):156–165.

66. Katz DJ, Nabulsi O, Tal R, Mulhall JP. Outcomes of clomiphene citrate treatment in young hypogonadal men. *BJU Int.* 2012;110(4):573–578.

67. Krzastek SC, Sharma D, Abdullah N, et al. Long-term safety and efficacy of clomiphene citrate for the treatment of hypogonadism. *J Urol.* 2019;202(5):1029–1035.

68. Wheeler KM, Sharma D, Kavoussi PK, Smith RP, Costabile R. Clomiphene citrate for the treatment of hypogonadism. *Sex Med Rev.* 2019;7(2):272–276.

69. Delemarre EM, Felius B, Delemarre-van de Waal HA. Inducing puberty. *Eur J Endocrinol.* 2008;159(Suppl. 1):S9–S15.

70. Buchter D, Behre HM, Kliesch S, Nieschlag E. Pulsatile GnRH or human chorionic gonadotropin/human menopausal gonadotropin as effective treatment for men with hypogonadotropic hypogonadism: a review of 42 cases. *Eur J Endocrinol.* 1998;139(3):298–303.

71. Raman JD, Schlegel PN. Aromatase inhibitors for male infertility. *J Urol.* 2002;167(2 Pt 1):624–629.

72. Dadhich P, Ramasamy R, Scovell J, Wilken N, Lipshultz L. Testosterone

versus clomiphene citrate in managing symptoms of hypogonadism in men. *Indian J Urol.* 2017;33(3):236–240.

73. Ramasamy R, Masterson TA, Best JC, et al. Effect of Natesto on reproductive hormones, semen parameters and hypogonadal symptoms: a single center, open label, single arm trial. *J Urol.* 2020;204(3):557–563.

74. Kavoussi PK MG, Gilkey M, Hunn C, et al. Converting men from clomiphene citrate to Natesto for hypogonadism improves libido, maintains semen parameters, and reduces estradiol. *Urology.* 2021;148:141–144.

75. Tanrikut C, Goldstein M, Rosoff JS, Lee RK, Nelson CJ, Mulhall JP. Varicocele as a risk factor for androgen deficiency and effect of repair. *BJU Int.* 2011;108 (9):1480–1484.

76. Li F, Yue H, Yamaguchi K, et al. Effect of surgical repair on testosterone production in infertile men with varicocele: a meta-analysis. *Int J Urol.* 2012;19(2):149–154.

77. Chen X, Yang D, Lin G, Bao J, Wang J, Tan W. Efficacy of varicocelectomy in the treatment of hypogonadism in subfertile males with clinical varicocele: a meta-analysis. *Andrologia.* 2017;49(10):e12778. https://doi.org/10.1111/and.12778.

78. Ahmed AF, Abdel-Aziz AS, Maarouf AM, Ali M, Emara AA, Gomaa A. Impact of varicocelectomy on premature ejaculation in varicocele patients. *Andrologia.* 2015;47(3):276–281.

79. Abdel-Meguid TA, Farsi HM, Al-Sayyad A, Tayib A, Mosli HA, Halawani AH. Effects of varicocele on serum testosterone and changes of testosterone after varicocelectomy: a prospective controlled study. *Urology.* 2014;84 (5):1081–1087.

80. Zohdy W, Ghazi S, Arafa M. Impact of varicocelectomy on gonadal and erectile functions in men with hypogonadism and infertility. *J Sex Med.* 2011;8 (3):885–893.

81. Najari BB, Introna L, Paduch DA. Improvements in patient-reported sexual function after microsurgical varicocelectomy. *Urology.* 2017;110:104–109.

82. Huggins C. Effect of orchiectomy and irradiation on cancer of the prostate. *Ann Surg.* 1942;115(6):1192–1200.

83. Morgentaler A, Traish A. The history of testosterone and the evolution of its therapeutic potential. *Sex Med Rev.* 2020;8(2):286–296.

84. Roddam AW, Allen NE, Appleby P, Key TJ. Endogenous sex hormones and prostate cancer: a collaborative analysis of 18 prospective studies. *J Natl Cancer Inst.* 2008;100(3):170–183.

85. Marks LS, Mazer NA, Mostaghel E, et al. Effect of testosterone replacement therapy on prostate tissue in men with late-onset hypogonadism: a randomized controlled trial. *JAMA.* 2006;296 (19):2351–2361.

86. Khera M, Bhattacharya RK, Blick G, Kushner H, Nguyen D, Miner MM. Changes in prostate specific antigen in hypogonadal men after 12 months of testosterone replacement therapy: support for the prostate saturation theory. *J Urol.* 2011;186(3):1005–1011.

87. Davidson E, Morgentaler A. Testosterone therapy and prostate cancer. *Urol Clin North Am.* 2016;43 (2):209–216.

88. Morgentaler A, Traish AM. Shifting the paradigm of testosterone and prostate cancer: the saturation model and the limits of androgen-dependent growth. *Eur Urol.* 2009;55(2):310–320.

89. Wallis CJ, Lo K, Lee Y, et al. Survival and cardiovascular events in men treated with testosterone replacement therapy: an intention-to-treat observational cohort study. *Lancet Diabetes Endocrinol.* 2016;4(6):498–506.

90. Thompson IM, Pauler DK, Goodman PJ, et al. Prevalence of prostate cancer among men with a prostate-specific antigen level < or =4.0 ng per milliliter. *N Engl J Med.* 2004;350(22):2239–2246.

91. Salonia A, Abdollah F, Capitanio U, et al. Serum sex steroids depict a nonlinear u-shaped association with high-risk prostate cancer at radical prostatectomy. *Clin Cancer Res.* 2012;18 (13):3648–3657.

92. San Francisco IF, Rojas PA, DeWolf WC, Morgentaler A. Low free testosterone levels predict disease reclassification in men with prostate cancer undergoing active surveillance. *BJU Int.* 2014;114(2):229–235.

93. Leon P, Seisen T, Cussenot O, et al. Low circulating free and bioavailable testosterone levels as predictors of high-grade tumors in patients undergoing radical prostatectomy for localized prostate cancer. *Urol Oncol.* 2015;33 (9):384.e21–27.

94. Ahlering TE, My Huynh L, Towe M, et al. Testosterone replacement therapy reduces biochemical recurrence after radical prostatectomy. *BJU Int.* 2020;126(1):91–96.

95. Sarosdy MF. Testosterone replacement for hypogonadism after treatment of early prostate cancer with brachytherapy. *Cancer.* 2007;109 (3):536–541.

96. Balbontin FG, Moreno SA, Bley E, Chacon R, Silva A, Morgentaler A. Long-acting testosterone injections for treatment of testosterone deficiency after brachytherapy for prostate cancer. *BJU Int.* 2014;114(1):125–130.

97. Pastuszak AW, Khanna A, Badhiwala N, et al. Testosterone therapy after radiation therapy for low, intermediate and high risk prostate cancer. *J Urol.* 2015;194(5):1271–1276.

98. Kacker R, Hult M, San Francisco IF, et al. Can testosterone therapy be offered to men on active surveillance for prostate cancer? Preliminary results. *Asian J Androl.* 2016;18(1):16–20.

99. Morgentaler A, Lipshultz LI, Bennett R, Sweeney M, Avila D, Jr., Khera M. Testosterone therapy in men with untreated prostate cancer. *J Urol.* 2011;185(4):1256–1260.

100. Debruyne FM, Behre HM, Roehrborn CG, et al. Testosterone treatment is not associated with increased risk of prostate cancer or worsening of lower urinary tract symptoms: prostate health outcomes in the Registry of Hypogonadism in Men. *BJU Int.* 2017;119(2):216–224.

101. Kohn TP, Mata DA, Ramasamy R, Lipshultz LI. Effects of testosterone replacement therapy on lower urinary tract symptoms: a systematic review and meta-analysis. *Eur Urol.* 2016;69 (6):1083–1090.

102. Yabe S, Kato H, Mizukawa S, et al. Predictive factors for outcomes of patients undergoing endoscopic therapy for bile leak after hepatobiliary surgery. *Dig Endosc.* 2017;29 (3):353–361.

103. LeBrasseur NK, Lajevardi N, Miciek R, Mazer N, Storer TW, Bhasin S. Effects of testosterone therapy on muscle performance and physical function in older men with mobility limitations (the TOM trial): design and methods. *Contemp Clin Trials.* 2009;30 (2):133–140.

104. Vigen R, O'Donnell CI, Baron AE, et al. Association of testosterone therapy with mortality, myocardial infarction, and stroke in men with low testosterone levels. *JAMA*. 2013;310(17):1829–1836.
105. Traish AM, Guay AT, Morgentaler A. Death by testosterone? We think not! *J Sex Med*. 2014;11(3):624–629.
106. Ho PM, Baron AE, Wierman ME. Deaths and cardiovascular events in men receiving testosterone: reply. *JAMA*. 2014;311(9):964–965.
107. Finkle WD, Greenland S, Ridgeway GK, et al. Increased risk of non-fatal myocardial infarction following testosterone therapy prescription in men. *PLoS ONE*. 2014;9(1):e85805.
108. Morgentaler A, Miner MM, Caliber M, Guay AT, Khera M, Traish AM. Testosterone therapy and cardiovascular risk: advances and controversies. *Mayo Clin Proc*. 2015;90(2):224–251.
109. Ohlsson C, Barrett-Connor E, Bhasin S, et al. High serum testosterone is associated with reduced risk of cardiovascular events in elderly men. The MrOS (Osteoporotic Fractures in Men) study in Sweden. *J Am Coll Cardiol*. 2011;58(16):1674–1681.
110. Araujo AB, Dixon JM, Suarez EA, Murad MH, Guey LT, Wittert GA. Clinical review: endogenous testosterone and mortality in men: a systematic review and meta-analysis. *J Clin Endocrinol Metab*. 2011;96(10):3007–3019.
111. Bojesen A, Juul S, Gravholt CH. Prenatal and postnatal prevalence of Klinefelter syndrome: a national registry study. *J Clin Endocrinol Metab*. 2003;88(2):622–626.
112. Fruhmesser A, Kotzot D. Chromosomal variants in Klinefelter syndrome. *Sex Dev*. 2011;5(3):109–123.
113. Hotaling JM. Genetics of male infertility. *Urol Clin North Am*. 2014;41(1):1–17.
114. Ross A, Bhasin S. Hypogonadism: its prevalence and diagnosis. *Urol Clin North Am*. 2016;43(2):163–176.
115. Loebenstein M, Thorup J, Cortes D, Clasen-Linde E, Hutson JM, Li R. Cryptorchidism, gonocyte development, and the risks of germ cell malignancy and infertility: a systematic review. *J Pediatr Surg*. 2020;55(7):1201–1210.
116. Rochira V, Diazzi C, Santi D, et al. Low testosterone is associated with poor health status in men with human immunodeficiency virus infection: a retrospective study. *Andrology*. 2015;3(2):298–308.
117. Zaid MIA, Menendez AG, Charif OE, et al. Adverse health outcomes in relationship to hypogonadism (HG) after platinum-based chemotherapy: a multicenter study of North American testicular cancer survivors (TCS). *J Clin Oncol*. 2017;35(18_suppl):LBA10012–LBA10012.
118. Dode C, Hardelin JP. Kallmann syndrome. *Eur J Hum Genet*. 2009;17(2):139–146.
119. Fechner A, Fong S, McGovern P. A review of Kallmann syndrome: genetics, pathophysiology, and clinical management. *Obstet Gynecol Surv*. 2008;63(3):189–194.
120. Hardelin JP, Dode C. The complex genetics of Kallmann syndrome: KAL1, FGFR1, FGF8, PROKR2, PROK2, et al. *Sex Dev*. 2008;2(4–5):181–193.
121. Smeets DF, Hamel BC, Nelen MR, et al. Prader-Willi syndrome and Angelman syndrome in cousins from a family with a translocation between chromosomes 6 and 15. *N Engl J Med*. 1992;326(12):807–811.
122. de Vries F, Bruin M, Lobatto DJ, et al. Opioids and their endocrine effects: a systematic review and meta-analysis. *J Clin Endocrinol Metab*. 2020;105(4):1020–1029.
123. Rasmussen JJ, Selmer C, Ostergren PB, et al. Former abusers of anabolic androgenic steroids exhibit decreased testosterone levels and hypogonadal symptoms years after cessation: a case-control study. *PLoS ONE*. 2016;11(8):e0161208.
124. Buvat J. Hyperprolactinemia and sexual function in men: a short review. *Int J Impot Res*. 2003;15(5):373–377.
125. Carter JN, Tyson JE, Tolis G, Van Vliet S, Faiman C, Friesen HG. Prolactin-screening tumors and hypogonadism in 22 men. *N Engl J Med*. 1978;299(16):847–852.
126. Patel SS, Bamigboye V. Hyperprolactinaemia. *J Obstet Gynaecol*. 2007;27(5):455–459.
127. Corona G, Monami M, Rastrelli G, et al. Testosterone and metabolic syndrome: a meta-analysis study. *J Sex Med*. 2011;8(1):272–283.
128. Wu FC, Tajar A, Pye SR, et al. Hypothalamic-pituitary-testicular axis disruptions in older men are differentially linked to age and modifiable risk factors: the European Male Aging Study. *J Clin Endocrinol Metab*. 2008;93(7):2737–2745.
129. Feldman HA, Longcope C, Derby CA, et al. Age trends in the level of serum testosterone and other hormones in middle-aged men: longitudinal results from the Massachusetts male aging study. *J Clin Endocrinol Metab*. 2002;87(2):589–598.
130. Fink HA, Ewing SK, Ensrud KE, et al. Association of testosterone and estradiol deficiency with osteoporosis and rapid bone loss in older men. *J Clin Endocrinol Metab*. 2006;91(10):3908–3915.
131. Diem SJ, Greer NL, MacDonald R, et al. Efficacy and safety of testosterone treatment in men: an evidence report for a clinical practice guideline by the American College of Physicians. *Ann Intern Med*. 2020;172(2):105–118.

Chapter 33: Selective Androgen Receptor Modulators in the Treatment of Hypogonadism and Men's Health

John T. Sigalos, Dyvon T. Walker, and Larry I. Lipshultz

33.1 Introduction

The androgen receptor (AR) is a member of a superfamily of nuclear receptors, which also includes the mineralocorticoid, glucocorticoid, and progesterone receptors. Once the endogenously produced ligand, for example, testosterone or 5α-dihydrotestosterone (DHT) for the AR, binds to its nuclear receptor, the ligand-receptor complex acts as a transcription factor by directly binding to DNA, which enacts transcriptional regulation of responsive genes. Additionally, this ligand-receptor complex also acts via protein-protein interactions to regulate gene expression [1]. The effects of the AR's transcriptional regulation are complex, and the downstream effects vary based on age, tissue type, gender, and hormonal status. The AR is classically known for its role in male sexual differentiation and preservation of the male phenotype. However, it also has effects on muscle mass and strength, bone density, hematopoiesis, cognition, and metabolism [2]. The AR not only has widespread effects, but it also is activated by diverse ligands, which include natural hormones, growth factors, peptides, or synthetic molecules [3]. This diversity of downstream effects makes the AR a potential target for many pathologies, including osteoporosis, cachexia or muscle wasting conditions, impairments in sexual differentiation, and hormone-responsive cancers.

The AR has become a popular target in the treatment of male hypogonadism. According to the Endocrine Society practice guidelines, hypogonadism is defined as "a clinical syndrome that results from failure of the testis to produce physiological levels of testosterone (T) (androgen deficiency) and a normal number of spermatozoa due to disruption of one or more levels of the hypothalamic-pituitary-testicular axis" [4, p. 2539]. Testosterone replacement therapy (TRT) in various forms, including gels, injections, pellets, intranasal formulations, and pills, is the mainstay of treatment for this condition to exogenously replace the deficiency of endogenously produced testosterone. The chronic use of TRT is known to have potential risks, including erythrocytosis, dyslipidemia, prostatic hypertrophy, hepatotoxicity, impaired fertility, aromatization of testosterone to estrogen, and testicular atrophy [5]. Since March 2015, the FDA has issued a black box warning regarding the potential increase of cardiovascular events with TRT. Of note, the American Urological Association guidelines from 2018 on the treatment of testosterone deficiency state "prior to initiating treatment, clinicians should counsel patients that, at this time, it cannot be stated definitively whether testosterone therapy increases or decreases the risk of cardiovascular events (e.g., myocardial infarction, stroke, cardiovascular-related death, all-cause mortality)" [6, p. 428]. Currently, randomized controlled trials are underway to better elucidate the relationship between TRT and cardiovascular events.

Given the widespread effects of TRT and its limitations, there is a desire for tissue-selective agonists of the AR to preserve the desirable effects such as increases in bone density and muscle mass while reducing effects where AR activation may not be desired such as the prostate, liver, heart, and bone marrow. These agonist molecules are known as selective androgen receptor modulators (SARMs) [3].

33.2 History and Development of SARMs

Hormone signaling is modulated by the expression of various enzymes, coactivators, corepressors, kinases, and growth factors, and leads to a myriad of hormone-specific downstream effects [3]. Estrogens, for example, have advantageous effects in both bone and the brain, while stimulating growth in the uterus and breast [7–9]. While the activation of the estrogen receptor by estradiol may result in the prevention and treatment of osteoporosis, it may also lead to uterine and mammary hyperplasia, thus increasing the risk for oncogenic processes. Therefore, the agonistic activities of estrogens that result in these growth-promoting effects may be considered beneficial or detrimental based on the tissue of action. In the 1990s, intending to bypass the global receptor activation that leads to nonspecific receptor activity, selective estrogen receptor modulators, such as clomiphene, tamoxifen, and raloxifene, became the first selective receptor modulators to be characterized and developed [10]. Decades later, nonsteroidal SARMs were developed to achieve tissue-selective modulation of ARs, thus minimizing adverse effects customarily attributed to steroidal androgens while capitalizing on anabolic effects [11]. This discovery was followed by that of selective glucocorticoid receptor modulators, selective progesterone receptor modulators, and others [12–14].

Tissue-selective activation of the AR was first evidenced in preclinical studies reporting increased muscle weight in the

AR-rich levator ani muscle in castrated rats to the level of sham-operated, eugonadal rats. This model became known as the "Hershberger assay," using the arylpropionamide class of SARMs [15,16]. SARMs have begun to be evaluated as therapy options in preclinical and clinical testing for various conditions, including cancer-related cachexia, benign prostatic hyperplasia (BPH), breast cancer, and hypogonadism [5]. With the addition of further studies over the subsequent few years, enobosarm emerged as the most clinically advanced SARM candidate [12,17]. Enobosarm has since been evaluated in several phase II and phase III clinical trials for multiple indications, and along with other arylpropionamide SARMs, has demonstrated beneficial effects on muscle as well as bone [18–21]. SARMs of various chemotypes, including quinolinone-based, bicyclic hydantoin-derived, aniline-based, and steroidal, have emerged over the decades, but require more data in order to address the regulatory and clinical challenges facing these novel therapeutics [11].

33.3 SARMs and Potential for Use in Hypogonadism

To date, no formal randomized controlled trial has used SARMs to treat hypogonadism specifically. However, there is evidence to suggest that SARMs may be useful in this setting. One of the most prominent symptoms of hypogonadism is loss of libido. SARMs have shown the ability to increase libido in the rat model. In one experiment, female rats who had their ovaries removed without SARM treatment showed no preference for spending time with castrate male rats versus sexually intact male rats, while those oophorectomized female rats with additional SARM treatment preferred spending time with sexually intact male rats [22]. Male rats having undergone orchiectomy when treated with the SARM LGD2226 showed increased desire (measured via number of mounts) and sexual performance (measured via number of intromissions and ejaculations) when compared to orchiectomized male rats without SARM treatment [23]. The third arm of this trial showed that the SARM LGD2226 had similar efficacy in increasing sexual desire and performance in male rats when compared to those treated with the synthetic androgen, fluoxymesterone.

Another common complaint of the hypogonadal male includes decreased muscle mass and strength. Studies in animal models including rats and monkeys have shown increases in muscle mass with SARM treatment [24,25]. In male cynomolgus monkeys treated with vehicle versus daily 10 mg/kg of SARM-2f versus daily 2 mg/kg testosterone enanthate (TE) for 28 days, lean body mass was significantly increased in the SARM-2f and TE groups when compared to the controls. Lean body mass increased by 11.8% from the start of treatment in the SARM-2f group [26]. These results have translated into human trials as well. A phase Ib trial of the investigational SARM, GlaxoSmithKline (GSK) 2881078, in healthy older men and women, showed an increase in mean lean body mass from a baseline of 1.76 kg (SE of 0.767) in males and 3.39 kg (SE of 0.406) in females after eight weeks of treatment. These increases in lean body mass were shown in a dose-responsive manner for both male and female subjects [27].

These findings are congruent with a phase II trial of the SARM GTx-024, also known as enobosarm. In this randomized, double-blind, placebo-controlled, and multicenter study, 115 elderly men and postmenopausal women were evaluated on changes in body composition and performance after 86 days of treatment. GTx-024 treatment led to a dose-dependent increase in total lean body mass. Subjects in the 3 mg dose group gained a statistically significant average of 1.3 kg of lean body mass compared to placebo. A statistically significant decrease in total fat mass was also observed at the 3 mg dose with a 0.6 kg relative fat loss compared to placebo. Additionally, performance was improved in a stair climb test. Stair climb time was reduced with a demonstrated dose-dependent decrease in the time required to climb 12 steps. Glucose levels were significantly decreased in the treatment group [19]. A randomized controlled trial with enobosarm in cancer patients with >2% weight loss in the six months preceding treatment showed increases in lean body mass for up to 113 days of treatment. The mean increase in lean body mass in the treatment group was 1.3–1.5 kg. Stair climb power was again demonstrated to be increased in the SARM-treated group. However, no improvement in grip strength or ECOG (Eastern Cooperative Oncology Group) status was noted [20]. The study drug was well tolerated in both these randomized controlled trials using enobosarm.

Based on the efficacy and results of the previously cited trials, enobosarm was subsequently tested in a phase III trial (POWER trial) to evaluate the effects on lean body mass as a treatment for muscle wasting in nonsmall cell lung cancer patients receiving chemotherapy [18]. The results of this trial have not been published. However, the company that makes enobosarm has publicly stated that the results of this trial failed to meet response criteria for its primary endpoints [28]. While enobosarm has been the most extensively studied SARM, MK-0773, a different SARM, has been evaluated in a phase IIa trial to assess ~170 sarcopenic, frail elderly women with respect to body composition and functional endpoints. The subjects showed a significant increase in lean body mass of 1.23 kg compared to controls over a six-month treatment cycle. This increase in lean body mass did not translate into more functional strength compared to placebo for endpoints such as stair climbing power, gait speed, and leg press capability [29].

The elusive connection between the increases seen in lean body mass and functional muscle outcomes seen in some of the studies involving SARMs is controversial and may limit what the clinician should expect with respect to its potential to treat other conditions such as hypogonadism. It is possible that exercise training may be a necessary component to convert the increase of lean body mass seen with SARMs use into functional improvements in muscle strength [30]. Furthermore, the subjects used in these initial trials contain confounding factors including advanced age, disease stage, baseline-impaired physical function, and chemotherapy that may diminish the response of SARMs as compared to the index hypogonadal patient that presents in middle age and without cancer.

33.4 SARMs and Men's Health

Given the properties of SARMs for selective agonism of the AR in muscle and bone with antagonism at the prostate, there has been growing interest in how SARMs may affect men's health related to prostatic conditions such as BPH. Unlike testosterone, SARMs are not converted to DHT by 5α reductase. In a rat model selected for BPH, this advantage has been used to demonstrate that prostatic weight is reduced in a dose-dependent manner using various SARMs [31,32]. In these experiments, levator ani weight was preserved to a higher degree with SARM use than when less selective global anti-androgens were used [31,32]. In humans, a phase II clinical trial was performed to study the efficacy and safety of the SARM OPK-88004 in men with BPH. Subjects were treated with placebo, 15, or 25 mg of OPK-88004 for 16 weeks duration. Endpoints were set to evaluate drug safety, plasma levels, effect on prostate size, and lower urinary tract symptoms. The trial was terminated without fully published results, which stated that the utilization of transrectal ultrasound for measuring prostate volume proved to be too imprecise to reliably determine the efficacy of the drug [33].

SARMs in the future may also be therapeutic for orally bioavailable male contraception. In male rats treated with the SARM C-6, the authors found significant reduction in the size of the prostate, seminal vesicles, testis, and epididymis to 68%, 83%, 60%, and 64% of control values, respectively. C-6 treated animals also had low testosterone values and sperm counts [34]. In a subsequent study, a different SARM known as S-23 was used in conjunction with estradiol benzoate, which led to four of six mice showing no sperm in the testis and zero pregnancies (zero of six) in mating trials. Infertility was fully reversible, with a 100% pregnancy rate observed after the recovery period [35].

33.5 Safety of SARMs

Although TRT is effective in treating hypogonadal symptoms and remains the "gold standard" of treatment, it is associated with potential adverse effects that require surveillance. These adverse effects include gynecomastia, acne, male pattern baldness, reduced spermatogenesis, and alterations in serum lipids, among others [36]. SARMs, in comparison with steroidal androgens such as testosterone (T), seem to be generally better tolerated with few serious adverse effects. Additionally, as SARMs are administered orally, they have a reduced risk of accidental exposure that may be seen with topical T, while improving ease of administration [5].

Clinical testing on enobosarm and novel SARMs that have undergone randomized controlled trials have shown them to be well tolerated with no increase in adverse events compared to placebo. These studies focused safety analysis on mechanism-related adverse events such as sebum production, female hirsutism, prostate-serum antigen (PSA) levels, serum hormone levels, serum lipid levels, and serum liver function biochemistry. The most consistent biological alterations reported among SARMs are decreases in high-density lipoprotein (HDL) and transient increases in alanine transaminase (ALT) [5]. The increase in ALT, though suggesting hepatocellular injury, requires further examination in relationship with SARM administration to determine whether there is a risk of significant hepatotoxicity [5]. Additionally, though a decrease in HDL is associated with increased risk of cardiovascular disease, studies have shown that the cardioprotective effects of HDL are related to the mechanism of HDL modification rather than changes in HDL levels. Thus, androgen-induced changes may not correspond to low baseline levels of HDL; nevertheless, long-term studies are required to determine the effects of SARMs on cardiovascular risk [37]. Other reported biological alterations associated with SARMs include expected decreases in sex hormone-binding globulin, decreases in total cholesterol and total testosterone in men, and increases in hematocrit [38]. Of note, most studies found no changes or differences from placebo regarding PSA levels, follicle-stimulating hormone and luteinizing hormone levels, or estradiol and dihydrotestosterone levels. Most of the other reported adverse events associated with SARMs were mild and infrequent, and include constipation, dyspepsia, nausea, headache, decreased appetite, dizziness, and upper respiratory infection [39,40]. Additionally, there has been reported infrequent development of moderate to severe adverse events with SARM use, including fatigue, anxiety leading to drug discontinuation, and maculopapular rash secondary to drug reaction [39,40].

Anabolic steroids are the most commonly abused appearance- and performance-enhancing drugs; however, the anabolic effects of SARMs and their lack of androgenic side effects make them appealing to the bodybuilding community and create the potential for abuse among competitive athletes [41,42]. This potential for abuse was acknowledged in 2008 by the World Anti-doping Agency, which banned SARMs in sports [41]. However, many SARMs are available for purchase online, despite the lack of approval by the US FDA. In response to this, Van Wagoner et al. conducted a systematic investigation of 44 products marketed and sold as SARMs online. They reported that only 52% of the products contained one or more SARMs, 39% contained another unapproved drug, and 25% contained substances not listed on the label. Additionally, only 41% of the products contained an amount of active compound matching that listed on the label [43]. These findings highlight the ease with which these unapproved drugs can be acquired as well as the safety uncertainties that accompany them.

33.6 Future Directions

Currently, there is limited randomized controlled data on human subjects on the effects of SARMs. Most work in this area has focused on use in muscle-wasting conditions and proving tolerability and safety of these currently investigational drugs. There are no currently available FDA uses for SARMs. More work will be needed to study these drugs in the hypogonadal male. Specifically, these trials should seek to evaluate improvement of symptoms such as low energy, low libido, erectile dysfunction, poor mood, poor concentration, and subjective well-being as endpoints. Additionally, body composition endpoints such as lean body mass, fat mass, and tests of muscular function will need to be evaluated with and without muscle-strengthening exercise programs compared to placebo treatment with and without these standard exercise regimens. Formal evaluation of parameters of male fertility will also be needed to see how negative feedback from ligand-AR binding affects or does not affect spermatogenesis. Unlike TRT, SARMs will likely not improve hormonal values in men as negative feedback from the downstream effects of AR ligand binding is likely to lead to negative feedback that will lead to paradoxically low values of testosterone. Safety measurements in larger studies with endpoints determining cardiovascular events, lower urinary tract symptoms, and prostate cancer will also be vital in showing benefits over TRT for hypogonadal men given the current controversies that exist in treating men with TRT.

33.7 Conclusions

SARMs offer an intriguing opportunity to target the AR specifically in the tissues where the effects of the AR are desired, such as bone and muscle, while sparing other tissues such as the prostate or bone marrow where these effects can cause potential unwanted side effects. Given the pathophysiology of hypogonadism, this condition is an area where SARMs may one day provide therapeutic benefit. Currently, no randomized controlled trials have used SARMs to treat hypogonadism. The available evidence suggests that SARMs may provide increases in lean body mass and reduce fat mass in humans. Animal models suggest that SARMs may increase libido, all while sparing the prostate from increased DHT levels. More scientific investigation needs to be done to study SARMs in human subjects as some men are already buying these products online, and physicians should be able to counsel these men on the risks and benefits of these compounds. Finally, continued drug development may find that SARMs become more useful as their potency and selectivity in tissues is increased.

References

1. Lu NZ, Wardell SE, Burnstein KL, et al. International Union of Pharmacology. LXV. The pharmacology and classification of the nuclear receptor superfamily: glucocorticoid, mineralocorticoid, progesterone, and androgen receptors. *Pharmacol Rev.* 2006;58(4):782–797.
2. Mooradian AD, Morley JE, Korenman SG. Biological actions of androgens. *Endocr Rev.* 1987;8(1):1–28.
3. Narayanan R, Coss CC, Dalton JT. Development of selective androgen receptor modulators (SARMs). *Mol Cell Endocrinol.* 2018;465:134–142.
4. Bhasin S, Cunningham GR, Hayes FJ, et al. Testosterone therapy in men with androgen deficiency syndromes: an Endocrine Society clinical practice guideline. *J Clin Endocrinol Metab.* 2010;95(6):2536–2559.
5. Solomon ZJ, Mirabal JR, Mazur DJ, et al. Selective androgen receptor modulators: current knowledge and clinical applications. *Sex Med Rev.* 2019;7(1):84–94.
6. Mulhall JP, Trost LW, Brannigan RE, et al. Evaluation and management of testosterone deficiency: AUA guideline. *J Urol.* 2018;200(2):423–432.
7. Burns KA, Korach KS. Estrogen receptors and human disease: an update. *Arch Toxicol.* 2012;86(10):1491–1504.
8. Dhandapani KM, Brann DW. Protective effects of estrogen and selective estrogen receptor modulators in the brain. *Biol Reprod.* 2002;67(5):1379–1385.
9. Rodan GA, Martin TJ. Therapeutic approaches to bone diseases. *Science.* 2000;289(5484):1508–1514.
10. Charles D, Barr W, Bell ET, Brown JB, Fotherby K, Loraine JA. Clomiphene in the treatment of oligomenorrhea and amenorrhea. *Am J Obstet Gynecol.* 1963;86:913–922.
11. Zhang X, Lanter JC Sui Z. Recent advances in the development of selective androgen receptor modulators. *Expert Opin Ther Pat.* 2009;19(9):1239–1258.
12. Dalton JT, Mukherjee A, Zhu Z, Kirkovsky L, Miller DD. Discovery of nonsteroidal androgens. *Biochem Biophys Res Commun.* 1998;244(1):1–4.
13. Link JT, Sorensen B, Patel J, et al. Antidiabetic activity of passive nonsteroidal glucocorticoid receptor modulators. *J Med Chem.* 2005;48(16):5295–5304.
14. Tabata Y, Iizuka Y, Shinei R, et al. CP8668, a novel orally active nonsteroidal progesterone receptor modulator with tetrahydrobenzindolone skeleton. *Eur J Pharmacol.* 2003;461(1):73–78.
15. Gao W, Reiser PJ, Coss CC, et al. Selective androgen receptor modulator treatment improves muscle strength and body composition and prevents bone loss in orchidectomized rats. *Endocrinology.* 2005;146(11):4887–4897.
16. Yin D, He Y, Perera MA, et al. Key structural features of nonsteroidal ligands for binding and activation of the androgen receptor. *Mol Pharmacol.* 2003;63(1):211–223.
17. Srinath R, Dobs A. Enobosarm (GTx-024, S-22): a potential treatment for cachexia. *Future Oncol.* 2014;10(2):187–194.
18. Crawford J, Prado CMM, Johnston MA, et al. Study design and rationale for the phase 3 clinical development program of enobosarm, a selective androgen receptor modulator, for the prevention and treatment of muscle wasting in cancer patients (POWER Trials). *Curr Oncol Rep.* 2016;18(6):37.
19. Dalton JT, Barnette KG, Bohl CE, et al. The selective androgen receptor modulator GTx-024 (enobosarm) improves lean body mass and physical function in healthy elderly men and postmenopausal women: results of a double-blind, placebo-controlled phase II trial. *J Cachexia Sarcopenia Muscle.* 2011;2(3):153–161.
20. Dobs AS, Boccia RV, Croot CC, et al. Effects of enobosarm on muscle wasting and physical function in patients with cancer: a double-blind, randomised

21. Kearbey JD, Gao W, Narayanan R, et al. Selective androgen receptor modulator (SARM) treatment prevents bone loss and reduces body fat in ovariectomized rats. *Pharm Res.* 2007;24(2):328–335.
22. Jones A, Hwang DJ, Duke CD 3rd, et al. Nonsteroidal selective androgen receptor modulators enhance female sexual motivation. *J Pharmacol Exp Ther.* 2010;334(2):439–448.
23. Miner JN, Chang W, Chapman MS, et al. An orally active selective androgen receptor modulator is efficacious on bone, muscle, and sex function with reduced impact on prostate. *Endocrinology.* 2007;148(1):363–373.
24. Chisamore MJ, Gentile MA, Dillon GM, et al. A novel selective androgen receptor modulator (SARM) MK-4541 exerts anti-androgenic activity in the prostate cancer xenograft R-3327G and anabolic activity on skeletal muscle mass & function in castrated mice. *J Steroid Biochem Mol Biol.* 2016;163:88–97.
25. Dubois V, Simitsidellis I, Laurent MR, et al. Enobosarm (GTx-024) modulates adult skeletal muscle mass independently of the androgen receptor in the satellite cell lineage. *Endocrinology.* 2015;156 (12):4522–4533.
26. Morimoto M, Yamaoka M, Hara T. A selective androgen receptor modulator SARM-2f activates androgen receptor, increases lean body mass, and suppresses blood lipid levels in cynomolgus monkeys. *Pharmacol Res Perspect.* 2020;8(1):e00563.
27. Neil D, Clark RV, Magee M, et al. GSK2881078, a SARM, produces dose-dependent increases in lean mass in healthy older men and women. *J Clin Endocrinol Metab.* 2018;103 (9):3215–3224.
28. GTx reports results for enobosarm POWER trials for the prevention and treatment of muscle wasting in patients with non-small cell lung cancer. *Businesswire.* April 16, 2020. Available from: www.businesswire.com/news/home/20130819005378/en/GTx-Reports-Results-Enobosarm-POWER-Trials-Prevention. Accessed November 10, 2022.
29. Papanicolaou DA, Ather SN, Zhu H, et al. A phase IIA randomized, placebo-controlled clinical trial to study the efficacy and safety of the selective androgen receptor modulator (SARM), MK-0773 in female participants with sarcopenia. *J Nutr Health Aging.* 2013;17(6):533–543.
30. Bhasin S. Selective androgen receptor modulators as function promoting therapies. *J Frailty Aging.* 2015;4 (3):121–122.
31. Nejishima H, Yamamoto N, Suzuki M, Furuya K, Nagata N, Yamada S. Anti-androgenic effects of S-40542, a novel non-steroidal selective androgen receptor modulator (SARM) for the treatment of benign prostatic hyperplasia. *Prostate.* 2012;72 (14):1580–1587.
32. Gao W, Kearby JD, Nair VA, et al. Comparison of the pharmacological effects of a novel selective androgen receptor modulator, the 5alpha-reductase inhibitor finasteride, and the antiandrogen hydroxyflutamide in intact rats: new approach for benign prostate hyperplasia. *Endocrinology.* 2004;145(12):5420–5428.
33. OPKO provides update on the development of OPK-88004, a selective androgen receptor modulator. *OPKO.* April 16, 2020. Available from: www.opko.com/news-media/press-releases/detail/351/opko-provides-update-on-the-development-of-opk-88004-a. Accessed November 10, 2022.
34. Chen J, Hwang DJ, Bohl CE, Miller DD, Dalton JT. A selective androgen receptor modulator for hormonal male contraception. *J Pharmacol Exp Ther.* 2005;312(2):546–553.
35. Jones A, Chen J, Hwang DJ, Miller DD, Dalton JT. Preclinical characterization of a (S)-N-(4-cyano-3-trifluoromethyl-phenyl)-3-(3-fluoro, 4-chlorophenoxy)-2-hydroxy-2-methyl-propanamide: a selective androgen receptor modulator for hormonal male contraception. *Endocrinology.* 2009;150(1):385–395.
36. Thirumalai A, Berkseth KE, Amory JK. Treatment of hypogonadism: current and future therapies. *F1000Res.* 2017;6:68.
37. Vignozzi L, Morelli A, Sarchielli E, et al. Testosterone protects from metabolic syndrome-associated prostate inflammation: an experimental study in rabbit. *J Endocrinol.* 2012;212 (1):71–84.
38. Choi SM, Lee BM. Comparative safety evaluation of selective androgen receptor modulators and anabolic androgenic steroids. *Expert Opin Drug Saf.* 2015;14(11):1773–1785.
39. Bhattacharya I, Tarabar S, Liang Y, Pradhan V, Owens J, Oemar B. Safety, pharmacokinetic, and pharmacodynamic evaluation after single and multiple ascending doses of a novel selective androgen receptor modulator in healthy subjects. *Clin Ther.* 2016;38(6):1401–1416.
40. Clark RV, Walker AC, Andrews S, et al. Safety, pharmacokinetics and pharmacological effects of the selective androgen receptor modulator, GSK2881078, in healthy men and postmenopausal women. *Br J Clin Pharmacol.* 2017;83(10):2179–2194.
41. Thevis M, Geyer H, Kamber M, Schänzer W. Detection of the arylpropionamide-derived selective androgen receptor modulator (SARM) S-4 (Andarine) in a black-market product. *Drug Test Anal.* 2009;1 (8):387–392.
42. Westerman ME, Charchenko CM, Ziegelmann MJ, Bailey GC, Nippoldt TB, Trost L. Heavy testosterone use among bodybuilders: an uncommon cohort of illicit substance users. *Mayo Clin Proc.* 2016;91(2):175–182.
43. Van Wagoner RM, Eichner A, Bhasin S, et al. Chemical composition and labeling of substances marketed as selective androgen receptor modulators and sold via the internet. *JAMA.* 2017;318(20):2004–2010.

Section 5 Medical and Surgical Management of Issues of Male Health

Chapter 34: Male Fertility and Testosterone Therapy

Juan Andino and James M. Dupree

34.1 Hypogonadism, Male Fertility, and Testosterone Therapy

There has been a rise in the use of testosterone therapy for men in their reproductive years. Unfortunately, many of these men are not counseled on the potential for infertility as a side effect of exogenous testosterone. In this chapter, we will first define hypogonadism and prevalence in populations of interest; second, we will describe the epidemiology of hypogonadism; third, we will review testosterone physiology and pathophysiology; fourth, we will provide historical context into the prescribing patterns of testosterone therapy; and finally, we will highlight relevant clinical data and synthesize these into clinical pathways used for patient counseling and management based on patients' timeline for desired fertility.

34.2 Defining Hypogonadism

The diagnosis of clinical hypogonadism requires patients to have signs and/or symptoms of hypogonadism in combination with low testosterone serum levels. The diagnosis of low testosterone requires two separate lab tests performed in the early morning. A total testosterone level <300 ng/dL (10.4 nmol/L) is a well-established cut-off [1]. Signs and symptoms associated with testosterone deficiency include physical manifestations, cognitive effects, and sexual dysfunction. Some men may experience loss of body hair, reduced beard growth, or decreased muscle mass while others report reduced energy, endurance, or decreased physical performance. Others notice poor memory, concentration, or motivation as well as depressive symptoms, cognitive dysfunction, and irritability. Furthermore, patients may present with reduced sex drive and erectile dysfunction. Men can present with a combination of these different concerns. A challenge in the diagnosis of hypogonadism is that many of the symptoms reported are nonspecific and can be impacted by other medical health conditions.

34.2.1 Workup of Hypogonadism

It is helpful to differentiate between hypergonadotropic (or primary/testicular) hypogonadism and hypogonadotropic (or secondary/pituitary-hypothalamic) hypogonadism. The American Urological Association (AUA) guidelines recommend measuring luteinizing hormone (LH) in patients with low testosterone levels and performing a reproductive health evaluation for men interested in fertility prior to initiation of exogenous testosterone. This includes evaluating testicular size, measuring follicle-stimulating hormone (FSH), and obtaining a baseline semen analysis (SA) to evaluate fertility potential [1]. In hypergonadotropic hypogonadism, LH and FSH are high and possible causes should be evaluated including cryptorchidism, history of testicular trauma or torsion, orchitis, chemotherapy, or testicular radiation. For hypogonadotropic hypogonadism, LH and FSH are low or inappropriately normal and causes can include genetic disorders such as Kallmann's syndrome, metabolic conditions including diabetes and liver failure, or reversible conditions such as chronic opioid use or prolactinoma.

34.3 Epidemiology of Hypogonadism

The proportion of men with hypogonadism who are interested in fathering children may continue to rise due to two different phenomena: rising rates of hypogonadism in younger men and higher rates of hypogonadism in older men who are growing their families.

34.3.1 Hypogonadism in Reproductive-Age Men

While hypogonadism is more common in older men, the prevalence of clinical hypogonadism in men 20–49 years of age ranges from 3% to 8% [2]. In 2010, men in this reproductive age group made up 42% of the male population in the United States [3]. In 2019, the entire male population of the United States was estimated to be 137,204,120 [4]. Assuming the prevalence of hypogonadism and proportion of men in their reproductive years remain stable, approximately 1,730,000–4,600,000 men age 20–49 may seek treatment for hypogonadal symptoms. The prevalence of hypogonadism will continue to rise due to increasing rates of diabetes, obesity, and chronic opioid use among younger men still interested in fertility [5].

34.3.2 Aging Fathers

The United States also has an aging population of fathers. In 2015, fertility rates for men 30–49 years old were the highest seen in 40 years. Meanwhile, fertility rates for men age 15–29 were at record lows [6]. Given that testosterone levels have been found to decrease by approximately 100 ng/dL (3.5 nmol/L) every 10 years, or an average rate of 1–2% per year beyond age

30, the aging population of men who still desire paternity is at increased risk of hypogonadism [5].

34.4 Testosterone Physiology and Pathophysiology

34.4.1 Testosterone Physiology

In healthy adult men, the hypothalamic-pituitary-gonadal (HPG) axis regulates testosterone levels. The hypothalamus secretes gonadotropin-releasing hormone (GnRH) in a pulsatile fashion stimulating the release of LH and FSH from the anterior pituitary. LH acts on Leydig cells to produce testosterone. FSH acts on Sertoli cells and seminiferous tubules to stimulate and support spermatogenesis. Aromatase in peripheral tissues, especially adipose tissues, converts testosterone into estradiol. Both testosterone and estradiol result in negative feedback suppression in the hypothalamic neurons and pituitary gland, thereby inhibiting additional release of GnRH, LH, and FSH [7].

34.4.2 The Role of Intratesticular Testosterone

Intratesticular testosterone (ITT) plays an important role in spermatogenesis. In the normal physiologic state, ITT levels are approximately 100 times higher than serum testosterone levels [8]. ITT works synergistically with FSH to stimulate Sertoli cell function [9]. This was discovered when FSH alone could not induce spermatogenesis in men with hypogonadotropic hypogonadism. Additional work has demonstrated that low ITT results in decreased proliferation of spermatogonia, defects in releasing mature spermatids from Sertoli cells, and accelerated apoptosis of spermatagonia [10].

34.4.3 Testosterone as a Contraceptive

Understanding the negative impact of exogenous testosterone on sperm production requires understanding how supplemental testosterone affects the HPG axis. Exogenous testosterone results in direct suppression of GnRH, FSH, and LH release at the level of the hypothalamus and anterior pituitary. The decrease in LH reduces endogenous testosterone production by Leydig cells, reducing ITT while serum testosterone remains elevated through replacement therapies. With low FSH and ITT levels, there is decreased spermatogenesis as well as decreased germ cell maturation and survival [9].

In fact, exogenous testosterone has been studied as a male contraceptive. In 1990, *The Lancet* published the results of a multicenter study coordinated by the World Health Organization (WHO) Task Force on methods for the regulation of male fertility [11]. A total of 271 healthy, fertile men were started on 200 mg testosterone enanthate weekly by intramuscular injection for one year. Suppression of spermatogenesis occurred in 98% of men and 40% of these men developed azoospermia. The mean time to azoospermia was 120 days and there was only one pregnancy without using other contraception during this 12-month study.

34.5 Trends in Prescribing Patterns

34.5.1 Testosterone Therapy Prescribing Patterns

Exogenous testosterone should be used with caution in men of reproductive age due to its impact on fertility. In a study of more than 600,000 men 40–49 years of age with commercial insurance, exogenous testosterone use rose from 3,370 (0.54%) to 15,900 (2.29%) between 2001 and 2012 [12]. During the same time period, exogenous testosterone use in 30–39 year-old men rose from less than 0.25–0.8% [13]. Over the time course of these studies, approximately 25% of men did not have a testosterone level measured in the year prior to initiating testosterone replacement [13]. Between 2013 and 2016, there was a decrease in proportion of men receiving testosterone prescriptions coinciding with the release of two published reports of adverse cardiovascular events associated with testosterone therapy and an FDA communication [12]. By 2016, rates in men 30–39 and 40–49 years of age dropped to 0.4% and 0.7%, respectively. However, these studies do not account for testosterone that is paid for with cash and not reimbursed through the patients' insurance plans. A 2020 study of 310 "men's health clinics" found that 91.1% of these clinics were not supervised by a urologist or endocrinologist and few were offering evidence-based, standard-of-care treatment options [14]. Therefore, it is challenging to understand the true number of men being offered exogenous testosterone and whether fertility concerns are appropriately discussed.

34.5.2 Anabolic Steroid Prescribing Patterns

In the 1950s, structural modifications to the testosterone model resulted in the creation of androgenic anabolic steroids (AASs) [15]. The mechanism of action of AASs is almost identical to testosterone and therefore also suppresses testicular function and spermatogenesis [16]. AASs were initially used primarily by body builders and athletes. More recently, men seeking the benefits of increased muscle development, enhanced athletic performance, and "rejuvenation" have resulted in estimates of up to 3 million AAS users in the United States [17,18]. In 2013, a retrospective review of 97 patients with profound hypogonadism (with total testosterone 50 ng/dL or less) revealed that 43% had a history of AAS use [19]. Some of these young men who use AAS may never recover normal endogenous testosterone levels.

34.6 Management of Hypogonadal Men Who Are Already on Testosterone and Now Want to Restore Fertility

We now provide an overview of management strategies that can be used to help men using exogenous testosterone who desire restoration of fertility. Understanding these different management strategies will allow providers to engage in shared decision-making and advise men based on how soon they are hoping to conceive children.

34.6.1 Testosterone Withdrawal

The most conservative approach for a man on testosterone therapy who is interested in restoring fertility is to stop testosterone and monitor for improvements in spermatogenesis. In the WHO study, healthy men who developed azoospermia on testosterone enanthate had a median time to recovery of 3.7 months to reach sperm concentration of at least 20 million/mL after stopping testosterone therapy. In a pooled analysis of 30 studies examining testosterone therapy as a short-term contraceptive, the probability of sperm concentration recovering to 20 million/mL was 67% within 6 months, 90% within 12 months, and 100% within 24 months [20]. Additional work has demonstrated that both advanced age and increased duration of exogenous testosterone prolong the time to recovery of spermatogenesis [21]. Similar studies in men who have used AAS have shown spontaneous return of sperm concentration to normal levels between 5 and 18 months after AAS cessation [22]. It is important to highlight that most of these time estimates are based off of studies in healthy, fertile men who were taking testosterone for contraception. It is possible that men with hypogonadism may not recover spermatogenesis as quickly or to the same degree without additional interventions. In some cases, recovery could take up to two years or more and sperm production may not return to pretreatment levels [20,23].

The major limitations to testosterone withdrawal include recurrence of bothersome hypogonadal symptoms and prolonged time before recovery of spermatogenesis. Furthermore, men who were started on testosterone therapy without a urologic or endocrinologic evaluation may have underlying endocrinologic disorders, such as hypogonadal hypogonadism, that impact both hypogonadal symptoms and spermatogenesis.

34.6.2 Testosterone Withdrawal and Lifestyle Modification

All hypogonadal men should be counseled on the importance of healthy weight loss, physical activity, and improving sleep hygiene to reduce signs and symptoms of testosterone deficiency [1]. An inverse relationship between testosterone and excess body weight has been reported in men of all ages, with lower testosterone levels found in subjects with higher body mass index (BMI) [24]. It is thought that at least 10% of weight loss is required to achieve increases in testosterone levels [25]. In an study of middle-aged, obese men with median testosterone levels of 199 ng/dL (6.9 nmol/L) randomized to testosterone or placebo in combination with intensive diet program, the placebo group lost 11% of their body weight and this was associated with modest increase in total testosterone by 84 ng/dL (2.9 nmol/L) [26]. However, at follow-up more than one year after completion of the study, many of these men had regained 66% of their weight. Testosterone levels fell back to their prestudy baseline. For morbidly obese patients who are considering bariatric surgery, there are small, nonrandomized studies that also support improvements in testosterone correlating with decreases in BMI [27]. Finally, while studies show conflicting results regarding the relationship between sleep and testosterone levels, most studies suggest a correlation between decreased sleep quality and worse symptoms of testosterone deficiency [28].

While the improvements in testosterone levels with weight loss appear modest, this approach helps optimize the overall health of men and could improve hypogonadal symptoms beyond the measured changes in testosterone levels. The limitations of this approach include prolonged time before recovery of spermatogenesis, likely similar to testosterone withdrawal alone, as well as the challenges associated with achieving and maintaining weight loss.

34.6.3 Testosterone Withdrawal and Selective Estrogen Receptor Modulators

Selective estrogen receptor modulators (SERMs) such as clomiphene citrate and tamoxifen have been used off-label since the 1970s for the treatment of male infertility [29]. These medications inhibit the negative feedback of estrogen at the level of the hypothalamus and pituitary thereby increasing LH and FSH secretion.

While there are no studies evaluating outcomes in men previously on testosterone therapy, the mechanism of action as well as limited data in hypogonadotropic hypogonadal patients [30] supports improvements in spermatogenesis with SERMs. This use of SERMs also reflects current practice patterns in the management of male infertility. Given its effect on the HPG axis, one can hypothesize that using clomiphene citrate would lead to quicker recovery in fertility potential over testosterone withdrawal alone in men without primary testicular failure. Using clomiphene citrate would also reduce hypogonadal symptoms compared to testosterone withdrawal. However, reassessing a hormonal profile at time of repeat SA is important as there have been rare reported cases of azoospermia with initiation of clomiphene citrate [31].

34.6.4 Testosterone Withdrawal and Anastrozole

Anastrozole is a nonsteroidal aromatase inhibitor. It causes reversible inhibition of the aromatase enzyme reducing peripheral conversion of testosterone to estradiol (E_2). The reduced negative feedback inhibition from estrogen on the pituitary and hypothalamus results in increased LH and FSH secretion. Anastrozole has the ability to increase testosterone levels without associated increase in estrogen levels that can sometimes be seen with clomiphene citrate [32]. There have been no studies evaluating the use of anastrozole for hypogonadal symptoms and spermatogenesis in men who have stopped testosterone therapy. However, treatment of infertile men with low serum testosterone levels with anastrozole has been associated with increased serum testosterone from 404 to 808 ng/dL (14–28 nmol/L), decreased E_2 levels, and improved sperm concentration from 5.5 to 15.6 million sperm/mL after three months of therapy [33].

Anastrozole provides another oral option for promoting gonadotropin secretion. Aromatase is present primarily in adipose tissues and thus may be particularly useful in obese men who convert a greater proportion of testosterone to estradiol. While not specifically studied in men previously on testosterone replacement, anastrozole may be helpful in men with increased estradiol levels or as an alternative agent for the rare case of azoospermia on clomiphine citrate [31,32]. Similar to SERMs, improvements in semen parameters have been seen within three months of initiating anastrozole in general infertility populations.

34.6.5 Testosterone Withdrawal and hCG

Human chorionic gonadotropin (hCG) has the biologic effects of LH and is used to stimulate Leydig cells to secrete testosterone, raising both serum and ITT [34]. By restoring ITT, hCG therapy should restore spermatogenesis for men with an intact HPG axis after cessation of testosterone. Studies in hypogonadal men demonstrate encouraging results for the off-label use of hCG in this setting. hCG has been used to treat hypogonadism associated with anabolic steroid use resulting in the recovery of ITT production with three times per week dosing ranging from 2,000 to 3,000 units [16,22]. In a case report of anabolic steroid–induced hypogonadism and azoospermia, hCG therapy improved testosterone levels and semen parameters with a pregnancy achieved after three months [35].

hCG therapy after testosterone withdrawal should be considered for three to six months. If semen parameters have not improved and pregnancy has not been achieved, combination therapy of hCG with other agents that increase FSH activity should be considered. The major limitations of using hCG include patient comfort with injection therapy and out-of-pocket costs as insurance coverage for hCG can vary.

34.6.6 Testosterone Withdrawal and hCG-Based Combination Therapy

While hCG addresses serum and ITT levels, it has no impact on FSH activity and Sertoli cell function. Therefore, there will be a subset of patients who will require concomitant therapies to increase FSH activity in order to optimize semen parameters. Options include SERMS, aromatase inhibitors, or FSH analogues.

In 2015, a retrospective review of 49 men highlighted the role of hCG-based combination therapy for managing infertility caused by exogenous testosterone use. All men were started on 3,000 units of hCG every other day after discontinuing exogenous testosterone. Supplemental medications were used to raise FSH levels and were based on clinician preference and clinical context. Thirty-five (71%) were prescribed clomiphene citrate, 28 (57%) were prescribed tamoxifen, 10 (20%) were prescribed anastrozole, and one (2%) was prescribed recombinant FSH. After starting hCG-combination therapy, return of spermatogenesis or improvement in sperm concentration to >1 million/mL was documented in 48 (98.0%) of men. Average testosterone levels were within the normal range when sperm first returned to the ejaculate. The average time to first sperm recovery in the ejaculate for men with azoospermia or improvement in sperm concentration above 1 million/mL for men with severe oligozoospermia was 4.6 months; the mean first sperm concentration was 22.6 million/mL. There did not appear to be a difference in time to sperm recovery based on type of testosterone supplementation previously used. Nineteen men (40%) achieved a clinically documented pregnancy during the mean 14 months of follow-up, with no significant difference by type of previous testosterone therapy or supplemental therapy used with hCG. No men discontinued therapy because of adverse effects [23].

Some experts treat with hCG alone for three to six months because many cases will demonstrate improvement in semen parameters during this time. In those without adequate spermatogenesis other agents including clomiphene, anastrozole, or recombinant FSH can be used to ensure both LH and FSH activity is present to optimize fertility potential [23,36]. The major limitations to this approach include the requirement for multiple pharmaceutical agents, costs of medications, and potential need for sperm extraction despite trying different medications.

34.7 Management of Hypogonadal Men Interested in Starting Testosterone Therapy and Maintaining Fertility

Both the AUA and the Endocrine Society published guidelines in 2018 that recommend against the use of exogenous testosterone in men wishing to preserve fertility [1,39]. However, there are patients who may be interested in starting testosterone therapy for hypogonadal symptoms while simultaneously maintaining fertility potential. There are emerging strategies that could allow for continued use of testosterone therapy when paternity is not a short-term goal.

34.7.1 Testosterone Therapy and hCG

In 2005, researchers demonstrated that exogenous testosterone caused ITT levels to drop by 94% in otherwise healthy, reproductive-aged men. In these men, adding hCG ranging from 250 IU to 500 IU every other day to testosterone therapy regimens maintained ITT levels [34]. However, this three-week study was too short to evaluate semen parameters or determine the short-term impact on spermatogenesis. A retrospective study in 2013 served to establish the idea of maintaining fertility while on exogenous testosterone. Twenty-six men initiating testosterone replacement therapy who desired fertility were simultaneously started on hCG. These men received 500 IU of hCG every other day while on different formulations of exogenous testosterone. Mean serum testosterone levels before initiating testosterone replacement and hCG were 207 ng/dL compared to 1,056 ng/dL on both agents. Mean pretreatment sperm concentration was 35 ± 30 million/mL. No differences in semen analysis parameters were observed during greater than one year of follow-up on testosterone and hCG. There were also no differences noted between sperm concentrations for men using different types of testosterone formulations [40]. Nine (35%) of these men achieved pregnancy at one year of follow-up. Of note, pregnancy information was incomplete as not all men were actively pursuing pregnancy during the study period.

More work is needed in this area to understand differences in outcomes across different testosterone formulations, varying duration of testosterone therapy, and impact on fertility potential based on semen parameters and pregnancy rates. The existing data suggests testosterone combined with hCG can address hypogonadal symptoms while maintaining fertility potential. The major limitations to this approach include potential for side effects of high testosterone levels, such as erythrocytosis; requiring two pharmaceutical agents and comfort with injection therapy; as well as costs of hCG and testosterone formulations that may not be covered by insurance.

34.7.2 Testosterone Therapy and hCG-Based Combination Therapy

In addition to maintaining ITT levels with hCG, some men will require Sertoli cell stimulation with FSH. Clomiphene citrate has been suggested as first-line combination therapy with hCG [41]. In three to six months, repeat semen analysis and hormonal evaluation should be performed to decide whether other oral agents or recombinant FSH should be used. Anastrozole should be employed instead of clomiphene if testosterone-to-estradiol ratio is less than 10:1. Finally, if little or no improvement in semen parameters and low FSH persists despite hCG-based combination therapy, then recombinant FSH every other day should be used for its direct gonadotropin action [16,42].

There are no studies summarizing the effect of testosterone and hCG-based combination therapy but physiologically these regimens should help promote spermatogenesis through simultaneous stimulation of Leydig and Sertoli cells. The major limitations to this approach include potential for side effects from multiple pharmaceutical agents, comfort with injection therapy, costs of medications, a lack of data for patient selection and counseling, and need for additional interventions despite maximal pharmacological therapy. Future studies should aim to evaluate impact on hormonal profile of these patients including testosterone, estradiol as well as long-term effects on spermatogenesis and pregnancy rates.

34.8 Recommended Treatment Algorithms

34.8.1 Our Recommended Pathway for Restoring Fertility

First, if a patient desires pregnancy within six months and has not yet started testosterone, they should abstain from initiating testosterone therapy until a pregnancy has been achieved. Otherwise, men who are actively trying for a pregnancy should stop taking testosterone and follow the recovery regimen detailed in Figure 34.1. After stopping testosterone, men can choose any of the management options already described through shared decision-making with their physician.

Men desiring the most efficient and data-driven management option should start a regimen consisting of 2,000–3,000 IU hCG every other day [42]. Clomiphene citrate 25 mg every day or 50 mg every other day should also be incorporated to help promote FSH production and pituitary function [23]. Repeat SA and hormonal evaluation should be repeated every three months. If pregnancy is not achieved and neither FSH levels or SA parameters show improvement, clomiphene should be discontinued and recombinant FSH 75–150 IU every other day should be added [42–44]. If this fails, testicular sperm retrieval with possible microdissection should be offered in conjunction with in vitro fertilization as a final chance for biologic paternity. Once pregnancy has been achieved, reinitiation of testosterone should be discussed with special consideration to future fertility goals [16].

34.8.2 Our Recommended Pathway for Maintaining Fertility While Initiating Exogenous Testosterone Therapy

All men wishing to preserve fertility should have a baseline SA prior to initiation of testosterone therapy. If a planned pregnancy is desired within the 6–12 month time frame, patient can be offered exogenous testosterone supplemented with hCG 500 IU every other day (Figure 34.2) [42]. Clomiphene citrate or anastrozole should be considered as optional throughout this time.

When planning for pregnancy in more than 12 months, testosterone therapy with adjuvant 500 IU hCG can be offered. These patients should be cycled off testosterone every six months given the increased risk of impaired fertility with prolonged, uninterrupted courses of exogenous testosterone [21]. Each off-cycle can involve a four-week cycle of 3,000 IU of hCG every other day and clomiphene citrate [21]. During any of these above regimens, anastrozole may be added and titrated in dose to address elevations in estradiol (Figure 34.3).

34.9 Future Directions

The idea of "fertility sustaining" testosterone therapy remains in its infancy and continues to be studied and refined. There are promising developments that may help with monitoring responses to therapy aimed at maintaining fertility as well as new therapeutic strategies.

34.9.1 17-hydroxyprogesterone as a Marker of Preserved Spermatogenesis

The changes in ITT levels with exogenous testosterone have historically relied on the association between preserved ITT and improvement in SA parameters. In the 2005 study already described, invasive testicular biopsies/aspiration were used to measure changes in ITT while on exogenous testosterone compared to the preservation of ITT with simultaneous testosterone and hCG administration [34]. Intratesticular steroids are comprised of approximately 70% testosterone, 20% 17-hydroxyprogesterone (17-OHP), and smaller percentages of other

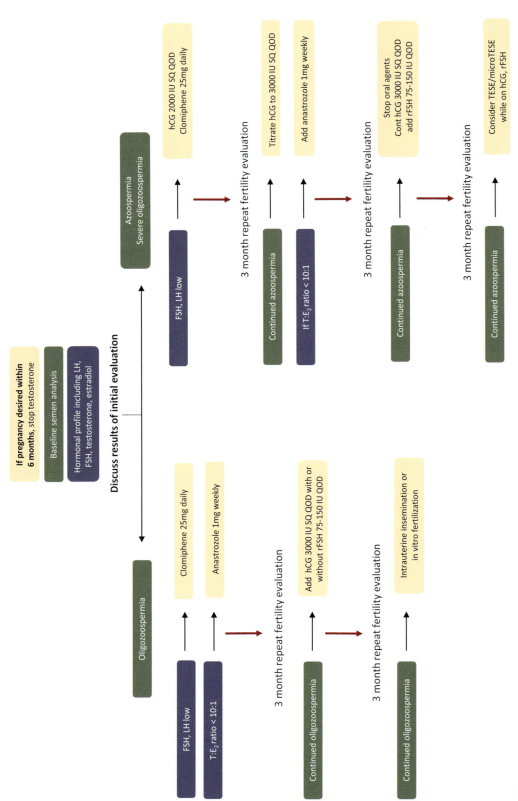

Figure 34.1 Pathway for restoring fertility after testosterone therapy

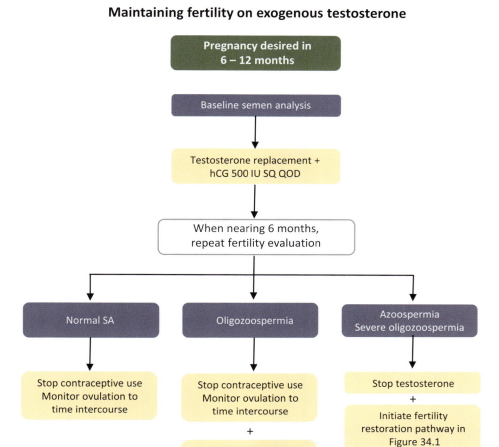

Figure 34.2 Maintaining fertility on exogenous testosterone

hormones. This intratesticular production contributes to the majority of serum testosterone and 17-OHP levels [45]. In 2018, Amory and colleagues found that serum 17-OHP decreased with exogenous testosterone, increased with hCG, and was strongly associated with end-of-treatment ITT levels [45,46]. They also found that other androgens such as androstenedione or dehydroepiandrosterone did not have this association.

17-OHP has the potential to function as a clinical biomarker used for counseling patients, tracking responses to therapy, and managing medications that support Leydig cell function and increase ITT. Future investigations should aim to identify minimal and optimal concentrations of ITT and 17-OHP for spermatogenesis.

34.9.2 Short-Acting Testosterone

Long-acting testosterone preparations including injections, topical gels, patches, and pellets suppress the HPG axis, reduce gonadotropin levels, and suppress ITT and spermatogenesis [7]. However, recent studies of an FDA-approved, short-acting testosterone nasal gel suggest that short-acting formulations of testosterone may not have the same impact on spermatogenesis [47].

A single-center, open-label, single-arm trial evaluated the effect of testosterone nasal gel on serum testosterone levels and semen parameters. A total of 38 out of 44 men (86.4%) and 30 out of 33 men (90.9%) achieved testosterone levels greater than 300 ng/dL at three and six months, respectively [47]. All men had normal FSH and LH levels prior to treatment. Fourteen (32.6%) and 16 (38.1%) men had levels of FSH and LH below normal levels at three months, respectively, while 6 (18.2%) and 9 (27.3%) were below lower limit of normal for FSH and LH at six months, respectively. At three and six months, there was no statistically significant difference in sperm concentration with mean difference of -4.1 million/mL at three months (p = 0.193) and -5.5 million/mL at six months (p = 0.081); similarly, there was no change in mean total motile sperm count. Of note, one patient (1.7%) developed azoospermia and three patients (5%) had SA with severe oligozoospermia [47].

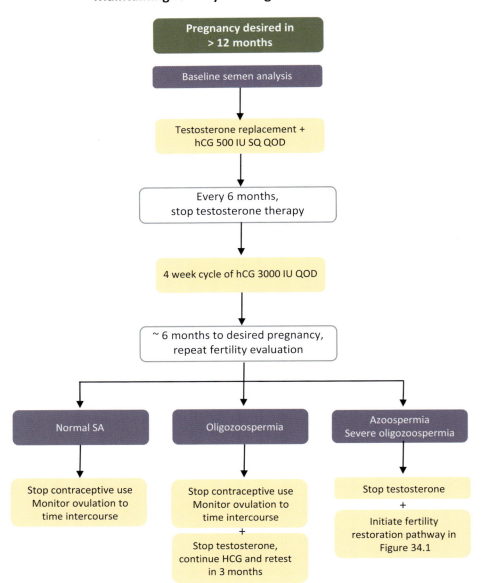

Figure 34.3 Maintaining fertility on exogenous testosterone

This early data is promising and short-acting testosterone formulations may offer hypogonadal symptom management with a less deleterious effect on fertility potential. However, while not statistically significant, the data suggests a possible decrease in sperm concentration over six months of follow-up. Long-term studies will be essential to determine whether this formulation can sustain spermatogenesis or result in quicker recovery of sperm concentration when stopping testosterone.

34.9.3 Leydig Stem Cell Injection

Animal models are now promising nonpharmacologic strategies for restoring testosterone without suppression of the HPG axis and its downstream effects on spermatogenesis. A 2019 study of castrate mice demonstrated that autografting of Leydig stem cells – a combination of Leydig, Sertoli, and peritubular smooth muscle cells – increased serum testosterone while simultaneously maintaining the production of FSH and LH [48]. This experiment was the first to show that ectopic grafting of Leydig stem cells in subcutaneous tissue resulted in testosterone production while preserving the HPG axis. However, this was a short study of four-week duration and the increase in testosterone was modest at best. Additional work will be required to determine the viability and sustainability of this approach and whether serum and ITT levels can be restored to eugonadal ranges.

This is not the only application of ectopic grafting of autologous tissues to address fertility concerns. In the same year, Fayomi and colleagues demonstrated successful autografting of cryopreserved prepubertal testicular tissues in Rhesus macaques with production of testosterone, spermatogenesis, and graft-derived sperm resulting in the birth of a healthy female macaque baby [49]. Testicular tissue grafting may be the next frontier in reproductive medicine that leverages native tissues to support Leydig and Sertoli cell function.

34.10 Conclusion

Over time, more men will need help managing hypogonadal symptoms while still wanting the option for future paternity. When these men present for evaluations, one of the most important aspects of the evaluation is the timing for desired pregnancy. For those interested in a pregnancy within six months, testosterone therapy should be stopped, and adjuncts should be used to stimulate Sertoli and Leydig function. For patients who have a longer timeline before pregnancy is desired, testosterone can be continued with hCG to support ITT levels and spermatogenesis.

In the future, improved serum biomarkers may help urologists monitor responses to therapy and predict pregnancy outcomes. New testosterone formulations may preserve spermatogenesis or lead to quicker recoveries in sperm counts. Finally, tissue grafting has the potential to revolutionize the management of male infertility.

References

1. Mulhall JP, Trost LW, Brannigan RE, et al. Evaluation and management of testosterone deficiency: AUA guideline. *J Urol.* 2018;200(2):423–432. doi:10.1016/j.juro.2018.03.115
2. Harman SM, Metter EJ, Tobin JD, Pearson J, Blackman MR. Longitudinal effects of aging on serum total and free testosterone levels in healthy men. *J Clin Endocrinol Metab.* 2001;86(2):724–731. doi:10.1210/jcem.86.2.7219
3. Howden LM, Meyer JA. *2010 Census Brief: Age and Sex Composition.* 2011. www.census.gov/population. Accessed March 16, 2020.
4. US Census. *Population QuickFacts.* 2019. www.census.gov/quickfacts/fact/table/US/LFE046218. Published 2020. Accessed July 19, 2020.
5. Cohen J, Nassau DE, Patel P, Ramasamy R. Low testosterone in adolescents & young adults. *Front Endocrinol (Lausanne).* 2020;10. doi:10.3389/fendo.2019.00916
6. Martin JA, Brady MPH, Hamilton E, Osterman MJK, Driscoll AK, Mathews TJ. Births final data for 2015. *Natl Vital Stat Rep.* 2017;66(1):1. www.cdc.gov/nchs/data_access/Vitalstatsonline.htm. Accessed March 16, 2020.
7. Basaria S. Male hypogonadism. *Lancet.* 2014;383(9924):1250–1263. doi:10.1016/S0140-6736(13)61126-5
8. Roth MY, Page ST, Lin K, et al. Dose-dependent increase in intratesticular testosterone by very low-dose human chorionic gonadotropin in normal men with experimental gonadotropin deficiency. *J Clin Endocrinol Metab.* 2010;95(8):3806–3813. doi:10.1210/jc.2010-0360
9. Walker WH. Non-classical actions of testosterone and spermatogenesis. *Philos Trans R Soc Lond B Biol Sci.* 2010;365(1546):1557–1569. doi:10.1098/rstb.2009.0258
10. Patel AS, Leong JY, Ramos L, Ramasamy R. Testosterone is a contraceptive and should not be used in men who desire fertility. *World J Mens Health.* 2019;37(1):45–54. doi:10.5534/wjmh.180036
11. World Health Organisation Task Force on Methods for the Regulation of Male Fertility. Contraceptive efficacy of testosterone-induced azoospermia in normal men. *Lancet.* 1990;336(8721):955–959. doi:10.1016/0140-6736(90)92416-F
12. Baillargeon J, Kuo Y-F, Westra JR, Urban RJ, Goodwin JS. Testosterone prescribing in the United States, 2002–2016. *JAMA.* 2018;320(2):200–202. doi:10.1001/jama.2018.7999
13. Baillargeon J, Urban RJ, Ottenbacher KJ, Pierson KS, Goodwin JS. Trends in androgen prescribing in the United States, 2001 to 2011. *JAMA Intern Med.* 2013;173(15):1465–1466. doi:10.1001/jamainternmed.2013.6895
14. Kansal JK, Dietrich PN, Doolittle J, et al. MP45-17: online marketing practices and characteristics of stand-alone men's health clinics. *J Urol.* 2020;203(4):e671. doi:10.1097/JU.0000000000000900.017
15. Dotson JL, Brown RT. The history of the development of anabolic-androgenic steroids. *Pediatr Clin North Am.* 2007;54(4):761–769. doi:10.1016/j.pcl.2007.04.003
16. Tatem AJ, Beilan J, Kovac JR, Lipshultz LI. Management of anabolic steroid-induced infertility: novel strategies for fertility maintenance and recovery. *World J Mens Health.* 2020;38(2):141–150. doi:10.5534/wjmh.190002
17. Silver MD. Use of ergogenic aids by athletes. *J Am Acad Orthop Surg.* 2001;9(1):61–70. doi:10.5435/00124635-200101000-00007
18. Kanayama G, Pope HG. History and epidemiology of anabolic androgens in athletes and non-athletes. *Mol Cell Endocrinol.* 2018;464:4–13. doi:10.1016/j.mce.2017.02.039
19. Coward RM, Rajanahally S, Kovac JR, Smith RP, Pastuszak AW, Lipshultz LI. Anabolic steroid induced hypogonadism in young men. *J Urol.* 2013;190(6):2200–2205. doi:10.1016/j.juro.2013.06.010
20. Ly LP, Liu PY, Handelsman DJ. Rates of suppression and recovery of human sperm output in testosterone-based hormonal contraceptive regimens. *Hum Reprod.* 2005;20(6):1733–1740. doi:10.1093/humrep/deh834
21. Kohn TP, Louis MR, Pickett SM, et al. Age and duration of testosterone therapy predict time to return of sperm count after human chorionic gonadotropin therapy. *Fertil Steril.* 2017;107(2):351–357.e1. doi:10.1016/j.fertnstert.2016.10.004
22. Rahnema CD, Lipshultz LI, Crosnoe LE, Kovac JR, Kim ED. Anabolic steroid-induced hypogonadism: diagnosis and treatment. *Fertil Steril.* 2014;101:1271–1279. doi:10.1016/j.fertnstert.2014.02.002
23. Wenker EP, Dupree JM, Langille GM, et al. The use of HCG-based combination therapy for recovery of

24. Chambers T, Anderson R. The impact of obesity on male fertility. *Hormones*. 2015;14(4):563–568. doi:10.14310/horm.2002.1621
25. Grossmann M. Hypogonadism and male obesity: focus on unresolved questions. *Clin Endocrinol (Oxf)*. 2018;89(1):11–21. doi:10.1111/cen.13723
26. Ng Tang Fui M, Prendergast LA, Dupuis P, et al. Effects of testosterone treatment on body fat and lean mass in obese men on a hypocaloric diet: a randomised controlled trial. *BMC Med*. 2016;14(1):153. doi:10.1186/s12916-016-0700-9
27. Rigon FA, Ronsoni MF, Hohl A, van de Sande-Lee S. Effects of bariatric surgery in male obesity-associated hypogonadism. *Obes Surg*. 2019;29(7):2115–2125. doi:10.1007/s11695-019-03829-0
28. Krzastek SC, Smith RP. Non-testosterone management of male hypogonadism: an examination of the existing literature. *Transl Androl Urol*. 2020;9(S2):S160–S170. doi:10.21037/tau.2019.11.16
29. Wheeler KM, Sharma D, Kavoussi PK, Smith RP, Costabile R. Clomiphene citrate for the treatment of hypogonadism. *Sex Med Rev*. 2019;7(2):272–276. doi:10.1016/j.sxmr.2018.10.001
30. Whitten SJ, Nangia AK, Kolettis PN. Select patients with hypogonadotropic hypogonadism may respond to treatment with clomiphene citrate. *Fertil Steril*. 2006;86(6):1664–1668. doi:10.1016/j.fertnstert.2006.05.042
31. Pasqualotto FF, Fonseca GP, Pasqualotto EB. Azoospermia after treatment with clomiphene citrate in patients with oligospermia. *Fertil Steril*. 2008;90(5):2014.e11–2014.e12. doi:10.1016/j.fertnstert.2008.03.036
32. Pavlovich CP, King P, Goldstein M, Schlegel PN. Evidence of a treatable endocrinopathy in infertile men. *J Urol*. 2001;165(3):837–841. www.ncbi.nlm.nih.gov/pubmed/11176482.
33. Raman JD, Schlegel PN. Aromatase inhibitors for male infertility. *J Urol*. 2002;98(6):624–629. doi:10.1097/00005392-200202000-00038
34. Coviello AD, Matsumoto AM, Bremner WJ, et al. Low-dose human chorionic gonadotropin maintains intratesticular testosterone in normal men with testosterone-induced gonadotropin suppression. *J Clin Endocrinol Metab*. 2005;90(5):2595–2602. doi:10.1210/jc.2004-0802
35. Turek PJ, Williams RH, Gilbaugh JHI, Lipshultz LI. The reversibility of anabolic steroid-induced azoospermia. *J Urol*. 1995;153(5):1628–1630. doi:10.1016/S0022-5347(01)67482-2
36. McBride JA, Coward R. Recovery of spermatogenesis following testosterone replacement therapy or anabolic-androgenic steroid use. *Asian J Androl*. 2016;18(3):373–380. doi:10.4103/1008-682X.173938
37. Buchter D, Behre H, Kliesch S, Nieschlag E. Pulsatile GnRH or human chorionic gonadotropin/human menopausal gonadotropin as effective treatment for men with hypogonadotropic hypogonadism: a review of 42 cases. *Eur J Endocrinol*. 1998;139(3):298–303. doi:10.1530/eje.0.1390298
38. Burgues S, Calderon MD. Subcutaneous self-administration of highly purified follicle stimulating hormone and human chorionic gonadotropin for the treatment of male hypogonadotrophic hypogonadism. Spanish Collaborative Group on Male Hypogonadotropic Hypogonadism. *Hum Reprod*. 1997;12(5):980–986. doi:10.1093/humrep/12.5.980
39. Bhasin S, Brito JP, Cunningham GR, et al. Testosterone therapy in men with hypogonadism: an Endocrine Society clinical practice guideline. *J Clin Endocrinol Metab*. 2018;103(5):1715–1744. doi:10.1210/jc.2018-00229
40. Hsieh T-C, Pastuszak AW, Hwang K, Lipshultz LI. Concomitant intramuscular human chorionic gonadotropin preserves spermatogenesis in men undergoing testosterone replacement therapy. *J Urol*. 2013;189:647–650. doi:10.1016/j.juro.2012.09.043
41. Lee JA, Ramasamy R. Indications for the use of human chorionic gonadotropic hormone for the management of infertility in hypogonadal men. *Transl Androl Urol*. 2018;7(Suppl. 3):S348–S352. doi:10.21037/tau.2018.04.11
42. Ramasamy R, Armstrong J, Lipshultz L. Preserving fertility in the hypogonadal patient: an update. *Asian J Androl*. 2015;17(2):197–200. doi:10.4103/1008-682X.142772
43. Liu PY, Turner L, Rushford D, et al. Efficacy and safety of recombinant human follicle stimulating hormone (Gonal-F) with urinary human chorionic gonadotrophin for induction of spermatogenesis and fertility in gonadotrophin-deficient men. *Hum Reprod*. 1999;14(6):1540–1545. doi:10.1093/humrep/14.6.1540.
44. Ishikawa T, Ooba T, Kondo Y, Yamaguchi K, Fujisawa M. Assessment of gonadotropin therapy in male hypogonadotropic hypogonadism. *Fertil Steril*. 2007;88(6):1697–1699. doi:10.1016/j.fertnstert.2006.11.022
45. Patel A, Patel P, Bitran J, Ramasamy R. Can serum 17-hydroxyprogesterone and insulin-like factor 3 be used as a marker for evaluation of intratesticular testosterone? *Transl Androl Urol*. 2019;8(S1):S58–S63. doi:10.21037/tau.2019.01.16
46. Amory JK, Coviello AD, Page ST, Anawalt BD, Matsumoto AM, Bremner WJ. Serum 17-hydroxyprogesterone strongly correlates with intratesticular testosterone in gonadotropin-suppressed normal men receiving various dosages of human chorionic gonadotropin. *Fertil Steril*. 2008;89(2):380–386. doi:10.1016/j.fertnstert.2007.02.059
47. Ramasamy R, Masterson TA, Best JC, et al. Effect of Natesto on reproductive hormones, semen parameters and hypogonadal symptoms: a single center, open label, single arm trial. *J Urol*. 2020;204(3):557–563. doi:10.1097/JU.0000000000001078
48. Arora H, Zuttion MSSR, Nahar B, Lamb D, Hare JM, Ramasamy R. Subcutaneous Leydig stem cell autograft: a promising strategy to increase serum testosterone. *Stem Cells Transl Med*. 2019;8(1):58–65. doi:10.1002/sctm.18-0069
49. Fayomi AP, Peters K, Sukhwani M, et al. Autologous grafting of cryopreserved prepubertal rhesus testis produces sperm and offspring. *Science*. 2019;363(6433):1314–1319. doi:10.1126/science.aav2914

Section 5 Medical and Surgical Management of Issues of Male Health

Chapter 35

Sleep and Men's Health

Vanessa Peña, Taylor P. Kohn, and Larry I. Lipshultz

35.1 Introduction

Although the myriad beneficial functions of sleep remain to be identified, it is widely accepted that sleep is essential for optimal health and well-being [1]. Despite its importance, over a third of American adults fail to achieve the 7–9 hours of sleep recommended by the American Academy of Sleep Medicine and the Sleep Research Society [2–3]. In addition to primary sleep disorders, such as sleep apnea, insomnia, and restless legs syndrome (RLS), many modern societal factors are also thought to contribute to the growing prevalence of chronic sleep deficiency [4]. Such factors include increased technology dependence, poor sleep hygiene, longer work hours, and shift work [4].

It is estimated that more than 21 million Americans, or 17.7% of the United States labor force, are nonstandard shift workers whose shifts at least partially fall outside the standard daytime shift range of 6 a.m. to 6 p.m. [5]. Nonstandard shift work interrupts the natural sleep–wake cycle and can result in poor sleep, impaired wakefulness, and, in severe cases, shift work disorder (SWD) [6]. According to the third edition of the *International Classification of Sleep Disorders*, SWD is defined as insomnia and/or excessive sleepiness associated with a work schedule that occurs during the habitual sleep phase for at least three months and causes significant distress or impairment in mental, physical, social, or occupational functioning [6–8]. The prevalence of SWD is not clear due to variable use of diagnostic criteria and heterogeneous study populations but has been reported to be as high as 23% [6,9].

Over the past several decades, researchers have investigated the consequences of nonstandard shift work, SWD, and overall poor sleep. In addition to the decreased productivity [10,11] and increased workplace accidents [12–14] seen in nonstandard shift workers, many studies have demonstrated a significant association between shift work and numerous chronic health conditions, including diabetes [15–17], hyperlipidemia [18], cardiovascular disease [19,20], hypertension [21–23], and depression [24,25]. Although far fewer studies have investigated the impact of nonstandard shift work on male reproductive health, a compelling association between sleep and male urogenital health has been demonstrated [26,27]. In this chapter, we will review the literature regarding the effects of shift work, SWD, and poor sleep on erectile dysfunction, lower urinary tract symptoms, hypogonadism, and male infertility, followed by a discussion of the important implications of these findings on the evaluation and management of these common urogenital conditions.

35.2 Sleep and Erectile Dysfunction

Erectile dysfunction (ED) is a common reproductive health problem that is estimated to affect over 50% of men to some degree in the United States [28]. Numerous risk factors for ED have already been identified, including diabetes, obesity, smoking, and hypertension [29]; in addition, multiple studies suggest poor sleep or sleep deprivation may be another important risk factor. Sleep disorders are a regular cause of sleep disturbance, and one of the most common and well-studied is obstructive sleep apnea (OSA), a condition characterized by repetitive upper airway obstruction resulting in oxygen desaturation and arousal from sleep [30]. Since the early 2000s, numerous cross-sectional studies have identified a significant association between OSA and ED [31–37]. A recent systematic review and meta-analysis of 10 collective studies by Kellesarian et al. found that the risk of ED was significantly lower in patients without OSA (OR 0.45, 95% CI: 0.18–0.71) [38].

Few studies have investigated the association between ED and other sleep conditions. One study by Bozorgmehri and colleagues in older men demonstrated a significant association between sleep-disordered breathing, defined using the Apnea–Hypopnea Index, and ED, defined using the Massachusetts Male Aging Study scale [39]. However, this association lost statistical significance after adjusting for BMI, socioeconomic status, and comorbidities, demonstrating the importance of confounding variables on ED. In another recent study investigating the role of insomnia on ED, Seehuus and Pigeon found a significant association between insomnia severity and ED, as assessed by the International Index of Erectile Function (IIEF) [40]. This association has been supported by several other studies [41,42]. In 2010, Gao et al. showed that men with RLS had greater odds of concurrent ED, and the odds increased with a higher frequency of symptoms per month [43]. In support of this, a follow-up prospective cohort study of over 10,000 men by Li et al. found that men with RLS were more likely to develop ED (risk ration [RR] 1.38 95% CI: 1.14–1.68) [44].

Given this strong association between sleep disorders and ED, many researchers have assessed the effects of sleep disorder treatments on ED that would further strengthen this association. One of the most well studied is continuous positive airway pressure (CPAP) for OSA in men with concurrent ED [36,45–49]. In a randomized controlled two-by-two factorial designed trial, Melehan and colleagues compared CPAP to sham-CPAP and 10 mg vardenafil to placebo for 12 weeks in 61 men with moderate-to-severe OSA and ED [47]. They found that while neither vardenafil nor CPAP improved IIEF scores compared to placebo and sham, respectively, there was a significant increase in overall sexual satisfaction and sleep-related erections in the CPAP group. In addition, after stratifying the CPAP group, they found that those who were adherent (used CPAP for >4 hours per night) had significantly improved erectile function compared to those who were nonadherent. In contrast, another randomized controlled trial (RCT) compared sildenafil (100 mg one hour prior to sexual intercourse) and nasal CPAP and found that sildenafil was superior based on successful attempts of sexual intercourse per week and satisfaction rate [48]. Given the conflicting results of trials and prospective studies, Li et al. recently conducted a meta-analysis, based on 4 RCTs and 11 observational studies, and concluded that while CPAP significantly improved IIEF scores, CPAP was inferior to phosphodiesterase type 5 inhibitors (PDE5i) in improving IIEF erectile function (IIEF-EF) and intercourse satisfaction subdomains [49]. In addition, although there was not enough evidence to recommend combination therapy, the combination of CPAP and PDE5i was superior to CPAP alone in improving the IIEF results [49].

In addition to those suffering from sleep disorders, nonstandard shift workers are another population at risk for sleep deprivation and have demonstrated higher rates of sexual dysfunction [26]. In 1990, one of the first studies to assess the relationship between ED and nonstandard shift workers failed to demonstrate a significant association compared to dayshift workers. However, the study was limited by a small sample size and lack of a validated questionnaire. Since then, multiple larger studies using validated measurement tools have been conducted. In a cross-sectional study of 182 men who worked nonstandard shifts, Pastuszak et al. found that participants who were "very dissatisfied" with their sleep quality had significantly lower IIEF scores than those who were "very satisfied" ($p = 0.001$) or "somewhat satisfied" ($p = 0.005$) [50]. In a follow-up study, Rodriguez et al. conducted a larger cross-sectional study of 802 men to examine the association between SWD and ED. While nonstandard shift work alone was not associated with worse IIEF-EF scores, men with SWD had statistically and clinically worse IIEF-EF scores compared to men without SWD [51]. In a similar study, Kohn et al. also found that shift work was not exclusively associated with worse IIEF-EF scores but those with worse global sleep quality, as measured by the Pittsburgh Sleep Quality Index (PSQI), had significantly worse IIEF-EF scores ($p = 0.003$). These authors also found a significant positive association between sleep hygiene and erectile function ($p = 0.02$). Overall, the evidence supporting the association between poor sleep and ED is continuing to grow, both in the setting of a sleep disorder and shift work. As a result, the importance of a sleep assessment at the time of ED evaluation will likely only continue to increase in significance.

35.3 Sleep and Lower Urinary Tract Symptoms

Lower urinary tract symptoms (LUTS), characterized by urinary frequency, urgency, weak stream, hesitancy, and/or nocturia, are another important and common condition in aging men [52]. Though LUTS is often attributed to benign prostatic hyperplasia, it is known that prostate volume poorly correlates with symptom severity [53]; rather, it has been suggested that multiple factors may contribute to the subjective experience of LUTS, including poor sleep [27].

Over the past decade, multiple cross-sectional studies have demonstrated a significant association between OSA and worsened LUTS [36,54–57]. In one of the largest studies, conducted by Martin et al., 708 randomly selected men in a community were invited to undergo in-home polysomnography testing to assess for OSA while nocturia, daytime sleepiness, and sleep quality were assessed with the American Urology Association-Symptom Index (AUA-SI), Epworth Sleepiness Scale (ESS), and the PSQI, respectively. In multiple adjusted models, they found that nocturia was significantly associated with OSA (OR 1.64, 95% CI: 1.03–2.55), poorer sleep quality (OR 1.65, 95% CI: 1.10–2.48), and excessive daytime sleepiness (OR 1.72, 95% CI: 1.01–2.93) [55]. Compared to daytime LUTS, nocturia is unique because the frequent urge to void overnight can lead to significant sleep disturbance, and many studies have demonstrated the strong impact of nocturia on sleep quality [58–60]. Thus, nocturia likely has a bidirectional relationship with sleep. In a recent study utilizing the National Health and Nutrition Examination Survey database between 2006 and 2008, Fantus et al. demonstrated that men with a sleep disorder (OSA, RLS, or insomnia) were more likely to report both nocturia (OR 1.23, 95% CI: 1.22–1.23) and daytime LUTS (OR 1.27, 95% CI: 1.26–1.27) [61].

Due to the compelling association between sleep disorders and LUTS, studies have assessed the effects of sleep disorder treatments on LUTS with largely positive results. Multiple prospective studies have demonstrated significant improvement in international prostate symptom score (IPSS) and frequency of nocturia in men with OSA and LUTS after one month, three months, and one year of CPAP [36,62,63]. In addition to medical management of OSA, one study by Park et al. of 66 patients diagnosed with OSA who underwent uvulopalatopharyngoplasty demonstrated the beneficial effects of surgical management of OSA on LUTS. They found that patients whose surgery was deemed a success (defined as greater than 50% reduction in snoring) experienced a significant decrease in nocturia episodes and total IPSS score while patients whose surgery failed saw no change [64]. One study by Shimizu et al. assessed the effects of ramelteon, an FDA-approved melatonin receptor agonist for insomnia, in 115 patients with insomnia and LUTS that demonstrated a significant reduction in total IPSS score in addition to insomnia severity [65]. While these studies all demonstrate the benefits of sleep disorder treatment on LUTS, other studies have demonstrated the benefits of LUTS management on sleep disorder [66,67]. In a prospective cohort study of 11 males with LUTS and insomnia, eight weeks of silodosin was associated with a significant improvement in IPSS total in addition to global PSQI score [66]. Although limited by a small sample size, such studies further demonstrate the bidirectional and complex association between LUTS and sleep.

Recent studies have also assessed the role of shift work and poor sleep quality on LUTS. In a cross-sectional study of 1,741 urologic clinic patients, Kim found that alternating shift workers reported increased nocturia frequency compared to nonshift workers, and though the study reached statistical significance (p<0.01), the clinical significance was questionable (2.38 ± 1.44 versus 2.18 ± 1.04) [68]. A larger (n = 2571) but similar study was recently conducted by Sigalos et al., and although they did not find a significant association between nonstandard shift work and LUTS, they did find that nonstandard shift workers diagnosed with SWD had significantly worse LUTS compared to those without SWD [69]. While studying 228 nonstandard shift workers, Scovell et al. found that it was those men with sleep difficulties, such as falling asleep or staying asleep, that had more severe LUTS [70]. These findings suggest that it is poor sleep rather than shift work alone that is linked to LUTS.

In addition to these cross-sectional studies, multiple large prospective cohort studies have also demonstrated a significant association between poor sleep quality and the incidence of LUTS [71–73]. In 2014, using the Boston Area Community Health survey database, Araujo et al. found that the odds of developing LUTS at five-year follow-up were increased for subjects who reported baseline poor sleep quality and sleep restriction, but the odds of developing sleep problems was only associated with baseline nocturia [72]. Of note, the addition of BMI to the multivariate logistic regression model reduced the association between sleep and incident irritative urinary symptoms, suggesting BMI may be a potential mediator of LUTS [72]. In 2018, Branche et al. conducted a similar study using data from the REDUCE (Reduction by Dutasteride of Prostate Cancer Events) trial. On multivariable analysis, men with worse baseline sleep problems, measured with the Medical Outcomes Study Sleep Scale, were at higher risk for both the development of LUTS at four-year follow-up if they were asymptomatic at baseline and the progression of LUTS if they were symptomatic [71]. An important limitation of these prospective studies was that they only considered baseline sleep scores and did not assess if the change in LUTS correlated with a change in sleep score over time. Despite this, it appears both poor sleep and sleep disturbance due to nonstandard shift work and sleep disorders significantly impact LUTS.

35.4 Sleep and Hypogonadism

Hypogonadism, also called testosterone deficiency, is defined by the AUA as a total testosterone level less than 300 ng/dL on at least two early morning serum samples combined with symptoms consistent with testosterone deficiency, including ED, decreased libido, fatigue, poor concentration, and/or sleep disturbance [74]. Although the relationship between ED alone and sleep is well supported by the evidence, the relationship between hypogonadism and sleep is less clear.

In 1971, Evans et al. first discovered that endogenous testosterone peaks in conjunction with periods of rapid eye movement (REM) sleep [75]. Since then, researchers have continued to investigate the association between testosterone and sleep. Multiple small randomized controlled studies in the 1980s found significant decreases in testosterone levels with extreme sleep deprivation (24 or 48 hours) [76–78]. Unfortunately, more recent controlled and cross-sectional studies assessing the effects of less extreme conditions have had less consistent results [79–88]. For instance, Leproult and Van Cauter found that daytime testosterone levels decreased by 10–15% after 1 week of sleep restriction to 5 hours per night in 10 healthy male volunteers [79]. In contrast, Smith et al. found that neither severe, acute sleep restriction (to 4 hours per night for 5 nights) or mild, chronic sleep restriction (habitual sleep minus 1.5 hours for 6 weeks) significantly affected plasma testosterone levels in 27 healthy men [80]. An important study by Schmid et al. found that while sleep restriction to four hours in the first half of the night (late bedtime) did not result in reduced testosterone, sleep restriction to four hours in the second half of the night (advanced awakening) did result in markedly reduced testosterone [85]. This finding suggests that sleep timing, rather restriction alone, may modulate the effect of sleep loss on testosterone and potentially explain the variation across these studies. In addition to these controlled studies, multiple cross-sectional studies have assessed the association between sleep disorders and testosterone, and it appears neither OSA nor insomnia significantly impact testosterone levels after adjusting for confounders [89–93].

Many researchers have also studied the effects of shift work on both testosterone levels and hypogonadal symptoms [50,94–99]. Despite one small case series of four oil refinery rotating shift workers that demonstrated a significant decrease in mean testosterone compared to dayshift workers [94], the majority of studies do not support an association between shift work alone and serum testosterone [50,96,97]. However, there are a few studies that suggest a potential indirect association. For instance, in a cross-sectional study of 42 male nonstandard shift workers, it was found that those who were dissatisfied with their schedule exhibited lower morning testosterone levels [95]. In an additional cross-sectional study of nonstandard shift workers conducted by Balasubramanian et al., those diagnosed with SWD had a significant lower serum testosterone compared to those without SWD [99]. These studies suggest dissatisfaction with shift schedule likely resulting in stress and SWD are potential mediators associated with serum testosterone.

While the evidence for the impact of sleep on testosterone level is conflicting, there appears to be a notable association between sleep and hypogonadal symptoms. One validated questionnaire frequently used to assess hypogonadal symptoms is the Androgen Deficiency in the Aging Male (ADAM) screening questionnaire [100]. In a cross-sectional study of 409 college-aged males, Charlier et al. found that 35% had a positive ADAM, or met the criteria for potential androgen deficiency, demonstrating an increased prevalence compared to previously established norms in young adult males [98]. Furthermore, by stratifying the participants by ADAM score, they found a significant association between a positive ADAM score and poor sleep quality, as measured by PSQI, in addition to stress levels [98]. Similar cross-sectional studies have also assessed the impact of sleep quality on hypogonadal symptoms in shift workers. Pastuszak et al. found that in a group of 182 men working nonstandard shifts, those who were "somewhat dissatisfied" with their sleep quality had significantly worse hypogonadal symptoms compared to those who were "very satisfied" [50]. In another cross-sectional study, Balasubramanian et al. found that nonstandard shift workers had significantly worse hypogonadal symptoms (ADAM score 1.12 points lower) than daytime workers ($p<0.01$), and nonstandard shift workers with SWD had even worse hypogonadal symptoms (ADAM score 5.47 points lower) than those without SWD [99]. These findings suggest poor sleep quality and SWD may contribute to more severe hypogonadal symptoms in a wide range of populations even if testosterone levels are largely unchanged.

35.5 Sleep and Male Infertility

Male factor infertility is suspected to contribute to approximately 50% of infertility cases worldwide [101]. One of the most important goals of any infertility evaluation is to identify potentially correctable conditions. Many recent studies demonstrate a significant association between sleep and fertility, suggesting poor sleep may be one of the most correctable conditions in male infertility. In contrast to the linear relationships seen between erectile dysfunction, LUTS, hypogonadal symptoms, and sleep, the relationship between fertility and sleep has been described as an inverted U-shape, with both reduced and excessive sleep linked to worse fertility outcomes, including fecundability and various semen parameters [102–105]. In a web-based prospective cohort study of 1,176 couples attempting to conceive, Wise et al. demonstrated a significant inverted U-shaped association between sleep duration and fecundability [102]. Compared to 8 hours of sleep per night, fecundability ratios in men who slept <6, 6, 7, and ≥9 hours were 0.62 (95% CI: 0.45–0.87), 1.06 (95% CI: 0.87–1.30), 0.97 (95% CI: 0.81–1.17), and 0.73 (95% CI: 0.46–1.15), respectively [102]. In a prospective cohort study of 796 male college students, Chen et al. demonstrated an inverse U-shaped association between sleep duration and total sperm number with 7–7.5 hours of sleep per day demonstrating the highest value compared to >9 hours and ≤6 hours. After 1 year, participants who altered their sleep duration toward 7–7.5 hours saw an increase in total sperm number from baseline [105]. In a cross-sectional study assessing sleep quality, Jensen et al. showed an inverted U-shape association between sleep disturbance, as measured by a modified four-item Karolinska Sleep Questionnaire, and semen parameters [104]. In addition, a cross-sectional study by Wang et al. demonstrated an inverted U-shaped association between sleep duration and sperm chromatin integrity [106]. This study not only supports the inverted U-shaped relationship between sleep and fertility, but it also proposes a possible mechanism. While many studies have demonstrated an inverted U-shaped relationship, some studies have instead found a significant linear association between sleep and fertility [88,107–110]. Regardless of the shape of the association, the link between sleep and fertility is clear.

Considering the significant effect shift work can have on sleep, many studies have also investigated the association between shift work and fertility. Although many early studies surveying women about their partners failed to show an association between fecundity and shift work in men [111,112], studies looking more closely at the nature of the work have provided more promising results. In a case-control study, El-Helaly et al. found that both shift work (OR 3.60, 95% CI: 1.12–11.57) and frequent work-related stress (OR 3.76, 95% CI: 1.96–7.52) were significantly increased in infertile males compared to fertile males [113]. In another case-control study, Sheiner et al. found that infertile men were more likely to work in industry and construction compared to fertile men and that industry and construction workers were more likely to work in shifts (OR 3.1, 95% CI: 1.2–8.3) and report physical exertion (OR 3.8, 95% CI: 1.4–7.8) compared to other workers. However, in a prospective cohort study, Eisenberg et al. did not find a significant association between shift work and semen quality but did find that heavy exertion at work was associated with lower semen concentration and total sperm count [114]. While additional longitudinal or interventional studies are needed to fully assess the impact of shift work on male fertility, the association between sleep and fertility is apparent and warrants investigation in fertility clinics.

Although the mechanism for sleep's effect on fertility has yet to be clearly elucidated, one proposed etiology is circadian disruption and changes in endogenous melatonin, a key circadian hormone. In addition to melatonin's indirect action on testicular function via its influence on the hypothalamic-pituitary-gonadal axis, recent studies also suggest a direct effect on testicular function [115]. To investigate the impact of melatonin on fertility, 18 men with idiopathic infertility and nonobstructive azoospermia underwent open testicular biopsy and subsequent histopathological studies. Rossi et al. found that melatonin testicular concentration was negatively correlated with macrophage concentration and inflammatory cytokine expression (TNFα, IL-1β) [116]. In addition, melatonin testicular concentration was positively correlated with antioxidant enzyme expression and decreased reactive oxygen species. Thus, this study supported the anti-inflammatory and antioxidant effects of melatonin. Based on these proposed effects, Bejarano et al. assessed the effects on long-term melatonin (6 mg daily) supplementation in 30 infertile men [117]. After 90 days, there was a significant increase in urinary and seminal antioxidant capacity in addition to a decrease in percentage of apoptotic sperm in ejaculate and sperm DNA fragmentation, and in vitro fertilization demonstrated significant embryo quality improvement [117]. These results suggest a potential beneficial role of melatonin in the treatment of male infertility although additional studies are needed. A potential future study could assess if these same beneficial effects of exogenous melatonin could be attained with endogenous changes in melatonin through light therapy.

35.6 Screening for Sleep Deficiency and Management

Given the increasing prevalence of sleep disturbance in today's modern society and the increasing evidence of a strong link between sleep and men's health, screening for sleep deficiency and sleep disorders has never been more important [118]. In fact, recent studies have found that approximately 50% of adult males presenting to a men's health clinic are considered at high risk for OSA or other sleep disorders and warrant further testing [119,120]. Based on this increased risk, men's health or andrology clinics provide an excellent opportunity to screen for unrecognized OSA and other sleep disorders.

Although one can evaluate for sleep disorders and sleep deficiency by simply asking "how are you sleeping?," a more objective assessment can be achieved with the use of standardized questionnaires. Multiple questionnaires can be used to identify individuals at high risk for sleep apnea. However, the STOP-Bang questionnaire has the highest sensitivity and is easily implemented in the clinic [121]. It is composed of eight dichotomous (yes/no) questions related to snoring, tiredness, observed apnea, high blood pressure, BMI, age, neck circumference, and male gender for a total score ranging from 0 to 8 [122]. Patients with a positive screening test should be referred to a primary care physician or sleep specialist for definitive diagnosis with polysomnography and management of OSA with CPAP. Treatment of OSA is essential due to the many potential adverse consequences of untreated OSA, including hypertension, diabetes, coronary heart disease, stroke, and increased all-cause mortality [123]. In addition, treatment of OSA may also improve ED and LUTS. Screening for other sleep disorders and sleep deficiencies can be accomplished with the PSQI. The PSQI is composed of 19 questions that generate seven "component" scores: subjective sleep quality, sleep latency, sleep duration, habitual sleep efficiency, sleep disturbances, use of sleep medication, and daytime dysfunction [124]. Each of the components is scored out of 3, providing an overall score ranging from 0 to 21 [124]. While individuals with more severe deficits can be referred to a primary care physician or sleep specialist for further assessment and treatment, those with less severe deficits may benefit from improved sleep hygiene alone.

Sleep hygiene is an important intervention for common sleep problems that do not meet the definition of clinical sleep disorder, including prolonged sleep onset latency, excessive wake after sleep onset, short total sleep time, low sleep efficiency, and poor sleep quality [125]. Sleep hygiene includes a variety of practices and habits that promote quality sleep and daytime alertness [27]. Such practices include increased daytime exposure to sunlight, regular exercise, avoiding daytime naps, avoiding caffeine before bed, maintaining a regular sleep schedule, limiting electronic screen light before bedtime, and relaxing activities before bedtime [125]. In addition to improving sleep quality, two recent studies have suggested an association between sleep hygiene and improved male urologic outcomes. In a cross-sectional study, Bates et al. demonstrated that men with better sleep hygiene had significantly improved LUTS compared to those with poor sleep hygiene [126]. In a similar cross-sectional study, Kohn et al. found a significant association between better sleep hygiene and improved erectile function [127]. Given these results and the importance of sleep on overall health, sleep hygiene education is a no-cost, no-risk intervention that can be easily incorporated into men's health clinics and may be beneficial in the management of common presenting symptoms.

35.7 Conclusions

In this chapter, we have reviewed the literature on the effect of sleep and shift work on ED, LUTS, hypogonadism, and male infertility. In all cases, poor sleep has demonstrated a negative impact. While some studies suggest shift work is associated with more severe presentations of these conditions, this is likely secondary to the quality of the work and sleep problems related to shift work, as men with SWD have demonstrated more significant symptoms compared to those without SWD. Given these findings and the increased risk of sleep disorders in men presenting to men's health clinics, universal screening for OSA, other sleep disorders, and overall poor sleep should be performed. Management of sleep disorders and improved sleep hygiene are important interventions that can improve sleep quality and possibly improve common men's health conditions.

References

1. Krueger JM, Frank MG, Wisor JP, Roy S. Sleep function: toward elucidating an enigma. *Sleep Med Rev.* 2016;28:46–54. doi:10.1016/j.smrv.2015.08.005.
2. Centers for Disease Control and Prevention. Short sleep duration among US adults. www.cdc.gov/sleep/data_statistics.html. Updated 2017. Accessed June 26, 2020.
3. Watson NF, Badr MS, Belenky G, et al. Joint consensus statement of the American Academy of Sleep Medicine and Sleep Research Society on the recommended amount of sleep for a healthy adult: methodology and

4. Luyster FS, Strollo PJ, Zee PC, Walsh JK. Sleep: a health imperative. *Sleep.* 2012;35(6):727–734. doi:10.5665/sleep.1846.
5. McMenamin TM. A time to work: recent trends in shift work and flexible schedules. *Mon Labor Rev.* 2007;130(12):3–15. www.scopus.com/inward/record.uri?eid=2-s2.0-39749201717&partnerID=40&md5=394413e24b44176f8bcdb03b6e58a218. Accessed June 27, 2020.
6. Åkerstedt T, Wright KP. Sleep loss and fatigue in shift work and shift work disorder. *Sleep Med Clin.* 2009;4(2):257–271. doi: 10.1016/j.jsmc.2009.03.001.
7. Sateia MJ. International classification of sleep disorders – third edition. *Chest.* 2014;146(5):1387–1394. doi:10.1378/chest.14-0970.
8. Drake CL, Roehrs T, Richardson G, Walsh JK, Roth T. Shift work sleep disorder: prevalence and consequences beyond that of symptomatic day workers. *Sleep.* 2004;27(8):1453–1462. doi:10.1093/sleep/27.8.1453.
9. Vanttola P, Puttonen S, Karhula K, Oksanen T, Härmä M. Prevalence of shift work disorder among hospital personnel: a cross-sectional study using objective working hour data. *J Sleep Res.* 2019;29(3):e12906. doi:10.1111/jsr.12906.
10. Fekedulegn D, Burchfiel CM, Hartley TA, et al. Shiftwork and sickness absence among police officers: the BCOPS study. *Chronobiol Int.* 2013;30(7):930–941. doi:10.3109/07420528.2013.790043.
11. Nätti J, Oinas T, Härmä M, Anttila T, Kandolin I. Combined effects of shiftwork and individual working time control on long-term sickness absence: a prospective study of Finnish employees. *J Occup Environ Med.* 2014;56(7):732–738. doi:10.1097/JOM.0000000000000176.
12. Lockley SW, Barger LK, Ayas NT, Rothschild JM, Czeisler CA, Landrigan CP. Effects of health care provider work hours and sleep deprivation on safety and performance. *Jt Comm J Qual Patient Saf.* 2007;33(Suppl. 11):7–18. doi:10.1016/S1553-7250(07)33109-7.
13. Keller SM. Effects of extended work shifts and shift work on patient safety, productivity, and employee health. *AAOHN J.* 2009;57(12):497–504. doi:10.3928/08910162-20091116-01.
14. Garbarino S, De Carli F, Nobili L, et al. Sleepiness and sleep disorders in shift workers: a study on a group of Italian police officers. *Sleep.* 2002;25(6):648–653. www.scopus.com/inward/record.uri?eid=2-s2.0-0037105031&partnerID=40&md5=ab041b7db1a8e5f30a104d7b96fe1b49. Accessed June 27, 2020.
15. Gan Y, Yang C, Tong X, et al. Shift work and diabetes mellitus: a meta-analysis of observational studies. *Occup Environ Med.* 2015;72(1):72–78. doi:10.1136/oemed-2014-102150.
16. Ika K, Suzuki E, Mitsuhashi T, Takao S, Doi H. Shift work and diabetes mellitus among male workers in Japan: does the intensity of shift work matter? *Acta Med Okayama.* 2013;67(1):25–33. doi:10.18926/AMO/49254.
17. Hansen AB, Stayner L, Hansen J, Andersen ZJ. Night shift work and incidence of diabetes in the Danish nurse cohort. *Occup Environ Med.* 2016;73(4):262–268. doi:10.1136/oemed-2015-103342.
18. Alefishat E, Abu Farha R. Is shift work associated with lipid disturbances and increased insulin resistance? *Metab Syndr Relat Disord.* 2015;13(9):400–405. doi:10.1089/met.2015.0052.
19. Kawachi I, Colditz GA, Stampfer MJ, et al. Prospective study of shift work and risk of coronary heart disease in women. *Circulation.* 1995;92(11):3178–3182. doi:10.1161/01.CIR.92.11.3178.
20. Vetter C, Devore EE, Wegrzyn LR, et al. Association between rotating night shift work and risk of coronary heart disease among women. *JAMA.* 2016;315(16):1726–1734. doi:10.1001/jama.2016.4454.
21. Ceïde ME, Pandey A, Ravenell J, Donat M, Ogedegbe G, Girardin JL. Associations of short sleep and shift work status with hypertension among black and white Americans. *Int J Hypertens.* 2015;2015:697275. doi:10.1155/2015/697275.
22. Ohlander J, Keskin M, Stork J, Radon K. Shift work and hypertension: prevalence and analysis of disease pathways in a German car manufacturing company. *Am J Ind Med.* 2015;58(5):549–560. doi:10.1002/ajim.22437.
23. Guo Y, Liu Y, Huang X, et al. The effects of shift work on sleeping quality, hypertension and diabetes in retired workers. *PLoS ONE.* 2013;8(8):e71107. doi:10.1371/journal.pone.0071107.
24. Lee HY, Kim MS, Kim O, Lee I, Kim H. Association between shift work and severity of depressive symptoms among female nurses: the Korea nurses' health study. *J Nurs Manag.* 2016;24(2):192–200. doi:10.1111/jonm.12298.
25. Park JN, Han MA, Park J, Ryu SY. Prevalence of depressive symptoms and related factors in Korean employees: The third Korean working conditions survey (2011). *Int J Environ Res Public Health.* 2016;13(4):424. doi:10.3390/ijerph13040424.
26. Deng N, Kohn TP, Lipshultz LI, Pastuszak AW. The relationship between shift work and men's health. *Sex Med Rev.* 2018;6(3):446–456. doi: S2050-0521(17)30150-6.
27. Kohn TP, Kohn JR, Haney NM, Pastuszak AW, Lipshultz LI. The effect of sleep on men's health. *Transl Androl Urol.* 2020;9:S178–S185. doi:10.21037/tau.2019.11.07.
28. Feldman HA, Irwin G, Hatzichristou DG, Krane RJ, McKinlay JB. Impotence and its medical and psychosocial correlates: results of the Massachusetts male aging study. *J Urol.* 1994;151(1):54–61. doi:10.1016/S0022-5347(17)34871-1.
29. Saigal CS, Wessells H, Pace J, Schonlau M, Wilt TJ. Predictors and prevalence of erectile dysfunction in a racially diverse population. *Arch Intern Med.* 2006;166(2):207–212. doi:10.1001/archinte.166.2.207.
30. American Academy of Sleep Medicine Taskforce. Sleep-related breathing disorders in adults: recommendations for syndrome definition and measurement techniques in clinical research. *Sleep.* 1999;22(5):667–689. doi:10.1093/sleep/22.5.667.
31. Margel D, Cohen M, Livne PM, Pillar G. Severe, but not mild, obstructive sleep apnea syndrome is associated with erectile dysfunction. *Urology.* 2004;63(3):545–549. doi:10.1016/j.urology.2003.10.016.
32. Heruti R, Shochat T, Tekes-Manova D, Ashkenazi I, Justo D. Association between erectile dysfunction and sleep

disorders measured by self-assessment questionnaires in adult men. *J Sex Med.* 2005;2(4):543–550. doi:10.1111/j.1743-6109.2005.00072.x.

33. Budweiser S, Enderlein S, Jörres RA, et al. Sleep apnea is an independent correlate of erectile and sexual dysfunction. *J Sex Med.* 2009;6(11):3147–3157. doi:10.1111/j.1743-6109.2009.01372.x.

34. Teloken PE, Smith EB, Lodowsky C, Freedom T, Mulhall JP. Defining association between sleep apnea syndrome and erectile dysfunction. *Urology.* 2006;67(5):1033–1037. doi:10.1016/j.urology.2005.11.040.

35. Zheng W, Chen X, Huang J, et al. Blood oxygen accumulation distribution area index is associated with erectile dysfunction in patients with sleep apnea: results from a cross-sectional study. *Sex Med.* 2020;8(1):36–44. doi:10.1016/j.esxm.2019.11.001.

36. İrer B, Çelikhisar A, Çelikhisar H, Bozkurt O, Demir Ö. Evaluation of sexual dysfunction, lower urinary tract symptoms and quality of life in men with obstructive sleep apnea syndrome and the efficacy of continuous positive airway pressure therapy. *Urology.* 2018;121:86–92. doi:10.1016/j.urology.2018.08.001.

37. Andersen ML, Santos-Silva R, Bittencourt LRA, Tufik S. Prevalence of erectile dysfunction complaints associated with sleep disturbances in Sao Paulo, Brazil: a population-based survey. *Sleep Med.* 2010;11(10):1019–1024. doi:10.1016/j.sleep.2009.08.016.

38. Kellesarian SV, Malignaggi VR, Feng C, Javed F. Association between obstructive sleep apnea and erectile dysfunction: a systematic review and meta-analysis. *Int J Impot Res.* 2018;30(3):129–140. doi:10.1038/s41443-018-0017-7.

39. Bozorgmehri S, Fink HA, Parimi N, et al. Association of sleep disordered breathing with erectile dysfunction in community dwelling older men. *J Urol.* 2017;197(3):776–782. doi:10.1016/j.juro.2016.09.089.

40. Seehuus M, Pigeon W. The sleep and sex survey: relationships between sexual function and sleep. *J Psychosom Res.* 2018;112:59–65. doi:10.1016/j.jpsychores.2018.07.005.

41. Le HH, Salas RME, Gamaldo A, et al. The utility and feasibility of assessing sleep disruption in a men's health clinic using a mobile health platform device: a pilot study. *Int J Clin Pract.* 2018;72(1):e12999. doi:10.1111/ijcp.12999.

42. Soterio-Pires JH, Hirotsu C, Kim LJ, Bittencourt L, Tufik S, Andersen ML. The interaction between erectile dysfunction complaints and depression in men: a cross-sectional study about sleep, hormones and quality of life. *Int J Impot Res.* 2017;29(2):70–75. doi:10.1038/ijir.2016.49.

43. Gao X, Schwarzschild MA, O'Reilly EJ, Wang H, Ascherio A. Restless legs syndrome and erectile dysfunction. *Sleep.* 2010;33(1):75–79. doi:10.1093/sleep/33.1.75.

44. Li Y, Batool-Anwar S, Kim S, Rimm EB, Ascherio A, Gao X. Prospective study of restless legs syndrome and risk of erectile dysfunction. *Am J Epidemiol.* 2013;177(10):1097–1105. doi:10.1093/aje/kws364.

45. Pascual M, Batlle Jd, Barbé F, et al. Erectile dysfunction in obstructive sleep apnea patients: a randomized trial on the effects of continuous positive airway pressure (CPAP). *PLoS ONE.* 2018;13(8):e0201930. doi:10.1371/journal.pone.0201930.

46. Jara SM, Hopp ML, Weaver EM. Association of continuous positive airway pressure treatment with sexual quality of life in patients with sleep apnea: follow-up study of a randomized clinical trial. *JAMA Otolaryngol Head Neck Surg.* 2018;144(7):587–593. doi:10.1001/jamaoto.2018.0485.

47. Melehan KL, Hoyos CM, Hamilton GS, et al. Randomized trial of CPAP and vardenafil on erectile and arterial function in men with obstructive sleep apnea and erectile dysfunction. *J Clin Endocrinol Metab.* 2018;103(4):1601–1611. doi:10.1210/jc.2017-02389.

48. Pastore AL, Palleschi G, Ripoli A, et al. Severe obstructive sleep apnoea syndrome and erectile dysfunction: a prospective randomised study to compare sildenafil vs. nasal continuous positive airway pressure. *Int J Clin Pract.* 2014;68(8):995–1000. doi:10.1111/ijcp.12463.

49. Li Z, Fang Z, Xing N, Zhu S, Fan Y. The effect of CPAP and PDE5i on erectile function in men with obstructive sleep apnea and erectile dysfunction: a systematic review and meta-analysis. *Sleep Med Rev.* 2019;48:101217. doi:S1087-0792(19)30185-6.

50. Pastuszak AW, Moon YM, Scovell J, et al. Poor sleep quality predicts hypogonadal symptoms and sexual dysfunction in male nonstandard shift workers. *Urology.* 2017;102:121–125. doi:10.1016/j.urology.2016.11.033.

51. Rodriguez KM, Kohn TP, Kohn JR, et al. Pd27-06 shift work sleep disorder and night shift work significantly impair erectile function. *J Urol.* 2018;199(4):e559. doi:10.1016/j.juro.2018.02.1357.

52. Taylor BC, Wilt TJ, Fink HA, et al. Prevalence, severity, and health correlates of lower urinary tract symptoms among older men: the MrOS study. *Urology.* 2006;68(4):804–809. doi:10.1016/j.urology.2006.04.019.

53. Lepor H. Pathophysiology of lower urinary tract symptoms in the aging male population. *Rev Urol.* 2005;7(Suppl. 7):S3–S11. www.ncbi.nlm.nih.gov/pubmed/16986059.

54. Bates J, Kohn T, Rodriguez K, et al. Pd65-08: poor sleep quality is associated with clinically significant lower urinary tract symptoms. *J Urol.* 2019;201:e1189–e1190. doi:10.1097/01.JU.0000557582.48673.b0.

55. Martin SA, Appleton SL, Adams RJ, et al. Nocturia, other lower urinary tract symptoms and sleep dysfunction in a community-dwelling cohort of men. *Urology.* 2016;97:219–226. doi.org/10.1016/j.urology.2016.06.022.

56. Arslan B, Gezmis CT, Çetin B, et al. Is obstructive sleep apnea syndrome related to nocturia? *Low Urin Tract Symptoms.* 2019;11(3):139–142. doi:10.1111/luts.12250.

57. Miyauchi Y, Okazoe H, Tamaki M, et al. Obstructive sleep apnea syndrome as a potential cause of nocturia in younger adults. *Urology.* 2020;143:42–47. doi:10.1016/j.urology.2020.04.116.

58. Everaert K, Anderson P, Wood R, Andersson FL, Holm-Larsen T. Nocturia is more bothersome than daytime LUTS: results from an observational, real-life practice database including 8659 European and American LUTS patients. *Int J Clin Pract.* 2018;72(6):e13091. doi:10.1111/ijcp.13091.

59. Doo SW, Lee HJ, Ahn J, et al. Strong impact of nocturia on sleep quality in patients with lower urinary tract

60. Obayashi K, Saeki K, Kurumatani N. Quantitative association between nocturnal voiding frequency and objective sleep quality in the general elderly population: the HEIJO-KYO cohort. *Sleep Medicine*. 2015;16(5):577–582. doi:10.1016/j.sleep.2015.01.021.

61. Fantus RJ, Packiam VT, Wang CH, Erickson BA, Helfand BT. The relationship between sleep disorders and lower urinary tract symptoms: results from the NHANES. *J Urol*. 2018;200(1):161–166. doi:10.1016/j.juro.2018.01.083.

62. Miyauchi Y, Okazoe H, Okujyo M, et al. Effect of the continuous positive airway pressure on the nocturnal urine volume or night-time frequency in patients with obstructive sleep apnea syndrome. *Urology*. 2015;85(2):333–336. doi:10.1016/j.urology.2014.11.002.

63. Fernández-Pello S, Gil R, Escaf S, et al. Síntomas de tramo urinario inferior y síndrome de apnea obstructiva del sueño: evolución urodinámica antes y después de un año de tratamiento con presión continua positiva de la vía aérea. *Actas Urológicas Españolas*. 2019;43(7):371–377. doi:10.1016/j.acuro.2019.03.004.

64. Park HK, Paick SH, Kim HG, et al. Nocturia improvement with surgical correction of sleep apnea. *Int Neurourol J*. 2016;20(4):329–334. doi:10.5213/inj.1632624.312.

65. Shimizu N, Nozawa M, Sugimoto K, et al. Therapeutic efficacy and anti-inflammatory effect of ramelteon in patients with insomnia associated with lower urinary tract symptoms. *Res Rep Urol*. 2013;5:113–119. doi:10.2147/RRU.S44502.

66. Takao T, Tsujimura A, Kiuchi H, Takezawa K, Nonomura N, Miyagawa Y. Improvement of nocturia and sleep disturbance by silodosin in male patients with lower urinary tract symptoms. *Int J Urol*. 2015;22(2):236–238. doi:10.1111/iju.12638.

67. Sakuma T, Sato K, Nagane Y, et al. Effects of α1-blockers for lower urinary tract symptoms and sleep disorders in patients with benign prostatic hyperplasia. *Lower Urin Tract Symptoms*. 2010;2(2):119–122. doi:10.1111/j.1757-5672.2010.00073.x.

68. Kim JW. Effect of shift work on nocturia. *Urology*. 2016;87:153–160. doi:10.1016/j.urology.2015.07.047.

69. Sigalos JT, Kohn TP, Cartagenova L, et al. Shift workers with shift work disorder have worse lower urinary tract symptoms. *Urology*. 2019;128:66–70. doi:10.1016/j.urology.2019.02.025.

70. Scovell JM, Pastuszak AW, Slawin J, Badal J, Link RE, Lipshultz LI. Impaired sleep quality is associated with more significant lower urinary tract symptoms in male shift workers. *Urology*. 2017;99:197–202. doi:10.1016/j.urology.2016.05.076.

71. Branche BL, Howard LE, Moreira DM, et al. Sleep problems are associated with development and progression of lower urinary tract symptoms: results from REDUCE. *J Urol*. 2018;199(2):536–542. doi:10.1016/j.juro.2017.08.108.

72. Araujo AB, Yaggi HK, Yang M, McVary KT, Fang SC, Bliwise DL. Sleep related problems and urological symptoms: testing the hypothesis of bidirectionality in a longitudinal, population based study. *J Urol*. 2014;191(1):100–106. doi:S0022-5347(13)04886-6.

73. Fukunaga A, Kawaguchi T, Funada S, et al. Sleep disturbance worsens lower urinary tract symptoms: the Nagahama study. *J Urol*. 2019;202(2):354. doi:10.1097/JU.0000000000000212.

74. Mulhall JP, Trost LW, Brannigan RE, et al. Evaluation and management of testosterone deficiency: AUA guideline. *J Urol*. 2018;200(2):423–432. doi:S0022-5347(18)42817-0.

75. Evans JI, MacLean AW, Ismail AA, Love D. Concentrations of plasma testosterone in normal men during sleep. *Nature*. 1971;229(5282):261–262. doi:10.1038/229261a0.

76. Åkerstedt T, Palmblad J, de la Torre B, Marana R, Gillberg M. Adrenocortical and gonadal steroids during sleep deprivation. *Sleep*. 1980;3(1):23–30. doi:10.1093/sleep/3.1.23.

77. Cortés-Gallegos V, Castañeda G, Alonso R, et al. Sleep deprivation reduces circulating androgens in healthy men. *Arch Androl*. 1983;10(1):33–37. doi:10.3109/01485018308990167.

78. González-Santos MR, Gajá-Rodríguez OV, Alonso-Uriarte R, Sojo-Aranda I, Cortés-Gallegos V. Sleep deprivation and adaptive hormonal responses of healthy men. *Arch Androl*. 1989;22(3):203–207. doi:10.3109/01485018908986773.

79. Leproult R, Van Cauter E. Effect of 1 week of sleep restriction on testosterone levels in young healthy men. *JAMA*. 2011;305(21):2173–2174. doi:10.1001/jama.2011.710.

80. Smith I, Salazar I, RoyChoudhury A, St-Onge MP. Sleep restriction and testosterone concentrations in young healthy males: randomized controlled studies of acute and chronic short sleep. *Sleep Health*. 2019;5(6):580–586. doi:S2352-7218(19)30139-1.

81. Jauch-Chara K, Schmid SM, Hallschmid M, Oltmanns KM, Schultes B. Pituitary-gonadal and pituitary-thyroid axis hormone concentrations before and during a hypoglycemic clamp after sleep deprivation in healthy men. *PLoS ONE*. 2013;8(1):e54209. doi:10.1371/journal.pone.0054209.

82. Arnal PJ, Drogou C, Sauvet F, et al. Effect of sleep extension on the subsequent testosterone, cortisol and prolactin responses to total sleep deprivation and recovery. *J Neuroendocrinol*. 2016;28(2). doi:10.1111/jne.12346.

83. Luboshitzky R, Zabari Z, Shen-Orr Z, Herer P, Lavie P. Disruption of the nocturnal testosterone rhythm by sleep fragmentation in normal men. *J Clin Endocrinol Metab*. 2001;86(3):1134–1139. doi:10.1210/jcem.86.3.7296.

84. Reynolds AC, Dorrian J, Liu PY, et al. Impact of five nights of sleep restriction on glucose metabolism, leptin and testosterone in young adult men. *PLoS ONE*. 2012;7(7):e41218. doi:10.1371/journal.pone.0041218.

85. Schmid SM, Hallschmid M, Jauch-Chara K, Lehnert H, Schultes B. Sleep timing may modulate the effect of sleep loss on testosterone. *Clin Endocrinol (Oxf)*. 2012;77(5):749–754. doi:10.1111/j.1365-2265.2012.04419.x.

86. Patel P, Shiff B, Kohn TP, Ramasamy R. Impaired sleep is associated with low testosterone in US adult males: results from the National Health and Nutrition Examination Survey. *World J Urol*. 2019;37(7):1449–1453. doi:10.1007/s00345-018-2485-2.

87. Penev PD. Association between sleep and morning testosterone levels in older men. *Sleep*. 2007;30(4):427–432. doi:10.1093/sleep/30.4.427.

88. Du C, Yang Y, Chen J, Feng L, Lin W. Association between sleep quality and semen parameters and reproductive hormones: a cross-sectional study in Zhejiang, China. *Nat Sci Sleep*. 2020;12:11–18. doi:10.2147/NSS.S235136.

89. Mohammadi H, Rezaei M, Sharafkhaneh A, Khazaie H, Ghadami MR. Serum testosterone/cortisol ratio in people with obstructive sleep apnea. *J Clin Lab Anal*. 2020;34(1):e23011. doi:10.1002/jcla.23011.

90. Mohammadi H, Rezaei M, Faghihi F, Khazaie H. Hypothalamic–pituitary–gonadal activity in paradoxical and psychophysiological insomnia. *J Med Signals Sens*. 2019;9(1):59–67. doi:10.4103/jmss.JMSS_31_18.

91. Auyeung TW, Kwok T, Leung J, et al. Sleep duration and disturbances were associated with testosterone level, muscle mass, and muscle strength: a cross-sectional study in 1274 older men. *J Am Med Dir Assoc*. 2015;16(7):630. e1–630.e6. doi:S1525-8610(15)00294-7.

92. Brigette MC, Andrew DV, Martin S, et al. Obstructive sleep apnea is not an independent determinant of testosterone in men. *Eur J Endocrinol*. 2020;183(1):31–39. doi:10.1530/EJE-19-0978.

93. Wittert G. The relationship between sleep disorders and testosterone in men. *Asian J Androl*. 2014;16(2):262–265. doi:10.4103/1008-682X.122586.

94. Touitou Y, Motohashi Y, Reinberg A, et al. Effect of shift work on the nighttime secretory patterns of melatonin, prolactin, cortisol and testosterone. *Eur J Appl Physiol Occup Physiol*. 1990;60(4):288–292. doi:10.1007/BF00379398.

95. Axelsson J, Åkerstedt T, Kecklund G, Lindqvist A, Attefors R. Hormonal changes in satisfied and dissatisfied shift workers across a shift cycle. *J Appl Physiol*. 2003;95(5):2099–2105. doi:10.1152/japplphysiol.00231.2003.

96. Smith AM, Morris P, Rowell KO, Clarke S, Jones TH, Channer KS. Junior doctors and the full shift rota – psychological and hormonal changes: a comparative cross-sectional study. *Clin Med*. 2006;6(2):174–177. doi:10.7861/clinmedicine.6-2-174.

97. Jensen MA, Hansen ÅM, Kristiansen J, Nabe-Nielsen K, Garde AH. Changes in the diurnal rhythms of cortisol, melatonin, and testosterone after 2, 4, and 7 consecutive night shifts in male police officers. *Chronobiol Int*. 2016;33(9):1280–1292. doi:10.1080/07420528.2016.1212869.

98. Charlier CM, Barr ML, Colby SE, Greene GW, Olfert MD. Correlations of self-reported androgen deficiency in ageing males (ADAM) with stress and sleep among young adult males. *Healthcare (Basel, Switzerland)*. 2018;6(4):121. doi:10.3390/healthcare6040121.

99. Balasubramanian A, Kohn TP, Santiago JE, et al. Increased risk of hypogonadal symptoms in shift workers with shift work sleep disorder. *Urology*. 2020;138:52–59. doi:10.1016/j.urology.2019.10.040.

100. Morley JE, Charlton E, Patrick P, et al. Validation of a screening questionnaire for androgen deficiency in aging males. *Metabolism*. 2000;49(9):1239–1242. doi:S0026-0495(00)25964-7.

101. Jarow JP, Sharlip ID, Belker AM, et al. Best practice policies for male infertility. *J Urol*. 2002;167(5):2138–2144. doi:S0022-5347(05)65109-9.

102. Wise LA, Rothman KJ, Wesselink AK, et al. Male sleep duration and fecundability in a North American preconception cohort study. *Fertil Steril*. 2018;109(3):453–459. doi:10.1016/j.fertnstert.2017.11.037.

103. Kohn TP, Pastuszak A. Shift work is associated with altered semen parameters in infertile men. *Fertil Steril*. 2017;108(3):E323–E324. doi:10.1016/j.fertnstert.2017.07.956.

104. Jensen TK, Andersson A, Skakkebæk NE, et al. Association of sleep disturbances with reduced semen quality: a cross-sectional study among 953 healthy young Danish men. *Am J Epidemiol*. 2013;177(10):1027–1037. doi:10.1093/aje/kws420.

105. Chen Q, Yang H, Zhou N, et al. Inverse U-shaped association between sleep duration and semen quality: longitudinal observational study (MARHCS) in Chongqing, China. *Sleep*. 2016;39(1):79–86. doi:10.5665/sleep.5322.

106. Wang X, Chen Q, Zou P, et al. Sleep duration is associated with sperm chromatin integrity among young men in Chongqing, China. *J Sleep Res*. 2018;27(4):e12615. doi:10.1111/jsr.12615.

107. Hvidt JEM, Knudsen UB, Zachariae R, Ingerslev HJ, Philipsen MT, Frederiksen Y. Associations of bedtime, sleep duration, and sleep quality with semen quality in males seeking fertility treatment: a preliminary study. *Basic Clin Androl*. 2020;30:5–7. doi:10.1186/s12610-020-00103-7.

108. Liu MM, Liu L, Chen L, et al. Sleep deprivation and late bedtime impair sperm health through increasing antisperm antibody production: a prospective study of 981 healthy men. *Med Sci Monit*. 2017;23:1842–1848. doi:10.12659/msm.900101.

109. Green A, Barak S, Shine L, Kahane A, Dagan Y. Exposure by males to light emitted from media devices at night is linked with decline of sperm quality and correlated with sleep quality measures. *Chronobiol Int*. 2020;37(3):414–424. doi:10.1080/07420528.2020.1727918.

110. Chen H, Sun B, Chen Y, et al. Sleep duration and quality in relation to semen quality in healthy men screened as potential sperm donors. *Environ Int*. 2020;135:105368. doi:10.1016/j.envint.2019.105368.

111. Bisanti L, Olsen J, Basso O, Thonneau P, Karmaus W. The European Study Group on Infertility, and Subfecundity. Shift work and subfecundity: a European multicenter study. *J Occup Environ Med*. 1996;38(4):352–358. doi:10.1097/00043764-199604000-00012.

112. Tuntiseranee P, Olsen J, Geater A, Kor-anantakul O. Are long working hours and shiftwork risk factors for subfecundity? A study among couples from Southern Thailand. *Occup Environ Med*. 1998;55(2):99–105. doi:10.1136/oem.55.2.99.

113. El-Helaly M, Awadalla N, Mansour M, El-Biomy Y. Workplace exposures and male infertility: a case-control study. *Int J Occup Med Environ Health*. 2010;23(4):331–338. doi:10.2478/v10001-010-0039-y.

114. Eisenberg ML, Chen Z, Ye A, Buck Louis GM. Relationship between physical occupational exposures and health on semen quality: data from the Longitudinal Investigation of Fertility and the Environment (LIFE) study. *Fertil Steril*. 2015;103(5):1271–1277. doi:10.1016/j.fertnstert.2015.02.010.

115. Palnitkar G, Phillips CL, Hoyos CM, Marren AJ, Bowman MC, Yee BJ. Linking sleep disturbance to idiopathic male infertility. *Sleep Med Rev*.

116. Rossi SP, Windschuettl S, Matzkin ME, et al. Melatonin in testes of infertile men: evidence for anti-proliferative and anti-oxidant effects on local macrophage and mast cell populations. *Andrology*. 2014;2(3):436–449. doi:10.1111/j.2047-2927.2014.00207.x.

117. Bejarano I, Monllor F, Marchena AM, et al. Exogenous melatonin supplementation prevents oxidative stress-evoked DNA damage in human spermatozoa. *J Pineal Res*. 2014;57(3):333–339. doi:10.1111/jpi.12172.

118. Colten HR, Altevogt BM, Institute of Medicine (US) Committee on Sleep Medicine and Research. Extent and health consequences of chronic sleep loss and sleep disorders. In: *Sleep Disorders and Sleep Deprivation: An Unmet Public Health Problem*. National Academies Press; 2006. www.ncbi.nlm.nih.gov/books/NBK19961/. Accessed July 2, 2020.

119. Walia AS, Lomeli, LJM, Jiang P, Benca R, Yafi FA. Patients presenting to a men's health clinic are at higher risk for depression, insomnia, and sleep apnea. *Int J Impotence Res*. 2019;31(1):39–45. doi:10.1038/s41443-018-0057-z.

120. Kalejaiye O, Raheem AA, Moubasher A, et al. Sleep disorders in patients with erectile dysfunction. *BJU Int*. 2017;120(6):855–860. doi:10.1111/bju.13961.

121. Pataka A, Daskalopoulou E, Kalamaras G, Fekete Passa K, Argyropoulou P. Evaluation of five different questionnaires for assessing sleep apnea syndrome in a sleep clinic. *Sleep Med*. 2014;15(7):776–781. doi:S1389-9457(14)00147-6.

122. Chung F, Abdullah HR, Liao P. STOP-Bang questionnaire: a practical approach to screen for obstructive sleep apnea. *Chest*. 2016;149(3):631–638. doi:10.1378/chest.15-0903.

123. Kim SD, Cho KS. Obstructive sleep apnea and testosterone deficiency. *W J Mens Health*. 2019;37(1):12–18. doi:10.5534/wjmh.180017.

124. Buysse DJ, Reynolds CF, Monk TH, Berman SR, Kupfer DJ. The Pittsburgh Sleep Quality Index: a new instrument for psychiatric practice and research. *Psychiatry Res*. 1989;28(2):193–213. doi:10.1016/0165-1781(89)90047-4.

125. Irish LA, Kline CE, Gunn HE, Buysse DJ, Hall MH. The role of sleep hygiene in promoting public health: a review of empirical evidence. *Sleep Med Rev*. 2015;22:23–36. doi:10.1016/j.smrv.2014.10.001.

126. Bates J, Kohn T, Rodriguez K, et al. PD65-08 poor sleep quality is associated with clinically significant lower urinary tract symptoms. *J Urol*. 2019;201:1189–1190. doi:10.21037/tau.2019.11.07.

127. Kohn TP, Rodriguez KM, Sigalos JT, et al. PD27-08 poor sleep quality is associated with clinically significant erectile dysfunction. *J Urol*. 2018;199:e560. doi:10.1016/j.juro.2018.02.1359.

Chapter 36

Molecular Biology and Physiology of Erectile Function and Dysfunction

James L. Liu, Arthur L. Burnett, and Amin S. Herati

36.1 Introduction

Erectile dysfunction (ED) refers to the inability to achieve or maintain an erection for satisfactory sexual performance. It is highly prevalent among aging men and can have significant impact on quality of life and interpersonal relationships [1]. It was estimated in 2000 that as many as 18 million Americans aged 40–70 have some degree of ED with a growing incidence rate of 26 new cases per 1,000 annually [1]. Similar projections suggest that by the year 2025, global prevalence may be as high as 322 million [2]. ED has well-established associations with poor general health including cardiovascular disease and diabetes, lifestyle factors, and even low socioeconomic status [3]. Therefore, identification of ED offers a glimpse into men's health, illuminating underlying illness and providing opportunities to intervene in otherwise asymptomatic men.

Over the last several decades there have been major advances in our understanding of erection physiology from the neural pathways of the sympathetic and parasympathetic nervous system down to the biochemical effectors such as nitric oxide (NO), Ras homologue A (RhoA), and cyclic adenosine monophosphate (cAMP). These discoveries have helped us better understand pathophysiology and develop a number of effective pharmacotherapies. The aim of this chapter is to summarize the anatomical and molecular biology of erectile function, highlighting the dynamic interplay of multiple neurochemical pathways that enable male potency.

36.2 Physiology of Erectile Function

Penile erection requires a highly coordinated process mediated by the nervous system, vascular smooth muscle tone regulation, and balancing pro-erectile and anti-erectile molecular mediators [3–4]. The penis is composed of three cylinders of erectile tissue: the corpus spongiosum that surrounds the urethra and is continuous with the glans penis and paired corpora cavernosa. The corpora cavernosa are found dorsally, encased by the dense tunica albuginea, and act as a vascular reservoir composed of trabeculae sinuses supplied by helicine arterioles from the deep penile cavernosal artery originating from the internal pudendal artery. The corpora cavernosal sinuses are drained by emissary venules into the circumflex or deep dorsal veins. These three cylinders are surround by Bucks fascia and Dartos fascia superficially [4–6] (Figure 36.1).

Generally, erections occur when neurotransmitters are released from cavernous nerve terminals leading to relaxation of tonically contracted cavernosal smooth muscle. This relaxation leads to dilation of the arterioles increasing blood flow into the trabeculae sinuses. Increased blood flow engorges the corpora cavernosa stretching the tunica albuginea to its capacity and compressing the venular plexus and restricting venous outflow, described as the veno-occlusive process. The summation of these events leads to increased pressure in the corpora cavernosa and tumescence of the penis. Detumescence is achieved when smooth muscles contract against the closed venous system leading to transient pressure increases. This triggers the venous channels to reopen with a return of basal arterial inflow and finally smooth muscle returning to its normal flaccid contracted state [6–7].

36.2.1 Neurophysiology

Physiologic erection relies on the integration of central, peripheral, and autonomic (sympathetic and parasympathetic) nervous systems. The sympathetic preganglia originate around the 10th to 11th thoracic to the 2nd to 3rd lumbar spinal cord segments. The sympathetic chain ganglia most commonly projecting to the penis are located in the sacral and caudal lumbar ganglia, though a few fibers will travel through the superior mesenteric and inferior hypogastric plexus and ultimately into the pelvic plexus [7–8]. The parasympathetic pathway originates from the second to fourth sacral spinal cord where the preganglionic fibers pass to the pelvic plexus and join sympathetic innervation from the superior hypogastric plexus to form the pelvic plexus. This plexus carries branches to the cavernosal nerves that innervate the penis. The somatic inputs, which comprise sensory and motor nerve signals, are driven via the pudendal nerve that innervates the bulbospongiosus and ischiocavernosus striated muscle, as well as the penile skin and urethra [7].

The parasympathetic pathway via the pelvic plexus activates physiologic erections. This is done by release of acetylcholine from cholinergic presynaptic nerve endings that promotes NO release from the endothelial cells as well as inhibits presynaptic adrenergic neurons. As will be discussed later, the activation of NO is a major driver of erectile function [4,9]. Penile detumescence is regulated by sympathetic release

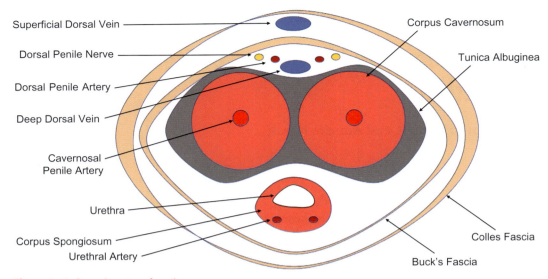

Figure 36.1 Coronal section of penile anatomy

of norepinephrine (NE) from adrenergic neurons stimulating alpha receptors in the penile vasculature and within the corpus cavernosum, ultimately leading to contraction of the arterioles and smooth muscle [8]. Additionally, endothelin, a vasoconstrictor also released by local endothelial cells, leads to long-lasting contractions throughout penile smooth muscle. Some studies suggest that endothelin maintains constriction in the basally flaccid penis, whereas norepinephrine plays an active role in acute detumescence [10].

There are three types of physiologic erections including psychogenic, reflexogenic, and nocturnal (sleep related). Psychogenic is driven by sexual stimulation from auditory, olfactory, visual, and mental erotic factors that activate supraspinal impulses. Animal studies have identified the medial preoptic area (MPOA), the paraventricular nucleus of the hypothalamus, and the hippocampus as some of the key integration centers for these sexual impulses [11]. These signals then travel down the spinal cord through the parasympathetic pathway to elicit penile erections. With regards to the supraspinal component of erections, imaging studies using positron emission tomography and MRI have been done to map brain activation patterns in males triggered by sexual stimuli [12–13]. This research is promising and may one day shed light on higher-level pathologies including sexual deviation, psychogenic ED, and orgasmic dysfunction.

In contrast to psychogenic, reflexogenic erections occur secondary to tactile stimulation of the external genitalia. Afferent sensory impulses travel through the pudendal nerve and either ascend the spinal column to become sensory perception or stimulate the reflexogenic pathways via interactions of the afferent signal with the inferior hypogastric plexus. Efferent signals from the inferior hypogastric plexus in turn stimulate cavernous nerves to elicit erections. This reflexive pathway explains how some patients with upper spinal cord injuries can lose psychogenic erections but have preserved reflexogenic erections. Erections of spinal cord injury men are often not strong enough for intercourse without pharmacologic stimulation [7]. Conversely, animal studies where the spinal cord is removed below the 4th or 5th lumbar can eliminate reflexogenic responses, but if presented with audio-visual stimuli psychogenic erections can occur [14].

Lastly, nocturnal penile tumescence (NPT) occurs during rapid eye movement (REM) sleep. The underlying pathway or evolutionary purpose of NPT is not completely clear; however, some studies suggest the central factors include activation of cholinergic neurons in the lateral pontine tegmentum, inhibition of adrenergic neurons in the locus ceruleus, and downplay of serotonergic neurons in the midbrain raphe [7]. Likewise, given the rise of testosterone during the early morning, some postulate there is an endocrine component in the mechanism as well [15].

36.2.2 Molecular Effectors

The regulation of penile erections depends on molecular transmitters that act at the level of the corporal smooth muscle. Smooth muscle relaxation and contraction is ultimately determined by the level of intracellular calcium. Sympathetic activation via NE causes ion channels to open releasing calcium from intracellular stores as well allowing influx of calcium from extracellular space. The increase in free calcium binds to the compound calmodulin forming a complex that phosphorylates myosin light chain kinase (MLCK). This activation triggers cross-bridging of the myosin filaments leading to muscle contraction [4,7] (Figure 36.2). Another pathway for smooth muscle contraction is altering the receptor sensitivity to calcium via RhoA, a small monomeric G protein. RhoA inhibits one of the regulatory subunits of myosin phosphatase, preventing deactivation of the myofilament and therefore promoting a contracted state [16]. Though both pathways lead to

Table 36.1 Classifications of erectile dysfunction

Organic
- I. Vasculogenic
- II. Neurogenic
- III. Anatomic
- IV. Endocrinologic

Psychogenic
- I. Generalized
- II. Situational

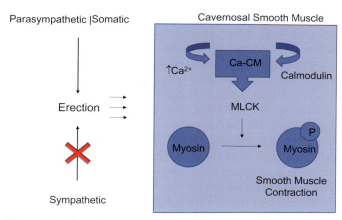

Figure 36.2 Physiology of penile erection and detumescence

smooth muscle contraction, it is believed that increases in cytosolic calcium cause the phasic contraction of penile smooth muscle, whereas the RhoA pathway regulating calcium sensitivity is key in maintaining the tonic contraction of a flaccid penis [17].

NO plays a similarly important role in erectile function. Parasympathetic activation of acetylcholine leads to the release of NO from the nonadrenergic noncholinergic (NANC) nerve fibers as well as from endothelial cells. NO release from the NANC fibers initiate smooth muscle relaxation for erections, whereas the NO from endothelial cells works to maintain the erection [18]. Furthermore, NO activates the secondary messenger cAMP and cyclic guanosine monophosphate (cGMP) that result in the opening of cytoplasmic potassium channels. The net effect is hyperpolarization of the cell, sequestration of intracellular calcium, and blockage of calcium influx [6–7]. As intracellular calcium decreases, fewer calmodulin complexes form and less cross-linking of myosin occurs. This results in smooth muscle relaxation. The process by which cGMP is deactivated is via phosphodiesterase type 5 (PDE5) hydrolysis. An entire class of erectogenic medications called PDE5 inhibitors block PDE5 function thereby promoting cGMP and drive cavernosal smooth muscle relaxation and erections [4].

36.3 Pathophysiology of Erectile Dysfunction

Erectile dysfunction has been classified though two prevailing paradigms: based on etiology, for example trauma, diabetes, drug induced, etc. versus blood flow/mechanism of action, for example failure to initiate (neurogenic/psychogenic), failure to fill (arterial), and failure to store (venous), etc. In the next part of this chapter, we aim to characterize the different pathologies leading to ED. This section has been organized based on the widely accepted classification espoused by the International Society of Impotence Research [19] (Table 36.1).

36.3.1 Vasculogenic

Erectile dysfunction secondary to underlying vascular disease is one of the most prevalent etiologies for organic dysfunction. Arterial insufficiency results in decreased perfusion of the hypogastric-cavernous-helicine arterial system leading to diminished intracavernosal pressures, longer filling times, and decreased penile rigidity. Furthermore, vasculogenic ED may feature veno-occlusive dysfunction (failure to occlude subtunical and emissary veins) either from traumatic injuries, venous shunts, or as degenerative/fibrotic from chronic poor arterial perfusion [7]. Arteriogenic ED is most often caused by atherogenic plaque of the internal pudendal, common penile, and cavernosal arteries [20]. Other focal arterial defects from vascular injury can be seen in men with history of trauma, surgery, and radiation to the pelvis. Arteriogenic ED may also be responsible for cycling-related ED; however, controversy remains whether cycling-related ED is due to neurogenic factors or ischemia [21–24].

Since vasculogenic ED is commonly due to chronic atherosclerotic disease, it often precedes significant cardiovascular and cerebrovascular disease [25]. Therefore, diagnosis of vasculogenic ED in otherwise asymptomatic men may warrant early cardiac and coronary artery disease workup [20].

The oxygen-poor environment of arteriogenic ED alters levels of several transmitters including prostaglandin E1 and transforming growth factor-B1 (TGF-B1) thereby increasing profibrotic and inflammatory cytokines [27,28]. The net effect is further collagen deposition, impaired endothelial vasodilation, and increased vascular resistance. A similar effect can occur with neurogenic ED. Endothelial damage, either through poor perfusion or lack of neurostimulation, leads to loss of smooth muscle and local fibrosis. Along with upregulated inflammatory markers, the endothelium becomes scarred, thereby restricting erectile function [7,27–28]. These changes can cause and worsen veno-occlusive dysfunction [7,28]. Arteriogenic ED often starts as a failure to fill (arterial), but with sustained fibrotic degeneration of cavernosal tissue, secondary veno-occlusive changes can develop.

36.3.2 Neurogenic

Neurologic deficits anywhere along the neuroaxis from brain to cavernosal nerves can lead to ED. An estimated 10–19% of

ED is neurologic in origin [29]. Ultimately, the end result from any neurologic deficit is diminished release of transmitters such as NO to penile smooth muscle. Similar to vascular ED, long-term neurologic ED results in apoptosis of smooth muscle cells and endothelial cells with collagenization of local tissue worsening penile inelasticity [30].

Starting at the level of the brain, the MPOA and hippocampus are the integration centers that translate sexual desire to penile erection. Therefore, neurologic damage, from such conditions as cerebrovascular disease, tumors, dementia, Alzheimer's, temporal lobe epilepsy, and trauma, can directly impact erectile function. Likewise, one study found that 53% of Alzheimer's patients in a study had ED, not related to depression, age of onset, or cognitive impairment, but correlated with the onset of Alzheimer's symptoms [31]. Likewise, many neurologic diseases that cause imbalance in brain neurotransmitters like serotonin and dopamine can cause ED. Classically, this is seen in Parkinson's disease where damage to the substania nigra kills cells producing dopamine and therefore disrupts a major neurotransmitter that potentiates the activation of erections [32]. At the same time serotonin when upregulated also causes ED by altering the central nervous system activation of erectile function. This effect can be seen in the increased rates of sexual dysfunction in patients taking selective serotonin reuptake inhibitors (SSRIs) [33]. Therefore, the balance of serotonin (inhibitory) and dopamine (facilitatory) is critical in normal sexual function [32–33].

Spinal cord injuries can result in variable degrees of ED depending on the level and extent of the injury. As previously discussed, reflexogenic erectile function can occur in patients with upper cord lesions due to an intact inferior hypogastric plexus. As many as 95% of spinal cord lesions above the tenth thoracic vertebral (T10) level have intact reflexogenic erection; however, lower spinal cord injuries preserve reflexogenic erectile function at lower rates. Twenty-five percent of men with spinal cord injury at the sacral spinal levels S2–S4 possess reflexogenic erectile function [29,34]. Disease that can impact the spinal cord includes trauma, disc herniation, tumors, multiple sclerosis, transverse myelitis, syringomeylia, and spina bifida [32–34].

At the level of the peripheral nerves, cavernous nerve injury can result in neurogenic ED in men with pelvic trauma or iatrogenic injury from pelvic surgery. Due to the limited pelvic space and close proximity to pelvic organs high rates of ED have been reported for radical prostatectomy (40–85% at varying centers of excellence [35]) and abdominal perineal resections (61.5% in one study [36]). Even with improved surgical technique, like cavernous nerve sparing radical prostatectomy, only two-thirds of patients undergoing pelvic oncologic surgery will preserve potency, depending on baseline function and extent of oncologic disease [37]. Likewise, patients can sometimes take up to 24 months to recover erectile function [37–38]. This has led to intense research in different medications and protocols for post pelvic surgery nerve rehabilitation [39]. Patients with pelvic trauma may also suffer from both vasculogenic and neurogenic ED given the close proximity of nerves with major blood vessels. This can explain the high level of sexual dysfunction in almost two-thirds of men after pelvic fractures [40].

Additionally, patients with diabetes represent a well-established risk group for ED. Diabetes ED is multifactorial and stems from endothelial dysfunction and neurogenic ED, with autonomic neuropathy and progressive demyelination of peripheral nerves [26].

36.3.3 Endocrine

Testosterone plays a critical role in men's health and male sexual behavior, enhancing sexual interest and increasing frequency of sex and nocturnal erections [41–42]. Additionally, testosterone has important roles in maintaining bone health, body composition, and cardiovascular health [42]. Therefore, testosterone is critical in erectile function. A 2017 meta-analysis inclusive of 14 studies and 2,298 patients showed that testosterone therapy used in hypogonadal men results in dose-dependent improvement in erectile function [43]. Using the validated International Index of Erectile Function Test (IIEF) the authors found that testosterone replacement therapy significantly improved erectile function when compared to placebo (mean difference = 2.31, $p<0.001$). The authors also found greater changes in IIEF score (mean difference 2.95 versus 1.4, $p = 0.02$) in severe hypogonadal men (total testosterone <8 nmol/L) compared to men with milder deficiency (total testosterone <12 nmol/L). Another group also performed a systematic review looking at hypogonadal men (total testosterone <10.4 nmol/L) who failed PDE5 monotherapy treated with PDE5 and testosterone replacement. Though the individual studies were heterogeneous, the authors found that the combination of the two medications may benefit patients who failed monotherapy alone [44]. These studies highlight the central theme that testosterone plays an important role for male sexual health and erectile function. However, this exact relationship is complex and far from linear since increasing testosterone in eugonadal men does not result in improved function [45]. Therefore, additional studies are needed, especially those that look at the correlation of testosterone with other known erectile regulators. For example, some are researching the role testosterone deficiency plays in downregulation of NO synthase via endothelial dysfunction [46]. By improving our understanding of the integration of these components we can seek to find new solutions for erectile dysfunction.

Dysfunction of endocrine hormones at other levels of the hypothalamic-pituitary gonadal axis can also impact erectile function. In patients with hyperprolactinemia, from medications (e.g., dopamine-receptor antagonists or depleting agents) to prolactin-secreting tumors, excess prolactin inhibits hypothalamic gonadotroponin-releasing hormone, which ultimately leads to low testosterone production and ED [41–42].

36.3.4 Psychogenic

Psychogenic ED was once believed to account for most forms of ED [4]. However, current belief is that organic ED is more common than previously thought and likely coexists in a large portion of psychogenic ED patients. In fact, studies in otherwise healthy men under 40 years of age found 15–72% had identifiable organic causes [47]. As discussed earlier, the brain processes sexual stimuli with input from stimulatory and inhibitory afferent signals. Anxiety and social stress can produce excessive sympathetic outflow. The increased circulatory catecholamine along with increased supra-sacral inhibition by sympathetic tracts can hamper erections. Some studies support this with higher levels of serum norepinephrine (sympathetic pathway) in patients with psychogenic ED compared to controls. A study looking at the level of catecholamines in penile blood during pharmacologic penile stimulation with papaverine showed levels of norepinephrine were higher in psychogenic ED than in those with vasculogenic ED ($p<0.01$), and it was higher in negative responders than in positive responders ($p<0.001$) [48].

A key feature of psychogenic ED is the situational and mental aspect. Components such as comfort with sexual partner, arousability, and higher inhibition due to conflict or threat all can lead to sexual anxiety and psychogenic ED. Therefore, psychogenic ED can be seen with other sexual dysfunctions such as premature ejaculation and also occur during periods of mental stress including death of loved ones and depression [49].

36.3.5 Drug-Induced

Drug-induced ED may contribute to ED in almost a quarter of affected men [50]. Though at times it can be difficult to differentiate between ED due to medication or an underlying disease, there are medications with well-established ED side effects. For instance, antihypertensives such as beta blockers can dampen the neurogenic impulses as well as inhibit the relaxation of the penile arteries. Diuretics can decrease the blood flow necessary to form a robust erection. Antidepressants such as SSRIs lead to excess serotonin, a known erectile inhibitor. Anti-androgen and several antifungal medications work by directly inhibiting testosterone, which as noted in the endocrine section are critical in erectile function [33,50]. Additionally, medications like digoxin, opiates, and H2 blockers have all been linked to ED. Recreational substances such as alcohol and marijuana have also been linked to ED [33]. Chronic alcoholism, for instance, can lead to decreased libido, alcoholic polyneuropathy, and liver dysfunction impacting testosterone levels. Therefore, a workup of ED should include a thorough reconciliation of a man's medication history.

36.4 Conclusion

In this chapter, we summarized the molecular biology and anatomy required to produce erectile function. Erectile function depends on the interactions between multiple body systems and can be influenced by molecular effectors that balance pro and anti-erectile function. The well-orchestrated steps result in smooth muscle dilation and improved vascular flow against venous drainage. Along this same route there are a number of ways erectile function can be disrupted. Erectile dysfunction can have tremendous impact on the male psyche and quality of life. Therefore, it is a critical area of research not only for symptomatic treatment, but durable long-lasting cures.

References

1. Johannes CB, Araju AB, Feldman HA, Derby CA, Kleinman KP, McKinlay JB. Incidence of erectile dysfunction in men 40–69 years old: longitudinal results from the Massachusetts Male Aging Study. *J Urol*. 2000;163(2):460–463.
2. Aytac IA, McKinlay JB, Krane RJ. The likely worldwide increase in erectile dysfunction between 1995 and 2025 and some possible policy consequences. *BJU Int*. 1999;84(1):50–56.
3. Yafi, FA, Jenkins L, Albertsen M, et al. Erectile dysfunction. *Nat Rev Dis Primers*. 2016;2:16003.
4. Hawksworth DJ, Burnett AL. Pharmacotherapeutic management of erectile dysfunction. *Clin Pharmacol Ther*. 2015;98(6):602–610.
5. Tanagho EA, Lue TF. Anatomy of the genitourinary tract. In: McAnich JW, Lue TF, eds. *Smith and Tanagho's General Urology*. 18th ed. The McGraw Hill Companies; 2013:Chapter 1.
6. Gratzke C, Angulo J, Chitaley K, et al. Anatomy, physiology, and pathophysiology of erectile dysfunction. *J Sex Med*. 2010;7(1 Pt 2):445–475.
7. Dean RC, Lue TF. Physiology of penile erection and pathophysiology of erectile dysfunction. *Urol Clin North Am*. 2005;32(4):379–395.
8. Andersson KE, Hedlund P, Alm P. Sympathetic pathways and adrenergic innervation of the penis. *Int J Impotent Res*. 2000;12(Suppl. 1):S5–S12.
9. Saenz de Tejada I, Kim N, Lagana I, et al. Regulation of adrenergic activity in penile corpus cavernosum. *J Urol*. 1989;142(4):1117–1121.
10. Saenz d Tejada I, Carson MP, de las Morenas A, et al. Endothelin: localization, synthesis, activity, and receptor types in human penile corpus cavernosum. *Am J Physiol*. 1991;261:H1078–H1085.
11. Sachs B, Meisel R. The physiology of male sexual behavior. In: Knobil E, Neill J, eds. *Physiology of Reproduction*. Raven Press; 1998:1393–1423.
12. Stoleru S, Redoute J, Costes N, et al. Brain processing of visual sexual stimuli in men with hypoactive sexual desire disorder. *Psychiatry Res*. 2003;124(2):67–86.
13. Ferrettti A, Caulo M, Del Gratta C, et al. Dynamics of male sexual arousal: distinct components of brain activation reveal by fMRI. *Neuroimage*. 2005;26(4):1086–1096.
14. Root W, Bard P. The mediation of feline erection through sympathetic pathway with some reference on sexual behavior after deafferentation of the genitalia. *Am J Physiol*. 1947;151:80–90.
15. Montorsi F, Oettel M. Testosterone and sleep-relate erections: an overview. *J Sex Med*. 2005;2(6):771–784.
16. Wang H, Eto M, Steers WD, et al. RhoA-mediated Ca2+ sensitization in

erectile function. *J Biol Chem.* 2002;277:30614–30621.
17. Cellk S, Rees RW, Kalsi J. A Rho-kinase inhibitor, soluble guanylate cyclase activator and nitric oxide-releasing PDE5 inhibitors: novel approaches to erectile dysfunction. *Expert Opin Investig Drugs.* 2002;11:1563–1573.
18. Hurt KJ, Musicki B, Palese MA, et al. Akt-dependent phosphorylation of endothelial nitric-oxide synthase meditate penile erection. *Proc Natl Acad Sci USA.* 2002;99(6):4061–4066.
19. Lizza EF, Rosen RC. Definition and classification of erectile dysfunction: report of the nomenclature committee of the International Society of Impotence Research. *Int J Impot Res.* 1999;11(3):141–143.
20. Levine FJ, Greenfield AJ, Goldstein I. Arteriographically determined occlusive disease within the hypogastric-cavernous bed in impotent patients following blunt perineal and pelvic trauma. *J Urol.* 1990;144(5):1147–1153.
21. Goldstein I, Feldman MI, Deckers PJ, et al. Radiation-associated impotence. a clinical study of its mechanism. *JAMA.* 1984;251(7):903–910.
22. Andersen KV, Bovim G. Impotence and nerve entrapment in long distance amateur cyclists. *Acta Neurol Scand.* 1997;95(4):233–240.
23. Gan ZS, Ehlers ME, Lin FC, Wright ST, Figler BD, Coward RM. Systematic review and meta-analysis of cycling and erectile dysfunction. *Sex Med Rev.* 2020;9(2):304–311.
24. Balasubramanian A, Yu J, Breyer BN, Minkow R, Eisenberg ML. The association between pelvic discomfort and erectile dysfunction in adult male bicyclists. *J Sex Med.* 2020;7(5):919–929.
25. Gupta N, Herati A, Gilbert BR. Penile Doppler ultrasound predicting cardiovascular disease in men with erectile dysfunction. *Curr Urol Rep.* 2015;16(3):16.
26. Heidler S, Temml C, Broessner C, et al. Is the metabolic syndrome an independent risk factor for erectile dysfunction? *J Urol.* 2007;177(2):651–654.
27. Moreland RB, Traish A, McMilin MA, Smith B, Goldstein I, Saenz de Tejada I. PGE1 suppressed the induction of collagen synthesis by transforming growth factor-beta 1 in human corpus cavernosum smooth muscle. *J Urol.* 1995;153(3):826–834.
28. Nehra A, Azadozi KM, Moreland RB, et al. Cavernosal expandability is an erectile tissue mechanical property which predicts trabecular histology in an animal model of vasculogenic erectile dysfunction. *J Urol.* 1998;159(6):2229–2236.
29. Steers WD. Neural control of penile erection. *Semin Urol.* 1990;8(2):66–79.
30. El-Sakka AI. Reversion of penile fibrosis: current information and a new horizon. *Arab J Urol.* 2011;9(1):49–55.
31. Zeiss AM, Davies HD, Wood M, Tinklenberg JR. The incidence and correlates of erectile problems in patients with Alzheimer's disease. *Arch Sex Behav.* 1990;19(4):325–331.
32. Nehra A, Moreland RB. Neurologic erectile dysfunction. *Urol Clin.* 2001;28(20):289–308.
33. Brock GB, Lue TF. Drug-induced male sexual dysfunction. An update. *Drug Saf.* 1993;8(6):414–426.
34. Eardley I, Kirby R. Neurogenic impotence. In: Kirby R, Carson C, Webster G, eds. *Impotence: Diagnosis and Management of Male Erectile Dysfunction.* Butterworth-Heinemann; 1991:227–231.
35. Nandipati KC, Raina R, Agarwal A, et al. Erectile dysfunction following radical retropubic prostatectomy: epidemiology, pathophysiology and pharmacological management. *Drugs Aging.* 2006;23(2):101–117.
36. Danzi M, Ferulano GP, Abate S, et al. Male sexual function after abdominoperineal resection for rectal cancer. *Dis Colon Rectum.* 1983;26(10):665–668.
37. Quinlan DM, Epstein JI, Carter BS, et al. Sexual function following radical prostatectomy: influence of preservation of neurovascular bundles. *J Urol.* 1991;145(5):998–1002.
38. Dean RC, Lue TF. Neuroregenerative strategies after radical prostatectomy. *Rev Urol.* 2005;7(2):26–32.
39. Bratu O, Oprea I, Marcu D, et al. Erectile dysfunction post-radical prostatectomy: a challenge for both patient and physician. *J Med Life.* 2017;10(1):13–18.
40. Metze M, Tiemann AH, Josten C. Male sexual dysfunction after pelvic trauma. *J Trauma.* 2007;62(2):394–401.
41. Mulligan T, Schmitt B. Testosterone for erectile failure. *J Gen Intern Med.* 1993;8(9):517–521.
42. Booth A, Johnson DR, Granger DA. Testosterone and men's health. *J Behav Med.* 1999;22(1):1–19.
43. Corona G, Rastrelli G, Morgentaler A, et al. Meta-analysis of results of testosterone therapy on sexual function based on international index of erectile function scores. *Eur Urol.* 2017;72(6):1000–1011.
44. Alhathal N, Elshal AM, Carrier S. Synergetic effect of testosterone and phosphodiesterare-5 inhibitors in hypogonadal men with erectile dysfunction: a systematic review. *Can Urol Assoc J.* 2012;6(4):269–274.
45. Buena F, Swerdloff RS, Steiner BS, et al. Sexual function does not change when serum testosterone levels are pharmacologically varied within the normal male range. *Fertil Steril.* 1993;59(5):1118–1123.
46. Hotta Y, Kataoka T, Kimura K. Testosterone deficiency and endothelial dysfunction: nitric oxide asymmetric dimethylarginine, and endothelial progenitor cells. *Sex Med Rev.* 2019;7(4):661–668.
47. Ludwig W, Phillips M. Organic causes of erectile dysfunction in men under 40. *Urol Int.* 2014;92(1):1–6.
48. Kim SC, Oh MM. Norepinephrine involvement in response to intracorporeal injection of papaverine in psychogenic impotence. *J Urol.* 1992;147(6):1530–1532.
49. Rosen RC. Psychogenic erectile dysfunction: classification and management. *Urol Clin North Am.* 2001;28(2):269–278.
50. Keene LC, Davies PH. Drug-related erectile dysfunction. *Adverse Drug React Toxicol Rev.* 1999;18(1):5–24.

Section 5 **Medical and Surgical Management of Issues of Male Health**

Chapter 37

Evaluation of the Male with Erectile Dysfunction

William T. Berg and Martin Miner

37.1 Introduction

The evaluation of the male who presents with erectile dysfunction (ED) can be one the most impactful visits in the long-term health for the patient. As illustrated in this chapter, ED has a number of important implications in overall men's health. ED may be the only symptom that convinces a man to seek medical advice, which he may have avoided for many decades. This can be described as a "delicate" or "sensitive" topic for many men as feelings of masculinity, vitality, and self-worth are often wrapped up in sexual performance. Furthermore, cultural norms have served to stifle open discussion of mores and sexual function. The issue of penetrative sex or intercourse is rarely discussed by men. It is important to remember that a man presenting to a physician's office with ED may have needed to build up a significant amount of courage to come forward, often not only needing to speak to the provider performing the evaluation, but also a number of other staff including call centers, schedulers, medical assistants, nurses, etc. The goal of the ED evaluation is to elucidate the emotional and physical well-being of the patient and to provide a safe and comfortable environment that allows the clinician to perform a proper and complete evaluation. Moreover, we have found many patients lack an understanding of the etiology of their ED, and part of the evaluation should include detailed patient education on how lifestyle and medical comorbidities contribute to ED.

37.1.1 Epidemiology

Worldwide prevalence studies estimate that approximately 20% of men will experience ED [1]. Prevalence increases as men age, with 1–10% of men younger than the age of 40 experiencing ED, ranging to up to 50–100% of men between the ages of 70 and 90 [2]. Projections estimate that the prevalence is increasing and will continue to increase in the coming decades as the boomer generation ages [3].

The increased prevalence of ED associated with age can be correlated to the increased prevalence of medical comorbidities. While the causes of ED can be multifactorial, there is strong evidence that specific comorbidities impacting blood flow and vascular endothelial function significantly increase the risk of having erectile dysfunction [4]. These comorbidities, which are increasing in the US population overall, include obesity, diabetes mellitus, hypertension, dyslipidemia, and cardiovascular disease.

Improvements in ED can be achieved by lifestyle changes, such as weight control, smoking cessation, a healthy diet, and exercise, which play a complementary role in ED management [5]. The management of specific comorbidities may also help improve ED. Treatment of obesity and hyperlipidemia have been associated with improved erectile function, whereas the impact of treating diabetes and depression is less clear [6,7].

Many of these comorbidities are more easily understood through the concept of metabolic syndrome. The risk factors associated with metabolic syndrome closely correlate with risk factors for cardiovascular disease, stroke, and heart attack, and significantly overlap with the most common conditions associated with ED. The defining characteristics of metabolic syndrome in men include an increased weight circumference greater than 102 cm (40 in), a triglyceride level greater than 150 mg/dL or being on a statin, a high-density lipoprotein (HDL) level less than 40 mg/dL, a blood pressure greater than 130/85 mmHg or being on an antihypertensive, and a fasting blood glucose level greater than 100 mg/dL. If a patient has three of the five listed criteria, a diagnosis of the metabolic syndrome can be made [8].

37.1.2 Public Health Implications

Erectile dysfunction has been found to be highly predictive of cardiovascular events in men less than 60 years old. Young men, who were not originally captured as part of the Framingham longitudinal heart study, are at risk as well. Younger patients presenting with ED should prompt screening for the presence or risk of cardiovascular disease, which might have otherwise have gone unevaluated. Erectile dysfunction can be considered both a marker of endothelial dysfunction, involving the nitric acid dependent vasodilation pathway, as well as a marker of atherosclerosis affecting penile blood flow. The manifestation of this dysfunction is then ED, which can be a harbinger for subclinical coronary artery disease (CAD) and a precursor for cardiovascular events [9]. While widespread invasive cardiac screening is not cost-effective for all patients, calculation of cardiovascular risk estimates based on known algorithms is important (atherosclerotic cardiovascular disease [ASCVD] risk calculator) [10]. Proper evaluation and screening has implications for overall societal well-being, quality of life, economic productivity, and formulation of public

Table 37.1 Erectile dysfunction risk factors

Condition	Multivariate adjusted odds ratio
Antidepressant use	9.1
Antihypertensive use	4.0
Diabetes mellitus	2.9
Obstructive urinary symptoms	2.2
Hypertension	1.6
Benign prostate enlargement	1.6
Current cigarette smoking	1.6
Increased body mass index	1.5
Physical inactivity	1.5
Cardiovascular disease	1.1
Hypercholesterolemia	1.0

Source: Reproduced from *Campbell–Walsh Urology*, 11th ed. [36].

health strategies to improve preventative medicine and decrease healthcare costs. Further, proper identification of ED, leading to treatment and management, has implications of mental health, and modifiable lifestyle factors.

37.2 Initial Detection

37.2.1 Screening

Erectile dysfunction can be understood as a complex blending between anatomic, physiologic, and behavioral processes that occurs through the context of a man's beliefs and values, which then informs the concept of sexuality overall and how it relates to sociocultural mores. This in turn is informed by the nature of the relationship with his partner, the quality of that partnership, and the partner's beliefs and values about sexual activity. In this complex human context, ED is conceptualized as the inability to attain and/or maintain sufficient penile rigidity for sexual satisfaction [11]. Understanding this definition can help to inform who needs to be treated but also how patients are evaluated.

The critical first step is simply asking patients about their sexual function. As mentioned previously, many male patients are reluctant to talk openly about issues of sexual dysfunction. The onus is on the healthcare provider to ask and screen for these issues. It is of upmost importance that providers take a proactive approach to sexual function rather a passive one. Likewise, patients with identifiable risk factors, such as in metabolic syndrome, are likely to experience ED (Table 37.1). These men in particular should be screened [12].

In summary, ED is a risk marker for the presence of treatable underlying medical conditions that, left untreated, reduce quality and length of life (e.g., undiagnosed diabetes and cardiovascular disease). In addition, ED can negatively affect a man's mental health, his relationship, and his general well-being. The presence of ED, therefore, provides an opportunity to potentially address multiple issues that affect a man's general health [11].

37.2.2 Sexual History

An important part of the initial evaluation is establishing a detailed baseline of sexual function and history, which will allow the healthcare practitioner to set goals and expectations. Erectile dysfunction may only be the one component of a complicated sexual history. Initial understanding should start with the context in which the ED occurs and determine if it is related to particular situations, or whether it occurs alone and/or with a sexual partner. Following this, an understanding of how the patient approaches his interpersonal and sexual relationships is imperative. One should determine the quality of the patient's current relationship and any new or long-standing relationship difficulties. Furthermore, exploring patient sexual interests and desires will help to tailor treatment options and dictate therapeutic pathways.

Often a patient's partner may blame the patient for lack of desire or interest. It can be very helpful to include the sexual partner in the discussion and education regarding ED. The partner may also provide either corroborating or differing information in the history. These questions may help determine if performance anxiety is playing a role in the ED. Often the extent of the partner's involvement in evaluation in treatment may help to predict treatment success or failure. Understanding the health of the partner and interest in improving the ED might provide significant insight into the nature of the problem.

Developing a safe space that emphasizes trust is an important component to building the physician–patient relationship in sexual medicine. The patient must understand that discussions are confidential. This allows the patient to be able to fully express the nature and extent of the dysfunction. This starts with a line of questioning from the practitioner that is non-judgmental and does not assume heteronormative behaviors. A clinician who is open and understanding will develop a more therapeutic relationship with the patient.

Basic questions characterizing the ED are paramount, including the circumstances in which erections do or do not occur, including inquiries regarding presence or absence of morning erections, and whether there is a difference in erections during self-stimulation and partnered interactions. Further inquiries should include timing of onset of ED, severity, and an assessment of self-understanding of causes of the ED. Additional inquiries should include attempted treatment options thus far, including both pharmacologic, mechanical, and over-the-counter supplements or naturopathic herbals [13].

Discussion over a period of several visits may be necessary in order to obtain clear understanding of the exact nature of the problem. Frequently, patients will generalize their complaints into a category of ED. Assessment of desire, orgasm, and ejaculation should be performed to determine if possibly another aspect of sexual function is truly the cause of distress. Frequently, men characterize premature ejaculation as ED. Clarification of this matter has important therapeutic implications.

37.2.3 Questionnaires

Validated questionnaires help to provide insight into the extent of the ED. Having baseline values for screening questionnaires provide clinicians and patients with measures of calculable success.

One of the mostly widely used questionnaires is the Index of Erectile Function (IIEF). This questionnaire has been decreased in length to five questions for more practical clinical use and is most commonly used in the form of the IIEF-5 or the Sexual Health Inventory for Men. This questionnaire uses a scale to classify ED as none, mild, mild to moderate, moderate, and severe. The Brief Male Sexual Function Inventory similarly scores the components of sexual function; sexual drive, erectile function, orgasmic function, problem assessment, and overall sexual satisfaction (Table 37.2) [14]. A number of other validated questionnaires exist to assist in the evaluation and management of ED. One is not necessarily better than the other, but practice consistency and longitudinal follow-up with repeated use of the questionnaires can provide useful treatment measures of success.

37.3 Medical History
37.3.1 Comorbidities and Medications

Metabolic syndrome, preexisting cardiovascular disease, and common disease conditions associated with aging may help point to etiologic causes of ED. Close scrutiny of medical comorbidities will identify modifiable lifestyle factors that, when corrected, may result in resolution or improvement in ED.

If the patient has diagnosed diabetes mellitus, a discussion of blood glucose control is necessary, as many patients do not correlate diabetes management with ED. Many have likely already been counseled on the long-term impact of diabetes on eyesight, coronary disease, and renal disease, but often are unaware of the sexual side effects of poor glucose control [15].

Detailed understanding of any preexisting CAD or peripheral vascular disease should be elucidated. This includes specific understanding of prior interventions of percutaneous coronary angioplasty, number, location, and type of coronary stents, endovascular aneurysm repair, peripheral vascular stenting, or open vascular bypass. Also, a review of systems focusing on an assessment of symptoms associated with congestive heart failure, CAD, shortness of breath with exertion, chest pain, or claudication-type pain is necessary [16]. Again, patients may be uninformed regarding the correlation of vascular disease and ED.

The presence of hypertension, dyslipidemia, or other endocrinopathies including hypogonadism or hypothyroidism should also be explored [17]. Compliance with the medical management of these conditions should be discussed and documented. This serves as another opportunity for patient education on the impact that these comorbidities have on ED. Patients may falsely believe that all ED is related to hypogonadism and that simple correction of low testosterone will result in normalized erectile function.

Further medical and surgical history should focus on identification of neurologic injury, spinal cord injury, or a history of trauma to the genitals, back, or pelvis. Also, a detailed accounting of spinal column surgery, pelvic surgery including prostate and rectal surgery, radiation treatments to the pelvis, as well as history of chemotherapy is compulsory. Understanding the nature of the possible cavernosal nerve injury will help guide treatment options.

A number of medications have been implicated as the cause or contribution to ED. The list of specific medications is long, but general classes of medications associated with ED include antihypertensives, antiarrhythmics, antidepressants, diuretics, antihistamines, Parkinson's disease medications, opiates, and muscle relaxants [18]. While many of these medications cannot be easily discontinued or substituted, patients should be educated on their impact on sexual function.

37.3.2 Social History/Lifestyle Factors

Modifiable lifestyle factors have been known to contribute significantly to ED. Patients should be questioned on their occupation, whether or not they perform shift work, their amount and extent of physical activity and exercise, sleep patterns, cigarette use, and drug use.

Obstructive sleep apnea is implicated in both ED and hypogonadism. Simple screening tools such as STOP-Bang are useful to determine whether a patient should be referred for sleep study [19]. This quick screening method stands for snoring, tired (feelings of daytime fatigue), observed (stopped breathing, choking, gasping), pressure (treated for high blood pressure), body mass index (of greater than 35 kg/m^2), age (greater than 50), neck (size larger than 40 cm), gender (male). Elevated scores determine the risk of obstructive sleep apnea. Patients should also be questioned on their quality and duration of sleep, as this influences energy, mood, and desire [20].

Patients should be counseled on the implications of cigarette smoking, alcohol intake greater than two drinks a day, as well as recreational drugs as this also is associated with worsening ED. The mechanisms of these lifestyle factors are likely related to endothelial injury resulting in damage to the vasodilatory mechanism of cavernosal arteries.

Sedentary lifestyle has been associated with ED as well as aerobic exercise linked to improvements in erectile function [21]. Changes in diet have also be shown to improve ED. A study of diabetic men demonstrated that the risk of ED was reduced with every additional serving of fruits and vegetables [22]. The Mediterranean diet has been associated with lower risk of ED and dietary counseling should be focused on increasing intake of fruit, vegetables, nuts, and whole grains, while reducing red meat and processed meats [23].

Table 37.2 The Brief Male Sexual Function Inventory

Section A. Interest

A1. Let's define sexual drive as a feeling that may include wanting to have sexual experience (masturbation or intercourse), thinking about having sex, or feeling frustrated due to lack of sex.
During the past 30 days, on how many days have you felt sexual drive?

A2. During the past 30 days, how would you rate your level of sexual drive?

A3. Consider a scale from zero to ten, where zero is no sex drive at all and ten is the best level of sex drive a person could have, what number would you give to your level of sex drive in the past 30 days?

Section B. Function

B1. During the past 30 days, how frequently did you awaken from sleep with at least a partial erection?
B2. During the past 30 days, how frequently did you awaken from sleep with a full erection?
B3. During the past 30 days, what is the most erect (or hard) your penis has become at any time?
  0 [ ] no erection at all
  1 [ ] partial erection – not capable of penetration even with manual assistance
  2 [ ] partial erection – capable of penetration with manual assistance
  3 [ ] nearly full erection – sufficient for penetration without manual assistance
  4 [ ] full erection
B4. Over the past 30 days, how often have you had partial or full sexual erections when you were sexually stimulated in any way
B5. Over the past 30 days, when you had erections, how often were they firm enough to have sexual intercourse?
B6. How much difficulty did you have getting an erection during the past 30 days?
B7. How much difficulty did you have keeping an erection during the past 30 days?

Section C. Ejaculation

C1. In the past 30 days, how much difficulty have you had ejaculating when you have been sexually stimulated?
C2. In the past 30 days, how much semen did you ejaculate when you climaxed?
C3. How much are you concerned about the amount of semen you ejaculate?
C4. In the past 30 days, how much did you consider the amount of semen you ejaculate to be a problem for you?

Section F. Summary

F1. In the past 30 days, to what extent have you considered a lack of sex drive to be a problem?
F2. In the past 30 days, to what extent have you considered your ability to get and keep and erections to be a problem?
F3. In the past 30 days, to what extent have you considered your ejaculation to be a problem?
F4. Overall, during the past 30 days, how satisfied have you been with your sex life?
F5. How did you feel about your level of sexual drive during the past 30 days?
  0 [ ] terrible   1 [ ] unhappy   2 [ ] mostly dissatisfied
  3 [ ] neutral or mixed (about equally satisfied and dissatisfied)
  4 [ ] mostly satisfied   5 [ ] pleased   6 [ ] delighted
F6. How did you feel about your ability to get and keep erections during the past 30 days?
F7. How did you feel about your ejaculation during the past 30 days?
F8. Overall, during the past 30 days, how have you felt about your sex life?

Source: Reproduced with permission from O'Leary M., et al., A Brief Male Sexual Function Inventory for urology. *Urology.* 1995;46(5):697–706.

37.4 Physical Exam

The cornerstone of any physical exam should include assessment of vital signs, including height, weight, and blood pressure, and calculation of body mass index. Waist circumference measurement has important implications as a risk factor for metabolic syndrome and a marker of cardiovascular risk [17].

A generalized head to toe exam should be performed with a focus on the cardiovascular system including auscultation of the heart, evaluation of the lower extremities for edema, and palpation of peripheral pulses. Additional auscultation of the carotid arteries and abdominal aorta and palpation of femoral arteries should be performed to evaluate for the presence of a bruit. Presence of any of these findings should prompt cardiac evaluation and point to a significant vasculogenic cause of the ED.

Particular focus should be paid to androgenization and evaluation of the presence of gynecomastia. This might point to pituitary derangements.

A detailed genitourinary exam should include an evaluation of testicular size, penile stretch length, and the palpation of the shaft of the penis for the presence of penile plaques associated with Pyronine's disease. Additionally, assessment should include penile sensation testing. Disorders of sensation or absence of bulbocavernosus reflex point to neurologic cause of ED. Abnormalities of genitalia would point to congenital causes of ED and sexual development including Klinefelter syndrome.

37.5 Diagnostic Testing
37.5.1 Laboratory Evaluation

The purpose of laboratory testing should be to identify and screen for any modifiable factors that may be contributing to ED. Furthermore, it will assist in risk stratification of patients for cardiovascular disease. A basic set of blood work includes a lipid panel with both total cholesterol and HDL level, total triglycerides, a fasting blood serum glucose, and a total testosterone level. We have found great benefit in measuring bioavailable testosterone and free testosterone. Many men will often have low or low normal total testosterone, but have disease states resulting in low levels of sex hormone binding globulin, which result in normal levels of bioavailable testosterone [24]. Testosterone levels should be drawn in the morning, preferable before 10 a.m. due to diurnal variation [25]. If the testosterone level is found to be less than 300 ng/dL, repeat levels should be drawn, along with luteinizing hormone and prolactin to help determine potential etiologic causes of hypogonadism [26].

37.5.2 Penile Function Evaluation

A helpful adjunct in the assessment of ED is specific vascular evaluation. This can help differentiate between psychogenic causes and vascular causes of ED. It may also differentiate between arterial insufficiency and venous leak. This adjunctive testing is often helpful in young, otherwise healthy men for which other identifiable causes for ED are not apparent.

The duplex doppler penile ultrasound is one such adjunctive measure of penile function. A rigid erection is induced by intracavernosal injection of vasodilatory medications such as prostaglandin, papaverine, and phentolamine. The type of medication, combination, and dosing should be adjusted so as to induce a full rigid erection. Erection quality should be measured and rated with the help of the patient. High-resolution ultrasound along with doppler ultrasonography is then used to measure the flow velocity within the cavernous arteries. Abnormal arterial peak systolic velocity less than 25 cm/second is suggestive of arterial insufficiency while veno-occlusive disease is suggested by an end diastolic velocity of greater than 5 cm/second. Additional measurements should include diameter of the cavernous arteries, the presence of penile curvature extent, and Peyronie's disease plaque calcification if present [27].

37.5.3 Cardiac Risk Assessment

As we have emphasized, the coexistence of ED and cardiovascular disease is strong, often in men without any overt symptoms of angina or shortness of breath with exercise. All men presenting with a complaint of ED should be regarded at potential risk for significant cardiovascular disease, therefore these patients should be particularly screened (Figure 37.1). New onset ED may precede symptoms of CAD particularly in younger men as vascular ED and CAD may be manifestations of the same disease. A flow limiting arterial plaque is more likely to manifest itself earlier in the penile caversonal arteries that are approximately 1–2 mm, while coronary arteries are 3–4 mm in diameter, and therefore more likely to manifest symptoms of a flow limiting plaque much later in the disease course [28]. Early identification and treatment may prevent future cardiac events [29].

The first step in a cardiac risk assessment is establishment of risk stratification. Evaluation and treatment should only be performed after quantitative risk assessment. We have found online risk calculators to be informative and easy to use. The calculator should be based on the 2019 American College of Cardiology/American Heart Association Guideline on the Assessment of Cardiovascular Risk [10]. This calculator estimates the 10-year risk of a first atherosclerotic cardiovascular disease event (e.g., stroke or myocardial infarction). The risk calculators utilize a combination of demographics (age, gender, and race), cholesterol levels (total cholesterol and HDL), blood pressure (systolic and diastolic), whether or not the blood pressure is treated with medication, and risk factors of diabetes mellitus and smoking history. The risk calculator can then stratify patients into categories of low risk (<5% risk of event),

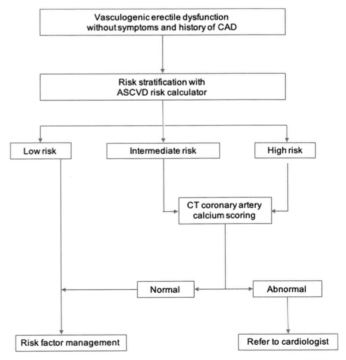

Figure 37.1 Algorithm for cardiovascular assessment in a patient with ED

Using 10-year ASCVD risk estimate plus coronary artery calcium (CAC) score to guide statin therapy				
Patient's 10-year atherosclerotic cardiovascular disease (ASCVD) risk estimate:	<5%	5–7.5%	>7.5–20%	>20%
Consulting ASCVD risk estimate alone	Statin not recommended	Consider for statin	Recommend statin	Recommend statin
Consulting ASCVD risk estimate + CAC				
If CAC score =0	Statin not recommended	Statin not recommended	Statin not recommended	Recommend statin
If CAC score >0	Statin not recommended	Consider for statin	Recommend statin	Recommend statin
Does CAC score modify treatment plan?	✗ CAC not effective for this population	✓ CAC can reclassify risk up or down	✓ CAC can reclassify risk up or down	✗ CAC not effective for this population

Figure 37.2 Coronary artery calcium Reproduced with permission from Greenland, et al. Coronary calcium score and cardiovascular risk. *Journal of the American College of Cardiology*, 2018;72(4):434–447.

borderline risk (5–7.5% risk of event), intermediate risk (7.5–20% risk of event), and high risk (>20% risk of event).

Men in the high-risk group should be referred to the cardiologist and would benefit from high-dose statin therapy. Men in the borderline and intermediate risk groups benefit from more intensive screening for CAD and benefit from treatment of cardiovascular risk factors, such as statin lipid-lowering medications and aspirin (Figure 37.2). These men are at risk of silent obstructive or future CAD. A noninvasive method of screening for these patients is the coronary artery calcium score. This is determined through a cardiac computed tomography (CT). A noncontrast CT of heart is obtained and the amount of calcified plaques is determined and converted into a scoring system. The coronary artery calcium score has been shown to closely correlate with risk of an atherosclerotic cardiovascular disease event [30]. Patients with elevated coronary calcium Agatston score (>100) should be referred to a cardiac specialist for further risk stratification and possible further diagnostic testing [31,32].

37.5.4 Psychological Evaluation

Comorbidities of depression and anxiety have strong correlations with ED [33]. Furthermore, the treatment of these conditions with pharmaceuticals can have strong effects on erectile function. A number of validated depression and anxiety questionnaires are available to assist in screening patients for comorbid psychological conditions. One such tool is the Patient Health Questionnaire [34]. This is a validated self-administered questionnaire that has been found to be a sensitive and specific measure for depressive disorders. The benefits of the questionnaire are in its relative brevity and reliable and valid measure of depression severity.

In-depth discussion and exploration of sexual performance anxiety is a valuable and necessary component of the evaluation of ED. It represents a large majority of ED complaints and can be independent or concomitant with vasculogenic ED. It occurs when anxiety about sexual performance leads to impairment of the sexual response in particular relaxed vasodilation penile blood flow. It is commonly associated with other anxiety disorders, including social anxiety, panic disorder, generalized anxiety disorder, obsessive compulsive disease, and body dysmorphic disorder.

If the patient has a regular partner, partner evaluation is a key part of a complete psychological evaluation. The partner can provide corroborating information and can often give additional insight into the nature and scope of the problem. It is also helpful to bring them into the therapeutic relationship as bridging understanding of the condition leading to ED will help manage treatment options and goals.

We have found sensate focus therapy, or structured touching exercises, to be both helpful in treatment of sexual performance anxiety but also in diagnosis. This therapy helps couples understand and explore the natural and physiological patterns of sexual responsiveness [35]. The techniques used in sensate focus help patients understand the fear of inadequacy that allows them to recognize their own anxious thoughts and feelings. After evaluation we recommend the couple work with a trained sexual therapist and continue a structured sensate therapy program.

37.6 Conclusions

Evaluating the male with ED includes a detailed and comprehensive patient history and a focal physical exam. Attention should be paid to development of a therapeutic relationship with the patient and with consideration paid to a shared decision-making process. Evaluation should be performed in a nonjudgmental atmosphere. This will allow for the patient to freely express the nature and extent of his ED and will allow for a more comprehensive treatment plan of available options and therapeutics. The physician–patient relationship should not be diminished, as this rapport will allow for a strong bond and a foundation for which to introduce, emphasize, and support the lifestyle changes that often drive ED and can improve it over time. This results in motivated patients who are committed and responsive to suggestions of regular exercise, efforts at weight loss, healthy eating, and smoking cessation.

Of utmost importance is the evaluation of cardiac risk factors. For many men, seeking care after the development of ED might be their first encounter with the healthcare system since their childhood. A properly balanced assessment will result in important long-term implications for the overall health of the patient and future morbidity. This is a unique opportunity to intervene in a patient's health and put them on a path to improved health and well-being.

References

1. McCabe MP, et al. Incidence and prevalence of sexual dysfunction in women and men: a consensus statement from the Fourth International Consultation on Sexual Medicine 2015. *J Sex Med.* 2016;13(2):144–152.
2. Lewis RW, et al. Definitions/epidemiology/risk factors for sexual dysfunction. *J Sex Med.* 2010;7(4 Pt 2):1598–1607.
3. Ayta IA, McKinlay JB, Krane RJ. The likely worldwide increase in erectile dysfunction between 1995 and 2025 and some possible policy consequences. *BJU Int.* 1999;84(1):50–56.
4. Guay AT. ED2: erectile dysfunction = endothelial dysfunction. *Endocrinol Metab Clin North Am.* 2007;36(2):453–463.
5. Kirby M. The circle of lifestyle and erectile dysfunction. *Sex Med Rev.* 2015;3(3):169–182.
6. DeLay KJ, Haney N, Hellstrom WJ. Modifying risk factors in the management of erectile dysfunction: a review. *World J Mens Health.* 2016;34(2):89–100.
7. Kostis JB, Dobrzynski JM. The effect of statins on erectile dysfunction: a meta-analysis of randomized trials. *J Sex Med.* 2014;11(7):1626–1635.
8. Grundy SM, et al. Definition of metabolic syndrome: report of the National Heart, Lung, and Blood Institute/American Heart Association conference on scientific issues related to definition. *Circulation.* 2004;109(3):433–438.
9. Feldman DI, et al. Subclinical vascular disease and subsequent erectile dysfunction: the multiethnic study of atherosclerosis (MESA). *Clin Cardiol.* 2016;39(5):291–298.
10. Lloyd-Jones DM, et al. Use of risk assessment tools to guide decision-making in the primary prevention of atherosclerotic cardiovascular disease: a special report from the American Heart Association and American College of Cardiology. *J Am Coll Cardiol.* 2019;73(24):3153–3167.
11. Burnett AL, et al. Erectile dysfunction: AUA Guideline. *J Urol.* 2018;200(3):633–641.
12. Selvin E, Burnett AL Platz EA. Prevalence and risk factors for erectile dysfunction in the US. *Am J Med.* 2007;120(2):151–157.
13. Hatzichristou D, et al. Recommendations for the clinical evaluation of men and women with sexual dysfunction. *J Sex Med.* 2010;7(1 Pt 2):337–348.
14. O'Leary MP, et al. A brief male sexual function inventory for urology. *Urology.* 1995;46(5):697–706.
15. Romeo JH, et al. Sexual function in men with diabetes type 2: association with glycemic control. *J Urol.* 2000;163(3):788–791.
16. Nehra A, et al. The Princeton III Consensus recommendations for the management of erectile dysfunction and cardiovascular disease. *Mayo Clin Proc.* 2012;87(8):766–778.
17. Ghanem HM, Salonia A, Martin-Morales A. SOP: physical examination and laboratory testing for men with erectile dysfunction. *J Sex Med.* 2013;10(1):108–110.
18. Saenz de Tejada I, et al. Pathophysiology of erectile dysfunction. *J Sex Med.* 2005;2(1):26–39.
19. Chung F, et al. High STOP-Bang score indicates a high probability of obstructive sleep apnoea. *Br J Anaesth.* 2012;108(5):768–775.
20. Liu PY. A clinical perspective of sleep and andrological health: assessment, treatment considerations, and future research. *J Clin Endocrinol Metab.* 2019;104(10):4398–4417.
21. Gerbild H, et al. Physical activity to improve erectile function: a systematic review of intervention studies. *Sex Med.* 2018;6(2):75–89.
22. Wang F, et al. Erectile dysfunction and fruit/vegetable consumption among diabetic Canadian men. *Urology.* 2013;82(6):1330–1335.
23. Esposito K, et al. Effect of lifestyle changes on erectile dysfunction in obese men: a randomized controlled trial. *JAMA.* 2004;291(24):2978–2984.
24. Jarecki P, et al. Can low SHBG serum concentration be a good early marker of male hypogonadism in metabolic syndrome? *Diabetes Metab Syndr Obes.* 2019;12:2181–2191.
25. Diver MJ, et al. Diurnal rhythms of serum total, free and bioavailable testosterone and of SHBG in middle-aged men compared with those in young men. *Clin Endocrinol (Oxf).* 2003;58(6):710–717.
26. Mulhall JP, et al. Evaluation and management of testosterone deficiency: AUA Guideline. *J Urol.* 2018;200(2):423–432.
27. Carson CC, et al. *Textbook of erectile dysfunction.* 2nd ed. Informa Healthcare; 2009.
28. Montorsi P, et al. Association between erectile dysfunction and coronary artery disease. Role of coronary clinical presentation and extent of coronary vessels involvement: the COBRA trial. *Eur Heart J.* 2006;27(22):2632–2639.
29. Miner MM. Erectile dysfunction and the "window of curability": a harbinger of cardiovascular events. *Mayo Clin Proc.* 2009;84(2):102–104.

30. Greenland P, et al. ACCF/AHA 2007 clinical expert consensus document on coronary artery calcium scoring by computed tomography in global cardiovascular risk assessment and in evaluation of patients with chest pain: a report of the American College of Cardiology Foundation Clinical Expert Consensus Task Force (ACCF/AHA Writing Committee to Update the 2000 Expert Consensus Document on Electron Beam Computed Tomography). *Circulation*. 2007;115(3):402–426.

31. Greenland P, et al. Coronary calcium score and cardiovascular risk. *J Am Coll Cardiol*. 2018;72(4):434–447.

32. Agatston AS, et al. Quantification of coronary artery calcium using ultrafast computed tomography. *J Am Coll Cardiol*. 1990;15(4):827–832.

33. Liu Q, et al. Erectile dysfunction and depression: a systematic review and meta-analysis. *J Sex Med*. 2018;15(8):1073–1082.

34. Kroenke K, Spitzer RL, Williams JB. The PHQ-9: validity of a brief depression severity measure. *J Gen Intern Med*. 2001;16(9):606–613.

35. Linschoten M, Weiner L, Avery-Clark C. Sensate focus: a critical literature review. *Sex Relatsh Ther*. 2016;21(2):230–247.

36. Wein AJ, Kavoussi LR, Campbell, MF. *Campbell–Walsh urology* [Wein AJ, ed.-in-chief; Kavoussi LR et al., eds.]. 10th ed. Elsevier Saunders; 2012.

Section 5 **Medical and Surgical Management of Issues of Male Health**

Chapter 38

Lifestyle Modifications for Erectile Dysfunction

Jeffrey S. Edman, Jade Warner, and Amy M. Pearlman

38.1 Introduction

Sexual health plays an important role in the lives of many men and, for some, erectile function, specifically, helps define one's sense of masculinity. Erectile dysfunction (ED), referring to the inability to attain and/or maintain an erection sufficient for sexual activity, is one component of sexual health. ED is common in the United States, affecting over 18% of men over the age of 20 with the risk of experiencing ED increasing as men age [1]. Moreover, the disease is often debilitating for men and can lead to significant psychosocial consequences [2]. ED results in decreased physical and emotional satisfaction from sexual activity as well as an overall decrease in quality of life. Fortunately, a variety of medical and surgical options exist to restore erectile function, including oral medications, vacuum erection devices, penile constriction rings, medicated urethral suppositories, intracavernosal injections, and penile implants.

Lifestyle modification, considered first-line therapy for many disease processes, is often overlooked and underdiscussed in the management of men presenting with ED. Early initiation of lifestyle changes can help improve function in these men, as well as reduce the risk of developing dysfunction [3]. Furthermore, some men prefer a less medicalized approach to the treatment of ED, as one study involving Mexican men demonstrated [4]. Modifications to lifestyle or initiation of alternative medicines were the preferred source of change in this subset of men who described their view of medications, such as phosphodiesterase 5 (PDE5) inhibitors, for the treatment of ED as physically dangerous due to the significant side effects mentioned on television commercials. Though pharmacologic and surgical interventions to restore erectile function are important tools in the armamentarium of the healthcare provider, the authors believe that discussions regarding pertinent lifestyle modification should play a role at time of patient presentation and throughout the treatment process.

The aim of this chapter is to review the literature assessing lifestyle modification for the treatment of ED. Medications for the treatment of ED are directly marketed to consumers via television with commercials for Viagra® and Cialis®, alone, exceeding $300 million a year [5]. The authors believe that behavioral modification should be marketed as a prevention strategy, standalone treatment strategy, and as an adjunct to current pharmacotherapy by healthcare providers who treat those with ED. We hope to clarify what is currently known about efficacy of lifestyle modification so as to improve the clinician's ability to educate patients on the importance of making healthier choices and to spawn ideas for future work to address gaps in knowledge.

38.2 Pathophysiology of Erection

Understanding the pathophysiology of obtaining and maintaining an erection is critical in order to comprehend the effects of lifestyle modification on both processes.

38.2.1 Nitric Oxide

Nitric oxide (NO) is a metabolite of L-arginine (catalyzed via nitric oxide synthases [NOS]) and is considered the principal neurotransmitter and vasoactive metabolite for erection [6]. Upon sexual arousal, NO is released by nerve terminals and endothelial cells where it activates guanylyl cyclase that increases intracellular concentrations of cyclic guanosine monophosphate (cGMP). This ultimately leads to smooth muscle relaxation, engorgement of corporal bodies, and, through tension on the tunic albuginea, creates an erection. Individual NO molecules are only transiently present before being metabolized to nitrate or nitrite in the blood as are intracellular cyclic GMP before being hydrolyzed to GMP by PDE5. Loss of erection occurs when NO-induced vasodilation terminates and blood is drained from the corporal bodies leaving less tension on the tunica and thus cessation of penile engorgement.

Sildenafil, vardenafil, tadalafil, and avanafil are all FDA-approved drugs to treat ED by blocking this PDE enzyme activity. By working on the cGMP pathway, these medications work indirectly on the NO pathway to promote erectile function, the same pathway impacted by nonpharmacologic interventions. As a result, these medications may have improved efficacy when combined with lifestyle modifications [7].

38.2.2 Reactive Oxygen Species

Reactive oxygen species (ROS) also play an important role in erectile function as they expedite NO destruction, thereby contributing to decreased effectiveness of both initiation and maintenance of erections [7]. ROS, including superoxide, peroxide, and peroxynitrite, are byproducts of normal bodily functions and can be heavily influenced by daily activities. Human bodies are protected from this biochemical process by antioxidants such as glutathione, which block the harmful effects of ROS. A study that demonstrates this association of vascular health and ROS assessed angiotensin receptor blockade and demonstrated the ability to reduce oxidative stress as a result of this blockade [8]. Those taking losartan had lower levels of 8-isoprostanes (a marker of oxidative stress) compared to those taking atenolol. While oxidative stress markers and the end point of flow-mediated dilation (FMD; a measurable variable suggestive of endothelial responsiveness to molecular triggers) of the brachial artery were affected, other contributing factors including hemoglobin A1c, c-reactive protein (CRP), and systolic blood pressure, remained unaffected suggesting that losartan's effect on ROS was significant enough to affect FMD and endothelial health. This mechanism and effect on dilation of systemic vasculature helps explain the improvement in erectile function noted in those taking losartan not seen with other antihypertensives. This study illustrates the important role of ROS in erectile function and suggests an underlying mechanism by which lifestyle changes can impact erections.

38.2.3 Cytokines

Cytokines such as tumor necrosis factor (TNF), interleukin 6 (IL-6), interleukin 8 (IL-8), and interleukin 18 (IL-18) are proinflammatory markers that affect serum NO throughout the body, including erectile tissue. Rats undergoing induction of periodontitis showed a decrease in NO expression in cavernosal tissue with concomitant increases in expression of TNF and CRP throughout the body [9]. Those with chronic systemic diseases, such as diabetes and/or obesity, have higher levels of these proinflammatory cytokines circulating throughout the body, which may help explain the higher rates of ED in these populations [10]. Presence of circulating proinflammatory markers also suggests a mechanism by which lifestyle changes addressing chronic diseases are effective in treating ED as suggested by endothelial dysfunction as a result of chronic low-level inflammatory states [11]. These chronic low-level inflammatory states refer to constant levels of mildly elevated inflammatory markers during which time the body has continued exposure. Proinflammatory markers are mildly increased in obesity and there is a direct relationship between acute phase (proinflammatory) markers and insulin resistance. As a result, acute phase markers may contribute to endothelial dysfunction in humans as described in the periodontitis study.

38.3 Lifestyle Changes

Proposed lifestyle modifications for those with ED closely resemble recommendations one might have to promote overall health and wellness.

38.3.1 Exercise

Coital and systemic exercise can improve erectile function. Exercise, in general, is considered to be the most significant single factor to improve erectile function as part of initial conservative management [12,13]. Coital exercise (i.e., getting and maintaining an erection) causes increased amount of blood to shunt to the penis and, when done repetitively, correlates with decreases in rates of ED by up to 50% in those 55–75 years old [12]. Increased blood flow to the penis, resulting in increased penile artery shear stress, has been shown to increase vascular NO levels with a suspected increase in FMD. Greater than one sexual episode per week was associated with reduced risk of developing ED. Systemic exercise (i.e., working multiple muscle groups throughout the body) also results in improved erectile function, thought secondary to increased systemic NO turnover that may lead to improvements in glucose disposal and insulin sensitivity [13]. Sedentary lifestyles have, conversely, been found to impair erectile function, though with moderate to high levels of exercise, improvement in erectile function may result. Forty minutes of moderate to high levels of aerobic exercise or 160 minutes of weekly exercise at the same moderate to high levels were effective in partially restoring erectile function for some patients. This association was demonstrated in 10 separate studies, all of which showed a statistically significant difference pre and post exercise initiation measuring erectile function using the International Index of Erectile Function (IIEF) questionnaire, a validated tool for evaluating erectile function [14]. Of note, extreme exercise, such as that performed by endurance athletes, increases muscular damage due to ROS, especially in those not accustomed to this level of exertion [15]. This is thought to be secondary to high oxidative damage from overwhelming typical physiologic barriers, namely glutathione, which is involved in many reduction-oxidation reactions throughout the body. This study, although not directly discussing erectile health, can act as a surrogate for suspected effects to erectile function with the superimposed variable of high ROS damage from extreme exercise.

38.3.2 Pelvic Floor Physical Therapy

Pelvic floor physical therapy (PFPT) may also improve erectile function mechanically, rather than chemically, by activating the ischiocavernosus and bulbocavernosus muscles that, when strengthened, can reduce venous outflow from the penis [16]. A randomized controlled study assessing pelvic floor exercises, in conjunction with lifestyle changes (subjects received counseling on weight loss, smoking cessation, reducing alcohol consumption, and avoiding bike saddle pressure) resulted in 40% of men returning to normal erectile function and another 35.5% of participants with improved erectile function as measured via the IIEF questionnaire. This study attempted to compare these lifestyle changes with PFPT plus lifestyle changes, but due to the overwhelming success of PFPT, all subjects were placed on PFPT. This study excluded men with known physical etiologies for ED such as those post prostatectomy or those with neurological conditions. Pelvic floor exercises included retraction of the penis and lifting the scrotum, gaining maximum contractions twice daily lying, sitting, or standing, submaximal work while walking, and tightening the bulbocavernosus muscle after urination to help eliminate urine.

Association between ED and postmicturition dribble caused by pelvic floor weakness has also been reported [17]. A similarly designed randomized controlled trial with a crossover arm of the same group of men showed that 65.5% of the men had postmicturition dribble (PMD) and pelvic floor exercises significantly improved this PMD. Men with PMD, in addition to ED, appear to experience improvements in both with PFPT. Presence of concomitant PMD may also help identify those presenting with ED who may benefit from PFPT although definitive data are lacking.

38.3.3 Weight Management

Weight management can also improve erectile function. Those who are overweight experience more systemic inflammation, increased ROS from increased caloric consumption, and decreased insulin sensitivity [18]. Similar to the effects of inflammation and ROS previously discussed, insulin sensitivity also impacts levels of endothelial NO. Decreased insulin sensitivity, demonstrated by increased circulating insulin, leads to less circulating NO [19]. Fortunately, erectile function can improve with weight loss. One study showed that a third of obese men reversed their ED after two years of behavior modifications aimed at losing weight [20]. Behavior modifications included personalized dietary, exercise, and counseling sessions aimed at a 10% reduction in weight over two years. Erectile function was measured using the IIEF and other parameters measured included inflammatory markers and endothelial responsiveness to the vasoactive molecule L-arginine. Even those who only lost a minimal amount of weight but participated in these weight-conscious behavior modifications had improved erectile function, suggesting that the modifications alone were enough to produce results regardless of achieving objective weight loss. Decreases in CRP and IL-6 levels, markers of reduced systemic inflammation elevated in obesity, are thought be the source of the improvement in endothelial function leading to improved erections.

38.3.4 Nutrition

Fat and sugar intake can affect erectile function. A high fat meal transiently decreases FMD of the brachial artery likely due to ROS and inflammatory molecules [21]. Active adults did not experience decreases in FMD with the bolus of a high fat meal, while inactive adults experienced significant decreases in responses to these boluses, suggesting that activity level may be protective from these inflammatory- and ROS-rich states. Furthermore, isolated increases in blood sugar result in increases of inflammatory factors such as TNF alpha and IL-6. Diabetes is a significant risk factor for ED both due to the pathophysiology of increased blood sugar but also the comorbidities (obesity, insulin resistance, sedentary lifestyle) typically associated with diabetes, which are independent risk factors for ED. Diabetics experience increases in ROS in response to even transient hyperglycemia, which can affect erectile function by shortening the half-life of NO within the penile vasculature [22].

38.3.5 Drug Use

Tobacco and alcohol can worsen erectile function. Cigarette smoke leads to increased systemic oxidative stress. Endothelial NO synthase is also uncoupled by cigarette smoke and leads to the production of superoxide (a free radical form of O_2) that may lead to additional systemic oxidative damage [23]. Fortunately, smoking cessation in both the short and long term can decrease the impact ROS have on NOS function and thus erectile function [24]. Mild to moderate alcohol intake (1–2 drinks per night) increases NO, though excess alcohol leads to decreased vascular NO [25]. The vasodilatory effects of minimal to moderate alcohol use can improve erections transiently, though heavy alcohol intake is associated with exacerbation of ED, for which the mechanism is not clearly understood. Levels of toxic alcohol metabolites, as well as cognitive impairment associated with heavy alcohol consumption, would be suspected sources of ED in this population.

38.3.6 Antioxidants

Inflammation and free radical formation are the most important molecular factors in erectile function and, therefore, it is not surprising that antioxidants can help prevent damage from free ROS and improve erectile function [26]. Important antioxidants, such as Vitamins C and E, are present in many foods such as broccoli, cauliflower, red bell peppers, pomegranate, nuts, and strawberries, and are present in high quantities (1,000 mg/day of Vitamin C and 800 IU of Vitamin E) in many supplements used to mitigate the effects of ROS on the body. FMD is one endpoint in the objective measurement of the effect of lifestyle modifications on ED and has been used as a dependent variable in studies assessing vascular health. FMD was measured in smokers and nonsmokers before and after steady-state levels of antioxidant supplementation with Vitamins C and E [27]. High levels of antioxidant supplementation (measured by steady-state levels above 100 microM of ascorbate or microM/total lipid of alpha-tocopherol) in smokers mitigated the effects on NO and led to improved FMD in the brachial artery (nearly 300% increase in FMD before and after supplementation, respectively [$p<0.05$]) whereas in nonsmokers, vitamin supplementation had no significant effect. This improvement in FMD highlights the importance of mitigating the consequences of ROS, especially in smokers, who have an elevated amount of ROS damage.

38.3.7 Treatment of Sleep Apnea

Obstructive sleep apnea (OSA) is another chronic medical condition commonly seen in men presenting with ED and has been demonstrated to worsen erectile function. Frequent pauses in breathing have been shown to impair endothelial function, resulting in decreased circulating NO, increased oxidative stress, and increased inflammation [28]. Men with OSA are more likely to have ED than the general population and this association holds true even when adjusting for other comorbidities. In two separate studies, ED was found in 51% and 48% of newly diagnosed OSA patients [29–31]. Continuous positive airway pressure (CPAP) therapy has been shown to improve erectile function (determined by IIEF questionnaire) along with gonadal function, orgasmic function, intercourse satisfaction, overall satisfaction, and overall sexual function when comparing outcomes before and after initiation of CPAP therapy in one study though a second study showed no significant difference. Therefore, limited research suggests possible improvement of ED with CPAP therapy for OSA.

38.3.8 Impact of Psychological Factors

One's emotional state also has implications on sexual function. One study using quality of life surveys found that emotional components led to a more profound impairment on erectile function compared to physical components [32]. The physical and emotional domains were assessed through a health-related quality of life (HRQOL) questionnaire with each domain scored separately from 0 to 100, with higher scores representing better HRQOL. A significant decrease in overall emotional well-being correlated with ED suggesting an association between the two, though causality cannot be determined.

Early viewpoints portrayed erectile problems to be principally physiologic in nature and thus there has been a substantial predilection toward medicalization of ED. The introduction of oral PDE5 inhibitors such as sildenafil also reinforced the notion of ED being a medical condition [33]. Even when presumptive medical factors are present, psychological distress may also be a contributing factor [34]. The prevalence of significant psychiatric pathology (major depression, substance abuse, anxiety disorders, and schizophrenia), excluding interview stress, was present in 33% of men with ED although only 16 of 40 cases were recognized and highlighted in the initial assessments by treating urologists. This psychogenic component of ED is important for healthcare providers to recognize so that these factors may be addressed alone or in combination with other therapies for ED.

38.3.9 Limitations

Few studies objectively assess changes in erectile function with various lifestyle modifications. Much of what we know about lifestyle interventions on the vascular system comes from its effect on the cardiovascular system with little objective data showing effects on cavernosal blood flow. Future research is warranted to better assess the effect of lifestyle modification behaviors on objective measurements of erectile function.

References

1. Selvin E, Burnett AL, Platz EA. Prevalence and risk factors for erectile dysfunction in the US. *Am J Med.* 2007;120(2):151–157.
2. Laumann EO, Paik A, Rosen RC. Sexual dysfunction in the United States. *JAMA.* 1999;281(6):537–544.
3. Derby CA, et al. Modifiable risk factors and erectile dysfunction: can lifestyle changes modify risk? *Urology.* 2000;56(2):302–306.
4. Wentzell E, Salmerón J. You'll "get Viagraed": Mexican men's preference for alternative erectile dysfunction treatment. *Soc Sci Med.* 2009;68(10):1759–1765.
5. Arnold DG, Oakley JL. Self-regulation in the pharmaceutical industry: the exposure of children and adolescents to erectile dysfunction commercials. *J Health Polit Policy Law.* 2019;44(5):765–787.
6. Rajfer J, et al. Nitric oxide as a mediator of relaxation of the corpus cavernosum in response to nonadrenergic, noncholinergic neurotransmission. *N Engl J Med.* 1992;326(2):90–94.
7. Meldrum DR, et al. The link between erectile and cardiovascular health: the canary in the coal mine. *Am J Cardiol.* 2011;108(4):599–606.
8. Flammer AJ, et al. Effect of losartan, compared with atenolol, on endothelial function and oxidative stress in patients with type 2 diabetes and hypertension. *J Hypertens.* 2007;25(4):785–791.
9. Zuo Z, et al. Effect of periodontitis on erectile function and its possible mechanism. *J Sex Med.* 2011;8(9):2598–2605.
10. Giugliano F, et al. Erectile dysfunction associates with endothelial dysfunction and raised proinflammatory cytokine levels in obese men. *J Endocrin Invest.* 2004;27(7):665–669.
11. Yudkin JS, et al. C-reactive protein in healthy subjects: associations with obesity, insulin resistance, and endothelial dysfunction. *Arterioscler Thromb Vasc Biol.* 1999;19(4):972–978.
12. Koskimäki J, et al. Regular intercourse protects against erectile dysfunction: Tampere Aging Male Urologic Study. *Am J Med.* 2008;121(7):592–596.
13. Gerbild H, et al. Physical activity to improve erectile function: a systematic review of intervention studies. *Sex Med.* 2018;6(2):75–89.
14. Rosen RC, et al. The International Index of Erectile Function (IIEF): a multidimensional scale for assessment of erectile dysfunction. *Urology.* 1997;49(6):822–830.
15. He F, et al. Redox mechanism of reactive oxygen species in exercise. *Front Physiol.* 2016;7:486.
16. Dorey G, et al. Pelvic floor exercises for erectile dysfunction. *BJU Int.* 2005;96(4):595–597.
17. Dorey G, et al. Pelvic floor exercises for treating post-micturition dribble in men with erectile dysfunction: a randomized controlled trial. *Urol Nurs.* 2004;24(6):490–497, 512.
18. Marseglia L, et al. Oxidative stress in obesity: a critical component in human diseases. *Int J Mol Sci.* 2014;16(1):378–400.
19. Russo GI, et al. Insulin resistance is an independent predictor of severe lower urinary tract symptoms and of erectile dysfunction: results from a cross-sectional study. *J Sex Med.* 2014;11(8):2074–2082.
20. Esposito K, et al. Effect of lifestyle changes on erectile dysfunction in obese men. *JAMA.* 2004;291(24):2978–2984.

21. Esposito K, et al. Effect of a single high-fat meal on endothelial function in patients with the metabolic syndrome: role of tumor necrosis factor-α. *Nutr Metab Cardiovasc Dis.* 2007;17(4):274–279.
22. Malavige LS, Levy JC. Erectile dysfunction in diabetes mellitus. *J Sex Med.* 2009;6(5):1232–1247.
23. Tostes RC, et al. Cigarette smoking and erectile dysfunction: focus on NO bioavailability and ROS generation. *J Sex Med.* 2008;5(6):1284–1295.
24. Kovac JR, et al. Effects of cigarette smoking on erectile dysfunction. *Andrologia.* 2015;47(10):1087–1092.
25. Abou-Agag LH, et al. Evidence of cardiovascular protection by moderate alcohol: role of nitric oxide. *Free Radic Biol Med.* 2005;39(4):540–548.
26. Ignarro LJ, et al. Pomegranate juice protects nitric oxide against oxidative destruction and enhances the biological actions of nitric oxide. *Nitric Oxide.* 2006;15(2):93–102.
27. Peluffo G, et al. Superoxide-mediated inactivation of nitric oxide and peroxynitrite formation by tobacco smoke in vascular endothelium: studies in cultured cells and smokers. *Am J Physiol Heart Circ Physiol.* 2009;296(6):H1781–H1792.
28. Atkeson A, et al. Endothelial function in obstructive sleep apnea. *Prog Cardiovasc Dis.* 2009;51(5):351–362.
29. Pascual M, et al. Erectile dysfunction in obstructive sleep apnea patients: a randomized trial on the effects of continuous positive airway pressure (CPAP). *PLoS ONE.* 2018;13(8):e0201930.
30. İrer B, et al. Evaluation of sexual dysfunction, lower urinary tract symptoms and quality of life in men with obstructive sleep apnea syndrome and the efficacy of continuous positive airway pressure therapy. *Urology.* 2018;121:86–92.
31. Hoekema A, et al. Sexual function and obstructive sleep apnea–hypopnea: a randomized clinical trial evaluating the effects of oral-appliance and continuous positive airway pressure therapy. *J Sex Med.* 2007;4(4):1153–1162.
32. Litwin MS, Nied RJ, Dhanani N. Health-related quality of life in men with erectile dysfunction. *J Gen Intern Med.* 1998;13(3):159–166.
33. Aghighi A, Grigoryan VH, Delavar A. Psychological determinants of erectile dysfunction among middle-aged men. *Int J Impot Res.* 2015;27(2):63–68.
34. Lee JC, et al. The prevalence and influence of significant psychiatric abnormalities in men undergoing comprehensive management of organic erectile dysfunction. *Int J Impot Res.* 2000;12(1):47–51.

Chapter 39: Medical and Surgical Management of Erectile Dysfunction

Mohit Khera and Skyler Howell

39.1 Introduction

Erectile dysfunction (ED) is defined as the inability to attain and/or maintain sufficient penile rigidity for sexual satisfaction. It is a complex, multifactorial condition that is part of the normal aging process, and thus most commonly affects middle-aged and elderly men. However, ED is seen in men of all ages, making it a common chief complaint in both primary care and urologic clinics. ED may result from several mechanisms: difficulty initiating erection (psychogenic, neurogenic, endocrinogenic), difficulty filling (arteriogenic), and/or difficulty maintaining blood flow (veno-occlusive) within the penis. This chapter will discuss medical and surgical management options for ED as well as psychosexual therapy, lifestyle modification, and hormone replacement therapy.

ED may be a manifestation of another condition and may resolve upon treatment of the underlying issue. In special cases including primary or predominantly psychogenic ED, poor overall health, or endocrinologic issues, specific management options are available and recommended.

39.1.1 Psychogenic ED

Most cases of ED involve a psychogenic component. Psychotherapy and psychosexual counseling are recommended in men with psychogenic ED as primary therapy or as an adjunct to organic ED treatment. Adjuvant psychosexual therapy may improve medical treatment efficacy [1] and adherence [2]. Counseling therapies assist patients and their partners with communication about sexual concerns, may reduce sexual anxiety, and allow discussion of strategies for integrating ED treatments into their sexual relationship.

39.1.2 Organic ED Secondary to Poor Overall Health

Lifestyle modification including changes to diet and exercise routines may have beneficial effects on erectile function in men with certain metabolic or cardiovascular comorbidities and may increase efficacy of ED treatments. Men with ED and metabolic or cardiovascular comorbidities have higher International Index of Erectile Function (IIEF) scores compared to counterparts who do not [3]. Smoking cessation may also lead to improved overall health and improvements in erectile function [4].

39.1.3 Organic ED Secondary to Hypogonadism

ED may present as a symptom of testosterone deficiency. While hormone replacement therapy alone is not an effective treatment for ED in these patients [5], testosterone-deficient men receiving combination hormone replacement and a phosphodiesterase type-5 (PDE5) inhibitor report better erectile function scores compared to men receiving either therapy alone [6]. Testosterone therapy in PDE5 inhibitor-nonresponsive patients results in improved erectile function [7], although testosterone monotherapy is not recommended in patients with normal testosterone levels. Optimum efficacy of PDE5 inhibitor medication is most likely to be achieved once testosterone levels are normalized [8].

39.2 Medical Management

Medical therapies for ED range from oral medications to locally acting agents to nonsurgical devices. We have already mentioned hormone replacement, a medical therapy useful in a specific population of men with ED, and will now discuss other significant medical ED therapies.

39.2.1 PDE5 Inhibitors

This class of oral medications remains the backbone of medical management for ED, and includes four FDA-approved agents – sildenafil, tadalafil, vardenafil, and avanafil – as well as several other PDE5 inhibitors approved for use in other countries. These medications assist with the arterial and venous mechanisms involved in erectile function, but notably do not affect the sexual arousal phase that relies on nervous input; they function by inhibiting the PDE5 enzyme, which breaks down cyclic guanosine monophosphate (cGMP). Inhibition of PDE5 results in elevated penile tissue cGMP concentrations, causing smooth muscle relaxation in the corpus cavernosum. Men receiving a PDE5 inhibitor should be educated regarding the need for sexual stimulation. Multiple medication trials may be required to establish efficacy, since medications differ in onset and duration of action. Men and partners should be counseled that initial nonresponse or inadequate response may be readily overcome with a dose increase just as adverse events may be ameliorated with a dose decrease. Treatment failure is largely attributable to incorrect use, and reeducation often leads to treatment success [9].

39.2.1.1 Use in the General ED Population

PDE5 inhibitor medications have been extensively studied in the general ED population, although the newer drug avanafil has been relatively less well-studied. PDE5 inhibitors appear to have similar efficacy in the general ED population, consistent across various measures of erectile function [3]. Differences in response rates between dose groups are small and usually not clinically significant. This is not true for many adverse events, which correlate directly with dose, supporting the recommendation that men use the lowest dose that produces acceptable outcomes. Dose titration and experimentation is a key step to optimize PDE5 inhibitor efficacy, so men may be offered dosing frequency changes [10] or an alternative PDE5 inhibitor [11]. Tadalafil is currently FDA-approved for daily dosing; all other PDE5 inhibitors were studied using on-demand dosing only.

39.2.1.2 Use in Special Populations

Not all PDE5 inhibitor have been evaluated in all special populations of men with ED (e.g., diabetes, benign prostatic hyperplasia [BPH]/lower urinary tract symptoms [LUTS], postprostatectomy, post spinal cord injury), but findings in general are similar to those reported in the general ED population, with data for avanafil generally limited [3]. For men with diabetes, sildenafil, tadalafil, and vardenafil appear equally effective. For men with BPH/LUTS and ED, sildenafil and tadalafil appear to have similar efficacy. For men with ED caused by radical prostatectomy (RP), efficacy also appears similar across the PDE5 inhibitors. For men post radiation therapy (RT) for prostate cancer, sildenafil and tadalafil appear to have similar efficacy. Dose-response effects in special populations have not been well-studied, but available data suggest that men with diabetes and men who are postprostatectomy have more severe ED at baseline and respond less robustly to PDE5 inhibitors; as a result, clinicians may consider initiating therapy at a higher dose.

39.2.1.3 Use in Post-RP/RT ED

Prostate cancer therapies including RP, RT, and systemic hormonal therapy may result in various degrees of ED, with the course of erectile function loss and recovery specific to the intervention. Post-RP ED involves either neuropraxia (temporary loss of nerve function) that may occur despite "nerve sparing," or complete nerve function loss following cavernous transection or removal. Concomitant penile vascular damage and cavernosal denervation also contribute [12]. Post-RT ED involves radiation-induced damage to the penile neurovascular supply [13]. Penile rehabilitation strategies following these treatments focus on sustaining and modulating nerve and vascular/cavernosal tissue function [14]. Due to their noninvasive nature and ease of administration, PDE5 inhibitors have been investigated most extensively for this purpose [15], although studies have yet to show a benefit over placebo in terms of restored erectile function. Lag time bias may be to blame; it is possible that a longer-term treatment schedule may be necessary to demonstrate erectile health recovery effects.

39.2.1.4 Contraindications

The clinician prescribing PDE5 inhibitors must be conversant with all potential disease state and medication contraindications. Nitrate medications taken with PDE5is can result in hypotension, so one medication should not be taken with the other prior to a washout period. Men using sublingual nitroglycerin for angina should not use this medication within 24 hours of PDE5 inhibitor use, or longer if using tadalafil, which has a longer half-life. Many other medications can also potentially interact with or influence the metabolism of PDE5 inhibitor, including antidepressants, antifungals, antihypertensives, and HIV/AIDS drugs [16]. PDE5 inhibitors should be used with caution in men with mild to moderate hepatic or renal impairment or men with spinal cord injury, given the potential for delayed metabolism; in men with severe renal or liver disease, use of PDE5 inhibitors is generally not recommended.

39.2.1.5 Adverse Events

Most adverse events associated with PDE5 inhibitor administration are mild to moderate, with dyspepsia, headache, flushing, back pain, nasal congestion, myalgia, visual disturbance, and dizziness most commonly reported. Rates of dyspepsia and dizziness were relatively similar across sildenafil, tadalafil, and vardenafil. Headache and flushing occur most commonly with sildenafil and vardenafil; back pain and myalgia with tadalafil; and nasal congestion with vardenafil. Sildenafil has the highest rates of visual disturbance [3]. Tadalafil is associated with lower rates of frequently reported adverse events – particularly headaches – due to daily dosing, which requires a lower dose compared to on-demand use, echoing the strong dose-response pattern seen in adverse events of PDE5 inhibitor therapy. Men post-RP and men post-RT reported substantially higher rates of adverse events than the general ED population; men post-RP reported higher rates in response to sildenafil in particular, while men post-RT reported higher rates across all PDE5 inhibitor as well as placebo groups. Men in this population may have heightened sensitivity to body sensations and/or increased needs for psychosocial support.

39.2.1.6 Other Concerns

Studies have suggested relationships between PDE5 inhibitor use and several conditions, notably nonarteritic anterior ischemic optic neuropathy [17], skin cancer [18], and prostate cancer recurrence [19], although the data supporting these conclusions is tenuous and contradicted by further investigation [20].

39.2.2 Local Therapies

Several locally acting options are available for assisted erection therapy. Intracavernosal injections (ICI) agents include alprostadil, or prostaglandin E1; papaverine, a nonspecific phosphodiesterase inhibitor; phentolamine, an alpha-adrenergic antagonist; and atropine. In addition, alprostadil may be delivered by intraurethral (IU) and topical administrations as well.

39.2.2.1 Use of ICI

Men with contraindications to PDE5 inhibitors, who find them ineffective, or who prefer no oral medications in general may choose ICI. Of the available injectable substances, only alprostadil is FDA-approved in the USA and is the only medication typically used as a single agent. Combinations of medications, such as bi-mix (papaverine + phentolamine) or tri-mix (papaverine + phentolamine + alprostadil) are also used to improve efficacy via synergistic effects and side-effect reduction via lower dose of individual agents. Combination medications require pharmacy compounding since they are not FDA approved, which may present a barrier to treatment. ICI medications are effective and highly satisfactory in men from the general ED population as well as those with diabetes, cardiovascular risk factors, men who are postprostatectomy, and men with spinal cord injuries [3]. Men considering ICI therapy should have an in-office injection test to determine the appropriate dose and medication(s), to help them achieve confidence with the technique and to facilitate adherence. At this visit, the risks of priapism and the proper course of action should be thoroughly explained, such as attempting ejaculation followed by oral pseudoephedrine and application of an ice pack to the penis, if unsuccessful. If the erection nevertheless persists, the importance of obtaining timely urgent or emergent intervention should be emphasized.

39.2.2.2 Adverse Events Associated with ICI

Rates of successful intercourse are similar across medications and medication combinations, but adverse event profiles differ. Priapism, pain, and penile fibrosis or plaque formation are of particular concern. Priapism, defined as a prolonged erection that requires intervention in order to resolve, is most serious. The lowest rates of priapism occur with alprostadil monotherapy, although prolonged or painful erections are actually more common. Pain is, as can be expected, a common consequence of ICI, and can result from pain from injection, penile pain, genital pain, or a combination. Pain with injection most commonly occurs with papaverine monotherapy, while pain during erection is most associated with alprostadil monotherapy; pain overall is most associated with bi-mix. Penile fibrosis or plaque as well as other penile deformities have been reported with use of ICI, although no single medication or medication combination is clearly associated with higher risk.

39.2.2.3 Intraurethral Alprostadil

IU erectile medications are recommended for patients in whom PDE5 inhibitors are contraindicated or men or partners who prefer to avoid oral medication in general. Urination is recommended prior to administration (since residual urine aids in dissolution and dispersal), which consists of applicator insertion through the urethral meatus as the penis is held upright and pulled taut. Alprostadil is deposited by depressing a button on the applicator, which is moved slightly to separate the pellet from the tip and then removed. The penis is kept upright and rolled to improve medication absorption. ICI alprostadil has had higher success rates than IU [21], but requires needles, which may cause men to prefer IU administration. Chronic IU alprostadil has only truly been studied in men who had erections firm enough for intercourse in response to in-office testing. Combined with a relatively lower treatment success rate, IU should not be prescribed until a man has undergone instruction in the method, an initial dose-titration in the office, and detailed counseling regarding possible adverse events and actions to take in response. A large proportion of men who have a positive in-office test will not be successful in the home environment [22]. IU alprostadil comes with its own adverse events, most commonly genital pain, minor urethral trauma, urethral pain or burning, and dizziness. Episodes of hypotension or syncope are rare, and prolonged or painful erection is less common compared to ICI [23]. Priapism is not reported, but patients should nevertheless be instructed on safe responses and maneuvers.

39.2.2.4 Alprostadil – Topical

Alprostadil cream is an effective and well-tolerated alternative to conventional treatment of ED and is safe in men undergoing therapy with alpha-blockers, antihypertensive agents, and/or nitrates. It can serve as second-line therapy for patients who fail to respond to, or are intolerant of, oral PDE5 inhibitors, and for those in whom these agents are contraindicated or may cause drug–drug interactions [24]. The lack of interference with food and alcohol is another advantage, as it allows for a higher degree of sexual spontaneity [25]. Alprostadil topical cream is less invasive and has fewer side effects compared to its injectable counterparts, a benefit that addresses many issues encountered with currently available ED therapy and may decrease the relatively high discontinuation rate [26].

39.2.3 Devices

For men who wish to avoid medications altogether, vacuum erection devices (VEDs) serve as an effective and low-cost alternative and are associated with high patient and partner satisfaction rates [3]. A pump is placed over the penis and suction induced, which draws blood into the penis. A ring is then placed at the base of the penis to prevent venous outflow. Vacuum limiters reduce the risk of penile injury. Nearly all patients successfully use the device to have intercourse [27]. However, studies examining patient satisfaction and efficacy for VEDs were carried out prior to the availability of PDE5 inhibitor medications, and men may prefer PDE5 inhibitors if given the option [28].

39.3 Surgical Management

Surgical options for men with ED have variable rates of success and satisfaction. Penile prostheses (both malleable and inflatable) have had great success, while vascular surgeries including arterial revascularization procedures and venous ligation surgery have significantly lower success rates.

39.3.1 Penile Prosthesis

Penile prosthesis implantation has been performed successfully in men from the general ED population as well as men from a variety of special populations [3]. Several devices are currently available, including malleable (noninflatable) models as well as two- or three-piece inflatable prostheses. Prostheses provide several advantages to medical therapy, including the ability to generate an erection on-demand for as long and as frequently desired. Potential risks and burdens include risks of infection, erosion, and device malfunction or failure. This treatment choice is essentially irreversible, since it is unlikely that a man's penis will be reliably responsive to other ED therapies after the prosthesis is removed.

39.3.1.1 Use of Penile Prostheses

Patients and partners generally prefer inflatable over malleable prostheses, depending on the specific model. Two-piece inflatable models are comprised of intracavernosal cylinders and a pump placed in the scrotum, whereas three-piece models add an intra-abdominal fluid reservoir. Two-piece models may be preferred for men in whom an abdominal reservoir may pose a risk (e.g., extensive scarring, kidney transplant) or those with poor manual dexterity. Malleable implants are more appropriate in certain situations including limited manual dexterity and cost concerns. A penile implant will not have a direct effect on libido; a man who is struggling with loss of libido should have this issue addressed separately. Although the penile implant will enhance shaft rigidity, it will not affect glans rigidity or enhance the processes of orgasm and ejaculation. Thorough explanation of the costs and benefits of each option are warranted, as more realistic preoperative expectations are associated with higher postoperative satisfaction [29]. Most adverse events are rarely serious and quickly resolve, such as penile edema or hematoma, corpus injury, urethral injury, acute urinary retention, and crura injury; postoperative pain usually resolves within three months. However, some adverse events are more serious and deserve further discussion, and include infection, erosion, and mechanical failure of the device.

39.3.1.2 Infection

Infection typically occurs within the first three months after surgery and usually requires removal of the prosthesis. Interestingly, there is no evidence currently that diabetic men are at higher risk of prosthesis infection than men from the general ED population [30]. Surgery should not be undertaken if there is evidence of systemic, cutaneous, or urinary tract infection. Perioperative antibiotic administration should include vancomycin or a first- or second-generation cephalosporin as well as an aminoglycoside before and after surgery. Use of antibiotic-coated prostheses [31] and the "no touch" technique reduce infection rates in the general ED population. "No touch" involves discarding all surgical instruments and changing all surgical gloves after the initial incision. Infected prostheses must be removed with antibiotic wash-out in the infected area. Systemic antibiotics are administered and the tissues allowed to heal. Once healing has occurred, a new prosthesis may be implanted; however, device placement may not be feasible due to scarring. If this occurs, penile shortening, change in penile shape, and loss of sensation are more likely. In men without evidence of sepsis or severe local infection, a new device may be placed immediately to avoid these complications. Antibiotic coatings appear to reduce infection rates during replacement [32].

39.3.1.3 Erosions

Erosion or cylinder extrusion occurs when the tissues at the tip of the penis are weakened, allowing the prosthetic cylinder to migrate into the head of the penis and through the skin, requiring surgical repair and reposition. Erosion rates are lower on average for inflatable models than for malleable models.

39.3.1.4 Mechanical Failure

Mechanical failure is more common with inflatable models and typically occurs when a component ruptures and leaks fluid. Refinements in design and materials have resulted in decreased failure rates; the majority of men will have a functioning prosthesis 10 years postsurgery [33]. More than half of mechanical failures involve pump malfunction followed by cylinder and reservoir malfunction. Device coating with parylene may protect against mechanical failure in certain models [34].

39.3.1.5 Managing Changes in Penile Length

Several strategies have been attempted to maximize penile length and girth after implant, including presurgical penile traction to maximize postoperative length [35], presurgical VED therapy to facilitate easier corporeal dilatation [36], or allowing longer cylinder placement at the time of surgery [37]. Preoperative VED use to soften corporeal fibrosis in men with a history of ischemic priapism or infection may facilitate successful implant of a device [38]. Several intra-operative techniques also have been examined, including ventral phalloplasty and suspensory ligament release [39]. Postoperatively, IU alprostadil [40] and PDE5 inhibitor medications [41] have been used to improve glans temperature, sensation, and enlargement. Successful penile dimension enhancement by using aggressive cylinder sizing and daily cylinder inflation postoperatively also has been reported [42]. There are insufficient data on specific approaches and techniques to constitute a reliable evidence base from which to provide clinical guidance regarding these approaches.

39.3.2 Vascular

Both arterial reconstruction and venous ligation surgeries have been attempted. Arterial reconstruction in certain candidates has had moderate success, but venous surgery has not been

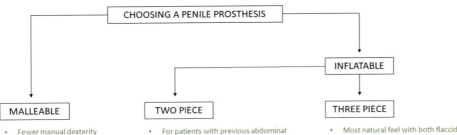

Figure 39.1 Benefits and costs associated with various options for penile prosthesis implantation

validated as an adequate treatment method even on those with solitary veno-occlusive ED.

39.3.2.1 Arterial

Penile arterial reconstruction surgery may be considered for the young man with ED without veno-occlusive dysfunction or evidence of generalized vascular disease or compromised vascular integrity. The long-term success of the procedure is not well established, although there is some evidence that surgery in ideal candidates leads to higher scores on erectile function questionnaires [43]. Patients respond well shortly after the procedure, but response rates decline over time. Predicting the long-term success of reconstructive surgery for a given man is extremely difficult, even in men without comorbidities and with good vascular health [44]. Frequently reported adverse events include penile hypervascularity, glans hyperemia, anastomosis occlusion, and postoperative edema or hematoma. Penile numbness, infection, shortening, bleeding, and inguinal hernia have also been reported.

39.3.2.2 Venous

Penile venous surgery is not recommended because of the lack of compelling evidence that it constitutes an effective ED management strategy in most men [3]. Even among men with pure veno-occlusive dysfunction, response rates vary over a wide range. Surgery is unlikely to result in long-term successful management of ED for the overwhelming majority of men and delays treatment with other more reliable options such as penile prosthesis surgery (Figure 39.1).

39.4 Future Direction and Experimental Therapy

Current therapies for ED are palliative in nature; future treatments are being developed that aim to restore erectile function rather than treat symptoms. However, treatments discussed in this section have not been studied sufficiently to be recommended for either general ED or special populations and should only be used in investigational settings.

39.4.1 Extracorporeal Shockwave Therapy

Low-intensity extracorporeal shockwave therapy functions by inducing cellular microtrauma, stimulating release of angiogenic factors that leads to neovascularization of the treated tissue [45]. The treatment's ability to restore normal erectile function is encouraging, but long-term duration of treatment effects is still being established [46]. Currently no serious adverse events have been reported.

39.4.2 Intracavernosal Stem Cell Therapy

Stem cell injection is well tolerated and appears to improve erectile function in men following radical prostatectomy [47] and diabetic ED [48] with no significant adverse reactions. However, the treatment's ability to restore normal erectile function in various populations of men with ED is still being investigated. Currently there are no randomized placebo-controlled trials assessing the efficacy of stem cells to treat erectile dysfunction. Long-term safety concerns include the risk of malignant degeneration, genomic or epigenetic changes, infection (especially with viral vector use), and potential immune reactions [49].

39.4.3 Platelet-Rich Plasma

Platelets play an important role in inflammation, tissue remodeling, and angiogenesis, leading to potential benefit of platelet-rich plasma (PRP) in vasculogenic ED. This treatment involves centrifugation of a blood sample to remove red and white blood cells and isolate platelets and plasma proteins in the supernatant, which is then injected into the corpus cavernosum [50]. Reliable information about potential benefits and risks/burdens of PRP therapy is not currently available.

39.5 Conclusion

ED is a multifactorial and complex condition affecting a wide range of male patients and is a common chief complaint in primary care and urologic clinics. A solid understanding of the many treatment options available will help physicians meet the needs of these patients.

References

1. Banner LL, Anderson RU. Integrated sildenafil and cognitive-behavior sex therapy for psychogenic erectile dysfunction: a pilot study. *J Sex Med.* 2007;4:1117–1125.
2. Hsu C, Sandford B. The Delphi technique: making sense of consensus. *Pract Assess Res Eval.* 2007;12:1–8.
3. Burnett AL, Nehra A, Breau RH, et al. Erectile dysfunction: AUA Guideline. *J Urol.* 2018;200:635–638.
4. Kovac JR, Labbate C, Ramasamy R, et al. Effects of cigarette smoking on erectile dysfunction. *Andrologia.* 2015;47:1087–1092.
5. Bolona ER, Uraga MV, Haddad RM, et al. Testosterone use in men with sexual dysfunction: a systematic review and meta-analysis of randomized placebo-controlled trials. *Mayo Clin Proc.* 2007;82:20–28.
6. Spitzer M, Basaria S, Travison TG, et al. Effect of testosterone replacement on response to sildenafil citrate in men with erectile dysfunction: a parallel, randomized trial. *Ann Intern Med.* 2012;157:681–691.
7. Kim JW, Oh MM, Park MG, et al. Combination therapy of testosterone enanthate and tadalafil on PDE5 inhibitor non-responders with severe and intermediate testosterone deficiency. *Int J Impot Res.* 2013;25:29–33.
8. Alhathal N, Elshal AM, Carrier S. Synergetic effect of testosterone and phophodiesterase-5 inhibitors in hypogonadal men with erectile dysfunction: a systematic review. *Can Urol Assoc J.* 2012;6:269–274.
9. Gruenwald I, Shenfeld O, Chen J, et al. Positive effect of counseling and dose adjustment in patients with erectile dysfunction who failed treatment with sildenafil. *Eur Urol.* 2006;50:134–140.
10. Kim ED, Seftel AD, Goldfischer ER, et al. A return to normal erectile function with tadalafil once daily after an incomplete response to asneeded PDE5 inhibitor therapy. *J Sex Med.* 2013;11:820–830.
11. Carson CC, Hatzichristou DG, Carrier S, et al. Erectile response with vardenafil in sildenafil nonresponders: a multicentre, double-blind, 12-week, flexible-dose, placebo-controlled erectile dysfunction clinical trial. *BJU Int.* 2004;94:1301–1309.
12. Salonia A, Adaikan G, Buvat J, et al. Sexual rehabilitation after treatment for prostate cancer – part 1: recommendations from the Fourth International Consultation for Sexual Medicine (ICSM 2015). *J Sex Med.* 2017;14:285–296.
13. Mahmood J, Shamah AA, Creed TM, et al. Radiation-induced erectile dysfunction: recent advances and future directions. *Adv Radiat Oncol.* 2016;1:161–169.
14. Weyne E, Castiglione F, Van der Aa F, et al. Landmarks in erectile function recovery after radical prostatectomy. *Nat Rev Urol.* 2015;12:289–297.
15. Salonia A, Adaikan G, Buvat J, et al. Sexual rehabilitation after treatment for prostate cancer – part 2: recommendations from the Fourth International Consultation for Sexual Medicine (ICSM 2015). *J Sex Med.* 2017;14:297–315.
16. Nehra A, Jackson G, Miner M, et al. The Princeton III consensus recommendations for the management of erectile dysfunction and cardiovascular disease. *Mayo Clin Proc.* 2012;87:766–778.
17. Pomeranz HD. The relationship between phosphodiesterase-5 inhibitors and nonarteritic anterior ischemic optic neuropathy. *J Neuroophthalmol.* 2016;36:193–196.
18. Pottegard A, Schmidt SA, Olesen AB, et al. Use of sildenafil or other phosphodiesterase inhibitors and risk of melanoma. *Br J Cancer.* 2016;115:895–900.
19. Michl U, Molfenter F, Graefen M, et al. Use of phosphodiesterase type 5 inhibitors may adversely impact biochemical recurrence after radical prostatectomy. *J Urol.* 2015;193:479–483.
20. Loeb S, Folkvaljon Y, Robinson D, et al. Phosphodiesterase type 5 inhibitor use and disease recurrence after prostate cancer treatment. *Eur Urol.* 2016;70:824–828.
21. Shabsigh R, Padma-Nathan H, Gittleman M, et al. Intracavernous alprostadil alfadex is more efficacious, better tolerated, and preferred over intraurethral alprostadil plus optional actis: a comparative, randomized, crossover, multicenter study. *Urology.* 2000;55:109–113.
22. Padma-Nathan H, Hellstrom WJ, Kaiser FE, et al. Treatment of men with erectile dysfunction with transurethral alprostadil. Medicated Urethral System for Erection (MUSE) Study Group. *N Engl J Med.* 1997;336:1–7.
23. Williams G, Abbou CC, Amar ET, et al. Efficacy and safety of transurethral alprostadil therapy in men with erectile dysfunction. MUSE Study Group. *Br J Urol.* 1998;81:889–894.
24. Padma-Nathan H, Yeager JL. An integrated analysis of alprostadil topical cream for the treatment of erectile dysfunction in 1732 patients. *Urology.* 2006;68(2):386–391.
25. Mehrotra N, Gupta M, Kovar A, Meibohm B. The role of pharmacokinetics and pharmacodynamics in phosphodiesterase-5 inhibitor therapy. *Int J Impot Res.* 2007;19(3):253–264.
26. Anaissie J, Hellstrom WJ. Clinical use of alprostadil topical cream in patients with erectile dysfunction: a review. *Res Rep Urol.* 2016;8:123–331.
27. Khayyamfar F, Forootan SK, Ghasemi H, et al. Evaluating the efficacy of vacuum constrictive device and causes of its failure in impotent patients. *Urol J.* 2013;10:1072–1078.
28. Chen J, Mabjeesh NJ, Greenstein A. Sildenafil versus the vacuum erection device: patient preference. *J Urol.* 2001;166:1779–1781.
29. Kramer AC, Schweber A. Patient expectations prior to Coloplast Titan penile prosthesis implant predicts postoperative satisfaction. *J Sex Med.* 2010;7:2261–2266.
30. Mulcahy JJ, Carson CC 3rd. Long-term infection rates in diabetic patients implanted with antibiotic-impregnated versus nonimpregnated inflatable penile prostheses: 7-year outcomes. *Eur Urol.* 2011;60:167–172.
31. Serefoglu EC, Mandava SH, Gokce A, et al. Long-term revision rate due to infection in hydrophilic-coated inflatable penile prostheses: 11-year follow-up. *J Sex Med.* 2012;9:2182–2186.
32. Nehra A, Carson CC 3rd, Chapin AK, et al. Longterm infection outcomes of 3-piece antibiotic impregnated penile

prostheses used in replacement implant surgery. *J Urol*. 2012;188:899–903.

33. Mirheydar H, Zhou T, Chang DC, et al. Reoperation rates for penile prosthetic surgery. *J Sex Med*. 2016;13:129–133.

34. Enemchukwu EA, Kaufman MR, Whittam BM, et al. Comparative revision rates of inflatable penile prostheses using woven Dacron® fabric cylinders. *J Urol*. 2013;190:2189–2193.

35. Levine LA, Rybak J. Traction therapy for men with shortened penis prior to penile prosthesis implantation: a pilot study. *J Sex Med*. 2011;8:2112–2117.

36. Canguven O, Talib RA, Campbell J, et al. Is the daily use of vacuum erection device for a month before penile prosthesis implantation beneficial? A randomized controlled trial. *Andrology*. 2017;5:103–106.

37. Pahlajani G, Raina R, Jones S, et al. Vacuum erection devices revisited: its emerging role in the treatment of erectile dysfunction and early penile rehabilitation following prostate cancer therapy. *J Sex Med*. 2012;9:1182–1189.

38. Tsambarlis PN, Chaus F, Levine LA. Successful placement of penile prostheses in men with severe corporal fibrosis following vacuum therapy protocol. *J Sex Med*. 2017;14:44–46.

39. Hakky TS, Suber J, Henry G, et al. Penile enhancement procedures with simultaneous penile prosthesis placement. *Adv Urol*. 2012;2012:314612.

40. Chew KK, Stuckey BG. Use of transurethral alprostadil (MUSE) (prostaglandin E1) for glans tumescence in a patient with penile prosthesis. *Int J Impot Res*. 2000;12:195–196.

41. Mulhall JP, Jahoda A, Aviv N, et al. The impact of sildenafil citrate on sexual satisfaction profiles in men with a penile prosthesis in situ. *BJU Int*. 2004;93:97–99.

42. Pryor MB, Carrion R, Wang R, et al. Patient satisfaction and penile morphology changes with postoperative penile rehabilitation 2 years after Coloplast Titan prosthesis. *Asian J Androl*. 2016;18:754–758.

43. Munarriz R, Uberoi J, Fantini G, et al. Microvascular arterial bypass surgery: longterm outcomes using validated instruments. *J Urol*. 2009;182:643–648.

44. Dabaja AA, Teloken P, Mulhall JP. A critical analysis of candidacy for penile revascularization. *J Sex Med*. 2014;11:2327–2332.

45. Gruenwald I, Appel B, Kitrey ND. Shockwave treatment of erectile dysfunction. *Ther Adv Urol*. 2013;5(2):95–99.

46. Sokolakis I, Hatzichristodoulou G. Clinical studies on low intensity extracorporeal shockwave therapy for erectile dysfunction: a systematic review and meta-analysis of randomised controlled trials. *Int J Impot Res*. 2019;31:177–194.

47. Yiou R, Hamidou L, Birebent B, et al. Safety of intracavernous bone marrow-mononuclear cells for postradical prostatectomy erectile dysfunction: an open dose-escalation pilot study. *Eur Urol*. 2016;69:988–991.

48. Al Demour S, Jafar H, Adwan S. Safety and potential therapeutic effect of two intracavernous autologous bone marrow derived mesenchymal stem cells injections in diabetic patients with erectile dysfunction: an open label phase I clinical trial. *J Urol Int*. 2018;101:358–365.

49. Chung E. A review of current and emerging therapeutic options for erectile dysfunction. *Med Sci (Basel)*. 2019;7(9):91.

50. Patel D, Pastuszak A, Hotaling J. Emerging treatments for erectile dysfunction: a review of novel, non-surgical options. *Curr Urol Rep*. 2019;20:44.

Section 5: Medical and Surgical Management of Issues of Male Health

Chapter 40: Surgical Management of Peyronie's Disease

Aron Liaw and Faysal Yafi

40.1 Introduction

Although nonsurgical treatments for Peyronie's disease have seen renewed interest in recent years, surgical correction of Peyronie's disease has proven efficacy and is often considered the gold standard for treatment [1]. The goals of surgical treatment should be cosmetic and functional correction of the deformity and preservation/restoration of sexual function.

Surgical planning begins with a thorough examination and history. The natural history of Peyronie's disease involves an early inflammatory phase, which may also include pain with erection, followed by a stable phase that is not typically symptomatic [2]. During the early phase, penile curvature is progressive, and thus no surgical intervention is recommended until after 12 months following disease onset, and once the penile curvature has been unchanged for at least 6 months. Surgical correction before this may fail due to disease progression.

Peyronie's disease is a disorder of sexual function and so it is imperative that surgeons assess the current degree of dysfunction. A patient with no interest in sexual activity needs no treatment, while someone with erectile dysfunction may need additional treatment beyond correction of curvature to achieve sexual function. Furthermore, surgical treatment of Peyronie's carries some risk of subsequent erectile dysfunction, so establishing baseline function is key to a satisfactory outcome [3].

Loss of function related to Peyronie's disease may arise from inability to achieve penetrative intercourse, either from physical limitations due to curvature or from pain with penetration for either the patient or his partner. In addition to other causes of erectile dysfunction, Peyronie's disease may cause veno-occlusive dysfunction, where the tunica is unable to expand and occlude the subtunical venules [4].

Routine preoperative workup for Peyronie's should therefore include a validated erectile function questionnaire, as well as examination of the erect penis after intracavernosal injection. Many surgeons also examine patients with a duplex Doppler penile ultrasound [5], which has the benefit of a direct assessment of both erectile function and of curvature, as well as possible diagnosis of any underlying vascular pathology.

Surgical correction of Peyronie's disease is done both for functional improvement and cosmesis, and it is thus crucial that patient expectations be clearly set and managed. It is important that the patient understand that the goal is not and should not be perfect straightness, or a penis that looks and functions as he may remember from his youth, especially since penile shortening is a common side effect of surgery. Plication procedures by necessity involve some shortening, but all surgical repairs can be associated with penile shortening [6]. Surgical risks, particularly any chance of new or worsened erectile dysfunction, must be clearly stated. We recommend that consent include the risks of persistence or recurrence of curvature, erectile dysfunction, loss of penile sensation, and loss of penile length [6].

40.2 Surgical Approaches

The surgical approach falls into three broad categories: shortening of the convex side of the curve, through plication or corporoplasty; lengthening of the concave side of the curve, through plaque incision, removal and/or grafting; and placement of a penile prosthesis with molding of the penis around the artificial device, which may also incorporate penile straightening techniques from the first two approaches. Mulhall et al. presented an algorithm wherein patients were assessed with dynamic infusion cavernosometry and cavernosography, as well as pharmacotherapy for those with erectile dysfunction [8]. Those that underwent plication reported significantly better postoperative erectile scores even without any surgical therapy for erectile dysfunction. Among the conclusions of this study were that not all patients with concomitant erectile dysfunction require penile prostheses. Notably, those that underwent plaque incision and grafting reported significantly worse erections, suggesting that this may be a poor treatment option for those with concomitant erectile dysfunction.

40.2.1 Plication Procedures

In part due to reported results like this, penile plication is a popular surgical treatment for Peyronie's disease. While a variety of techniques exist, the underlying principle is the same – shortening of the convex side of the curvature, to pull the penis into alignment. Although this involves surgery on a healthy area of the penis, away from the pathology causing curvature, and also involves a theoretical shortening of the penis, high satisfaction rates with plication indicate that the functional improvement in well-selected patients outweighs these limitations.

Most plication surgeries have common critical steps. Inducing an artificial erection during the procedure is a key step, to replicate the curvature in a controlled setting and test for correction. This can be done through injection of injectable saline or through erectogenic medication. Mobilization of adjacent structures is also critical. Dorsal curvature is common, but the urethra does not generally require mobilization. If it does, small perforator vessels can be ligated or cauterized without complication. Ventral curvature is less common, but requires careful dissection on the dorsal side to avoid the neurovascular bundles that lie deep to Buck's fascia alongside the deep dorsal vein. Many surgeons will test correction with easily reversible steps, such as using Allis clamps or suture to simulate the effect of plication before excising a wedge or taking a similar irreversible step [9]. Frequently, a circumcising incision is performed to expose the tunica, but in some cases with less complex curvature, typically dorsal or lateral curvature, a longitudinal incision over the surgical site may suffice [10]. In cases of ventral curvature, the neurovascular bundles must be carefully identified and avoided, and so a circumcising incision is recommended for better exposure but a small localized incision has also been described [11]. Plication of a severe, long, or complex curvature is best done through multiple small plications, rather than one large one, to prevent a hinging effect or indentation deformity in the penis.

The earliest published plication technique is the Nesbit plication [12], originally employed for the correction of congenital curvature. This technique involves excision of an elliptical portion of tunica at the point of maximal curvature and suturing it closed, thereby pulling the penis into alignment. Sutures should be either permanent or slow-dissolving, such as polydioxanone. Outcomes of the procedure when used for Peyronie's disease show high success and satisfaction rates, and a Nesbit plication or modified version thereof is the preferred option of most surgeons for Peyronie's correction. Syed et al. published data with a median follow-up of seven years using this procedure, with a 90.5% rate of curvature correction and a 76.2% satisfaction rate [13].

Variations on the Nesbit procedure involve modifying the nature of the incision into the tunica and/or how it is closed. Yachia published a variation that does not involve excising a wedge of tunica, but rather making vertical incisions and closing them in a horizontal fashion, that is, a Heineke–Mikulicz maneuver [14]. Schwarzer and Steinfatt described a technique involving an incised U-shaped flap that is advanced under the intact tunica and secured, thus theoretically reinforcing the closure with a double layer of tunica albuginea [15]. Similarly, Duckett and Baskin described a variation, initially used for the correction of congenital curvature in hypospadias, much like the original Nesbit procedure [16]. In this, only the outer layer of tunica albuginea is excised, after approximating the correction with clamps, as already described. Levine later published his series of a similar procedure, the tunica albuginea plication procedure [17]. In this, two transverse incisions are made in the outer layer of tunica albuginea while leaving the inner layer intact, and these are then sutured together. For ventral curvature, the deep dorsal vein is carefully dissected and can be excised at no risk to the penile blood flow, to leave the neurovascular bundles intact. For dorsal curvature, the excision and plication is done on either side of the urethra. In this series of 154 patients, 99% showed improvement to curvature less than 20 degrees.

As an alternative to the excisional and incisional plication techniques already described, many surgeons have published on plications without incision. Essed and Schroeder published a short series in 1985 describing imbricating stitches on the convex side of the curvature [18]. The same year, Ebbehoj published a slightly larger series describing one or more four-point imbricating stitches into the tunica, similar to a figure of eight stitch [19]. In 1994, Klevmark et al. published a similar four-point stitch in a figure of eight, plicating together an area 5 mm in width over a 1 cm length [20].

Gholami and Lue published a large series in 2002 [21] describing the 16-dot plication technique. This involves two or three pairs of stitches in a linear fashion at the point of maximal curvature, rather than a crossed stitch in the manner of the Ebbehoj and Klevmark techniques. This allowed for sutures to be placed adjacent to midline structures such as the urethra and deep dorsal vein more easily. In this series, 15% of patients had some recurrence at 2.6 years mean follow-up, but overall satisfaction was extremely high at 96% (Figure 40.1).

Broadly, then, plication procedures can be divided into excisional techniques, such as the Nesbit; incisional techniques where no tunica is removed, such as the Yachia or Schwarzer techniques; and plication-only procedures, such as the Lue 16-dot plication technique. Comparative studies on plication procedures tend to be comparisons of a more recent technique or modification to historical data of an older technique. Mufti et al. compared Nesbit procedures to both Heineke–Mikulicz-type incisional procedures and plication-only techniques in a small study, and found no significant difference between the three approaches [22]. The failure rate in this study was comparatively high, especially in those with pain at time of procedure, suggesting that patient selection of those with persistent disease may have been a factor. By contrast, Schultheiss et al. compared the Nesbit procedure with plication-only techniques such as that described by Essed and Schroeder using data from multiple studies [23]. Their conclusion was that the Nesbit procedure provided better outcomes and that their institution would change its approach as a result. Licht and Lewis reported a comparison of their modified incisional technique to both a standard Nesbit procedure and a plaque excision with graft technique [24]. There were no significant differences in success rate or patient satisfaction between the incisional and excisional plication procedures, but plaque excision and grafting resulted in much lower rates of satisfaction (30% vs. ~80%), success (61% vs. 80–90%), and postoperative erectile dysfunction (18% vs. 0–2%).

Plication procedures benefit from relative ease and shorter operative times compared to other curvature correction

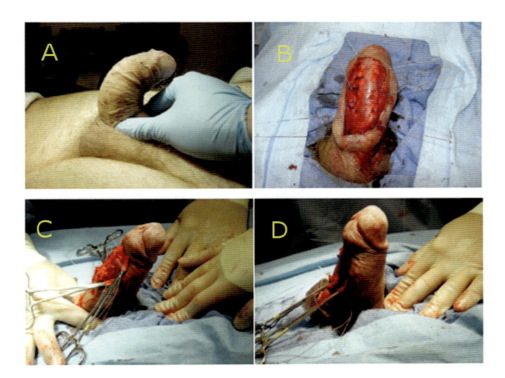

Figure 40.1 Lue 16-dot plication. (A) Initial curvature. (B) Placement of periurethral plication sutures longidutinally. (C) Penile straightening after tying of the sutures. (D) Final result after reapproximation of Buck's fascia. (Courtesy of Dr William Brant, MD FACS FECSM)

procedures. The major potential downside is that some degree of penile shortening is unavoidable. In practice, high satisfaction rates suggest that for a majority of patients, the restoration of function is preferable to a small amount of shortening. In recent years, some practitioners are offering postoperative traction therapy with a penile traction device [9]. A retrospective analysis of 52 patients who underwent penile traction for two or more hours per day, starting three to four weeks after surgery, showed preservation of length and, in some cases, gain of length after plication [25]. Another concern is palpable nodules from sutures, especially in the case of permanent suture material. A retrospective review of 81 patients found that reduced use of permanent suture reduced nodularity and pain at the suture sites, without significant return of curvature after absorbable sutures dissolved [26].

40.2.2 Plaque Incision and Grafting

Plication procedures, whether excisional/incisional or not, remain the simplest and most popular methods of correcting Peyronie's curvature. However, a common point to all these surgeries is that they do not address the diseased tissue and instead shorten the healthy part of the penis to produce a functional improvement. As such, an alternative is to instead lengthen the part of the penis affected by the plaque, through incising or removing the plaque and replacing it with a graft. Removing the entire plaque results in very high rates of erectile dysfunction [3] and this method is generally no longer pursued or recommended.

These procedures follow the same general principles of exposure and assessment of curvature as plication procedures. Following exposure and mobilization, the plaque is then incised or partially excised, typically with a modified H- or double Y-incision to create a rectangular defect in the tunica. This defect must then be covered with some sort of graft.

No definitive evidence exists that favors any one graft material over others, save that synthetic grafts should not be used due to increased risks of fibrosis, infection, and compromised functional outcomes. Ideally, graft material should be easily available, simple to work with, inexpensive, and have a low risk of infection or antigenicity. Its physical properties are also vital given that normal tunica is expected to expand with erection yet maintain rigidity.

Autologous grafts were the earliest grafts used for this purpose, starting in 1974 with Devine and Horton publishing their technique of a 1 mm thickness dermal graft harvested from the lower abdomen [27]. Their subsequent outcomes report showed 84% of patients were able to resume sexual activity, with 24% showing some recurrence of curvature, at follow-up of at least 12 months. Similar results are reported in multiple series, with the largest reporting some recurrence of curvature in 17% of patients, as well as a 20% rate of erectile dysfunction [28].

Saphenous vein grafts have theoretical advantages as a graft material in that they incorporate a muscular coat and elastic fibers with thin vascular walls, allowing for perfusion, graft take, and good compliance. The first large series with this technique involved incision of the plaque and addition of a saphenous vein graft, and showed 92% patient satisfaction with short-term follow-up (maximum 18 months), as well as a 12% rate of decreased erectile function and 17% rate of penile shortening [29].

Less frequently used are deeper fascial tissues, such as fascia lata and rectus sheath, or buccal mucosa grafts. Deeper fascial grafts may have a role in grafting with simultaneous placement of a penile prosthesis, to avoid contamination. Only small series exist using these tissues [30].

While synthetic graft materials have thus far proven unsuitable, tissue engineering has provided a variety of extracellular matrix (ECM) tissues that cause minimal fibrosis due to their acellular and immunocompatible nature. Through intelligent remodeling, a graft of ECM repopulates the wound with local tissue, and the graft tends to increase in tensile strength over time. Current practice favors off-the-shelf allografts such as bovine or human pericardium, small intestinal submucosa, or collagen fleece. Porcine small intestinal submucosa (SIS) has achieved good success rates of up to 90% resolution of curvature [31], but a number of studies have also reported a higher rate of complications, as well as high rates of recurrence of both curvature and plaques [32].

A more recent development in ECM allografts is the use of collagen fleece, which will stick to the tunical defect without any suturing or precise measurement of graft needed, representing a considerable time saving. A very recent multicenter study reviewed 51 patients from three sites who underwent plaque incision and grafting for complex (mean compound curvature 69.6 degrees) Peyronie's disease with a mean follow-up of 10.6 months [33]. Only 12% of patients reported mild residual curvature, and no patients reported significant erectile dysfunction. Matched-pair analysis of 43 patients who underwent collagen-fleece grafting indicated no relapse of curvature in these patients and improved erectile function when compared with patients with SIS grafts, at a mean follow-up of 39 months [34]. Long-term follow-up of this technique over a mean of 37 months indicated a very high success rate of 97.5% with 10% reporting worsened erectile function and 5.9% reporting a change in glans sensation [35] (Figure 40.2).

Overall, plaque incision and grafting is a more complex and time-consuming procedure than plication. Autologous grafts require harvesting and preparation of a graft and have a small risk of complications at the harvest site, though allografts avoid these concerns. The purported advantage is that lengthening the affected side of the curve should avoid any penile shortening, which is inherent to plication. However, most studies on Peyronie's graft surgeries report a percentage of patients who do experience penile shortening even with an otherwise technically successful surgery [30]. The reasons for this are hard to clearly identify. Graft contracture has been reported with many materials, both autologous and allograft, and progressive erectile dysfunction and fibrosis are associated with Peyronie's disease itself [3]. Plaque incision and grafting surgeries do carry increased risk of erectile dysfunction when

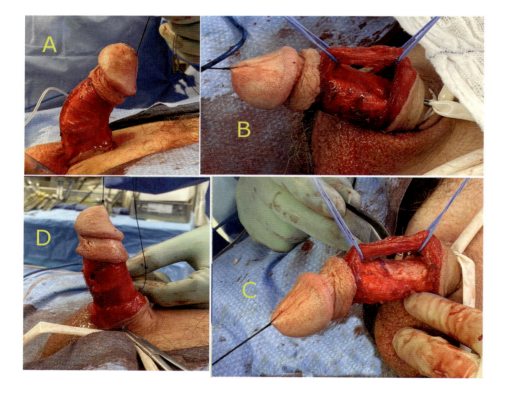

Figure 40.2 Plaque incision and grafting with collagen fleece. (A) Initial curvature with artificial erection. (B) Following dissection of Buck's fascia and elevation of neurovascular bundles to expose the plaque. (C) Following incision of the plaque and placement of collagen fleece. Note that the fleece is in place and requires no sutures. (D) Repeat artificial erection after closure of Buck's fascia. (Courtesy of Dr Faysal Yafi)

compared to plications, and for these reasons, most practitioners use plaque incision and grafting judiciously in carefully selected patients. Grafting techniques are most indicated for severe penile curvature (>60 degrees), hourglass deformity, or severe penile shortening [36].

40.2.3 Prosthetic Implantation

Peyronie's disease and erectile dysfunction commonly occur together, and the risk of postoperative erectile dysfunction, as well as worse outcomes for patients with preexisting erectile dysfunction, often lead surgeons and patients to address both simultaneously after shared decision-making. Both the American Urological Association and International Society of Sexual Medicine guidelines state that surgeons may offer penile prosthesis and adjunctive procedures such as plication, grafting, and modeling for patients with disabling curvature and/or erectile dysfunction. Semirigid prostheses are no longer used for patients that may require curvature correction as there are low satisfaction and success rates with these devices, and inflatable devices are thus recommended [36]. The AMS Ultrex and its successor, the LGX, are not recommended as they are not as successful at straightening the Peyronie's penis [37], and thus the AMS CX or Coloplast Titan devices should be employed, as no appreciable difference exists between the two in terms of penile straightening [38].

In the majority of cases, placement of the device alone is sufficient to achieve a functionally straight penis. Mulhall et al. noted that no patients with curvature <30 degrees required any further manipulation other than prosthetic placement to achieve straightness [39]. If implantation alone is insufficient, manual modeling should be attempted, in which the cylinders are maximally inflated, the pump tubing is shodded to protect it from back pressure, and the cylinders are then forcibly flexed opposite to the curvature. The corporotomies should be protected with fingers to prevent further rupture, and downward pressure on the end of the glans should be avoided to prevent distal urethral perforation, as there is an approximately 3% risk of urethral injury with these techniques. This forcible bending is intended to crack or deform the plaque and facilitate straightening. Once straightened, the penis should be held in this position for around 90 seconds, and if this fails, a second attempt at manual modeling is recommended. If more than two attempts are needed, surgeons should consider other maneuvers to achieve functional straightness [40] (Figure 40.3).

Most of the previously described techniques of plication, with or without incision/excision, or grafting are applicable and can be done concurrently with a prosthesis implantation. When grafts are used, dermal grafts are not recommended due to concerns for infection, and thus allografts or rectus fascia should be preferred [41]. If a surgeon anticipates needing to perform additional straightening procedures, plication sutures can be placed before placement of the cylinders to avoid risking damage to the cylinders from a needle [38].

Techniques to incise the plaque without the need for a graft have also been attempted, following the same principle behind manual modeling – breaking up the fibrotic plaque to allow it to reshape around a prosthetic implant. These techniques involve scratching or breaking up the plaque from within the corpora through the corporotomy, after dilation, but keeping the outer layer of tunica intact to avoid the need for grafting, and also to avoid needing to mobilize structures such as the

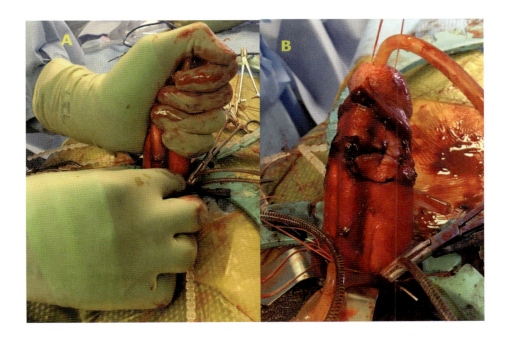

Figure 40.3 Correction of Peyronie's curvature with penile prosthesis. (A) Manual modeling. Note compression of both urethral meatus and the corporotomies. (B) Curvature correction after plication sutures placed ventrally. Note that this patient has a circumcising incision for planned concurrent circumcision, and the prosthesis has been placed via a subcoronal approach. (Courtesy of Dr Faysal Yafi)

neurovascular bundles. A 12-blade scalpel can be used with the scratch technique, as described by Perito and Wilson [42], or endoscopic techniques as described by Shaeer [43].

Penile shortening can occur after any Peyronie's surgery, but is especially problematic in those patients who undergo prosthetic implantation. This is likely due to the concomitant erectile dysfunction, as well as the limitations of a prosthetic device when compared to a natural erection, but some practitioners have attempted techniques during implantation to increase penile length. Among the simpler of these is penile degloving after a circumcising incision, releasing the dartos fascia that may be restricting maximal extension. Shaeer et al. recently reported on a technique of dorsal phalloplasty, where the dermis at the dorsal juncture of penis and pubis is tacked down to the pubic periosteum, revealing more visible length of penis [44].

More invasive techniques involve incising the corpora circumferentially, stretching the penis, and grafting the resulting defect. Sansalone et al. described a technique involving circumcising and penoscrotal incisions followed by aggressive mobilization of both neurovascular bundles and the urethra away from the corpora, followed by a circumferential incision [45]. Rolle et al. used a sliding technique, using longitudinal incisions on the lateral side of each corpora, then joining them with hemicircumferential incisions before sliding the corpora apart along the plane of the longitudinal incision and grafting the defect with SIS [46]. Similarly, Egydio and Kuehhas published a modification of this technique, where only a circumcising incision is used and multiple smaller hemicircumferential incisions are used to make smaller defects that are then not grafted [47]. These techniques are highly invasive and should thus be considered only with caution and by experienced practitioners, as they may be associated with serious complications such as glans ischemia, from damage to the neurovascular bundles during mobilization [48]. To minimize dissection of these bundles, a proposed alternative is to do a ventral incision and free up the urethra, as well as mobilizing Buck's fascia away from the corpora with the penile skin before performing a sliding technique [49].

40.3 Key Points

- Surgical correction of Peyronie's disease remains a safe and highly successful method of treatment. Prior to any surgery, patients must be carefully counseled on risks and realistic expectations of surgery. It is important to assess sexual function and degree of curvature to select the right approach.
- Surgical steps that are common to any approach include intraoperative assessment of curvature through induced or artificial erection, as well as careful mobilization of adjacent structures, particularly the dorsal neurovascular bundles and the urethra.
- For most cases, plication techniques offer a safe, easy method of curvature correction. Plication is preferred for the majority of Peyronie's cases and can be done with excision or incision of the tunica albuginea, or through plication alone. Most comparisons of techniques show little difference, though some studies favor excisional plication.
- Plaque incision and grafting is indicated for severe or complex curvatures but carries a higher risk of erectile dysfunction and should not be used alone for patients with preexisting erectile dysfunction. Modern allograft materials are commonly used, while autologous grafts are less commonly used due to increased operative time and the low chance of harvest site morbidity. No strong evidence exists that favors any one type of graft material. Synthetic grafts should not be used.
- Placement of a penile prosthetic should be considered for a patient with erectile dysfunction as well as curvature. In some cases, prosthetic placement alone is sufficient to correct curvature. If not, manual modeling or additional plication or grafting can be attempted.
- There is a risk of postoperative erectile dysfunction with any Peyronie's surgery, as well as penile shortening. Careful preoperative assessment of erectile function is important. Penile traction may be of benefit to counteract penile shortening in the absence of a prosthesis.

References

1. Levine LA, Burnett AL. Standard operating procedures for Peyronie's disease. *J Sex Med*. 2013;10(1):230–244.
2. Hatzichristodoulou G, Lahme S. Peyronie's disease. In: Merseburger A, Kuczyk M, Moul J, eds. *Urology at a Glance*. Springer-Verlag; 2014:225–236.
3. Segal RL, Burnett AL. Surgical management for Peyronie's disease. *World J Mens Health*. 2013;31(1):1–11.
4. Chung E, De Young L, Brock GB. Penile duplex ultrasonography in men with Peyronie's disease: is it veno-occlusive dysfunction or poor cavernosal arterial inflow that contributes to erectile dysfunction?. *J Sex Med*. 2011;8(12):3446–3451.
5. Ralph D, Gonzalez-Cadavid N, Mirone V, et al. The management of Peyronie's disease: evidence-based 2010 guidelines. *J Sex Med*. 2010;7(7):2359–2374.
6. Yafi FA, Hatzichristodoulou G. Surgical reconstruction for Peyronie's disease. *AUA Update Ser*. 2018;37(11–15):11.
7. Chen R, McCraw C, Lewis, R. Plication procedures – excisional and incisional corporoplasty and imbrication for Peyronie's disease. *Transl Androl Urol*. 2016;5(3):318–333.
8. Mulhall J, Anderson M, Parker M. A surgical algorithm for men with combined Peyronie's disease and erectile dysfunction: functional and satisfaction outcomes. *J Sex Med*. 2005;2(1):132–138.
9. Chung E, Wang R, Ralph D, Levine L, Brock G. A worldwide survey on Peyronie's disease surgical practice patterns among surgeons. *J Sex Med*. 2018;15(4):568–575.
10. Adibi M, Hudak SJ, Morey AF. Penile plication without degloving enables effective correction of complex Peyronie's deformities. *Urology*. 2012;79(4):831–835.

11. Chung PH, Tausch TJ, Simhan J, Scott JF, Morey AF. Dorsal plication without degloving is safe and effective for correcting ventral penile deformities. *Urology*. 2014;84(5):1228–1233.
12. Nesbit RM. The surgical treatment of congenital chordee without hypospadias. *J Urol*. 1954;72(6):1178–1180.
13. Syed AH, Abbasi Z, Hargreave TB. Nesbit procedure for disabling Peyronie's curvature: a median follow-up of 84 months. *Urology*. 2003;61(5):999–1003.
14. Yachia D. Modified corporoplasty for the treatment of penile curvature. *J Urol*. 1990;143(1):80–82.
15. Schwarzer JU, Steinfatt H. Tunica albuginea underlap – a new modification of the Nesbit procedure: description of the technique and preliminary results. *J Sex Med*. 2012;9(11):2970–2974.
16. Baskin LS, Duckett JW. Dorsal tunica albuginea plication for hypospadias curvature. *J Urol*. 1994;151(6):1668–1671.
17. Levine LA. Penile straightening with tunica albuginea plication procedure: TAP procedure. In: Levine LA, ed. *Peyronie's Disease: A Guide to Clinical Management*. Humana; 2006:151–159.
18. Essed E, Schroeder FH. New surgical treatment for Peyronie disease. *Urology*. 1985;25(6):582–587.
19. Ebbehøj J, Metz P. New operation for "krummerik" (penile curvature). *Urology*. 1985;26(1):76–78.
20. Klevmark B, Andersen M, Schultz A, Talseth T. Congenital and acquired curvature of the penis treated surgically by plication of the tunica albuginea. *Br J Urol*. 1994;74(4):501–506.
21. Gholami SS, Lue TF. Correction of penile curvature using the 16-dot plication technique: a review of 132 patients. *J Urol*. 2002;167(5):2066–2069.
22. Mufti GR, Aitchison M, Bramwell SP, Paterson PJ, Scott R. Corporeal plication for surgical correction of Peyronie's disease. *J Urol*. 1990;144(2 Pt 1):281–282.
23. Schultheiss D, Meschi MR, Hagemann J, Truss MC, Stief CG, Jonas U. Congenital and acquired penile deviation treated with the Essed plication method. *Eur Urol*. 2000;38(2):167–171.
24. Licht MR, Lewis RW. Modified Nesbit procedure for the treatment of Peyronie's disease: a comparative outcome analysis. *J Urol*. 1997;158(2):460–463.
25. Rybak J, Papagiannopoulos D, Levine L. A retrospective comparative study of traction therapy vs. no traction following tunica albuginea plication or partial excision and grafting for Peyronie's disease: measured lengths and patient perceptions. *J Sex Med*. 2012;9(9):2396–2403.
26. Papagiannopoulos D, Phelps J, Yura E, Levine LA. Surgical outcomes from limiting the use of nonabsorbable suture in tunica albuginea plication for Peyronie's disease. *Int J Impot Res*. 2017;29(6):258–261.
27. Devine CJ, Horton CE. Surgical treatment of Peyronie's disease with a dermal graft. *J Urol*. 1974;111(1):44–49.
28. Austoni E, Colombo F, Mantovani F, Patelli E, Fenice O. Radical surgery and conservation of erection in Peyronie's disease. *Arch Ital Urol Androl*. 1995;67(5):359–364.
29. El-Sakka AI, Rashwan HM, Lue TF. Venous patch graft for Peyronie's disease. Part II: outcome analysis. *J Urol*. 1998;160(6 Pt 1):2050–2053.
30. Kadioglu A, Sanli O, Akman T, Ersay A, Guven S, Mammadov F. Graft materials in Peyronie's disease surgery: a comprehensive review. *J Sex Med*. 2007;4(3):581–595.
31. Knoll LD. Use of small intestinal submucosa graft for the surgical management of Peyronie's disease. *J Urol*. 2007;178(6):2474–2478.
32. Breyer BN, Brant WO, Garcia MM, Bella AJ, Lue TF. Complications of porcine small intestine submucosa graft for Peyronie's disease. *J Urol*. 2007;177(2):589–591.
33. Hatzichristodoulou G, Yang DY, Ring JD, Hebert KJ, Ziegelmann MJ, Köhler TS. Multicenter experience using collagen fleece for plaque incision with grafting to correct residual curvature at the time of inflatable penile prosthesis placement in patients with Peyronie's disease. *J Sex Med*. 2020;17(6):1168–1174.
34. Rosenhammer B, Sayedahmed K, Fritsche HM, Burger M, Kübler H, Hatzichristodoulou G. Long-term outcome after grafting with small intestinal submucosa and collagen fleece in patients with Peyronie's disease: a matched pair analysis. *Int J Impot Res*. 2019;31(4):256–262.
35. Hatzichristodoulou G, Fiechtner S, Gschwend J, Lahme S. Long-term results after partial plaque excision and grafting with collagen fleece in Peyronie's disease. *J Sex Med*. 2016;13(5):S103.
36. Nehra A, Alterowitz R, Culkin DJ, et al. Peyronie's disease: AUA guideline. *J Urol*. 2015;194(3):745–753.
37. Montague DK, Lakin MM. Early experience with the controlled girth and length expanding cylinder of the American Medical Systems Ultrex penile prosthesis. *J Urol*. 1992;148(5):1444–1446.
38. Chung PH, Francis Scott J, Morey AF. High patient satisfaction of inflatable penile prosthesis insertion with synchronous penile plication for erectile dysfunction and Peyronie's disease. *J Sex Med*. 2014;11(6):1593–1598.
39. Mulhall J, Ahmed A, Anderson M. Penile prosthetic surgery for Peyronie's disease: defining the need for intraoperative adjuvant maneuvers. *J Sex Med*. 2004;1(3):318–321.
40. El-Khatib, FM, Huynh LM, Yafi FA. Intraoperative methods for residual curvature correction during penile prosthesis implantation in patients with Peyronie's disease and refractory erectile dysfunction. *Int J Impot Res*. 2020;32(1):43–51.
41. Levine LA, Becher EF, Bella AJ, et al. Penile prosthesis surgery: current recommendations from the International Consultation on Sexual Medicine. *J Sex Med*. 2016;13(4):489–518.
42. Perito P, Wilson SK. The Peyronie's plaque "scratch": an adjunct to modeling. *J Sex Med*. 2013;10(5):1194–1197.
43. Shaeer O. Trans-corporal incision of Peyronie's plaques. *J Sex Med*. 2011;8(2):589–593.
44. Shaeer O, Shaeer K, AbdelRahman IFS, Raheem A. Dorsal phalloplasty accompanying penile prosthesis implantation minimizes penile shortening and improves patient satisfaction. *Int J Impot Res*. 2019;31(4):276–281.
45. Sansalone S, Garaffa G, Djinovic R, et al. Simultaneous total corporal

reconstruction and implantation of a penile prosthesis in patients with erectile dysfunction and severe fibrosis of the corpora cavernosa. *J Sex Med*. 2012;9(7):1937–1944.

46. Rolle L, Ceruti C, Timpano M, et al. A new, innovative, lengthening surgical procedure for Peyronie's disease by penile prosthesis implantation with double dorsal-ventral patch graft: the "sliding technique". *J Sex Med*. 2012;9(9):2389–2395.

47. Egydio PH, Kuehhas FE. Penile lengthening and widening without grafting according to a modified "sliding" technique. *BJU Int*. 2015;116(6):965–972.

48. Wilson SK, Mora-Estaves C, Egydio P, et al. Glans necrosis following penile prosthesis implantation: prevention and treatment suggestions. *Urology*. 2017;107:144–148.

49. Clavell-Hernández J, Wang R. Penile size restoration with nondegloving approach for Peyronie's disease: initial experience. *J Sex Med*. 2018;15(10):1506–1513.

Section 5 Medical and Surgical Management of Issues of Male Health

Chapter 41

Medical Management of Benign Prostatic Hyperplasia

Christopher Martin, Laurel Mast, and Stephen Summers

41.1 Introduction

Benign prostatic hyperplasia (BPH) is the most common benign neoplasm in males in the United States [1]. There appears to be a genetic component to BPH, suggesting a heritable form of the disease, as well as a sporadic form [2].

Clinically significant BPH is characterized by the development of lower urinary tract symptoms (LUTS): weak stream, urinary frequency and urgency, incomplete emptying, urinary hesitancy, nocturia, acute urinary retention. Note that LUTS includes both storage (frequency, nocturia, urgency) and voiding dysfunction. Presentation of men with LUTS secondary to BPH is variable and any combination of the LUTS may be present [3].

LUTS may be due to pathology other than BPH: the lower urinary tract is made up of the bladder, prostate, sphincter complex, and urethra, and aberrant functioning of any of these structures, or their underlying peripheral and central nervous system controls, can lead to LUTS [3].

LUTS due to causes other than enlargement of the prostate due to BPH is known as "LUTS independent of BPH" [3].

LUTS secondary to BPH is commonly experienced in men 30 years of age and older, with approximately 90% of men between the ages of 45 and 80 years experiencing some degree of LUTS. The prevalence as well as the severity of LUTS increases with increasing age [1,2].

Estimates of prevalence and incidence in population-based studies of LUTS use the presence of moderate to severe LUTS, as defined by a score greater than or equal to 8 on the American Urological Association Symptom Score (AUASS) survey (see Section 41.3 for a full description of the AUASS) [1].

Nocturia is the most prevalent and the most bothersome LUTS.

Urinary retention is the most progressive form of LUTS and the risk of retention rises with age, more severe LUTS, and increased prostate size [1].

Risk factors associated with BPH and LUTS include non-modifiable factors – increasing age, genetics – and modifiable factors, which include metabolic syndrome, cardiovascular disease, obesity, and diabetes [4].

41.2 Pathophysiology

The prostate is anatomically divided into four regions: the transition zone, which encases the urethra proximal to the paired ejaculatory ducts; the central zone, which surrounds the ejaculatory ducts and extends toward the base of the prostate; the peripheral zone, which composes the apex and the majority of the gland distal to the verumontanum; and the fibromuscular stroma, located anteriorly [5]. Enlarged lateral prostatic lobes seen on cystoscopy are due to growth of the transition zone, while an enlarged median lobe arises from central zone growth [6].

BPH is a histologic diagnosis that is the result of proliferation of the epithelial and smooth muscle components of transition zone of the prostate gland [6].

Biochemically, BPH is primarily driven by androgens, although BPH growth is multifactorial. Within the prostate gland, 5-alpha-reductase metabolizes testosterone to dihydrotestosterone (DHT). DHT binds to androgen receptors within the prostate and triggers genetic modulations that promote epithelial and smooth muscle growth [7].

Longitudinal studies have found an annual prostate growth rate of 1.6–2.5% using transrectal ultrasonography [1,8].

BPH can cause LUTS via two mechanisms: first, bladder outlet obstruction due to the enlarged gland and, second, increased smooth muscle tone within the prostatic urethra leading to increased resistance. BPH can also indirectly result in LUTS due to changes to the detrusor muscle caused by chronic obstruction, such as increased bladder wall thickening and decreased bladder compliance [9].

Comorbid conditions seen with LUTS secondary to BPH include hypertension (postulated to share underlying age-related increase in sympathetic tone) and erectile dysfunction (ED) [10,11].

41.3 Diagnosis and Evaluation

Evaluation of men presenting with LUTS begins with a medical history and physical exam, which should include a digital rectal exam to evaluate the prostate for size and any abnormal features.

The AUASS is a standard questionnaire used to quantify and measure a patient's LUTS. The components of the AUASS capture both voiding and storage dysfunction; assessing incomplete emptying, frequency, urgency, intermittency, weak stream, straining, and nocturia. The International Prostate Symptom Score is also used, and is nearly identical to the AUASS, with an additional question evaluating quality of life [3]. A change of three points on the AUASS is considered a meaningful change in symptomatology [3].

A voiding diary can be useful, especially if nocturia or storage symptoms are the primary bothersome symptoms. The voiding diary, also called a frequency-volume chart, is used to assess for polyuria, which is defined as greater than three liters of urine output over 24 hours, or nocturnal polyuria, in which greater than 33% of daily urine output is produced at night [12].

Urinalysis should also be performed for every patient presenting for initial evaluation of LUTS to screen for underlying infection, hematuria resulting in irritative voiding symptoms, or other potential disorders that can lead to worsening urinary symptoms [3].

Prostate specific antigen (PSA) level should be obtained for any presenting patient greater than 50 years old with an expected life span greater than 10 years who has not had a recent PSA in the last year [3].

Postvoid residual can be a useful objective outcome to complement the subjective measure captured by the AUASS.

Uroflowmetry can be helpful in determining whether LUTS is due to obstruction, and is another objective measure to accompany the AUASS. A peak flow value less than 10mL/sec is indicative of an obstructive component [13].

Urodynamics is another modality that may be used to definitively diagnose the presence of obstruction, or further elucidate voiding function in a patient presenting with overlapping LUTS. Urodynamics is helpful when the diagnosis is unclear or in patients who are not responding appropriately to therapy [3].

Evaluation of the size of the prostate with imaging can be helpful prior to initiation of medical therapy, although it is not required. This may be performed with transrectal or abdominal ultrasonography in the clinic, computed tomography, or magnetic resonance imaging. Similarly, cystoscopy is not routinely performed for initial presentation of LUTS secondary to BPH, but may become useful for the evaluation of patients not responding to medical therapy or when deciding on surgical intervention [3,14].

LUTS may be due to pathology other than BPH and a wide range of differential diagnoses can be considered, including but not limited to bladder calculi, urinary tract infection (UTI), bladder neck contracture, urethral stricture, overactive bladder, severe ED, prostate cancer, neurodegenerative disorders such as multiple sclerosis, and medication side effects [3].

41.4 Treatment

The goal of treatment of LUTS and underlying BPH is improvement in quality of life and the prevention of disease progression and the development of related complications, such as changes to bladder architecture, UTIs, bladder stones, acute urinary retention, or renal insufficiency and failure [1].

Behavioral modifications are the cornerstone and starting point of management of LUTS secondary to BPH, and there are multiple interventions that may be of utility, depending on individual patient factors at time of presentation.

Dietary modifications such as increased total caloric intake are linked to increased risk of BPH, as is higher intake of protein in general and specifically red meat, dairy products, cereals, and starches. Conversely, fruits, vegetables, linoleic acid, vitamins D and E, and polyunsaturated fatty acids may decrease the risk of BPH [2,15,16]. Recommendations regarding alcohol intake are less clear, as alcohol consumption is associated with a decreased risk of BPH but an increased risk of LUTS [2,17]. As a diuretic, caffeine should be avoided, especially in the evening. Certain foods are known to irritate the bladder and thereby worsen irritative symptoms. These foods include alcohol and carbonated drinks, apples, bananas, cantaloupes, cheese, spicy foods, chocolate, citrus, coffee (including decaffeinated), cranberries, dairy products, fava beans, grapes, lentils, nuts, raw onions, peaches, pineapples, plums, prunes, soy sauce, strawberries, tomatoes, and vinegar [18].

Fluid restriction, especially in the evening, is particularly useful for patients with nocturia and storage symptoms.

Increased physical activity has been linked to decreased risk of LUTS and BPH [2,15,19,20].

Weight loss itself, separate from increased physical activity, can also be beneficial as body mass index, weight, and waist circumference have been associated with increased prostate size, and obesity increases the risk of progression of LUTS severity [2,20,21].

Double voiding, in which the patient voids as normal, allows several minutes to pass and changes positions, and then returns and attempts to void again, helps to ensure that the bladder is emptied completely and can decrease urgency and frequency and improve incomplete emptying. Timed voiding, in which attempts to void are determined by time interval instead of basing on sensation of needing to void, can be used to prevent overfilling of the bladder and improve urgency symptoms [22]. Timed voiding also includes voiding immediately prior to going to sleep.

If a patient is taking diuretics, these medications should be taken in the morning rather than the evening to reduce nocturia.

Some common medications can contribute to LUTS and should be avoided if possible. These medications include antidepressants, decongestants, antihistamines, bronchodilators, anticholinergics, and sympathomimetics [23].

Treatment options for LUTS secondary to BPH also include several categories of oral supplements and medications.

Herbal therapy has been centered on two predominant herbal supplements: saw palmetto (Serenoa repens) and stinging nettle (Urtica dioica). The efficacy of saw palmetto has been more rigorously evaluated. While early evidence suggested that saw palmetto may modestly improve LUTS secondary to BPH, more recent data fail to show saw palmetto as an effective therapy [24]. Currently, there are inadequate data to recommend strongly against herbal therapies but they are not routinely recommended for patient care [3].

Medication therapy for treatment of LUTS secondary to BPH has multiple therapeutic pathways that work both independently and synergistically. The general categories, based on mechanism of action, are alpha blockers, 5-alpha reductase inhibitors (5-ARIs), anticholinergic and beta-3 agonist therapy, and phosphodiesterase 5 inhibitors (PDEi-5s) [25]. Alpha blockers act as smooth muscle relaxants to improve the flow rate of urine across the prostate and proximal urethra [25]. 5-ARIs act via a hormonal blockade to reduce prostatic gland hypertrophy [25]. Anticholinergic and beta-3 agonist therapy act via the muscarinic receptor and beta-3 receptor, respectively, to reduce bladder muscular contractions and hypertonicity [25,26]. PDEi-5s increase nitric oxide synthesis to reduce muscular tone at the bladder trigone, bladder neck, and prostatic fossa [25]. These medications may be used alone or in combination, as discussed later.

Alpha blockers (alfuzosin, doxazosin, tamsulosin, silodosin, prazosin, and terazosin) are one of the most common classes of medications for treatment of LUTS secondary to BPH. These medications can be subclassified into prostate-selective and nonselective alpha blockers [27]. Tamsulosin's status as first-line therapy is likely due to the favorable side-effect profile of these medications. Notable side effects of the selective alpha blockers are retrograde ejaculation and orthostatic hypotension (5–17%) [27]. While retrograde ejaculation is bothersome for some men, this side effect is not constant or consistent across each of the selective alpha blockers. As such, clinicians can consider switching between different medications in this class as the rates of retrograde ejaculation are variable, with alfuzosin showing the lowest rate among the selective alpha blockers [27]. Orthostatic hypotension is most commonly encountered when patients are also taking PDEi-5s [28]. This can typically be managed by having the patient take these two medications at opposite times of the day, although separation by only a few hours is likely adequate. Orthostatic hypotension as a side effect generally improves with time and most patients tolerate this better when taking the alpha blocker prior to bedtime. The nonselective alpha blockers are typically used when patients also have concomitant hypertension, PTSD, or another medical condition where nonselective alpha blockade is desired for clinical outcomes [27]. These medications act to inhibit smooth muscle within the prostate to improve flow rates and thus improve LUTS but do not have a notable improvement in reduction of urinary retention compared to placebo [29]. Combination of selective and nonselective alpha blockade is not recommended and unlikely to improve clinical efficacy [3].

While alpha blockers are typically well tolerated, there is one concerning association with intraoperative floppy iris syndrome (IFIS). This can result in posterior capsule rupture, postoperative intraocular pressure spikes, and iris prolapse. It is suspected to be most common with tamsulosin, but it can occur with most of the alpha blockers [30]. It is also unclear if discontinuing the alpha blocker prevents this risk in the future, or if there should be considered a lifetime risk for IFIS for anyone placed on an alpha blocker [30]. More contemporary cataract surgery has been less influenced by the use of alpha blockers; however, this is an important consideration that patients should discuss with their ophthalmic surgeon prior to these cases [30].

The clinical utility of 5-ARIs in treating LUTS secondary to BPH has been established with multiple clinical trials. These medications act as inhibitors of 5-alpha reductase, thereby preventing the conversion of testosterone to dihydrotestosterone [29,31,32]. The main benefit of 5-ARIs is in reduction of prostate size, with a total reduction in volume typically 25–30% [33]. Compared to alpha blockers, which have a very quick onset, 5-ARIs require weeks to months to have a noticeable response. While the improvement in flow rates is slightly reduced compared to an alpha blocker, there is a notable decrease in rates of urinary retention and reduction in progression to bladder outlet surgery with 5-ARIs. Importantly, patients must have prostatic enlargement to derive a benefit from prostatic size reduction. This evidence comes in part from the exclusion of patients with small prostates from a number of trials, as well as data from the Medical Therapy of Prostatic Symptoms (MTOPS) study [29]. While there is no strict definition of prostatic enlargement, the CombAT trial's inclusion criteria of prostate size 30 mL or greater is commonly used [32]. Conversely, meta-analysis of multiple of the clinical trials suggested a cutoff of 40 g to best define the efficacy of finasteride therapy [34].

The mechanism of action of the two most commonly used 5-ARIs, finasteride and dutasteride, differ in the isoform of the 5-alpha reductase enzyme that undergoes blockade. Dutasteride blocks both type 1 and 2 isoforms, while finasteride blocks type 2 only [33]. While this has some theoretical implications on side-effect profile associated with these medications and efficacy, the difference in mechanism of action has not resulted in consistent outcome differences in clinical trials, and as such finasteride and dutasteride are effectively clinically equivalent [33].

Postfinasteride syndrome is a purported condition associated with finasteride and other 5-ARIs [35]. The syndrome consists of decreased libido, ED, worsening LUTS, gynecomastia, cognitive impairment, and depression, which persist beyond discontinuation of the agent. While this has not been confirmed on meta-analyses of clinical data [35], it is important for the clinician to be aware of this reported condition, as this can be a finding of concern for patients after independent research on their medications.

Another application of 5-ARIs is the management of BPH-associated hematuria. Though malignancy is the most concerning potential cause of gross hematuria, one of the most common underlying etiologies of gross hematuria is BPH [36,37]. Hypertrophic blood vessels associated with the prostatic mucosa can rupture and cause profound bleeding. Finasteride has been shown to clinically reduce hematuria episodes in patients with BPH-associated hematuria [3,38]. While hematuria resolution does not obviate the need for evaluation of patients for additional underlying etiologies, 5-

ARI use can be an effective management strategy for relieving one of the more unsettling sequelae of BPH [3].

5-ARIs impact both PSA kinetics and prostate cancer. The general rule is that the PSA value can be expected to halve following initiation of a 5-ARI [33]. This effect is expected to be seen 3–6 months after starting a 5-ARI as the PSA achieves a new steady state. Two trials have studied the effect of 5-ARIs on the risk of development of prostate cancer. In the Prostate Cancer Prevention Trial (PCPT), seven years of finasteride was associated with a reduction in the prevalence of prostate cancer by 24.8%, while the Reduction by Dutasteride of Prostate Cancer Events (REDUCE) trial found that dutasteride therapy for four years was associated with a prevalence reduction of 22.8% [39,40]. However, while the overall risk decreased, the proportion of high-risk disease increased. There have been varying interpretations of these trials. The most optimistic interpretation is that 5-ARIs truly reduce low-risk prostate cancer without affecting high-risk prostate cancer, with a relative increase in proportion of high-risk cancer only as a result of the decrease in low-risk cases. The more pessimistic interpretation is that 5-ARIs increase the risk of high-risk prostate cancer while decreasing PSA, and thus lower detection of all prostate cancers. The middle ground interpretation is that 5-ARIs have little meaningful effect on any prostate cancer and that the low-risk prostate cancer detection decrease is due to a decrease in PSA values. These conclusions are complicated by more recent literature suggesting that 5-ARIs are associated with higher adjusted PSA values at prostate cancer diagnosis, delayed presentation, and increased prostate cancer mortality. This has resulted in an FDA warning stating that 5-ARIs may increase the risk of development of high-grade prostate cancer [33]. The American Urologic Association has no defined position statements for 5-ARIs with regard to prostate cancer prevention or risk but it is included as a primary medication in the BPH algorithm.

PDEi-5s are another adjunctive therapy that have been shown to improve LUTS secondary to BPH. Although the exact mechanism by which improvement to LUTS occurs remains debated, the predominant theory is that current good manufacturing practice production and nitric oxide synthesis results in further smooth muscle relaxation of the bladder neck, prostate, and possibly trigone with resultant improvement in LUTS [28]. The only FDA-approved PDEi-5 for use in treating LUTS is daily tadalafil due to its prolonged half-life. Other PDEi-5s are used by urologists and other clinicians to treat LUTS; however, this use is considered off label.

Anticholinergic medications can improve LUTS in select cases. These medications predominantly work by inhibiting the muscarinic receptor to reduce detrusor activation [41]. While it is somewhat counterintuitive to start a patient having symptoms related to an obstructing prostate on medication to decrease detrusor contraction or activation, anticholinergics can be very helpful for patients with predominant storage issues: urinary frequency, urgency, and nocturia. Bladder remodeling from obstruction results in bladder wall thickening and collagen deposition with a resultant poor storing, irritated bladder. In men without urinary retention or significant post-void residual, utilization of an anticholinergic can reduce incontinence episodes and improve storage rates by approximately 40–60 mL [41]. Side effects associated with anticholinergic therapy are due to antagonism of other muscarinic receptors, resulting in blurry vision, dry eyes, dry mouth, constipation, and delirium and confusion [42].

The cognitive side-effect profile is the most concerning adverse effect associated with anticholinergic therapy. While anticholinergics have historically been associated with delirium or other temporary cognitive side effects, there is newer data linking anticholinergic therapy to dementia [43]. However, this evidence is based on correlation studies, which may produce false associations. First, LUTS secondary to BPH increases with age at a similar time horizon at which dementia occurs [43]. Secondly, nocturia results in poor sleep patterns, which is a known and important association with the development of dementia [44]. Lastly, family members and providers may have increased vigilance in identifying cognitive decline in patients on anticholinergic therapy due to its known cognitive side effects, thus more readily identifying the development of dementia in patients on anticholinergic therapy. Regardless of the underlying relationship, these correlated findings warrant further study and prospective evaluation is required.

Beta-3 agonist therapy acts in a similar fashion to anticholinergics by reducing detrusor activation. This results in improved bladder capacity and decreased bladder overactivity. While the beta-3 receptor is fairly specific to the bladder, this medication can nonetheless result in worsening hypertension related to systemic beta-3 receptor activation. On average, patients have an increase of about 0.4 mmHg each in diastolic and systolic blood pressures [26]. While this may not appear significant, a smaller proportion of patients have a more substantial blood pressure elevation: about 5% of patients have a blood pressure increase of 10–15 mmHg [26]. The indications for beta-3 agonists and responses are very similar to those of the anticholinergic class. In patients with particularly severe bladder overactivity and irritative symptoms, anticholinergics and beta-3 agonists can be combined.

Combination therapy is one of the most important approaches in the management of LUTS secondary to BPH. Major trials including MTOPS, PREDICT, and CombAT have established that combined therapy is superior to monotherapy for symptom improvement, peak urinary flow, prevention of urinary retention, and overall progression of disease [29,31,32]. Urinary retention rates between monotherapy on 5-ARIs and combination therapy in these studies have been found to be equivalent, suggesting the majority of this benefit is derived from the 5-ARI portion of the combination therapy [29,31,32].

A large number of patients with LUTS secondary to BPH who are initially managed with medical therapy will progress on to need surgical treatment of their bladder outlet obstruction. Indications for surgery include: symptoms inadequately managed with oral medications, refractory urinary retention, recurrent urinary tract infections (particularly in those with elevated postvoid residual), recurrent bladder stones, bladder diverticuli, upper tract changes (typically presents with a thickened bladder and bilateral hydronephrosis), those who cannot tolerate medications, or those who do not want to take medications [45]. Certainly, patients with true clinical manifestations related to bladder outlet obstruction warrant closer follow-up, more aggressive early therapy, specifically earlier initiation of dual medical therapy, and a lower threshold to consider operative interventions. It is paramount to realize that much of the pathophysiology of BPH symptoms is related to irreversible changes to the bladder wall that can occur with prolonged disease.

41.5 Conclusions

Future directions in the medical management of LUTS secondary to BPH include expanded utilization of beta-3 agonists in clinical practice, prospective study of anticholinergic medications and their link with dementia, additional clinical trials of triple therapy (the combination of an alpha blocker, a 5-ARI, and an anticholinergic or beta-3 agonist), and improved tools for early identification of patients with LUTS refractory to medical therapy or at risk of developing detrusor failure to guide earlier recommendation of surgical intervention.

References

1. Wei JT, Calhoun E, Jacobsen SJ. Urologic diseases in America project: benign prostatic hyperplasia. *J Urol.* 2005;173 (4):1256–1261.
2. Lim KB. Epidemiology of clinical benign prostatic hyperplasia. *Asian J Urol.* 2017;4(3):148–151.
3. McVary KT, et al. Update on AUA guideline on the management of benign prostatic hyperplasia. *J Urol.* 2011;185 (5):1793–1803.
4. Patel ND, Parsons JK. Epidemiology and etiology of benign prostatic hyperplasia and bladder outlet obstruction. *Indian J Urol.* 2014;30 (2):170–176.
5. Villers A, Steg A, Boccon-Gibod L. Anatomy of the prostate: review of the different models. *Eur Urol.* 1991;20 (4):261–268.
6. McNeal JE. Normal histology of the prostate. *Am J Surg Pathol.* 1988;12 (8):619–633.
7. Carson C, 3rd, Rittmaster R. The role of dihydrotestosterone in benign prostatic hyperplasia. *Urology.* 2003;61(4 Suppl. 1):2–7.
8. Loeb S, et al. Prostate volume changes over time: results from the Baltimore Longitudinal Study of Aging. *J Urol.* 2009;182 (4):1458–1462.
9. Bellucci CHS, et al. Increased detrusor collagen is associated with detrusor overactivity and decreased bladder compliance in men with benign prostatic obstruction. *Prostate Int.* 2017;5(2):70–74.
10. Aslan G, et al. Association between lower urinary tract symptoms and erectile dysfunction. *Arch Androl.* 2006;52(3):155–162.
11. McVary KT. BPH: epidemiology and comorbidities. *Am J Manag Care.* 2006;12(Suppl. 5):S122–S128.
12. Weiss JP, Everaert K. Management of nocturia and nocturnal polyuria. *Urology.* 2019;133s:24–33.
13. Reynard JM, et al. The ICS-'BPH' Study: uroflowmetry, lower urinary tract symptoms and bladder outlet obstruction. *Br J Urol.* 1998;82 (5):619–623.
14. Stone BV, et al. Prostate size, nocturia and the digital rectal examination: a cohort study of 30 500 men. *BJU Int.* 2017;119(2):298–304.
15. Parsons JK. Modifiable risk factors for benign prostatic hyperplasia and lower urinary tract symptoms: new approaches to old problems. *J Urol.* 2007;178(2):395–401.
16. Kristal AR, et al. Dietary patterns, supplement use, and the risk of symptomatic benign prostatic hyperplasia: results from the prostate cancer prevention trial. *Am J Epidemiol.* 2008;167(8):925–934.
17. Parsons JK, Im R. Alcohol consumption is associated with a decreased risk of benign prostatic hyperplasia. *J Urol.* 2009;182(4):1463–1468.
18. Abrams P, et al. Evaluation and treatment of lower urinary tract symptoms in older men. *J Urol.* 2009;181(4):1779–1787.
19. Fowke JH, et al. Association between physical activity, lower urinary tract symptoms (LUTS) and prostate volume. *BJU Int.* 2013;111 (1):122–128.
20. Parsons JK, et al. Obesity increases and physical activity decreases lower urinary tract symptom risk in older men: the Osteoporotic Fractures in Men study. *Eur Urol.* 2011;60 (6):1173–1180.
21. Parsons JK, et al. Obesity and benign prostatic hyperplasia: clinical connections, emerging etiological paradigms and future directions. *J Urol.* 2013;189(Suppl. 1):S102–S106.
22. Wein AJ. Diagnosis and treatment of the overactive bladder. *Urology.* 2003;62 (5 Suppl. 2):20–27.
23. Wuerstle MC, et al. Contribution of common medications to lower urinary tract symptoms in men. *Arch Intern Med.* 2011;171(18):1680–1682.
24. Bent S, et al. Saw palmetto for benign prostatic hyperplasia. *N Eng J Med.* 2006;354(6):557–566.
25. Lepor H. Medical treatment of benign prostatic hyperplasia. *Rev Urol.* 2011;13 (1):20–33.
26. Bragg R, et al. Mirabegron: a beta-3 agonist for overactive bladder. *Consult Pharm.* 2014;29(12):823–837.
27. Lepor H. The evolution of alpha-blockers for the treatment of benign prostatic hyperplasia. *Rev Urol.* 2006;8 (Suppl. 4):S3–S9.
28. Laydner HK, et al. Phosphodiesterase 5 inhibitors for lower urinary tract symptoms secondary to benign prostatic hyperplasia: a systematic review. *BJU Int.* 2011;107 (7):1104–1109.
29. McConnell JD, et al. The long-term effect of doxazosin, finasteride, and combination therapy on the clinical progression of benign prostatic hyperplasia. *N Engl J Med.* 2003;349 (25):2387–2398.
30. Christou CD, et al. Intraoperative floppy iris syndrome: updated perspectives. *Clin Ophthalmol.* 2020;14:463–471.
31. Kirby RS, et al. Efficacy and tolerability of doxazosin and finasteride, alone or in combination, in treatment of

symptomatic benign prostatic hyperplasia: the Prospective European Doxazosin and Combination Therapy (PREDICT) trial. *Urology.* 2003;61(1):119-126.

32. Roehrborn CG, et al. The effects of combination therapy with dutasteride and tamsulosin on clinical outcomes in men with symptomatic benign prostatic hyperplasia: 4-year results from the CombAT study. *Eur Urol.* 2010;57(1):123-131.

33. Nickel JC. Comparison of clinical trials with finasteride and dutasteride. *Rev Urol.* 2004;6(Suppl. 9):S31-S39.

34. Boyle P, Gould AL, Roehrborn CG. Prostate volume predicts outcome of treatment of benign prostatic hyperplasia with finasteride: meta-analysis of randomized clinical trials. *Urology.* 1996;48(3):398-405.

35. Liu L, et al. Effect of 5α-reductase inhibitors on sexual function: a meta-analysis and systematic review of randomized controlled trials. *J Sex Med.* 2016;13(9):1297-1310.

36. Gonzalez AN, et al. The prevalence of bladder cancer during cystoscopy for asymptomatic microscopic hematuria. *Urology.* 2019;126:34-38.

37. Davis R, et al. Diagnosis, evaluation and follow-up of asymptomatic microhematuria (AMH) in adults: AUA guideline. *J Urol.* 2012;188(6 Suppl.):2473-2481.

38. Puchner PJ, Miller MI. The effects of finasteride on hematuria associated with benign prostatic hyperplasia: a preliminary report. *J Urol.* 1995;154(5):1779-1782.

39. Andriole GL, et al. Effect of dutasteride on the risk of prostate cancer. *N Engl J Med.* 2010;362(13):1192-1202.

40. Thompson IM, et al. Long-term survival of participants in the prostate cancer prevention trial. *N Engl J Med.* 2013;369(7):603-610.

41. Herbison P, et al. Effectiveness of anticholinergic drugs compared with placebo in the treatment of overactive bladder: systematic review. *BMJ.* 2003;326(7394):841-844.

42. Feinberg M. The problems of anticholinergic adverse effects in older patients. *Drugs Aging.* 1993;3(4):335-348.

43. Gray SL, et al. Cumulative use of strong anticholinergics and incident dementia: a prospective cohort study. *JAMA Intern Med.* 2015;175(3):401-407.

44. Wennberg AMV, et al. Sleep disturbance, cognitive decline, and dementia: a review. *Semin Neurol.* 2017;37(4):395-406.

45. Foster HE, et al. Surgical management of lower urinary tract symptoms attributed to benign prostatic hyperplasia: AUA Guideline Amendment 2019. *J Urol.* 2019;202(3):592-598.

Section 5 Medical and Surgical Management of Issues of Male Health

Chapter 42

Evidence-Based Management of Chronic Orchialgia and Chronic Prostatitis/Chronic Pelvic Pain Syndrome

Sharon P. Lo and Kelli X. Gross

42.1 Background

Testicular pain is a common complaint that can have a wide variety of different causes, and thus it has been difficult to standardize its workup and treatment. Testicular pain can be either acute, subacute, or chronic. Chronic orchialgia is defined as pain to the testis, scrotum, epididymis, paratesticular structures, and/or spermatic cord lasting at least three months. Chronic orchialgia makes up 2.5–4.8% of all urology clinic visits [1]. There is some overlap with this condition and chronic prostatitis/chronic pelvic pain syndrome (CP/CPPS), given that 57–63% of men with this diagnosis also complain of testicular pain [2]. CP/CPPS is defined as chronic pain or discomfort in the pelvic region for at least three of the past six months, and is often associated with lower urinary tract symptoms [2]. The term "prostatitis" is vague and can refer to acute or chronic symptomatology as well as asymptomatic histologic findings.

Chronic orchialgia can undoubtedly be distressing, and has been associated with somatization disorder, chronic pain syndromes, major depression, chemical dependency, low social support, and social isolation [3]. Men with chronic orchialgia may experience loss of productivity [4], social changes, or decreases in sexual function [5]. Many men see medical providers seeking care for chronic orchialgia, but both practice patterns and varying patient responses limit consistent outcomes.

42.2 Anatomy and Pathophysiology

Pain of the scrotal contents can arise from any number of organs in the scrotal and pelvic region. The sensory innervation of the pelvic region involves a number of nerve roots in a relatively small area (Figure 42.1). The testis (T10–T12) and epididymis (T12–L1) mainly have sympathetic innervation [6]. The anterior scrotum is innervated via the genital branch of the genitofemoral and ilioinguinal nerve, arising from L1 and L2 (Figure 42.2). The posterior scrotum is innervated by the scrotal branches of the superficial perineal nerve via the pudendal nerve (S2–S4) [7]. The inferior portion of the scrotum is innervated by the long scrotal branches of the posterior femoral cutaneous nerve (S1–S3) [6]. Any part of the body with a shared neural pathway can refer pain to this area [6].

With a painful stimulus, nociceptors are activated, which then transmit the pain sensation via nerve fibers to the spinal

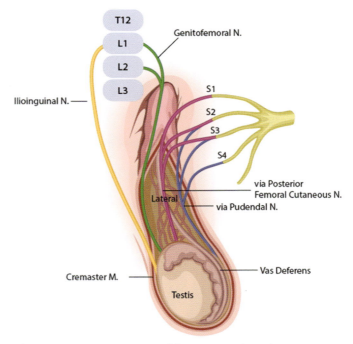

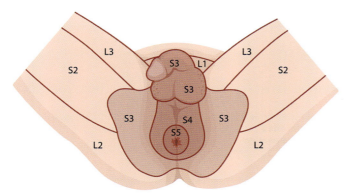

Figure 42.1 Sensory innervation of the pelvic region

Figure 42.2 Sensory innervation of the scrotum and testicle

cord [6]. Inflammatory chemicals can also activate nociceptors and elicit a pain response. This is mediated by neuropeptides such as substance P and calcitonin gene-related peptide (CGRP). Nerve injury may also lead to Wallerian degeneration, which is a destructive change to the neuron after injury (Figure 42.3) [6]. Wallerian degeneration appears to be more common in men with chronic orchialgia, as it has been seen in 84% of men undergoing microsurgical spermatic cord denervation compared to only 20% of controls (Figure 42.4) [8]. This was mainly found in nerves of the cremasteric muscle fibers, around the vas deferens, and posterior periarterial lipomatous tissues [8].

42.3 Workup

Every patient should have a careful assessment of history as well as a physical exam. The location of pain should be assessed. Abnormalities such as hydrocele, varicocele, or pain that localizes to a particular structure can be telling. Evaluation of the scrotal contents and groin, with and without Valsalva may provide diagnostic information. A digital rectal exam can discern any abnormalities to the prostate, as well as any tenderness to the prostate or pelvic floor. At times, exam can replicate the patient's pain.

Laboratory tests, including urinalysis and urine culture, may be helpful. Semen culture or urine culture after a prostatic massage using a two- or four-glass test may also be used [9]. If there are concerns of scrotal pathology, ultrasound may be helpful. Compared to ultrasound, a physical exam was 71.4% sensitive and 90.9% specific, with a negative predictive value of 88.2% in identifying pathology in chronic testicular pain without swelling [10]. Lau et al. found that all clinically significant abnormalities were identified on clinical examination as well. Abnormalities identified by ultrasound alone did not affect the clinical management. Thus, scrotal ultrasound is an option but not necessary in the evaluation of chronic scrotal pain. Depending on the differential diagnosis, other tests or imaging may be useful.

42.4 Differential Diagnosis

Any number of things may refer pain to the testes, and thus there is a relatively broad differential diagnosis of scrotal content pain. Within the scrotum itself, epididymitis, testicular torsion, malignancy, varicocele, hydrocele, spermatocele, and infection may cause pain [1]. Pain may be referred to the scrotum from pathology such as a ureterolithiasis, irritable bowel syndrome, aortic or iliac aneurysm, interstitial cystitis, inguinal hernia, musculoskeletal sources, or nerve entrapment [1,5]. Approximately 25–50% of chronic orchialgia is idiopathic in nature [11].

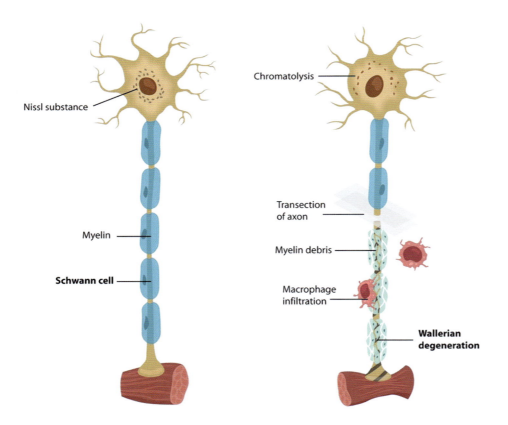

Figure 42.3 Wallerian degeneration

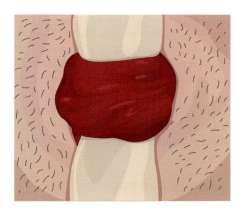 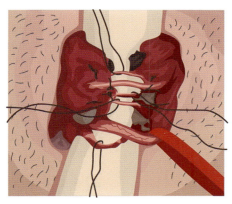

Figure 42.4 Before and after microsurgical denervation of the spermatic cord

42.5 Treatment of Idiopathic Chronic Orchialgia

42.5.1 Behavioral and Conservative Measures

As first-line therapy, patients should attempt to modify any causative factors such as postural habits or aggravating activities. The help of a knowledgeable pelvic floor physical therapist can be indispensable in identifying and adjusting any such factors. Compressive underwear can be helpful for some patients. Stress relief techniques and treating any underlying psychological conditions can be beneficial.

42.5.2 Pharmacologic Therapies

Chronic testicular pain is considered part of a more complex urogenital focal pain syndrome and it is empirically helped by medication used to treat neuropathic pain syndromes like anticonvulsant drugs (gabapentin and carbamazepine) or nonsteroidal anti-inflammatory drugs (NSAIDs).

42.5.3 Microsurgical Denervation of the Spermatic Cord

Microsurgical denervation of the spermatic cord (MDSC) was developed to divide all nerve fibers to the testicle, while still preserving the testicle and often the vas deferens. Originally described in 1996 by Levine et al., six of seven patients had complete relief of pain after MDSC [12]. Typically, the surgery is done with an operating microscope but has been described using robot assistance [13]. All structures in the spermatic cord are divided except the arterial supply, a few lymphatics, and in some cases the vas deferens. Division of the vas deferens remains surgeon preference as well as the fertility concerns of the patient.

A positive response to a cord block has been used as an indicator of response to MDSC [14]. Positive outcomes have been confirmed by numerous additional studies [15,16]. Risks include hydrocele (which may be reduced by preserving lymphatic vessels), testicular atrophy, and increased pain [15].

42.5.4 Ultrasound-Guided Microcryoablation of Spermatic Cord

Ultrasound guided targeted microcryoablation of the spermatic cord can be done after MDSC as men who fail MDSC may still have residual nerve fibers around the spermatic cord as the source of persistent pain. One study found a 75% significant reduction in pain and sustained results including 64% reduction at five years in patients who had failed microsurgical denervation [17].

42.5.5 Injection Therapies

Onabotulinumtoxin-A has been thought to reduce neurogenic inflammation, potentially due to decreased release of substance P and CGRP [18].

Amniotic fluid injection directly to the spermatic cord may also be used in refractory cases. In 14 patients who did not have a sufficient response to MDSC, 50% had a response to amniotic fluid injection.

42.5.6 Epididymectomy and Orchiectomy

Epididymectomy and orchiectomy have had mixed results in the treatment of chronic orchialgia. Data are limited, but may be more successful in post-vasectomy pain syndrome (93.3% success) than with chronic epididymitis or idiopathic epididymalgia (43–50% success) [19,20]. Orchiectomy may be a last resort for men with continued pain; however, men need to be counseled on a strong likelihood on continued pain and potential risks of infertility and hypogonadism. If the patient elects for orchiectomy, an inguinal approach may be associated with better success (73% pain relief) compared to a scrotal approach (55%).

42.5.7 Spinal Cord Stimulation

Spinal cord stimulation has been used for a number of chronic pain conditions and has likewise been shown to be effective for chronic orchialgia.

42.6 Notable Causes of Chronic Orchialgia

42.6.1 Varicocele

Varicoceles are relatively common, with an incidence of 10–20%, with 2–10% of these men being symptomatic regarding pain [21]. Pain related to a varicocele tends to be dull or throbbing, worse at the end of the day, and worsens with activity [21]. Multiple studies have shown improvement of orchialgia after varicocelectomy, with a complete response rate of 72–91% after varicocelectomy [22,23].

42.6.2 Post-Vasectomy Pain Syndrome

There are multiple studies, albeit of relatively low quality, that show that chronic scrotal pain is more common after vasectomy compared to controls. After vasectomy, 1–2% of men report new pain severe enough to affect their quality of life, and 14.7% of men report any pain [24]. A prospective trial showed 0.9% of men will have pain this severe at seven months after vasectomy [25]. A comparative study with 3.9 years of follow-up showed that 6.0% of men sought medical care for pain compared to 2.0% of men without vasectomy [26]. Post-vasectomy pain syndrome is included in the American Urological Association guidelines as one of the minimum and necessary concepts to counsel patients on prior to vasectomy [24]. Treatment for post-vasectomy pain syndrome includes conservative measures such as addressing predisposing musculoskeletal factors, scrotal support, NSAIDs, and treating concurrent psychiatric and chronic pain conditions. Vasectomy reversal has been shown to be quite effective in treating post-vasectomy pain, with satisfaction or pain-free rates of 69–100% in five separate studies [27]. However, this may not be covered by insurance companies as it is seen as a treatment for infertility. MSCD has also been shown to be effective, with a success rate of 71% even in the setting of prior vasectomy reversal and epididymectomy [28]. Epididymectomy may also be an option, with improvement in pain in up to 93.3% of men after vasectomy, but data are limited [20]. Orchiectomy has not been rigorously studied for post-vasectomy pain syndrome but may be an option in otherwise refractory cases.

42.6.3 Chronic Prostatitis/Chronic Pelvic Pain Syndrome

Chronic prostatitis/chronic pelvic pain syndrome (CP/CPPS) is a common cause of chronic scrotal pain [2]. Additional symptoms that may suggest CP as a cause of chronic orchialgia may include pelvic pain, urinary symptoms, bilateral nature of pain, or tenderness of the prostate or pelvic floor on physical exam [29]. The National Institutes of Health (NIH) CP/CPPS classification system categorizes CP to clarify how the term "prostatitis" is used. Type I prostatitis is an acutely symptomatic, infectious prostatitis. Type II is a chronic infectious prostatitis, which only makes up 5–10% of prostatitis. Type III prostatitis is synonymous with CP/CPPS. Type 4 is asymptomatic histologic findings of prostatitis.

CP/CPPS syndrome has been shown to have a negative effect on quality of life [2]. Increased stress burden, stress response, pain catastrophizing, poor social functioning, and psychiatric comorbidity have been shown to contribute [30]. It is associated with syndromes such as irritable bowel syndrome, interstitial cystitis, chronic fatigue syndrome, and fibromyalgia [2].

Patients may be monitored using the NIH Chronic Prostatitis Symptom Index (CPSI), which is a validated nine-question survey evaluating pain, urinary function, and quality of life.

42.6.4 Pathophysiology of CP/CPPS

There are many theories regarding the etiology and pathogenesis of CP/CPPS. A common theory is that it has a psycho-neuromuscular etiology, with pelvic floor guarding and tension paired with psychosocial stress. Pelvic floor hypertonicity develops as a result, causing a cycle of chronic pelvic floor irritation and worsening stress [31]. Though the isolation of uropathogenic bacteria in prostatic fluid occurs at similar rates in men with CP/CPPS when compared to controls, there may be some relation to infection [32]. Bacterial DNA may be detected more frequently in men with CP/CPPS [33], and a history of sexually transmitted infection has been reported to be more common in those with CP/CPPS [34]. There may also be difference in the urinary microbiome in patients with CP/CPPS [35]. Gram positive isolates from CP/CPPS may induce tactile allodynia compared to similar gram-positive strains from healthy controls [36].

Other theories include autoimmune processes [37], adrenal axis abnormalities [38], pelvic floor muscle dysfunction [29], pelvic nerves entrapment [39], genetic predisposition to inflammation [40], dyssynergic voiding with bladder neck hypertrophy [41], intraprostatic urinary reflux [42], and oxidative stress [43]. Given the varied presentation and response to treatment, it could certainly be a multifactorial etiology.

42.6.5 Treatment of CP/CPPS

42.6.5.1 Lifestyle Changes

A number of lifestyle factors, a number of which are modifiable, have been shown to play a role in CP/CPPS. Risk has been shown to be related to age, shift work, stress, smoking, alcohol use, water intake, dietary factors, sexual activity, delaying ejaculation, and delaying urination [44]. A sedentary lifestyle, intake of caffeinated beverages, and insufficient fluid intake were associated with severe pain. Treating underlying psychiatric and chronic pain conditions is also recommended [30].

42.6.5.2 Alpha Blockers and 5-Alpha-Reductase Inhibitors

Alpha blockers reduce sympathetic tone in the bladder neck and prostate, improving urinary flow and lower urinary tract symptoms. 5-alpha-reductase inhibitors reduce the production of dihydrotestosterone and, consequently, the size of the prostatic gland dependent on the stimulation of this hormone and likewise can treat voiding symptoms. Side effects of alpha blockers include hypotension, ejaculatory dysfunction, headache, dizziness, and nasal congestion. Side effects of 5-alpha-reductase inhibitors include decreased libido, impotence, and potentiation of hypotension (in combination with alpha blockers).

42.6.5.3 NSAIDs

NSAIDs are antagonists to the cyclooxygenases enzymes (COX) type 1 and 2 and their proinflammatory subproducts. Both nonselective and selective (COX-2) inhibitors could therefore decrease inflammatory mediated pain in CP/CPPS. Side effects of NSAIDs include peripheral edema, rash, dyspepsia, peptic ulcer and bleeding, renal and hepatic injury, and increased risk of adverse cardiovascular events.

42.6.5.4 Phytotherapy

Phytotherapy includes such over-the-counter therapies as bioflavonoids such as quercetin and bee pollen extract. These therapies have been thought to have anti-inflammatory properties, decreasing proinflammatory cytokines [45]. Quercetin has been shown to be associated with significant symptomatic improvement in men with CP/CPPS [46]. Likewise, there are a number of studies that show improvement in symptoms with bee pollen extract; a 2009 study by Wagenlehner showed a decrease in the NIH CPSI score by at least six points in 70.6% of men given bee pollen extract compared with 50% of controls [47]. Side effects of phytotherapy are rare, but include gastrointestinal discomfort and allergic reactions.

42.6.5.5 Antibiotics

Even if CP/CPPS is defined when no bacterial cause can be identified, antibiotics have been used to treat it under the assumption of the existence of an occult or undertreated infection [33]. The most commonly used antibiotics include quinolones and tetracyclines. Side effects of quinolones include gastrointestinal discomfort, headache, dizziness, rash, and tendinopathy. Side effects of tetracyclines include gastrointestinal discomfort, rash, teeth discoloration, and hepatotoxicity.

42.6.5.6 Botulinum Toxin A

Botulinum toxin A has denervating properties and also causes reduction in pain mediators when applied to the prostate in animal models. It also causes apoptosis and involution of the prostate gland [48].

42.6.5.7 Allopurinol

Allopurinol reduces the prostatic secretions of purine and pyrimidine base containing metabolites in urine. These metabolites could be responsible for prostatic inflammation through urinary reflux [49].

42.6.5.8 Nonpharmacologic Therapy

Acupuncture is an ancient eastern practice that utilizes fine needles inserted into the body. Electric current may be added (electroacupuncture). In animal models, electroacupuncture has anti-inflammatory properties and activates analgesic neurotransmitters [50]. Locally induced hyperthermia, or using transrectal or transurethral methods to apply heat in the prostate, has been postulated to decrease oxygen free radicals and thus potentially prostate inflammation [51].

Myofascial trigger points release targets pelvic floor musculature dysfunction as a potential cause or contributor to CP/CPPS [52]. Biofeedback also addresses the pelvic floor muscles through initial contraction in order to achieve further relaxation [45].

42.6.5.9 Low-Intensity Shockwave Therapy

Extracorporeal shockwave therapy has long been utilized in urology as treatment for urolithiasis. Low-intensity shockwave therapy (Li-SWT) uses this technology in lower intensity. Multiple randomized trials comparing Li-SWT to sham treatment showed it to be relatively effective with few side effects [53].

42.7 Conclusions

Chronic orchialgia can have a number of different causes and phenotypes, and careful evaluation of the symptomatology of these men is often more of an art than a science.

References

1. Sigalos JT, Pastuszak AW. Chronic orchialgia: epidemiology, diagnosis and evaluation. *Transl Androl Urol.* 2017;6: S37–S43.
2. Wagenlehner FM, van Till JW, Magri V, et al. National Institutes of Health Chronic Prostatitis Symptom Index (NIH-CPSI) symptom evaluation in multinational cohorts of patients with chronic prostatitis/chronic pelvic pain syndrome. *Eur Urol.* 2013;63:953–959.
3. Schover LR. Psychological factors in men with genital pain. *Cleve Clin J Med.* 1990;57:697–700.
4. Costabile RA, Hahn M, McLeod DG. Chronic orchialgia in the pain prone patient: the clinical perspective. *J Urol.* 1991;146:1571–1574.
5. Ciftci H, Savas M, Gulum M, Yeni E, Verit A, Topal U. Evaluation of sexual function in men with orchialgia. *Arch Sex Behav.* 2011;40:631–634.
6. Patel AP. Anatomy and physiology of chronic scrotal pain. *Transl Androl Urol.* 2017;6:S51–S56.
7. Hunter CW, Stovall B, Chen G, Carlson J, Levy R. Anatomy, pathophysiology and interventional therapies for chronic pelvic pain: a review. *Pain Physician.* 2018;21:147–167.
8. Chaudhari R, Sharma S, Khant S, Raval K. Microsurgical denervation of spermatic cord for chronic idiopathic orchialgia: long-term results from an institutional experience. *World J Mens Health.* 2019;37:78–84.
9. Nickel JC, Shoskes D, Wang Y, et al. How does the pre-massage and post-massage 2-glass test compare to the Meares-Stamey 4-glass test in men with chronic prostatitis/chronic pelvic pain syndrome? *J Urol.* 2006;176:119–124.
10. Lau MW, Taylor PM, Payne SR. The indications for scrotal ultrasound. *Br J Radiol.* 1999;72:833–837.

11. Davis BE, Noble MJ, Weigel JW, Foret JD, Mebust WK. Analysis and management of chronic testicular pain. *J Urol.* 1990;143:936–939.
12. Levine LA, Matkov TG, Lubenow TR. Microsurgical denervation of the spermatic cord: a surgical alternative in the treatment of chronic orchialgia. *J Urol.* 1996;155:1005–1007.
13. Parekattil SJ, Gudeloglu A, Brahmbhatt JV, Priola KB, Vieweg J, Allan RW. Trifecta nerve complex: potential anatomical basis for microsurgical denervation of the spermatic cord for chronic orchialgia. *J Urol.* 2013;190:265–270.
14. Benson JS, Abern MR, Larsen S, Levine LA. Does a positive response to spermatic cord block predict response to microdenervation of the spermatic cord for chronic scrotal content pain? *J Sex Med.* 2013;10:876–882.
15. Oliveira RG, Camara C, Alves JMAF, Coelho RF, Lucon AM, Srougi M. Microsurgical testicular denervation for the treatment of chronic testicular pain initial results. *Clinics (Sao Paulo).* 2009;64:393–396.
16. Marconi M, Palma C, Troncoso P, Dell Oro A, Diemer T, Weidner W. Microsurgical spermatic cord denervation as a treatment for chronic scrotal content pain: a multicenter open label trial. *J Urol.* 2015;194:1323–1327.
17. Calixte N, Kartal IG, Tojuola B, et al. Salvage ultrasound-guided targeted cryoablation of the perispermatic cord for persistent chronic scrotal content pain after microsurgical denervation of the spermatic cord. *Urology.* 2019;130:181–185.
18. Calixte N, Brahmbhatt J, Parekattil S. Chronic testicular and groin pain: pathway to relief. *Curr Urol Rep.* 2017;18:83.
19. Padmore DE, Norman RW, Millard OH. Analyses of indications for and outcomes of epididymectomy. *J Urol.* 1996;156:95–96.
20. Hori S, Sengupta A, Shukla CJ, Ingall E, McLoughlin J. Long-term outcome of epididymectomy for the management of chronic epididymal pain. *J Urol.* 2009;182:1407–1412.
21. Peterson AC, Lance RS, Ruiz HE. Outcomes of varicocele ligation done for pain. *J Urol.* 1998;159:1565–1567.
22. Park HJ, Lee SS, Park NC. Predictors of pain resolution after varicocelectomy for painful varicocele. *Asian J Androl.* 2011;13:754–758.
23. Kim HT, Song PH, Moon KH. Microsurgical ligation for painful varicocele: effectiveness and predictors of pain resolution. *Yonsei Med J.* 2012;53:145–150.
24. Sharlip ID, Belker AM, Honig S, et al. Vasectomy: AUA guideline. *J Urol.* 2012;188:2482–2491.
25. Leslie TA, Illing RO, Cranston DW, Guillebaud J. The incidence of chronic scrotal pain after vasectomy: a prospective audit. *BJU Int.* 2007;100:1330–1333.
26. Morris C, Mishra K, Kirkman RJ. A study to assess the prevalence of chronic testicular pain in post-vasectomy men compared to non-vasectomised men. *J Fam Plann Reprod Health Care.* 2002;28:142–144.
27. Smith-Harrison LI, Smith RP. Vasectomy reversal for post-vasectomy pain syndrome. *Transl Androl Urol.* 2017;6:S10–S13.
28. Tan WP, Tsambarlis PN, Levine LA. Microdenervation of the spermatic cord for post-vasectomy pain syndrome. *BJU Int.* 2018;121:667–673.
29. Shoskes DA, Berger R, Elmi A, et al. Muscle tenderness in men with chronic prostatitis/chronic pelvic pain syndrome: the chronic prostatitis cohort study. *J Urol.* 2008;179:556–560.
30. Riegel B, Bruenahl CA, Ahyai S, Bingel U, Fisch M, Lowe B. Assessing psychological factors, social aspects and psychiatric co-morbidity associated with chronic prostatitis/chronic pelvic pain syndrome (CP/CPPS) in men – a systematic review. *J Psychosom Res.* 2014;77:333–350.
31. Anderson RU, Wise D, Nathanson BH. Chronic prostatitis and/or chronic pelvic pain as a psychoneuromuscular disorder: a meta-analysis. *Urology.* 2018;120:23–29.
32. Nickel JC, Alexander RB, Schaeffer AJ, et al. Leukocytes and bacteria in men with chronic prostatitis/chronic pelvic pain syndrome compared to asymptomatic controls. *J Urol.* 2003;170:818–822.
33. Hou DS, Long WM, Shen J, Zhao LP, Pang XY, Xu C. Characterisation of the bacterial community in expressed prostatic secretions from patients with chronic prostatitis/chronic pelvic pain syndrome and infertile men: a preliminary investigation. *Asian J Androl.* 2012;14:566–573.
34. Pontari MA, McNaughton-Collins M, O'Leary MP, et al. A case-control study of risk factors in men with chronic pelvic pain syndrome. *BJU Int.* 2005;96:559–565.
35. Shoskes DA, Altemus J, Polackwich AS, Tucky B, Wang H, Eng C. The urinary microbiome differs significantly between patients with chronic prostatitis/chronic pelvic pain syndrome and controls as well as between patients with different clinical phenotypes. *Urology.* 2016;92:26–32.
36. Murphy SF, Anker JF, Mazur DJ, Hall C, Schaeffer AJ, Thumbikat P. Role of gram-positive bacteria in chronic pelvic pain syndrome (CPPS). *Prostate.* 2019;79:160–167.
37. Pontari MA, Ruggieri MR. Mechanisms in prostatitis/chronic pelvic pain syndrome. *J Urol.* 2004;172:839–845.
38. Anderson RU, Orenberg EK, Chan CA, Morey A, Flores V. Psychometric profiles and hypothalamic-pituitary-adrenal axis function in men with chronic prostatitis/chronic pelvic pain syndrome. *J Urol.* 2008;179:956–960.
39. Antolak SJ, Hough DM, Pawlina W, Spinner RJ. Anatomical basis of chronic pelvic pain syndrome: the ischial spine and pudendal nerve entrapment. *Medical Hypotheses.* 2002;59:349–353.
40. Shoskes DA, Albakri Q, Thomas K, Cook D. Cytokine polymorphisms in men with chronic prostatitis/chronic pelvic pain syndrome: association with diagnosis and treatment response. *J Urol.* 2002;168:331–335.
41. Dellabella M, Milanese G, Muzzonigro G. Correlation between ultrasound alterations of the preprostatic sphincter and symptoms in patients with chronic prostatitis-chronic pelvic pain syndrome. *J Urol.* 2006;176:112–118.
42. Mehik A, Hellström P, Nickel JC, et al. The chronic prostatitis-chronic pelvic pain syndrome can be characterized by prostatic tissue pressure measurements. *J Urol.* 2002;167:137–140.
43. Arisan ED, Arisan S, Kiremit MC, et al. Manganese superoxide dismutase polymorphism in chronic pelvic pain syndrome patients. *Prostate Cancer Prostatic Dis.* 2006;9:426–431.

44. Chen X, Hu C, Peng Y, et al. Association of diet and lifestyle with chronic prostatitis/chronic pelvic pain syndrome and pain severity: a case-control study. *Prostate Cancer Prostatic Dis.* 2016;19:92–99.

45. Capodice JL, Bemis DL, Buttyan R, Kaplan SA, Katz AE. Complementary and alternative medicine for chronic prostatitis/chronic pelvic pain syndrome. *Evid Based Complement Alternat Med.* 2005;2:495–501.

46. Shoskes DA, Zeitlin SI, Shahed A, Rajfer J. Quercetin in men with category III chronic prostatitis: a preliminary prospective, double-blind, placebo-controlled trial. *Urology.* 1999;54:960–963.

47. Wagenlehner FM, Schneider H, Ludwig M, Schnitker J, Brahler E, Weidner W. A pollen extract (Cernilton) in patients with inflammatory chronic prostatitis-chronic pelvic pain syndrome: a multicentre, randomised, prospective, double-blind, placebo-controlled phase 3 study. *Eur Urol.* 2009;56:544–551.

48. Chuang YC, Tu CH, Huang CC, et al. Intraprostatic injection of botulinum toxin type-A relieves bladder outlet obstruction in human and induces prostate apoptosis in dogs. *BMC Urol.* 2006;6:12.

49. McNaughton Collins M, Wilt TJ. Allopurinol for chronic prostatitis. *Cochrane Database Syst Rev.* 2002;2002 (4):CD001041.

50. Kim HW, Roh DH, Yoon SY, et al. The anti-inflammatory effects of low- and high-frequency electroacupuncture are mediated by peripheral opioids in a mouse air pouch inflammation model. *J Altern Complement Med.* 2006;12:39–44.

51. Gao M, Ding H, Zhong G, et al. The effects of transrectal radiofrequency hyperthermia on patients with chronic prostatitis and the changes of MDA, NO, SOD, and Zn levels in pretreatment and posttreatment. *Urology.* 2012;79:391–396.

52. Fitzgerald MP, Anderson RU, Potts J, et al. Randomized multicenter feasibility trial of myofascial physical therapy for the treatment of urological chronic pelvic pain syndromes. *J Urol.* 2013;189: S75–S85.

53. Mykoniatis I, Pyrgidis N, Sokolakis I, et al. Low-intensity shockwave therapy for the management of chronic prostatitis/chronic pelvic pain syndrome: a systematic review and meta-analysis. *BJU Int.* 2021;128 (2):144–152.

Index

Numbers in **bold** = tables, *italics* = figures

abortive apoptosis, 180, 183
accountable care organizations (ACO), 10, 12
acetylcholine, 289
achondroplasia, 88
acrosin, *27*, 29
acrosomal development, 28
acrosome, 27, 28, 29
   definition, 27
   development phases, 27
acrosome development, 28
acrosome exocytosis, 193
acrosome function assays, 193
acrosome reaction, 179, 180, 193, 207
acrosome response to ionophore challenge (ARIC), 171
active stem cells, 26
activin-inhibin B-follistatin system, 41
activins, 40
acupuncture, 333
acute lymphoblastic leukemia (ALL), 93
Ad spermatogonia
   distinction abandoned (versus Ap spermatogonia), 30
   nuclear morphology, 30
   nuclei, 26
   reserve stem cells, 26
Adamopoulos DA, 108
adenylyl cyclase (AC), 38
adhesion G-protein-coupled receptor G2 (ADGRG2) gene, 68
adhesion molecules, 36
adipocytes, 259
adiposity, 83, 84
Ad-p spermatogonia
   small proportion recruited into differentiation pathway, 30
adrenergic neurons, 290
advanced paternal age (APA), 176, 184
Affordable Care Act, 2
agarose, 55, 234, 247

agarose plugs, 56, *57*
Agatston score, 300
age, 161, 176, 255, 266, 269, 270, 295, 297, 323
age group, 2, 18
aging, 9, 83, 269, 280, 289, 297, 308, See also paternal age
   alterations (epigenetic and genetic) in sperm, 87–88
   effect on offspring health, 92–93
   effects on male fertility and health of offspring, 87–93
   sperm DNA damage, 184
aging process, 79
agonadal humans, 36
agouti-related peptide (AgRP), 38
Ahlering TE, 257
air pollution, 185
Aitken RJ, 199
albumin, 45
alcohol, 98, 185, 293, 297, 305, 324
alginate, 247
aliquots, 160, 162, 166
allopurinol, 333
alpha agonists, 144
alpha blockers, 325
alpha reductase inhibitors, 185, 325, 326, 332
alprostadil, 135, 310
alprostadil topical cream, 310
Alzheimer's patients, 292
American Academy of Pediatrics, 147
American Academy of Sleep Medicine, 279
American Association of Tissue Banks (AATB), 224
American College of Cardiology/American Heart Association Guideline on Cardiovascular Risk, 299
American College of Physicians, 259
American Congress of Obstetricians and Gynecologists, 148

American Medical Association (AMA), 148
American Oncofertility consortium, 231
American Society for Reproductive Medicine (ASRM), 124, 143, 149, 224
American Society of Clinical Oncology (ASCO), 147, 149
American Society of Reproductive Medicine (ASRM), 12, 143, 147, 206
American Urological Association (AUA), 3, 9, 10, 11, 18, 108, 124, 210, 252, 257, 264, 269, 272, 319, 326, 332
American Urological Association Symptom Score (AUASS), 323, 324
American Urology Association-Symptom Index (AUA-SI), 280
amino acid sequence, 35
Amory JK, 275
amphibians, 41
AMS CX device, 319
Amsterdam, 151
anabolic androgenic steroid (AAS), 259
anabolic steroids, 266, 272
   prescribing patterns, 270
anastomosis, 114
anastrozole, 109, 271, 272, 273
Androgen Binding Protein (ABP), 46
androgen concentrations, 257
androgen deficiency, 264
androgen deficiency in aging male (ADAM), 282
androgen deprivation therapy (ADT), 253, 257
androgen receptor (AR), 47, 130
   definition, 264
   effects, 264
   role, 264
androgenic anabolic steroids (AAS), 19, 270, 271

androgens, 40, 251, 323
   definition, 35
andrology, 8
Andrology Research Consortium (ARC), 72
androstenedione, 275
anejaculation, 88
aneuploidy rates, 201
annexin V (AV), 205, 214
anorchia, 44
anorgasmia, 100
anoscopy, 137
anosmia, 36, 130, 259
antegrade ejaculation, 161
antibiotics, 333
anticholinergic therapy, 326
anti-Müllerian hormone (AMH), 43, 45, 48, 99
Antinori M, 200
antioxidant therapy
   sperm DNA treatment, 187
antioxidants, 180–181, 304
   erectile dysfunction (lifestyle modifications), 305
antisperm antibodies (ASAB), 101, 163, 169, 185
anxiety, 300
Ap spermatogonia, 26, 30
   active stem cells, 26
   nuclear morphology, 30
   nuclei, 26
Ap-d spermatogonia, 30, 31
   clonal expansion, 30
   divides only once every three epithelial cycles, 30
   mitotic, 30
   most if not all are single cells, 30
   proliferate throughout cycle, 30
Apert syndrome, 88, 177
apnea-hypopnea index (AHI), 279
aquablation (novel technique), 64
Araujo AB, 281
Argonaute (AGO), 82

Index

ARIs. *See* alpha reductase inhibitors
aromatase, 46, 98, 252, 270
   enzyme expressed in Sertoli cells, 40
aromatase inhibitors (AIs), 109, 255, 271, 272
array comparative genomic hybridization (aCGH), 132
artificial intelligence, 199
   sperm selection, 206
Ashkenzani J, **121**, 122
aspermia, 100
assisted conception
   spermatozoa selection, 204–208
assisted reproduction, 224, 225
assisted reproductive technology (ART), 4, 61, 65, 87, 89, 97, 100, 101, 102, 116, 120, 124, 127, 138, 160, 167, 183, 191, 218
   benefits of prior varicocelectomy, 120–121
   effect of paternal age, 91–92
   outcomes (impact of oxidative stress), 180
   outcomes (impact of sperm DNA fragmentation), 177–178
asthenospermia, 101
asthenozoospermia, 104, 204, 207
Aston KI, 79
atherosclerotic cardiovascular disease (ASCVD) risk calculator, 295
attention deficit hyperactivity disorder (ADHD), 92
autism, 224
autism spectrum disorders (ASD), 92
autonomic dysreflexia (AD), 138
   definition, 137
autonomic neuropathy, 63
avanafil, 308, 309
Avon Longitudinal Study of Pregnancy and Childhood (ALSPAC Study Team), 90
Awaga HA, 200
azoospermia, 32, 76, 99, 100, 103, 113, 115, 124, 127, 226
   accounts for 10% of male infertility cases, 101
   definition, 210
   IVF/ICSI outcomes, *123*
   prevalence, 210
azoospermia (DAZ) gene, 103
azoospermia factor (AZF), 67, 69
azoospermia factor (AZF) regions, 103, 128, 129, 132
   maps, *130*

B spermatogonia, 30
   almost half "not actively in cell cycle," 30
   generations, 30
   intensively stained chromatin clumps, 26
   nuclei, 26
   three generations, 26
Balasubramanian A, 17, 19, 20, 282
Barnes R, 115
Bartoov B, 200
base excision repair (BER), 30
Baskin LS, 316
Bates J, 283
Baukloh V, 211
Baunacke M, 18
bee pollen extract, 333
Beebe DJ, 212
Beeder L, 17
Beguería R, 91
Bejarano I, 283
Bella AJ, 20
benign prostatic hypertrophy (BPH), 2, 88, 185, 255, 265, 266, 280, 309
   diagnosis and evaluation, 323–324
   epidemiology, 323
   hypogonadism and, 257
   pathophysiology, 323
   treatment, 324–327
Berendsen JTW, 214
Bernie AM, 206
beta-3 agonists, 326, 327
Bianchi PG, 197
bilateral orchiectomy, 44
biology
   male reproduction and infertility, 23–32
bipolar disorder, 87, 92, 177
birds, 197
birefringence, 200, 206, 207
birth defects, 191
   effect of paternal age, 92
bladder, 323, 324
   double voiding, 324
bladder neck, 61
bladder neck closure, 63, 64
bladder neck incompetence, 63, 64
Bland & Altman plots, 171
blood glucose control, 297
blood pressure, 295, 297, 304, 326
blood vessels, 46
blood-testis barrier, 23, 24, 45, 239
   cyclical rearrangements, 25
BMI, 180, 252, 271, 279, 281, 283, 297, 324
body mass index. *See* BMI
Boman JM, 121
bone, 46, 251, 265, 292
bone marrow, 264, 267
bone morphogenetic protein (BMP), 247
Borges E, 177

Boston Area Community Health (BACH), 281
Boston Medical Group, 10
botulinum toxin A, 333
bovine serum albumin (BSA), **236**
Bozorgmehri S, 279
brachial artery, 304
brain, 46, 251, 253, 264, 291, 293
Branche L, 281
breast, 46, 264
breast cancer, 2, 128, 265
Brief Male Sexual Function Inventory (BMSFI), 297
Brinster RL, 246
Brody JP, 212
BTB. *See* blood-testis barrier
buccal testosterone tablet, 254
Buck's fascia, 316, *318*, 320
buffalo, **237**
bulbocavernosus muscle, 304
bulbospongiosus muscle, 61
bulbourethral glands, 61
Butola A, 199

cachexia, 264
calcitonin gene related peptide (CGRP), 330
calcium, 290, 291
cAMP response element-binding protein (CREB), 38
cancer
   case distribution (young people), *142*
   sperm DNA damage, 184
cancer diagnosis, 148, 149
cancer therapy
   sequelae on male reproductive function, *142*
cancer treatment, **230**
Cap-Score values, 192
carbamazepine, 331
cardiovascular disease, 1, 8, 10, 257–258, 266, 279, 291, 295, 297
cardiovascular risk factors, 310
Caroppo E, 210
catecholamines, 293
caudal lumbar ganglia, 289
causative genetic variants, 32
cavernosography, 315
cavernosometry, 315
cavernous nerve injury, 292
Cayan S, 120
CC. *See* clomiphene citrate
cell cytoplasm, 27
Centers for Disease Control, 197
Centers for Medicare & Medicaid Services (CMS), 8
central nervous system, 61, 253, 323
cervical mucus, 99, 162, 167, 172, 193, 197
Chargaff E, 67

Charlier CM, 282
chemotherapy, 184, **230**, 231, 252, 259, 265, 297
   mechanisms of toxic therapies, 143–144
Chen Q, 282
chicken, 35
childhood cancer, 93, 141, 244
   benign and malignant conditions (epidemiology), 143
childlessness, 156, 160
China, 89, 91
chlamydia trachomatis, 184
cholesterol, 44, 251, 299
   C27 steroid, *44*
cholinergic neurons, 290
chromatids, 26
chromatin architecture, 27
chromatin modifications, 81
chromatin rarefaction zone, 26
chromodomain protein, Y linked (CDY), 129
chromomycin A3, 194, 199
chromosomal abnormalities, 92
chromosome synapsis, 26
chromosomes, 39
   translocations and inversions, 129
chronic epididymitis, 331
chronic orchialgia, 330
   causes, 332
   definition, 329
   symptoms, 329
chronic orchialgia (treatment), 331
   behavioral and conservative measures, 331
   epididymectomy and orchiectomy, 331
   injection therapies, 331
   microsurgical denevation of spermatic cord, 331
   pharmacologic therapies, 330
   spinal cord stimulation, 331
   ultrasound-guided microcryoablation of spermatic cord, 331
Chronic Prostatitis Symptom Index (CPSI), 332
chronic prostatitis/chronic pelvic pain syndrome (CP/CPPS), 332–333
   definition, 329
   pathophysiology, 332
chronic prostatitis/chronic pelvic pain syndrome (CP/CPPS) (treatment), 332–333
   allopurinol, 333
   alpha blockers, 332
   antibiotics, 333
   botulinum toxin A, 333
   lifestyle changes, 332
   Li-SWT, 333

Index

non-pharmacologic therapy, 333
NSAIDs, 333
phytotherapy, 333
chronic testicular pain, 3
Chua ME, 108
ciliary dyskinesia, 162
Claycombe-Larson KG, 84
Clermont Y, 30, 244
clinical andrology
  pillars, xi
Clinical Genome Resource Initiative (ClinGen), 73
clinical pregnancy rate (CPR), 204
clomiphene citrate (clomid), 108, 255, 271, 272, 273
clostridium collagenase histolyticum (CCH), 11
clustered regulatory interspaced short palindromic repeats-associated protein 9 (CRISPR-Cas9), 71, 72, 247
cocaine- and amphetamine-regulated transcript (CART), 38
Cochrane reviews, 181, 198, 200, 201, 205, 206, 208
coital exercise, 304
collagen fleece grafting, 318, *318*
collagenases
  definition, 211
Coloplast Titan, 319
COMET assays, 59
computed tomography (CT), 300, 324
computer-assisted semen analysis (CASA), 4, 159, 165–172, 193
  clinical applications (validation strategies), 171
  current status, 166–168
  early era (1988-1999), 171
  kinematics (non-comparability issues), 168–169
  limitations, 165
  need, 165
  research benefits, 165
  sperm concentration, 166–168
  sperm function assessment, 170
  sperm morphology, 170
  sperm motility, 166–168
  sperm vitality assessment, 170
  validation strategy, 171–172
conception rates, 91
congenital bilateral absence of vas deferens (CBAVD), 74, 100, 101, 103, 117, 130, 210
congenital hypogonadotropic hypogonadism (CHH), 130
  genes associated with, **129**
congenital unilateral absence of vas deferens (CUAVD), 131

congenital adrenal hyperplasia (CAH), 229
continuous positive airway pressure (CPAP), 280, 283, 306
contraceptive options, 1, 5
conventional testicular sperm extraction (cTESE), 206
Convery N, 218
Copenhagen Sperm Analysis Laboratory, 89
copy number variants (CNVs), 68, 69, 132
Corona G, 253
coronary artery calcium (CAC), *300*
coronary artery disease (CAD), 295, 299
corpora cavernosa, 289
corporotomy, 319
corpus cavernosum, 312
corpus spongiosum, 289
corticotropin-releasing hormone (CRH), 38
Costello syndrome, 88
COVID-19 vaccine, xi
Cowper's glands, 61, 161
c-reactive protein (CRP), 304
Crick F, 67
Crouzon syndrome, 177
cryopreservation
  barriers, 147–148
  consent, 146, 225
  freeze thaw process (survival rate), 146
  insurance coverage, 146
  loss of sperm motility (acceptable levels), 226
  options, 144
  practical concerns, 225–226
  time before starting therapy, 146
cryopreservation process, 225–226
cryopreservation rates (USA, Canada), 141
cryptorchidism, 97, 128, **230**, 258, 269
cryptozoospermia, 207
CVD. *See* cardiovascular disease
cycle of seminiferous epithelium, 28
cyclic adenosine monophosphate (cAMP), 38, 291
cyclic guanosine monophosphate (cGMP), 291, 303, 308, 326
cyclooxygenases enzymes (COX), 333
cyclophosphamide, 142, 143
cylinder extrusion, 311
cystic fibrosis gene mutation, 103, 130–131
cystic fibrosis transmembrane conductance regulator (CFTR), 67, 101, 103, 127

cystoscopy, 323, 324
cytokines, 304, 333
cytometry, 167
cytosine phosphate guanine dinucleotides (CpGs), 76, 77

Dadi (sperm bank), 12
Daitch JA, **121**, 121
Darwin CR, 197
de la Rochebrochard E, 91
de Wagenaar B, 213
DEAD box protein 3, Y-chromosomal (DBY) gene, 129
deep neural networks (DNN), 200
deeper fascial tissues, 318
dehydroepiandrosterone (DHEA), 44, 275
deleted in azoospermia (DAZ) genes, 129
dementia, 326, 327
Denmark, 93
density gradient centrifugation (DGC), 204, 210
depression, 279, 300
desensitization, 36, 39
deterministic lateral displacement (DLD), 219
Devine CJ, 317
Di Persio S, 30
diabetes, 63, 269, 279, 292, 297, 305, 309, 310
dielectrophoresis (DEP), 213
diet, 83–84, 107, 176, 180, 271, 295, 297, 305, 308, 324
differentiating spermatogonia, 25, 28, 30, 31, **237**, 246
dihydrotestosterone (DHT), 40, 46, 47, 254, 257, 264, 266, 267, 323, 325, 332
diploidy, 102, 184
direct-to-consumer (DTC), 10, 11, 17, 18
discrepancy analysis, 171
disease targeted sequencing, 131
disorders of sexual development (DSD), 68
DNA, 67
  protection from nucleases by protamines, 56
DNA damage, 175–178
  etiology, 183–185
  impact of lifestyle and male age, 175–177
  induced by ROS (types), *176*
  SCD, 175
  SCSA, 175
  single celled gel electrophoresis assay, 175
  testing for, 175
  testing methods (pros and cons), **176**
  TUNEL, 175

DNA damage repair, 177
DNA double-strand breaks (DSBs), 26
DNA fragmentation, 98, 102
DNA fragmentation index (DFI), 200
DNA methylation, 76–77, 81, 83, 87
DNA methyltransferases (DNMTs), 81
DNA replication
  single round of, 26
DNA-binding domain (DBD), 47
dopamine, 36, 109, 253, 259, 292
Doppler ultrasound, 100, 299, 315
Drosophila melanogaster, 72
dry ejaculation, 161
DSM-V, 62
Dubin and Amelar grading system, 115
Duchenne muscular dystrophy, 177
Duckett JW, 316
dutasteride, 325, 326
dynorphin, 37
dyslipidemia, 11, 297

Ebbehøj J, 316
economies of scale, 12
ED. *See* erectile dysfunction
EDTA, 54, 56, 59
  arrests luminal nuclease activity, 57
Egydio PH, 320
Eisenberg ML, 282
ejaculate examination
  assessments of questionable value, 162–163
  cells other than spermatozoa, 163
  development, 159–160
  exactness, 160
  normality versus abnormality, 160
  purposes, 159–160
  standardization, 160
  techniques for reliable results, 161–162
  theory and techniques, 159–163
ejaculate physiology, 160–161
  contribution of accessory sex glands, 161
  ejaculation sequence, 161
  sperm content, 160–161
  sperm production, 160–161
ejaculate volume, 61, 99, 159, 161
ejaculation, 61–65, 311
  cerebal control and neurotransmission, 62
  clinical concerns, 61
  emission phase (secretion of semen), 61

339

Index

ejaculation (cont.)
  expulsion phase (propulsion of semen), 62
  pathophysiology, 62
  physiology, 61–62
ejaculatory disorders, 61, 67, 88, 139, 155
ejaculatory duct obstruction (correction), 114–115
  background and preoperative considerations, 114
  outcomes and complications, 115
  procedure notes, 115
ejaculatory duct obstruction (EDO), 100, 101, 161
ejaculatory dysfunction (EjD), 88
  diagnosis, 62
ejaculatory physiology
  semen characteristics and age, 161
electroejaculation (EEJ), 64, 136–138, 144
  illustration, 136
electrophoresis, 205
El-Helaly M, 282
Eliasson R, 159
embryogenesis, 78, 79
endocrine evaluation, 99
  hormone profiles (interpretation), 100
Endocrine Society, 253, 264, 272
endocrinology, 34–48
endoplasmic reticulum, 46
endothelin, 290
enobosarm, 265
enzymes, 46
eosin, 244
Eosin Y-Nigrosin staining test, 162
epididymal luminal fluid, 57
epididymal luminal nuclease, 55
epididymal obstruction (correction)
  background and pre-operative considerations, 113–114
  outcomes and complications, 114
epididymectomy, 3, 331, 332
epididymis, 3, 54, 59, 61, 98, 117, 161, 329
  site, 231
epididymitis, 330
epididymosomes, 78, 82
epigenetics, 131
  definition, 81
epipidymal obstruction (correction)
  procedure notes, 114
epithelial cycle
  six germ cell associations, 28
Eppworth Sleepiness Scale (ESS), 280
equatorial division, 26

erectile dysfunction, 3–4, 88, 98, 154, 281
  arteriogenic, 291
  business landscape, 8–11
  cardiovascular assessment algorithm, 296
  classification, **296**
  definition, 18, 289, 308
  drug-induced, 293
  endocrine hormones (failure), 292
  global prevalence, 289
  incidence in USA, 279
  men with spinal cord injury, 135–136
  neurogenic, 291–292
  online content landscape, 18–19
  organic, 308
  pathophysiology, 291–293
  psychogenic, 292, 308
  risk factors, **296**
  screening, 296
  sleep and, 279–280
  vasculogenic, 291, 296, 300, 312
  worldwide prevalence, 18
erectile dysfunction (future direction)
  extracorporeal shock-wave therapy, 314
  intracavernosal stem cell therapy, 312
  platelet-rich plasma, 312
erectile dysfunction (lifestyle modifications), 303–306
  antioxidants, 305
  drug use, 305
  exercise, 304
  nutrition, 305
  pelvic floor physical therapy, 304
  psychological factors (impact), 306
  sleep apnea treatment, 305
  weight management, 305
erectile dysfunction (medical management), 308–310
  devices, 310
  local therapies, 309–310
  PDE-5i, 308–309
erectile dysfunction (surgical management), 310–312
  arterial reconstruction, 312
  penile prosthesis, 311
  vascular surgery, 311
  venous surgery, 312
erectile dysfunction evaluation, 295–301
  cardiac risk assessment, 299
  comorbidities and medications, 297
  diagnostic testing, 299–300
  epidemiology, 295
  goal, 295

  initial detection, 296–297
  laboratory work, 299
  lifestyle improvements, 295
  medical history, 297
  penile function, 299
  physical examination, 298
  psychological issues, 300
  public health implications, 295
  social history (lifestyle factors), 297
erectile function
  molecular effectors, 290
  neurophysiology, 293
  physiology, 289–291
erection
  pathophysiology, 303–304
erythrocytes, 163, 207, 211, 214
erythrocytosis, 273
ESHRE Andrology SIG, 167
Essed E, 316
Esteves SC, **121**, 122
estradiol, 37, 40, 44, 109, 251, 254, 255, 259, 264, 270, 271
estradiol benzonoate, 266
estrogens, 37, 40, 46, 109, 252, 264, 271
euploidy rates, 201
Europe, 91
European Association of Andrology, 130
European Association of Urology (EAU), 3, 11, 124, 127
European Molecular Genetics Quality Network, 130
European Society for Human Reproduction and Embryology (ESHRE), 231
European Union, 231
Eutherian sperm motility, 165
Evans JI, 281
Evenson DP, 197
exercise, 295, 297, 304, 308
exome sequencing, 68, 68
extracellular matrix (ECM), 233, 318
extracellular N-terminal domain (ECND), 42
extracorporeal shockwave therapy (ESWT), 312

failure of emission (FE), 63–64
  treatment, 64–65
family planning, 1
Fanconi Anemia genes, 72
Fantus R, 18
Farley S, 115
Fayomi AP, 277
female genital tract, 35, **179**, 191
female infertility, xi
female life expectancy, 1
female reproductive tract, 28, 88, 178, 191, 197, 205, 208, 212
feminizing hormone therapy (FHT), 143
FertiCare 2.0 medical vibrator, 138

fertility, 4–5
fertility preservation
  approaches, 147
  barriers to access, 147–148
  clinical decision, 141–151
  ethics, 148–149
  female oncologic patients, 151
  future strategies (pre-pubertal patients), 149–150
  transgender female patients, 150–151
fertility work up, 97
fertily preservation
  decision making, 147
fetus
  HPT axis, 39
fibroblast growth factor receptor-1 (FGFR1), 36
fibroblasts, 23
finasteride, 325, 326
Finkle WD, 258
fish, 41
flagellum, 27
flies, 72
flow mediated dilation (FMD), 304, 305
fluorescence activated cell sorting (FACS), 215
fluorescent in situ hybridization (FISH), 102, 128
folic acid, 84
follicle-stimulating hormone (FSH), 35, 38, 39–41, 45, 48, 89, 99, 106, 107, 108, 109, **235**, 269, 270
  actions, 42–43
  definition, 39
follicle-stimulating hormone receptor (FSHR), 42, 43
follistatin, 41
Food and Drug Administration (FDA), 3, 9, 171, 185, 224, 253, 254, 264, 266, 275, 309, 326
forhims.com (Hims™), 18
FP. See fertility preservation
Framingham longitudinal heart study, 295
Franklin R, 67
free hormone hypothesis, 46

gabapentin, 331
Gadegaard N, 218
gamma-aminobutyric acid (GABA), 36, 38, 62
gender, 297
gender differences
  preventive-care services, 1
gender dysphoria, 148, 151
  definition, 143
gender health gap, 8
gender nonconformity
  definition, 143
gene editing, 73
gene transcription, 47

340

Index

genetic abnormalities, 92
genetic analysis
  tools, 67
genetic disorders, **230**
genetic polymorphisms, 62
genetic testing
  indications, 127, *127*
  non-obstructive azoospermia and oligozoospermia, 127–130
Genetics of Male Infertility Initiative (GEMINI), 72
genital tract infection
  sperm DNA damage, 184
Genome Aggregation Database (gnomAD), 71
genotype-phenotype mismatch, 128
Genotype-Tissue Expression (GTEx), 69
germ cell associations, 28
  heterogeneously mixed, 28
  histological arrangement, 28
  incomplete, 28
germ cell development, 25–28, 231, 233
  factors, **233**
germ cells, 23, 24, 25, 129
  development, *25*
  types, 25
Germany, 90, 155, 207
germ-cell development, 247
germline mutations, 30
getroman.com (Roman™), 18
GFRA1, 30
Gholami SS, 316
glans penis, 289
glial cell line-derived neurotrophic factor (GDNF), 245
Global Burden of Disease, 8
globozoospermia, 69
glucocorticoids, 38
glucose, 265, 304
glutamine, **235**
glutathione, 304
glycosylation, 39
GnRH. *See* gonadotropin-releasing hormone
GnRH-associated peptide (GAP), 35
Gode F, 199
Gokce A, 122
Gold RZ, 165
Goldstein M, 120
gonadotoxicity
  risk, **145**
  severity, **150**
gonadotrophs, 35
gonadotropin therapy, 107
gonadotropin-inhibitory hormone (GnIH), 38, 41
gonadotropin-releasing hormone, 35, 106, 107, 108, 127, 251, 270
  actions, 38–39

encoded by gene, 35
kisspeptin-neurokinin B-dynorphin system, 36–37
metabolic signals, 38
neurons (neuroanatomy and embryology), 35–36
pulse frequency, 39, 40
secretion, 36
secretion regulation, 36–37
structure and synthesis, 35
sub-types, 35
gonadotropin-releasing hormone receptor (GnRHR), 38
gonadotropins, 35, 39–43
  actions, 42–43
  glycosylation, 39
  role of GnIH/RFRP, 41
  role of inhibin, activins, follistatin, 40–41
  secretion, 39–41
  secretion regulation, 40–41
  sex steroids (role), 40
  structure and synthesis, 39
gonocytes
  definition, 246
Goodman L, 147
Gosling R, 67
GPCR kinases (GRK), 42
G–protein-coupled receptor-54 (GPR54), 36
Gregoriou O, 109
Guay AT, 255
Guillemin R, 35
guinea pigs, 234
Guo J, 245
gynecomastia, 128, 298

haemochromatosis, 230
haemocytometer, 162
haemocytometry, 167
Hamilton Thorne IVOS platforms, 167, 168
haploid cells, 26, **236**
Harris G, 35
Hassan M, 90
Haydardedeoglu B, 123
health care
  drivers for seeking, 1–2
health disparities, 1
health literacy, 16
healthcare utilization, 16
health-related quality of life (HRQOL), 306
heart, 264
Heineke-Mickulicz manoeuvre, 316
hematocrit, 255, 266
hematoma, 311, 312
hematoxylin, 244
hematuria, 324, 325
hemizona assay index, 193
hepatocellular injury, 266
hepatocyte growth factor (HGF), 36
herbal therapy, 324

Hershberger assay, 265
high density lipoprotein (HDL), 266, 295, 299
high-resolution light microscopy (HRLM), 26
Hims, 10, 11, 14, 18
hippocampus, 290, 292
histology
  spermatogenesis, 23–32
histology of human testis parenchyma, *24*
histone modification, 77
histone proteins, 77
histones, 57, *58*, 81, 87
histone-to-protamine transition, 28
HIV/AIDS, 16, 224, **230**, 252, 258, 309
Hodgkin's lymphoma, 184
Holmium laser enucleation of prostate (HoLEP), 64
homologous chromosomes, 26
hormonal deficiency, 186, **230**
  sperm DNA damage, 184
hormonal therapy
  sperm DNA damage treatment, 186
Horton CE, 317
HPG. *See* hypothalamic-pituitary-gonadal
Huang S, 213
human chorionic gonadotropin (hCG), 39, 255, 272, 273
human follicle stimulating hormone (hFSH), 107
human genome, 69
Human Genome Project, 67
human genome sequence data, 67
Human Protein Atlas, 69, 71, 73
hyaluronic acid (HA), 187
  binding selection, 205
hydrogen peroxide (H_2O_2), 178, 179, 180, 200
hydroxypregnenolone, 44
hydroxyprogesterone, 273
hypergonadotropic hypogonadism (primary testicular failure), 99, 269
hyperlipidemia, 279, 295
hyperprolactinemia, 109, 259, 292
hypertension, 279, 323
hypogonadal men
  fertility maintenance (recommended pathway), 273
  fertility restoration, 270–272
  fertility restoration (recommended pathway), 273
  testosterone therapy (fertility maintenance), 273
  treatment algorithms, 273

hypogonadism, 8–9, 89, 109, 160, **230**
  cardiovascular disease, 257–258
  comorbidities, 259
  definition (AUA), 281
  definition and diagnosis, 252–253
  diagnosis, 269
  Endocrine Society definition, 264
  endocrinopathy (specific etiologies), 258–259
  epidemiology, 269
  evaluation and treatment, 251–259
  men with spinal cord injury, 138
  online content landscape, 19
  organic ED secondary to, 308
  primary, 258
  reproductive age group, 269
  secondary, 259
  sleep and, 281–282
  testosterone and sexual function, 253
  testosterone replacement therapy, 253–255
  treatment in fertility preserving manner, 255–256
  varicocele and, 256
hypogonadism treatment
  SARMs, 264–267
hypogonadotropic hypogonadism (HH), 67, 68, 129–130, 138, 269
  secondary testicular failure, 99
hypoosmotic swelling test (HOST), 207
hypospadias, 316
hypospermatogenesis (HS), 123
hypothalamic-pituitary-gonadal axis, 23, 44, 149, 270, 271, 275, 276, 292
  anatomy and physiology, 251–252
hypothalamic-pituitary-testicular (HPT) axis
  hypothalamus (GnRH and kisspeptin networks), 35–39
  organization (anatomical and functional), 35
  physiology, 35–43
  pre-pubertal suppression, 36
  testicular function, 43–48
hypothalamus, 292

idiopathic conditions, 129
idiopathic epididymalgia, 331
idiopathic hypogonadotropic hypogonadism (IHH), 259
Ignarro, Louis, 16
imipramine, 64
immunofluorescence (IF)
  detection of acrosin, 29

immunohistochemical (IHC) detection of acrosin, 29
immunoregulatory and immunosuppressive factors, 23
in vitro culture strategies
  advantages and disadvantages, 232
in vitro fertilization (IVF), 4, 12, 79, 91, 100, 101, 102, 107, 109, 113, 116, 117, 138, 144, 147, 154, 169, 180, 186
  after varicocelectomy, 122
  failure rate, 204
  IVF/ICSI era, 120–124
  sperm selection, 201
in vitro spermatogenesis, 233–238, 247
  scenarios (research and clinical applications), 238–239
  timeline, 232
in vitro systems
  challenges, 231–233
Inci K, 121
induced pluripotent stem cell (iPSC), 149
infants, 39
infertility, 12
  definition (WHO), 141
  distress in man and couple, 154
  impact on sexual dysfunction, 154–156
  incidence, 97
  men with spinal cord injury, 138
infertility phenotype, 67
inflatable penile prostheses (IPP), 3
informed consent, 148, 149, 151, 225
inhibin, 40, 48, 99, 251
  clinical importance, 45
innervation, 61
inositol-trisphosphate (IP3), 38
insomnia, 281
insulin, 304
insulin-like factor 3 (INSL3), 23, 44
insulin-like growth factor-1 (IGF1), 38, 236
insurance coverage, 148
International Classification of Sleep Disorders, 279
International Index of Erectile Function (IIEF), 135, 253, 256, 279, 280, 292, 297, 304, 305, 306, 308
International Male Infertility Genomics Consortium (IMIGC), 68, 72
International Prostate Symptom Score (IPSS), 280, 281, 323
International Society of Sexual Medicine (ISSM), 8, 62, 296, 319

internet
  exaggerated product efficacy claims, 19
  urologic men's health, 16–20
interpersonal relationships, 289
intracavernosal injections (ICI), 3, 135
  adverse events, 310
  use, 310
intracavernosal stem cell therapy, 312
intracytoplasmic morphologically selected sperm injection (IMSI), 198, 200, 205
intracytoplasmic sperm injection (ICSI), 4, 61, 91, 102, 103, 107, 113, 116, 117, 138, 149, 162, 163, 169, 177, 180, 183, 186
  after varicocelectomy, 122
  IVF/ICSI era, 120–124
  men with sperm DNA fragmentation, 187
intraoperative floppy iris syndrome (IFIS), 325
intra-testicular testosterone (ITT), 270, 272, 273
  role, 270
intraurethral alprostadil, 310
intrauterine insemination (IUI), 4, 91, 100, 101, 102, 120, 124, 138, 144, 147, 177, 186
  after varicocelectomy, 121–122
  outcomes (effect of conventional sperm preparation), 204
  pregnancy outcomes, 121
intravaginal ejaculatory latency time (IELT), 62, 63
ipsilateral renal agenesis, 98
ipsilateral vasal agenesis, 99
Ireland, 103
ischiocavernosus muscle, 304
ISO, 171
Ivanov N, 19
IZUMO gene, 194

JAMA, 258
James ER, 78
Jan SZ, 27
Japanese quail, 41
Jensen TK, 282
Jin M, 193
Jodar M, 79
Johnsen's score, 24
Johnson SL, 89
June Men's Health Month, 16
JUNO, 194

Kaarouch I, 91
Kallmann syndrome, 36, 127, 130, 230, 259, 269
Kandel ME, 200

Karolinska Sleep Questionnaire, 282
karyotype analysis, 67, 127
karyotype testing, 127–129, 132
karyotype-associated abnormalities, 103
Kashaninejad N, 218
Katz DJ, 255
Keye W, 154
Khandwala Y, 89, 92
Kheirollahi-Kouhestani M, 199
Khera M, 257
Ki67 index, 30
Kidd SA, 89
kidney, 311
Kirby EW, 122, 123
kisspeptin
  definition, 36
  neuropeptide, 35
kisspeptin-neurokinin B-dynorphin system, 36–37
KIT marker, 30
Klevmark B, 316
Klinefelter syndrome, 67, 69, 103, 127–128, 229, 244, 247, 258, 299
  resulting from extra maternal X chromosome, 128
  resulting from paternal X chromosome, 129
Kohn TP, 257, 280, 283
Krawetz SA, 197
Krzastek SC, 255
KS. See Klinefelter syndrome
Kuehhas FE, 320

laboratory evaluation, 248
Lambrot R, 83
lamina propria, 24
  thickening, 24
Lancet, 270
Large Urology Group Practices (LUGPA), 9, 10
lateral pontine tegmentum, 290
Layton JB, 9
LDL receptor-related protein (LRP) family, 47
lean body mass, 265
Lee R, 124
Legacy (sperm bank), 12
Leproult R, 281
leptin, 38
Letorneau J, 148
letrozole, 109
leukemia inhibitory factor (LIF), 36
leukocytospermia
  WHO definition, 101
Levene P, 67
Levine H, 12
Levine LA, 316, 331
Lewis RW, 316
Leydig cell dysfunction, 184
Leydig cell hypoplasia, 258

Leydig cells, 35, 42, 46, 106, 108, 115, 236, 251, 259, 270, 272, 273
  development phases, 23
  function, 43–45, 275
Leydig stem cell injection, 276
Leydig-cell tumors, 42
Li Y, 279
Li Z, 280
libido, 98, 265, 267, 281, 293, 311
Licht MR, 316
Life Events Scale, 154
life expectancy, 83
life goals, 141
ligand-binding domain (LBD), 47
lipid peroxidation, 179
Liu W, 213
live birth rates, 121, 123, 124, 177, 178, 200, 204
  treated versus untreated varicoceles, 121
liver, 46, 251, 264, 269, 293, 309
  testosterone metabolism, 46
local therapies (erectile dysfunction), 309–310
  alprostadil (intraurethral), 310
  alprostadil (topical), 310
  use of ICI, 309
locus ceruleus, 290
long non-coding RNAs (lncRNAs), 82
low T. See low testosterone, See
low testosterone, 2, 9, 11
lower urinary tract symptoms (LUTS), 88, 257, 266, 279, 309, 323–327, 329
  sleep and, 280–281
low-intensity extracorporeal shock wave therapy (LI-ESWT), 4
low-intensity shock wave therapy (Li-SWT), 10, 11, 333
Lue TF, 316
lumen, 28
luminal nuclease, 54, 59
  active in SDS for short time, 54–55
luminal nuclease digestion
  in situ, 56, 58
  two steps, 56
  unprotected, 56, 58
luteinizing hormone (LH), 35, 36, 38, 39–41, 44, 88, 99, 106, 108, 109, 236, 269, 270
  actions, 42
  definition, 39
  pulse frequency, 44
  secretion, 44
luteinizing hormone receptor (LHR/LHCGR), 42
luteinizing hormone-releasing hormone (LH-RH), 35
lymphoma, 93

Index

machine learning, 206
MacLeod J, 159, 165
macrophages, 23
MAGEA4 marker, 30
magnetic activation cell sorting (MACS), 198, 205, 214
Makler chambers, 167
male factor infertility, 79, 80, 91, 113, 127, 156, 175, 226, 229, 282
   cause (most common), 120
   coverage in states with laws related to infertility coverage, 13
male fertility
   effects of aging, 87–93
   testosterone therapy, 269–277
male fertility disorders, 31
male fertility preservation
   reasons, 224
   regulatory issues, 224
male gametes (spermatozoa), 43
   fertility preservation (potential options), 143
male germ cell differentiation, 25
male health issues
   medical and surgical management, 251–259
male infertility, xi
   biology, 23–32
   CASA, 165–172
   clinical evaluation and treatment, 97–104
   clinical pathologies (by age groups), 230
   evaluation and treatment (prospects), 103
   genetic analysis (advances), 67
   genetic aspects, 67–73
   global market size, 12
   laboratory evaluation and treatment, 248
   online content landscape, 17–18
   sleep and, 282–283
   surgical management, 113–118
male infertility (genetic evaluation), 102–103
   CVABD, 103
   cystic fibrosis gene mutations, 103
   karyotype-associated abnormalities, 103
   Y chromosome microdeletions, 103
male infertility (genetic factors)
   qualitative sperm defects, 69
   quantitative sperm defects, 68–69
male infertility (medical management), 106–109
   aromatase inhibitors, 109
   gonadotropin therapy, 107–108
   lifestyle factors, 106–107

prolactin modulators, 109
   selective estrogen modulators, 108–109
male infertility genetic factors, 68–69
   obstructive azoospermia, 68
   pre-testicular infertility, 68
male infertility genetic studies
   challenges, 69
   ClinGen Initiative, 73
   collaborative approaches, 72
   data resources, 69–71
   gene curation efforts, 72–73
   model systems, 71–72
   resources, 69
male infertility genetics
   history, 67–68
male life expectancy, 1
male pseudohermaphroditism, 42
male reproduction and infertility biology, 23–32
male reproductive endocrinology, 34–48
Male Reproductive Health Initiative (MRHI), 72
male reproductive potential, 89
   unassisted conception (oldest age), 89
male reproductive system (MRS), 35
male sex hormones (androgens), 43
Male Sexual Health Questionnaire, 256
Mallidis C, 200
mammals, 29, 35, 37, 41, 72, 76, 81, 82, 83, 161, **167**
mammary hyperplasia, 264
manchette, 28
   definition, 28
Marie Curie International Training Network "GROWSPERM," 231
marker analysis, 31
Marmar JL, **121**, 121
marmoset, 246
Martin SA, 280
Massachusetts Male Aging Study (MMAS), 155, 279
maternal age, 87, 89, 124, 176, 197
Mati E, 18
matrix attachment regions (MARs), 58
maturation arrest (MA), 123
maturation depletion process, 143
mature male gametes, 23
Mayo Clinic, 20
McBride JA, 19
measurement uncertainty (MU), 171, 172
meatus, 61, 98, 310

medial preoptic area (MPOA), 35, 290, 292
Medicaid, 148
medical management
   male infertility, 109
Medical Outcomes Study Sleep Scale (MOS-Scale), 281
Medicare, 11
meiosis, 26–27, 68, 71, 90, 129, 160, 175, **236**, 246
   critical step, 26
   etymology (Greek μείωσις, lessening), 26
meiosis I division, 26
meiosis II division, 26
meiotic arrest, 27
   types, 27
meiotic checkpoints, 26
Meischer F, 67
Meistrich M, 143
melatonin, 282
Melehan KL, 280
men's health, 2, 16–20
   business landscape, 8–14
   change over past two decades, 1–5
   emergence as distinct discipline, 1
   progress and achievements, 5
   sleep, 279–283
men's health centers, 2, 13
Mendel G, 67
Meng MV, 124
menopause, 89
menstrual cycle, 37
   pre-ovulatory phase, 36
mental health, 154–156
messenger RNA (mRNA), 28, 30, 81
metabolic disorders, 38
metabolic syndrome, 295, 296, 297, 298
mice, 31, 54, 71, 72, 77, 83, 84, 103, 150, 184, 193, 233, 237, 245, 246, 247
   spermatogonial stem cells (human comparison), 246
microarray technology, 132
microbiological cultures, 163
microcinematography, 165
microcryoablation of spermatic cord
   ultrasound guided targeted, 331
microdissection testicular sperm extraction (microTESE), 4, 103, 117, **117**, 123, 124, 206, 210, 211, 214, 215
microfluidic sperm selection (MSS), 206, 207
microfluidic system, **232**
microfluidics, 199, 211–214, 218
   definition, 218
   sperm identification, 219–221
   sperm sample preparation, 218–219
   spiral, 214

microRNAs (miRNAs), 81
microscopy, 200
microsurgical advances, 4
microsurgical denervation of spermatic cord, 331
microsurgical epididymal sperm aspiration (MESA), 117, 206
microsurgical spermatic cord denervation, 3, 330, 331, 332
microvascular disease, 88
milodrine, 64
mini-puberty, 36, 40, 48
miRNA-induced silencing complex (miRISC), 82
miRNAs, 83, 84
miscarriage, 103, 177, 200, 201
miscarriage rates, 91, 204
mitochondria, 27, 44
mitogen-activated protein kinase (MAPK), 38
mitotic cells
   peaks, 30
mitotic compartment, 30
mitotic KIT, 30
mitotic peaks, 30
mitotic spermatogonia
   topographical arrangement, 30
mobile phone exposure, 107
molecular biology
   erectile function and dysfunction, 289–293
molecular genetics, 67
molecular makeup
   interstitial immune cells, 23
monkeys, 184, 234, 244, 265
   epithelial cycle, 29
monocytes, 23, 43
morphological development of acrosome in spermatids, 28
mortality
   gender gap, 8
motile sperm, 145
Movember Foundation, 16
   established in 2006, 2
MRI, 100, 109, 290, 324
mTESE. *See* microdissection testicular sperm extraction
Mufti GR, 316
Mulhall J, 315, 319
Multiple Morphological Abnormalities of the Sperm Flagella (MMAF), 69
multiple sclerosis, 324
mumps orchitis, **230**, 258
muscle, 61, 264, 265, 267, 269, 270, 289, 290, 292, 304
myosin light chain kinase (MLCK), 290
myosin phosphatase, 290

nasal embryonic LHRH factor (NELF), 36
National Center for Health Statistics, 197

Index

National Health and Nutrition Examination Survey (NHANES), 280
National Institutes of Health (NIH), 73, 332
Nätt D, 84
natural conception, 89–91, 183, 191
natural pregnancy (NP), 120, 128
ncRNAs, 82
Nesbit plication, 316
neurobiology, 62
neurodevelopmental disorders, 92
neurokinins, 37
neuropeptide Y (NPY), 36
neuropeptides, 330
neuropraxia, 309
neurotransmitters, 62, 253, 289
neurovascular bundles, 316, 320
next-generation DNA sequencing (NGS), 131
nifedipine, 137
nitric oxide, 289, 291, 292, 303, 325, 326
nitric oxide synthases (NOS), 303
nitroglycerin, 309
NO. See nitric oxide
nocturia, 280, 281, 323, 324, 326
nocturnal penile tumescence (NPT), 293
non-adrenergic non-cholinergic (NANC), 291
non-coding RNA (ncRNA), 78, 81
non-growing follicles (NGFs), 89
non-Hodgkin lymphoma, 93
non-homologous end joining (NHEJ), 177
non-obstructive azoospermia (NOA), 68, 69, 99, 101, 102, 103, 113, 117, 124, 206, 210, 282
   definition, 210
   IVF-ICSI after varicocelectomy, 122–123
non-progressive motility (NPM), 167
norepinephrine (NE), 36, 290, 293
NSAIDs, 184, 332, 333
nuclear condensation, 27, 28
nuclear proteins, 77–78
nucleases
   protection of DNA by protamines, 56
nucleotide excision repair (NER), 30
nucleus of Onuf, 62
nutraceuticals, 19, 102
nutrition
   erectile dysfunction (lifestyle modifications), 305

obesity, 1, 11, 83, 98, 252, 269, 279, 295, 305, 324
obstructive azoospermia (OA), 5, 68, 101, 117, 206
   definition, 210

obstructive sleep apnea (OSA), 280, 281, 283, 297, 305
   definition, 279
office evaluation of infertile male
   defects in isolated semen parameters, 100–101
   endocrine evaluation, 99
   history, 97–98
   imaging, 100
   initial evaluation (interpretation), 100
   initial laboratory assessment, 98–99
   physical examination, 97
   semen analysis, 98–99
offspring health
   birth defects, 92
   childhood cancer and mortality, 93
   chromosomal and genetic abnormalities, 92
   effect of paternal age, 92–93
   neurodevelopmental disorders, 92
   perinatal, neonatal, and obstetric outcomes, 92
Ohlsson C, 258
Ohta AT, 213
Oldereid NB, 92
oligoasthenospermia, 100
oligoasthenoteratospermia (OAT), 101
oligospermia, 115, 124
   definition, 103
   IUI and IVF/ICSI outcomes, *122*
   IVF-ICSI after varicocelectomy, 122–123
   WHO definition, 100
oligozoospermia, 68, 69, 108, 127, 129, 226
Onabotulinumtoxin-A, 333
Oncofertility Consortium (OC), 143
oocyte fertilization process, *192*
oocyte quality, 178
oocyte zona pellucida, 179
oocytes, 201
opioid use, 269
opioids, 98, 259, 269
orchialgia, 3
orchiectomy, 3, 144, 259, 265, 331, 332
organoid culture, **232**
orgasm, 61, 155, 161, 311
orofacial abnormalities, 92
orthostatic hypotension, 325
Osadchiy V, 17
osteoporosis, 259, 264
ovarian reserve, 89
over the counter (OTC) medications, 185
ovulatory monthly cycles, 89
oxidative stress, 10, 84, 102, **179**, 180, 183, 184, 186, 187, 215, 256, 304, 305
   impact on ART outcomes, 180

pain, 310
Papanicolaou staining, 162
papaverine, 293, 299, 310
paracrine regulation, 25
parasympathetic pathway, 289, 290
paraventricular nucleus (PVN), 290
parents, 149
Park HK, 280
Parkinson's Disease, 292, 297
Parrella A, 199
Pasqualotto FF, **121**, 123
Pastuszak AW, 257, 280, 282
paternal age, 76, 87, 197
   effect on ART conception, 91–92
   effect on fertility, 89–92
   effect on natural conception, 89–91
   effect on offspring health, 92–93
   semen parameters (changes), 89
paternal age affect (PAE), 88, 177
Patient Health Questionnaire (PHQ-9), 300
peanut agglutinin (PNA), 171
pelvic floor, 330
pelvic floor physical therapy (PFPT), 304
pelvic fractures, 292
penile erection and detumescence physiology, *291*
penile prosthesis, 311
   erosions, 311
   infection, 311
   managing changes in penile length, 311
   mechanical failure, 311
   options (benefits and costs), *312*
   use, 311
penile prosthesis implantation, 136, 319–320
penile tunica albuginea, 20
penile vibratory stimulation (PVS), 64, 136–138, 144
   illustration, *136*
penis
   coronal section, *290*
   cylinders of erectile tissue, 289
percutaneous epididymal sperm aspiration (PESA), 117, **117**, 206
percutaneous testicular biopsy (PercBiopsy), 206
periodic acid-Schiff (PAS) staining method, 28
periodontitis, 304
peripheral nerves, 292
Perito P, 320
peritubular cells (PTC), 24
peritubular layer, *27*

Pew Research Center, 16
Peyronie's Disease (PD), 11–12, 13, 14, 299
   correction of curvature with penile prosthesis, *319*
   definition, 19
   natural history, 315
   online content landscape, 20
   routine preoperative workup, 315
   surgical correction, 315
Peyronie's Disease (surgical approaches), 315–320
   plaque incision and grafting, 317–319
   plication procedures, 315–317
   prosthetic implantation, 319–320
Pfeiffer syndrome, 177
pharmaceutical industry, 18
pharmaceuticals, 300
   global market, 10
pharmacotherapy, 315
phentolamine, 299, 310
phimosis, 98
phosphatidylserine, 205, 214
   definition, 214
phosphodiesterase-5 (PDE-5), 292
phosphodiesterase-5 inhibitors (PDE-5i), 3, 8, 10, 18, 135, 280, 291, 303, 306, 308, 310, 325, 326
   adverse events, 309
   contraindications, 309
   erectile dysfunction, 308–309
   other concerns, 309
   use in general ED population, 309
   use in post-RP/RT ED, 309
   use in special populations, 309
phosphorylation, 42
phosphotyrosine phosphatase (Shp2), 43
photo-selective vaporization of prostate (PVP), 64
physiologic erections
   types, 290
physiological intracytoplasmic sperm injection (PICSI), 205, 211
physiology
   HPT axis, 35–43
phytotherapy, 333
pinched flow fractionation, 213
Pinktober campaign, 2
Pittsburgh Sleep Quality Index (PSQI), 280, 281, 282
pituitary gland, 39, 109
pituitary hormones, 108, **235**
piwiRNAs (piRNAs), 82
plaque incision and grafting, 317, 320
plasma testosterone, 281

Index

platelet-rich plasma (PRP), 4, 10, 11, 12, 312
plication procedures, 315–317, 320
　Lue 16-dot plication, *317*
plumage, 197
pluripotent stem cells
　transformation into SSCs, 247
polarization microscopy, 206
polychlorinated biphenyls (PCBs), 185
polydimethylsiloxane (PDMS), 212
polymerase chain reaction (PCR), 67, 129
polymorphisms, 68, 77, 130
　androgen receptor, 130
polysialic acid form of neural adhesion molecule (PSA-NCAM), 36
polysomnography (PSG), 280
polyuria, 324
　definition, 324
positron emission tomography (PET), 290
posterior peri-arterial lipomatous tissues, 330
post-finasteride syndrome, 325
post-masturbatory urinalysis, 63, 64
postmicturition dribble (PMD), 305
post-testicular disorders, 67
post-vasectomy pain syndrome, 331, 332
Prader-Willi syndrome, 259
pregnancy, 76, 77, 79, 83, 87, 113
　maternal age, 92
　separation of maternal and paternal genomes, 177
　time to, 91
pregnancy loss, 132
pregnancy rates, 89, 90, 91, 102, 107, 108, 114, 116, 120, 121, 122, 123, 124, 128, 138, 147, 176, 199, 226, 272, 273
　treated versus untreated varicoceles, **121**
pregnenolone, 44, 251
preleptotene spermatocytes, 26
premature ejaculation (PE), 62
　diagnosis, 62
　etiologies, 62
　primary versus secondary, 62
　treatment, 62–63
pre-testicular disorders, 67
pre-testicular infertility, 68
preventable disease, 1
priapism, 310, 311
　definition, 310
Priapus shot, 10
Primary Ciliary Dyskinesia (PCD), 69, 99, 101
primates, 31, 36, 231, 238, 245, 246

primordial germ cells (PGCs), 244, 247
Priskorn L, 89
progesterone, 37, 38, 39, 44, 191, 192, 193, 264
Progesterone Receptor Modulators (SPRMs), 264
prokineticin-2 (PROK2), 36
prolactin, 38, 259, 292, 299
　definition, 109
prolactin modulators, 109
prolactinomas, 130, 259, 269
proopiomelanocortin (POMC), 38
prophase I, 26
prostaglandin, 3, 45, 61, 204, 225, 291, 299, 309
prostate, 61, 88, 264, 267, 323, 330
　function, 231
prostate cancer, 2, 253, 309, 324, 326
　hypogonadism and, 256–257
Prostate Cancer Active Surveillance initiative, 2
Prostate Cancer Prevention Trial (PCPT), 326
prostate specific antigen (PSA), 9, 61, 252, 257, 266, 324, 326
prostatectomy, 3, 292, 304, 309, 310, 312
prostatic urethra, 61, 63, 64, 161, 323
prostatitis, 329, 332
prosthetic urology, 4
protamine 1 (PRM1) gene, 28
protamine 2 (PRM2) gene, 28
protamine deficiency, 183
protamine extraction, 59
protamine loop domain model
　sperm chromatin structure and luminal nuclease digestion, *58*
protamines, 28, *58*, 77, 81
　protection of DNA from nucleases, 56
protein kinase A (PKA), 38, 42
protein kinase C (PKC), 38
protein-coding (PRY) genes, 129
pseudoephedrine, 310
pseudotime trajectory analysis, 31
psychogenic erections, 135, 290
puberty, 48, 130
Pubmed citations
　whole genome and whole exome sequencing, *68*
pulsatile gonadotropin-releasing hormone, 255
pulsed-field gel electrophoresis (PFGE), 54

quality of life, 289, 293, 324, 332
　gender gap, 8
quantitative laboratory medicine, 159
questionnaires, 297, 300, 315, 323
quinolones, 333

rabbit, 233
radiation
　mechanisms of toxic therapies, 143–144
radiation therapy (RT), 184, 252, 259, 297, 309
radical prostatectomy (RP), 309
Raman Spectroscopy, 200, 215
Ramasamy R, 256
randomized clinical trial (RCT), 84
rapid eye movement (REM) sleep, 281, 290
rat, 234, 253, 265, 304
reactive oxygen species (ROS), 4, 88, 101–102, 120, 178–181, 283, 303
　antioxidants, 180–181
　consequences in sperm, *179*
　consequences of excess, 179
　damage to DNA (means), 180
　definition, 178
　impact on ART outcomes, 180
　necessary for normal sperm function, 178
　source, 178
Read J, 18
reciprocal translocations, 129
recreational drugs, 98, 176, 180, 297
　erectile dysfunction (lifestyle modifications), 305
recurrent pregnancy loss (RPL), 177
Reddit, 17, 18
Reduction by Dutasteride of Prostate Cancer Events (REDUCE), 281, 326
reduction division, 26
reflex ejaculation, 137
reflex erections, 135
reflexogenic erectile function, 292
reflexogenic erections, 290
religion, 148
reproductive female potential, 89
reproductive outcomes
　paternal effects, 197
reproductive tract obstruction
　correction, 113–115
　epididymal obstruction, 113–114
　vasal obstruction, 113–114
reserve stem cells, 26
restless legs syndrome (RLS), 279
retinoids, **235**
retinol, 236
retrograde ejaculation (RE), 63–64, 88, 100, 161, 325
　treatment, 64–65

retroperitoneal lymphadenectomy (RPLND), 63
RFamide-related peptides (RFRP), 41
rhesus monkey, 36, 149, **235**, 246, 277
RhoA, 290
RNAs
　sperm epigenetic landscape, 78
Robertshaw I, 91
Robertsonian translocations, 129
Roddam AW, 257
rodents, 30, 234, **238**
　epithelial cycle, 29
Rodriguez M, 280
Rolle L, 320
Rossi SP, 282
round cells, 99

SA. *See* semen analysis
Said TM, 198
Saleh RA, 155
Samplaski MK, 17, 120
Samuel R, 215, 218
Sanger sequencing, 67, 72
Sansalone S, 320
saphenous vein grafts, 317
Sato T, 247
saw palmetto (*Serenoa repens*), 324
Saylam B, 109
Scarselli F, 200
Schally AV, 35
schizophrenia, 87, 92, 177, 224
Schmid SM, 281
Schover L, 141, 148
Schroeder FH, 316
Schwarzer JU, 316
SCI. *See* spinal cord injury
Scovell JM, 281
scrotal pain, 332
scrotum, 329, 330
SDS, 55, 56, *57*, 59
　sperm luminal nuclease active for short time, 54–55
　time course in activation of luminal nuclease, *55*
sedentary lifestyle, 107, 297
Seehuus M, 279
Segré-Silberberg Effect, 167
selective androgen receptor modulators (SARMs), 264–267
　future directions, 266
　history and development, 264–265
　men's health, 266
　potential for use in hypogonadism, 265–266
　safety, 266
selective estrogen receptor modulators (SERMs), 108–109, 255, 264
　testosterone withdrawal, 271

Index

Selective Glucocorticoid Receptor Modulators (SGRMs), 264
Selective Receptor Modulators (SRMs), 264
selective serotonin reuptake inhibitors (SSRIs), 63, 185, 292, 293
self-priming, 39
sella turcica, 130
semen (additional tests), 101–102
  DNA fragmentation, 102
  fluorescent in situ hybridization, 102
  reactive oxygen species, 101–102
semen analysis, 4, 98–99, 100, 106, 107, 159–163, 175, 191, 195, 210
  azoospermia, 99
  biological and technical issues, 167
  ejaculate volume, 99
  main diagnostic tool, 89
  round cells, 99
  seminal viscosity, 99
  sperm concentration, 99
  sperm motility, 99
semen banking
  practical concerns, 224–227
semen collection, 155
semen parameters, 89, 100–101, 120, 121, 122, 124, 127, 129, 132, 272
  volume disorders, 100
semen quality, 92, 193
seminal fluid
  composition, 61
seminal vesicles, 61, 64, 115
seminiferous epithelium, 24, 28
  adluminal compartment, 24, 28
  basal compartment, 24, 28
  somatic cells, 24
seminiferous epithelium cycle
  comparison between six- and twelve-stage models, 29
  re-definition, 28–29
seminiferous tubules, 27, 99, 200, 234, 244, 270
  whole mounted, 26
Sensate Focus therapy, 300
September National Prostate Cancer (PCa) Awareness Month, 16
serotonin, 36, 292
Sertoli cell only syndrome (SCOS), 68
Sertoli cells, 23, 24, 35, 40, 41, 43, 48, 106, 129, 184, 211, **235**, 259, 270, 273
  cytoplasm highly branched, 24
  ectoplasmic specialization, 24
  endocrine function, 45
  niche, 25
  prominent nucleolus, 24
  tubulobulbar complex, 24
sex glands, 161
sex hormone-binding globulin (SHBG), 45, 252, 266, 299
  conditions associated with increased or decreased concentrations, **46**
  definition, 46
sex hormones, 1, 23
sex steroids, 37, 40
sex-determining region (SRY), 128
sexual difficulty
  three areas, 154
sexual dysfunction
  impact of infertility, 154–156
  in couple, 155–156
  in men, 155–156
  psychosocial implications, 156
  treatment, 156
sexual function, 253
Sexual Health Inventory for Men (SHIM), 297
sexual history, 296–297
Sexual Medicine Society of North America (SMSNA), 10
Seymour F, 89
Shaeer O, 320
Shahinyan R, 18
Sherman JK, 224
shift work disorder (SWD), 280, 281, 282, 283
  definition, 279
Shimizu N, 281
Shirota K, 199
short-acting testosterone, 275
Shuchat S, 213
Sigalos JT, 281
sildenafil, 3, 16, 135, 280, 303, 308, 309
silodosin, 88, 281, 325
simple periodic array for trapping and isolation (SPARTAN), 219
single nucleotide polymorphisms (SNPs), 68
single nucleotide variations (SNV), 132
single-cell gel electrophoresis (COMET), 102, **175**, 175, 177, 178, 181, 194
single-cell RNA sequencing (scRNAseq), 29, 30, 31, 71
single-cell transcriptome analysis, 31
skin, 46, 251
sleep, 176, 271, 297
  erectile dysfunction, 279–280
  hypogonadism, 281–282
  LUTS, 280–281
  male infertility, 282–283
  men's health, 279–283
sleep apnea treatment, 305
sleep deficiency, 283
sleep hygiene, 283
Sleep Research Society, 279
sliding technique, 320
small intestinal submucosa (SIS), 318, 320
smallpox vaccine, xi
Smith ED, 72, 73
Smith GD, 199
Smith I, 281
smoking, 106, 107, 180, 183, 185, 279, 295, 297, 305
  sperm epigenome, 84
smooth muscle, 24, 325
social media
  exaggerated product efficacy claims, 19
  urologic men's health, 16–20
socioeconomic status, 148, 279, 289
Sohni A, 30
somatic cell types, 77
somatic fibers, 61
Son J, 214
spectroscopy, 200
sperm
  age prediction model, 79
  components (diagrammatic representation), 198
  DNA damage, 87
  DNA fragmentation (impact of lifestyle and male age), 175–177
  DNA fragmentation repair, 177
  fresh vs frozen (practical concern), 226
  image after acid denaturing, 102
  oxidative stress in (causes), **179**
  production and maturation period, 99
  size, shape, speed, **220**
  testicular (use in cases without azoospermia), 207
  with high DNA integrity (isolation), 178
sperm abnormalities, **230**
sperm aneuploidy, 102, 128, 129
sperm banking
  future, 226–227
  overview, 224
sperm capacitation assays, 191–192
sperm chromatin, 183, 187
  anomalies, 194–195
  most highly condensed DNA known, 54
sperm chromatin dispersion (SCD), 102, 170, 175, **176**, 178
sperm chromatin packaging, 54–59
sperm chromatin structure, 57
  toroid loop model (revised), 54
sperm chromatin structure assay (SCSA), 102, 175, **176**, 177, 178
sperm concentration, 89
  CASA, 166–168
sperm counts, 76, 83, 99, 109, 160
sperm defects
  qualitative, 69
  quantitative, 68–69
sperm delivery improvement, 113–115
sperm DNA, 59
sperm DNA damage
  environmental factors, 185
  etiology, 183–185
  lifestyle factors, 185
  medications, 184
  treatment, 186–187
sperm DNA damage assays, 59
sperm DNA damage treatment
  advanced sperm processing techniques, 187
  short abstinence, 187
sperm DNA fragmentation, 4, 170, 194
  impact on ART outcomes, 177–178
sperm DNA fragmentation tests
  clinical value, 183–188
sperm DNA tests
  clincial aspects, 186
  results (relationship with reproductive outcomes), 186
sperm epigenetic landscape, 76–78
  DNA methylation, 76–77
  nuclear proteins, 77–78
  RNAs, 78
sperm epigenetics
  clinical utility, 78–79
  mechanistic and predictive utility, 76–80
sperm epigenome, 81–83
  adiposity, 83
  aging and environmental interactions, 81–84
  aging effects, 83
  DNA methylation, 81
  histone and chromatic modifications, 81
  IncRNAs, 82
  lifestyle and environmental factors, 83–84
  miRNAs, 81
  non-coding RNAs, 81
  piRNAs, 82
  tRFs, 82
sperm factor, 191
sperm fertilizing ability tests, 171

Index

sperm function assessment, 170
sperm function assays, 191–195
sperm hyperactivation assays, 192–193
sperm identification microfluidic techniques, **219**
sperm kinematics, 165, **166**
   derivation and calculation, *165*
sperm methylome, 77
sperm morphology, 101, 162
   assessment, 170
sperm motility, 61, 69, 99, 101, 161, **219**
   CASA, 166–168
   categorization, 162
   hyperactivated (HA), 168
   prime factor in semen analysis, 165
sperm number, 162
sperm parameters, 197
sperm populations
   washed and capacitating, 168
sperm quality, 107
sperm retrieval, 113, 117, 123, 129, 206
   background and pre-operative considerations, 117–118
   procedural notes and outcomes, 117–118
   techniques, **117**
sperm retrieval rate (SRR), **121**, 123, 215
sperm selection, *201*
   advanced, 205–206
   conventional, 204
   sophisticated, 205–206
sperm selection strategies
   artificial intelligence, 199
   charges, 199
   in vitro fertilization, 197
   membrane properties, 198–199
   microfluidics, 199
   microscopy, 200
   morphology, 200
   spectroscopy, 200
sperm sorting, 178
   conventional techniques (limitations), 210–211
sperm sub-populations identification (clinical value), 170
sperm tail, 28
sperm track, *166*
   kinematic values, **170**
   perceived (effect of frame rate), *168*
   perceived (influence of smoothing), *169*
sperm tracks, **166**
sperm transport, 61–65, 68, 99, 161
sperm vitality, 162
   assessment, 170
sperm wash method, 178, 204, 211
spermatic cord
   pampiniform venous plexus, 120
spermatid development
   six-step versus 12-step classifications, 29
spermatid shaping, 28
spermatids, 27, 29, **236**
   elongated, 26
   nucleus, 28
   round, 26
   six morphological types, 28
spermatocytes, 25, **236**
spermatogenesis, 35, 40, 43, 67, 69, 97, 233
   crosstalk between somatic and germ cells, 31
   defective, 183
   histology, 23–32
   in vitro, 233–238
   in vitro studies (lack of tools), 69
   location, 23
   normal and pathological conditions, 32
   novel classification, 29
   stem cell hierarchy (current model), 26
   widespread transcription "reduces germline mutations," 30
spermatogenesis (kinetics), 28–31
   seminiferous epithelium cycle (re-definition), 28–29
   spermatogonial compartment (current knowledge), 29–31
spermatogenesis (phases), 25–28
   (1) mitotic phase, 25–26
   (2) meiotic phase, 26–27
   (3) spermiogenesis, 27
   (4) spermiation, 26
spermatogonia, 31, **235**
   cell clusters, 29, 31
   cell types, 26
   intermediate morphology, 26
   models, 244–246
spermatogonia detection methodological approaches, 27
spermatogonia types, 26
spermatogonial cell subsets, 30
spermatogonial clones expansion, 30
spermatogonial expansion kinetics, 30
spermatogonial layer, 27
spermatogonial stem cells (SSCs), 23, 30, 31, 226
   approaches (strengths and limitations), 246–247
   clinical significance, 244–248
   current understanding, 244–246
   future perspectives, 247–248
   gene editing, 247
   human and mouse comparison, 246
   in vitro expansion, 246
   low rate of proliferation, 30
   maturation (generating functional niche), 247
   transplantation, 246–247
spermatogonial subsets identification by scRNAseq, *31*
spermatozoa, 23, 26, 28
   definition, 35
   epidydimal, 206
   main epigenetic factors, *82*
   rapid progressive, 167
   surgically retrieved (preparation and selection), 206–207
   testicular, 206
   testicular (selection methods), 207
spermatozoa selection assisted conception, 204–208
spermiation
   definition, 43
spermiogenesis, 27, 175
   steps, 28
   twelve different steps, 28
   unique chromatin remodeling process, 28
sperm-oocyte fusion assays, 194
sperm-zona pellucida binding, 193–194
sphincter complex, 323
spinal cord, 290
spinal cord injury, 64, 292, 297
   andrological care, 135–139
spinal cord stimulation, 331
spinal interneurons, 62
stages (germ cell associations), 28
Steinfatt H, 316
stem cells (spermatogonia), 160
steroid hormones, 44
steroid receptor co-activator (SRC), 47
steroidogenesis, 42, 43, 44, *45*
steroidogenic acute regulatory (STAR) protein, 42, 44, 251
stillbirth, 91, 92
stinging nettle (*Urtica dioica*), 324
STOP-BANG questionnaire, 283, 297
stress, 38, 62, 141, 149, 156, 244, 282, 293, 332
structural protein transport, 28
substania nigra, 292
surface charge selection methods, 205
surgical management
   male infertility, 113–118
swim-up (SU) method, 204, 211
Syed AH, 316
sympathetic chain ganglia, 289
sympathetic preganglia, 289
systemic exercise, 304

tachykinin family of peptides, 37
tactile allodynia, 332
tadalafil, 303, 308, 309
Takagi J, 214
Takayama S, 199, 212
tamoxifen, 108, 255, 264, 272
tamsulosin, 63, 88, 325
Tanrikut C, 256
telemedicine websites, 18
teleost fish, 35
temperature, **235**
teratospermia, 101
teratozoospermia, 197, 207
Teratozoospermia Index (TZI), 169, 170
terminal de-oxynucleotide transferase dUTP nick end labelling (TUNEL), 175, **175**, 177, 194
testicles, 98
   radiation-sensitivity, 143
testicular cancer, 144, 184
testicular cell transplantation (TCT), 149
testicular disorders, 67
testicular fine needle aspiration, 229
testicular function, 43–48
   different phases of lifespan, 47–48
   Leydig cell function, 43–45
   optimization (varicocele repair), 117
   Sertoli cell endocrine function, 45
   testosterone actions, 46–47
   testosterone metabolism, 46
   testosterone transport, 45–46
testicular germ cell tumors (TGCTs), 244
testicular hormones, 35
testicular hyperthermia
   sperm DNA damage, 185
testicular pain, 330, 331
   types, 329
testicular sperm
   generally non-motile, 211
testicular sperm aspiration (TESA), 117, 138, 206, 210
   percutaneous procedure, 210
testicular sperm extraction (TESE), 102, 117, 123, 124
testicular tissue, 108, **117**, 117, 149, 211, 218, 227, **230**, 231, 233, 234
   degradation, 211
   laboratory processing, 207
testicular tissue grafting, 246
testicular ultrasound, *101*
testis, 117, 329
   immune privileged site, 23
   interstitial compartment, 23, 43

Index

testis (cont.)
  most transcriptionally diverse tissue, 69
  role, 43
  seminiferous tubules, 23, 24–25
  transcriptional and translational complexity, 69
  transcriptome analysis (single cell level), 31–32
  tubular compartment, 43, 45
testis function, 231–233
testis parenchyma
  histology, *24*
testis-specific Y-encoded protein 1 (TSPY), 129
testolactone, 109
testosterone, 23, 37, 43, 99, 108, 109, 251, 253
  actions, 46–47
  C19 steroid, *44*
  conversion to active metabolites, *45*
  critical role in male sexual behavior, 292
  main inhibitor of LH secretion, 40
  most important androgen, 35
testosterone as contraceptive, 270
testosterone boosting supplements (T-Boosters), 19
testosterone clinics, 2
testosterone deficiency, 292
  same as 'hypogonadism' (*qv*), 281
testosterone enanthate (TE), 265
testosterone enanthate subcutaneous autoinjector, 254
testosterone gels
  intranasal, 254, 255
  transdermal, 254
testosterone injections
  intramuscular, 254
testosterone levels, 299
testosterone metabolism, 46
testosterone patches, 254
testosterone pellets (subcutaneous), 254
testosterone physiology, 270
testosterone replacement therapy, 136, 253–255, 264
  benefits and risks, 255
  cardiovascular disease, 257–258
  men with spinal cord injury, 138
testosterone sales, 2, 8
testosterone therapy, 19, 269–277
  future directions, 273–277
  human chorionic gonadotropin, 272–273
  hypogonadal men (fertility maintenance), 273
  prescribing patterns, 270
testosterone transport, 45–46

testosterone undecanoate, 253, 254
testosterone withdrawal, 271–272
  anastrozole, 271
  human chorionic gonadotropin (hCG), 272
  lifestyle modification, 271
  SERMs, 271
testosterone/estradiol (T/E) ratios, 109
tetracyclines, 333
Thompson IM, 257
thyroid-stimulating hormone (TSH), 39
TIME magazine, 3
tissue culture, **232**
topoisomerase II, 54
toroid linker DNA
  definition, *58*
toroid linker model (revised), 54
toroid loop model (revised) methods, 54
total motile count (TMC), 146
  cryopreservation strategies, *146*
total motile sperm count (TMSC), 120, 121, 124
total sperm concentration, 167
  importance, 167
tramadol, 63
transcription activator-like effector nucleases (TALENs), 247
transcription factors, 36
transcriptional scanning, 30
transcriptional silencing, 28
transcriptional-coupled repair (TCR), 30
transcriptome analysis, 31–32
transcriptome profile, 30
transduceosome complex, 42
transforming growth factor-α (TGF-α), **236**
transforming growth factor-β (TGF-β) superfamily, 40, 45
transgender females
  mechanisms of gonadal suppression in, *146*
transgender population, 148
translational sciences, xi
translocator protein (TSPO), 42
transplantation, 232
transrectal ultrasound (TRUS), 99, 100, 115, 266, 323
transurethral incision of prostate (TUIP), 64
transurethral resection of ejaculatory ducts (TURED, 115
transurethral resection of the prostate (TURP), 64, 88
tRNA fragments (tRFs), 82
Trowell's method, 234
TRT. *See* testosterone replacement therapy

trust
  physician-patient relationship, 296
Trypan blue cells, 213
tubular fluid, 25
tubule culture, **232**
Tukey windows, 168
tumor necrosis factor (TNF), 304, 305
tunica albuginea, 289, 316, 320
tunica albuginea plication (TAP), 316
Turek PJ, 210
Turgut H, 120
Twitter, 17, 20
Tygerberg strict criteria, 162

ubiquitin specific peptidase 9 Y-linked (USP9Y) gene, 129
UCHL1, UTF1 and GFRA1 markers, 30
ultrasonography, 100, 324
ultrasound, 120, 330
undifferentiated spermatogonia collectively defined as Ap-d, 30
undifferentiated spermatogonial subsets
  histological identification, 31
United Kingdom, 9, 90
United States, 93, 99, 124, 197, 244, 269, 270, 279, 323
  birth analysis (paternal age factor), 89
  cancer (young people), 141
  life expectancy, 16
  transgender rate, 143
upregulation, 39
urethra, 289, 316, 320, 323
urethral injury, 319
urinalysis, 324, 330
urinary retention, 323
urinary tract infection (UTI), 324
urodynamics, 324
uroflowmetry, 324
urologic men's health, 16–20
urology, 2
  functional disorders, 88–89
uterine hyperplasia, 264
uterus, 208, 264
uvulopalatopharyngoplasty, 280

vacuum erection devices (VED), 310, 311
Valsalva, 98, 100, 115, 120, 330
van Leeuwenhoek A, 159
van Wagoner RM, 266
vancomycin, 311
vardenafil, 280, 303, 308, 309
variants of uncertain significance (VUS), 73
varicocele repair, 113, 115–117, 120–124, 175
  background and pre-operative considerations, 115

  outcomes and complications, 116–117
  procedure notes, 115
varicocelectomy, 4, 113, 115, 116, 117, 120, 124, 332
  approaches, **116**
  ART considerations, 124
  before IUI, 121–122
  before IVF-ICSI, 122
  benefits prior to ART, 120–121
  treatment of sperm DNA damage, 186
varicoceles, 98, 100, 101, 113
  and hypogonadism, 256
  definition, 120
  most frequent cause of male infertility, 180
  sperm DNA damage, 184
  treated versus untreated, **121**
vas deferens, 54–59, 61, 98, 115, 127, 330, 331
  definition, 231
  luminal nuclease inhibited by prolonged exposure to SDS, *55*
vasal obstruction (correction)
  background and pre-operative considerations, 113–114
  outcomes and complications, 114
  procedure notes, 114
vasectomy, 113, 114
vasectomy reversal, 5, 113, 332
vasoactive intestinal peptide (VIP), 38
vasoepididymostomy (VE), 113, 114, 206
vasography, 100
vasovasostomy (VV), 3, 5, 113, 114, 206
Veltman JA, 68, 72
venular plexus, 289
verumontanum, 64, 115, 323
Veterans Health Administration, 9
viagra. *See* sildenafil
Vigen R, 258
vinca alkaloids, 143
Vitamin C, 305
Vitamin D, 83
Vitamin E, 305
voltage-dependent anion channel-1 (VDAC1), 42

Waddington C, 81
Wagenlehner FM, 333
Waldeyer H, 67
Wallerian degeneration, 3, 330, *330*
Wallis CJ, 257
Wang C, 108
Wang R, 93
Wang X, 282

washed sperm track segments, **166**
Watkins AJ, 84
Watson J, 67
weight loss, 271
WHO, 16, 89, 99, 100, 108, 141, 159, 160, 161, 162, 167, 195, 210, 270, 271
WHO manual, 162, 169
whole-exome sequencing (WES), 69, 92, 131
whole-genome sequencing (WGS), 68, *68*, 131
Wilkins M, 67
Wilson SK, 320
Wise LA, 282
Wolffian duct developmental abnormalities, 98
women, 46, 154, 156, 186, 198, 265
World Anti-Doping Agency, 266
World Professional Association for Transgender Health (WPATH), 143, 147
Worrilow KC, 198

X chromosome, 26, 47, 67, 130, 244
X-ray imaging, 67
XX male, 127, 128, 229, 258

Y chromosome, 26, 69, 128, 132
Y chromosome map, *130*
Y chromosome microdeletions, 101, 103, 127, 129, 132, 160, 244
Yachia D, 316
Yidiz K, 199
YouTube, 18
Yu JH, 72
Yuksel S, 199

Zaila KE, 17
zebrafish (*Danio rerio*), 72
Zenker-formal-fixed testis, 26
zeta potential, 199, 205
Zhang K, 18
Zimmermann JW, 246
zona pellucida, 27, 102, 162, 180, *192*, 193–194, 226
ZP. *See* zeta potential
Zymot, 219